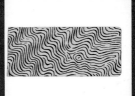

SLEEP AND BREATHING DISORDERS

SLEEP AND BREATHING DISORDERS

From *Principles and Practice of Sleep Medicine*

Meir Kryger, MD, FRCP(C)

Professor of Medicine (Pulmonary)
and Clinical Professor of Nursing
Yale University School of Medicine
New Haven, Connecticut

ELSEVIER

ELSEVIER

1600 John F. Kennedy Blvd.
Ste 1800
Philadelphia, PA 19103-2899

Sleep and Breathing Disorders   ISBN: 978-0-323-47675-1

Cover: Bottom right image courtesy of Inspire Medical Systems, Inc.

Library of Congress Cataloging-in-Publication Data

Kryger, Meir H., editor.
Sleep and breathing disorders / [edited by] Meir Kryger.
First edition. | Philadelphia, PA : Elsevier, [2017] | Includes bibliographical references and index.
LCCN 2016012135 | ISBN 9780323476751 (hardcover : alk. paper)
| MESH: Sleep Wake Disorders | Sleep Apnea Syndromes | Sleep–physiology | Comorbidity
LCC RC737.5 | NLM WL 108 | DDC 616.2/09–dc23 LC record available at
   http://lccn.loc.gov/2016012135

Content Strategist: Russell Gabbedy
Senior Content Development Specialist: Laura Schmidt
Publishing Services Manager: Patricia Tannian
Project Manager: Stephanie Turza
Design Direction: Amy Buxton

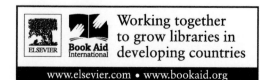

Last digit is the print number: 9 8 7 6 5 4 3 2 1

Contributors

Fernanda R. Almeida, DDS, PhD
Associate Professor
Division of Orthodontics
Oral Health Sciences
University of British Columbia
Vancouver, British Columbia, Canada
Obstructive Sleep Apnea: Oral Appliance Therapy

Alon Y. Avidan, MD
Director, University of California, Los Angeles Sleep
    Disorders Center
Director, University of California, Los Angeles Neurology
    Clinic
Professor of Neurology
Department of Neurology
David Geffen School of Medicine at University of
    California, Los Angeles
Los Angeles, California
Physical Examination in Sleep Medicine

M. Safwan Badr, MD
Professor and Chief
Division of Pulmonary, Critical Care, and Sleep Medicine
Wayne State University School of Medicine
Detroit, Michigan
Anatomy and Physiology of Upper Airway Obstruction

Bilgay Izci Balserak, PhD
Assistant Professor
Department of Women, Children, and Family Health
    Science
Center for Narcolepsy, Sleep, and Health Research
UIC College of Nursing
Chicago, Illinois
Sleep-Disordered Breathing in Pregnancy

Claudio L. Bassetti, MD
Chairman and Head
Neurology Department
University Hospital of Bern
Bern, Switzerland
Stroke

Mark B. Berger, MD
Chief Medical Officer
Precision Pulmonary Diagnostics, LLC
Houston, Texas
Obstructive Sleep Apnea in the Workplace

Richard B. Berry, MD
Professor of Medicine
Division of Pulmonary, Critical Care, and Sleep Medicine
University of Florida
Gainesville, Florida
Sleep-Related Breathing Disorders: Classification

Luis Buenaver, PhD
Assistant Professor
Psychiatry and Behavioral Sciences
The Johns Hopkins University and Hospital School of
    Medicine
Baltimore, Maryland
*Obstructive Sleep Apnea: Alternative, Adjunctive, and
    Complementary Therapies*

Jane E. Butler, PhD
Principal Research Fellow
Neuroscience Research Australia;
Senior Research Fellow
National Health and Medical Research Council of Australia;
Associate Professor
School of Medical Sciences
University of New South Wales
Sydney, Australia
*Respiratory Physiology: Understanding the Control of
    Ventilation*

Michelle T. Cao, DO
Clinical Assistant Professor
Psychiatry and Behavioral Sciences
Sleep Medicine Division
Stanford University School of Medicine
Stanford, California
Neuromuscular Diseases

Maria Clotilde Carra, DMD, PhD
Assistant Professor
Department of Periodontology
Hospital Rothschild;
Faculty of Odontology
Paris Diderot University
Paris, France
Obstructive Sleep Apnea: Oral Appliance Therapy

Santiago J. Carrizo, MD
Senior Consultant
Respiratory Service
Hospital Universitario Miguel Servet
Zaragoza, Spain
Overlap Syndromes of Sleep and Breathing Disorders

Ronald D. Chervin, MD
Professor of Neurology
Michael S. Aldrich Collegiate Professor of Sleep Medicine
Director, Sleep Disorders Center
University of Michigan Health System
Ann Arbor, Michigan
Use of Clinical Tools and Tests in Sleep Medicine

Peter Anthony Cistulli, PhD, FRACP
ResMed Chair in Sleep Medicine
Sydney Medical School
University of Sydney
Sydney, Australia;
Director
Centre for Sleep Health and Research
Royal North Shore Hospital
St. Leonards, Australia
Obstructive Sleep Apnea: Oral Appliance Therapy

Anita P. Courcoulas, MD, FACS
Professor of Surgery
Minimally Invasive Bariatric and General Surgery
University of Pittsburgh Medical Center
Pittsburgh, Pennsylvania
Obstructive Sleep Apnea, Obesity, and Bariatric Surgery

O'Neill F. D'Cruz, MD
Chief Medical Officer
Cyberonics
Houston, Texas
Cardinal Manifestations of Sleep Disorders

Peter R. Eastwood, PhD
Winthrop Professor and Director
Centre for Sleep Science
School for Anatomy, Physiology, and Human Biology
University of Western Australia;
Senior Scientist
West Australian Sleep Disorders Research Institute
Department of Pulmonary Physiology and Sleep Medicine
Sir Charles Gairdner Hospital
Perth, Australia
Obstructive Sleep Apnea: Anesthesia for Upper Airway Surgery

Danny J. Eckert, PhD
Principal Research Fellow
Neuroscience Research Australia;
R.D. Wright Fellow
National Health and Medical Research Council of Australia;
Associate Professor
School of Medical Sciences
University of New South Wales
Sydney, Australia
Respiratory Physiology: Understanding the Control of Ventilation

Francesca Facco, MD
Assistant Professor
Department of Obstetrics, Gynecology, and Reproductive Sciences
University of Pittsburgh School of Medicine
Magee-Womens Hospital of UPMC
Pittsburgh, Pennsylvania
Sleep-Disordered Breathing in Pregnancy

Karl A. Franklin, MD, PhD
Associate Professor
Surgical and Perioperative Science, Surgery
Umeå University
Umeå, Sweden
Coronary Artery Disease and Obstructive Sleep Apnea

Neil Freedman, MD
Division of Pulmonary and Critical Care Medicine
Department of Medicine
NorthShore University Healthsystem
Evanston, Illinois
Obstructive Sleep Apnea: Positive Airway Pressure Therapy

Avram R. Gold, MD
Associate Professor of Clinical Medicine
Pulmonary, Critical Care, and Sleep Medicine
Stony Brook University School of Medicine
Stony Brook, New York;
Staff Physician
Pulmonary Section, Medical Service
DVA Medical Center
Northport, New York
Snoring and Pathologic Upper Airway Resistance Syndromes

Cathy A. Goldstein, MD
Assistant Professor of Neurology
Sleep Disorders Center
University of Michigan Health System
Ann Arbor, Michigan
Use of Clinical Tools and Tests in Sleep Medicine

Harly Greenberg, MD
Professor of Medicine
Pulmonary, Critical Care, and Sleep Medicine
Hofstra North Shore LIJ School of Medicine
New Hyde Park, New York
Obstructive Sleep Apnea: Diagnosis and Management

Christian Guilleminault, MD
Professor
Psychiatry and Behavioral Sciences
Sleep Medicine Division
Stanford University School of Medicine
Stanford, California
Neuromuscular Diseases

Jan Hedner, MD, PhD
Professor
Department of Sleep Medicine
Respiratory Medicine and Allergology
Sahlgrenska University Hospital
Gothenburg, Sweden
   Coronary Artery Disease and Obstructive Sleep Apnea

Raphael Heinzer, MD
Director
Center for Investigation and Research in Sleep
University Hospital of Lausanne;
Senior Lecturer
University of Lausanne
Lausanne, Switzerland
   Physiology of Upper and Lower Airways

David R. Hillman, MBBS, FANZCA
Medical Director, Research Scientist
West Australian Sleep Disorders Research Institute
Department of Pulmonary Physiology and Sleep Medicine
Sir Charles Gairdner Hospital
Perth, Australia
   Obstructive Sleep Apnea: Anesthesia for Upper Airway Surgery

Max Hirshkowitz, PhD
Consulting Professor
Division of Public Mental Health and Population Sciences
Stanford University School of Medicine
Stanford, California;
Professor (Emeritus)
Department of Medicine
Baylor College of Medicine
Houston, Texas
   Monitoring Techniques for Evaluating Suspected Sleep-Disordered Breathing

Aarnoud Hoekema, MD, DMD, PhD
Associate Professor
Academic Centre for Dentistry Amsterdam
Amsterdam, Netherlands;
Doctor
Department of Oral and Maxillofacial Surgery
University Medical Center Groningen
Groningen, the Netherlands;
Staff Surgeon
Department of Oral and Maxillofacial Surgery
Tjongerschans Hospital
Heerenveen, the Netherlands
   Upper Airway Surgery to Treat Obstructive Sleep Apnea

Mary Sau-Man Ip, MD
Mok Hing Yiu Endowed Professor and Chair
Department of Medicine
Li Ka Shing Faculty of Medicine
University of Hong Kong
Hong Kong, China
   Obstructive Sleep Apnea and Metabolic Disorders

Shahrokh Javaheri, MD
Medical Director
SleepCare Diagnostics, Inc.
Cincinnati, Ohio
   Cardiovascular Effects of Sleep-Related Breathing Disorders
   Heart Failure
   Systemic and Pulmonary Hypertension in Obstructive Sleep Apnea

Stefanos N. Kales, MD
Associate Professor of Medicine
Harvard Medical School
Associate Professor and Program Director
Occupational Medicine Residency
Harvard School of Public Health
Boston, Massachusetts;
Division Chief
Occupational Medicine
Cambridge Health Alliance
Cambridge, Massachusetts
   Obstructive Sleep Apnea in the Workplace

Eliot S. Katz, MD
Assistant Professor of Pediatrics
Division of Respiratory Diseases
Boston Children's Hospital
Harvard Medical School
Boston, Massachusetts
   Central Sleep Apnea: Definitions, Pathophysiology, Genetics, and Epidemiology

Melissa Pauline Knauert, MD, PhD
Assistant Professor
Pulmonary, Critical Care, and Sleep Medicine
Department of Internal Medicine
Yale University School of Medicine
New Haven, Connecticut
   Sleep-Disordered Breathing in Pregnancy

Meir Kryger, MD, FRCP(C)
Professor of Medicine (Pulmonary) and Clinical Professor of Nursing
Yale University School of Medicine
New Haven, Connecticut
   Approach and Evaluation of the Patient
   Monitoring Techniques for Evaluating Suspected Sleep-Disordered Breathing
   Physical Examination in Sleep Medicine

Viera Lakticova, MD
Assistant Professor of Medicine
Hofstra North Shore LIJ School of Medicine
New Hyde Park, New York
   Obstructive Sleep Apnea: Diagnosis and Management

Christopher J. Lettieri, MD
Professor of Medicine
Uniformed Services University;
Program Director, Sleep Medicine
Pulmonary, Critical Care, and Sleep Medicine
Walter Reed National Military Medical Center
Bethesda, Maryland
Obstructive Sleep Apnea: Oral Appliance Therapy

Judette Louis, MD
Assistant Professor
Department of Obstetrics and Gynecology
College of Medicine
Assistant Professor
Department of Community and Family Health
College of Public Health
University of South Florida
Tampa, Florida
Sleep-Disordered Breathing in Pregnancy

Madalina Macrea, MD, PhD
Associate Professor of Medicine
Salem Veterans Affairs Medical Center
Salem, Virginia;
Associate Professor of Medicine
University of Virginia
Charlottesville, Virginia
Central Sleep Apnea: Definitions, Pathophysiology, Genetics, and Epidemiology

Atul Malhotra, MD
Professor of Medicine
Division Chief, Pulmonary and Critical Care Medicine
Director of Sleep Medicine
Kenneth M. Moser Professor
Department of Medicine
University of California, San Diego
San Diego, California
Central Sleep Apnea: Definitions, Pathophysiology, Genetics, and Epidemiology
Obstructive Sleep Apnea in the Workplace

Beth A. Malow, MD
Professor and Director, Sleep Disorders Division
Neurology and Pediatrics
Vanderbilt University
Nashville, Tennessee
Approach and Evaluation of the Patient

Jose M. Marin, MD
Head, Respiratory Sleep Disorders Unit
Hospital Universitario Miguel Servet;
Associated Professor of Medicine
Department of Medicine
University of Zaragoza
Zaragoza, Spain
Overlap Syndromes of Sleep and Breathing Disorders

Reena Mehra, MD
Associate Professor of Medicine
Sleep Center, Neurologic Institute
Cleveland Clinic Lerner College of Medicine
Case Western Reserve University
Cleveland, Ohio
Sleep Breathing Disorders: Clinical Overview

Babak Mokhlesi, MD
Director, Sleep Disorders Center and Sleep Medicine
Fellowship Program
Department of Medicine
Section of Pulmonary and Critical Care
University of Chicago
Chicago, Illinois
Obesity-Hypoventilation Syndrome

Mary J. Morrell, PhD
Professor of Sleep and Respiratory Physiology
National Heart and Lung Institute
Imperial College
London, United Kingdom
Obstructive Sleep Apnea and the Central Nervous System

Douglas E. Moul, MD
Sleep Psychiatrist, Staff Physician
Sleep Disorders Center, Neurological Institute
Cleveland Clinic
Cleveland, Ohio
Sleep Breathing Disorders: Clinical Overview

F. Javier Nieto, MD, PhD
Professor and Chair of Population Health Sciences
School of Medicine and Public Health
University of Wisconsin–Madison
Madison, Wisconsin
Systemic and Pulmonary Hypertension in Obstructive Sleep Apnea

Eric J. Olson, MD
Associate Professor of Medicine
Mayo Clinic College of Medicine
Division of Pulmonary and Critical Care Medicine
Co-Director, Center for Sleep Medicine
Mayo Clinic
Rochester, Minnesota
Obstructive Sleep Apnea, Obesity, and Bariatric Surgery

Susheel P. Patil, MD, PhD
Assistant Professor of Medicine
The Johns Hopkins University and Hospital School of Medicine
Baltimore, Maryland
Obstructive Sleep Apnea: Alternative, Adjunctive, and Complementary Therapies

Yüksel Peker, MD, PhD
Professor
Department of Pulmonary Medicine
Marmara University
Istanbul, Turkey;
Department of Molecular and Clinical Medicine/
    Cardiology
Sahlgrenska Academy, University of Gothenburg
Gothenburg, Sweden
    Coronary Artery Disease and Obstructive Sleep Apnea

Thomas Penzel, PhD
Professor
Department of Cardiology
Interdisciplinary Sleep Medicine Center
Charité–Universitätsmedizin Berlin
Berlin, Germany
    Home Sleep Testing

Paul E. Peppard, PhD
Associate Professor
Population Health Sciences
University of Wisconsin–Madison
Madison, Wisconsin
    Systemic and Pulmonary Hypertension in Obstructive Sleep Apnea

Barbara A. Phillips, MD, FCCP
Professor
Division of Pulmonary, Critical Care, and Sleep Medicine
University of Kentucky College of Medicine
Lexington, Kentucky
    Obstructive Sleep Apnea in Older Adults

Susan S. Redline, MD
Farrell Professor of Sleep Medicine
Harvard Medical School
Brigham and Women's Hospital
Beth Israel Deaconess Medical Center
Boston, Masachusetts
    Obstructive Sleep Apnea: Phenotypes and Genetics

Albert Rielly, MD
Physician
Department of Medicine
Cambridge Health Alliance
Cambridge, Massachusetts;
Clinical Instructor
Harvard Medical School
Boston, Massachusetts
    Obstructive Sleep Apnea in the Workplace

Ivana Rosenzweig, MD, PhD, MRCPsych
Wellcome Research Fellow and Consultant
    Neuropsychiatrist
Sleep and Brain Plasticity Centre
Department of Neuroimaging
King's College London;
Sleep Disorders Centre
Guy's and St. Thomas' Hospital
London, United Kingdom
    Obstructive Sleep Apnea and the Central Nervous System

James A. Rowley, MD
Professor of Medicine
Division of Pulmonary, Critical Care, and Sleep Medicine
Wayne State University School of Medicine
Detroit, Michigan
    Anatomy and Physiology of Upper Airway Obstruction

Steven M. Scharf, MD, PhD
Professor of Medicine
University of Maryland
Baltimore, Maryland
    Obstructive Sleep Apnea: Diagnosis and Management

Frédéric Sériès, MD
Centre de Recherche
Institut Universitaire de Cardiologie et de Pneumologie de
    l'Université Laval
Quebec City, Quebec, Canada
    Physiology of Upper and Lower Airways

Michael T. Smith, PhD
Professor
Psychiatry and Behavioral Sciences
The Johns Hopkins University and Hospital School of
    Medicine
Baltimore, Maryland
    *Obstructive Sleep Apnea: Alternative, Adjunctive, and
        Complementary Therapies*

Virend K. Somers, MD, PhD
Professor of Medicine
Department of Internal Medicine
Division of Cardiovascular Diseases
Mayo Medical School/Mayo Clinic
Rochester, Minnesota
    Cardiovascular Effects of Sleep-Related Breathing Disorders

Riccardo Stoohs, MD
Director
Sleep Disorders Clinic
Somnolab
Doermund, Germany
    Snoring and Pathologic Upper Airway Resistance Syndromes

Kingman P. Strohl, MD
Professor of Medicine and Anatomy
University Hospitals of Cleveland
Cleveland Veterans Affairs Medical Center
Case Western Reserve University
Cleveland, Ohio
    Sleep Breathing Disorders: Clinical Overview

Robert Joseph Thomas, MD
Associate Professor of Medicine
Pulmonary, Critical Care, and Sleep Division
Beth Israel Deaconess Medical Center
Boston, Massachusetts
    Central Sleep Apnea: Diagnosis and Management

Olivier M. Vanderveken, MD, PhD
Consultant ENT, Head and Neck Surgeon
Antwerp University Hospital;
Professor
Faculty of Medicine and Health Sciences
University of Antwerp
Antwerp, Belgium
Obstructive Sleep Apnea: Anesthesia for Upper Airway Surgery
Upper Airway Surgery to Treat Obstructive Sleep Apnea

Bradley V. Vaughn, MD
Professor of Neurology
University of North Carolina School of Medicine
Chapel Hill, North Carolina
Cardinal Manifestations of Sleep Disorders

Edward M. Weaver, MD
Professor
Otolaryngology/Head and Neck Surgery
Co-Director
Sleep Center
University of Washington;
Staff Surgeon
Surgery Service
VA Puget Sound Healthcare System
Seattle, Washington
Upper Airway Surgery to Treat Obstructive Sleep Apnea

Terri E. Weaver, PhD, RN, FAAN
Professor and Dean
UIC College of Nursing
Chicago, Illinois
Obstructive Sleep Apnea and the Central Nervous System

Ephraim Winocur, DMD
Senior Lecturer in Orofacial Pain
Oral Rehabilitation
Tel Aviv University
Tel Aviv, Israel
Obstructive Sleep Apnea: Alternative, Adjunctive, and Complementary Therapies

Terry Young, PhD
Professor of Population Health Sciences
School of Medicine and Public Health
University of Wisconsin–Madison
Madison, Wisconsin
Systemic and Pulmonary Hypertension in Obstructive Sleep Apnea

Chunbai Zhang, MD
University of Washington
Valley Medical Center
Renton, Washington
Obstructive Sleep Apnea in the Workplace

Andrey V. Zinchuk, MD
Fellow
Pulmonary, Critical Care, and Sleep Medicine
Yale University School of Medicine
New Haven, Connecticut
Central Sleep Apnea: Diagnosis and Management

Preface

Sleep medicine is a fairly new field. Before 1975, nobody had heard of sleep apnea. The term had not even been coined. Now, everybody knows someone on a CPAP machine, and all clinicians (whether they know it) have patients in their practice who have sleep disorders. In the past 40 years, the management of sleep breathing disorders has changed. In the decade after the birth of sleep medicine, patients with sleep breathing disorders were diagnosed and treated only at academic medical centers. Now, in most cases, diagnosis can be done in a patient's own bed, and management can be done in many types of clinics by different types of practitioners. The efficacy and adherence to treatment can be monitored remotely.

It is now expected that most pulmonary specialists and otolaryngologists be able to diagnose and manage sleep breathing disorders. Other specialists may have many patients with sleep breathing disorders as well. For example, patients seen by cardiologists frequently have sleep apnea, and many dentists see patients who seek oral appliance treatment for their snoring or sleep apnea. Many primary care practitioners and physician extenders (mid-levels) are now following sleep apnea patients.

Every patient with a sleep breathing disorder is unique. In some, diagnosis is straightforward and can be done in the home, and the patient is placed on an autotitrating CPAP machine. In others, diagnosis and management guidance requires in-lab testing, and treatment may require different interfaces, more complex devices, or even surgery.

Sleep and Breathing Disorders is composed of chapters from the sixth edition of *Principles and Practice of Sleep Medicine*, and we believe it will be helpful to practitioners who manage patients with sleep breathing disorders. This volume is divided into the following sections.

Assessment and Pathophysiology

This section covers what is needed to make a diagnosis: taking the history, performing the physical examination, conducting in-lab and home sleep testing, and reviewing the pathophysiological mechanisms that underlie the clinical assessment.

Sleep Apnea Syndromes

This section provides an overview of sleep breathing disorders and focuses on the two most common sleep breathing disorders: central and obstructive sleep apnea.

Management

This section covers the treatment modalities, including positive airway pressure devices, oral appliances, and different types of surgery (upper airway and bariatric).

Consequences

Patients with sleep breathing disorders present with many abnormalities that involve cardiovascular, endocrine, and neurological function. These are reviewed in detail.

Special Populations

Groups of patients that require special consideration are reviewed here: those with overlap syndromes or obesity hypoventilation, the elderly, the pregnant, and those whose disorder impacts the workplace.

Sleep breathing disorders are very common throughout medicine, and we hope that clinicians will find *Sleep and Breathing Disorders* helpful in treating their patients.

Meir Kryger, MD, FRCP(C)
2016

Contents

Video Contents

Abbreviations

AASM: American Academy of Sleep Medicine
AHI: apnea-hypopnea index
AIM: ancestry informative marker
AMS: acute mountain sickness
ANS: autonomic nervous system
AVAPS: average volume assured pressure support
BAC: blood alcohol content
BMI: body mass index
BPD: biliopancreatic diversion
BPDDS: biliopancreatic diversion with duodenal switch
BzRA: benzodiazepine receptor agonist
CAD: coronary artery disease
CAPS: cyclic alternating pattern sequence(s)
CHF: congestive heart failure
CI: confidence interval
COPD: chronic obstructive pulmonary disease
CPAP: continuous positive airway pressure
DMD: Duchenne muscular dystrophy
DSISD: Duke Structured Interview for Sleep Disorders
DSM-V: *Diagnostic and Statistical Manual of Mental Disorders,* fifth edition
ECG: electrocardiogram, electrocardiographic
EDS: excessive daytime sleepiness
EEG: electroencephalogram, electroencephalographic
EMG: electromyogram
EOG: electrooculogram
ESS: Epworth Sleepiness Scale
FEV_1: forced expiratory volume in 1 second
FFT: fast Fourier transform
FOSQ: Functional Outcomes of Sleep Questionnaire
FRC: functional residual capacity
GABA: gamma-aminobutyric acid
GAD: generalized anxiety disorder
GAHMS: genioglossus advancement, hyoid myotomy, and suspension
GWA: genome-wide association
Hcrt: hypocretin
5-HIAA: 5-hydroxyindole acetic acid
HIF: hypoxia inducible factor
HIV: human immunodeficiency virus
HRV: heart rate variability
HVA: homovanillic acid
ICD: International Classification of Diseases
ICD-9-CM: *International Classification of Diseases*, ninth revision, Clinical Modification
ICD-10: *International Classification of Diseases*, tenth revision
ICSD3: *International Classification of Sleep Disorders*, third edition
ILD: interstitial lung disease
iVAPS: intelligent volume assured pressure support
LAUP: laser-assisted uvulopalatoplasty
LOC: left outer canthus
LSAT: lowest oxyhemoglobin saturation
LTIH: long-term intermittent hypoxia
MI: myocardial infarction
MMO: maxillary and mandibular osteotomy

MPA: medroxyprogesterone acetate
MRA: mandibular repositioning appliance
MSA: multiple system atrophy
MSLT: Multiple Sleep Latency Test
MWT: Maintenance of Wakefulness Test
NASH: nonalcoholic steatohepatitis
NFLD: nonalcoholic fatty liver disease
NFLE: nocturnal frontal lobe epilepsy
NPPV: noninvasive positive-pressure ventilation
NREM: non–rapid eye movement, non-REM
OHS: obesity-hypoventilation syndrome
OR: odds ratio
OSA: obstructive sleep apnea
OSAHS: obstructive sleep apnea–hypopnea syndrome
OSAS: obstructive sleep apnea syndrome
PACU: postanesthesia care unit
PCOS: polycystic ovary syndrome
PEEP: positive end-expiratory pressure
PLMS (or PLM): periodic limb movements during sleep
PSG: polysomnography, polysomnographic
PSQI: Pittsburgh Sleep Quality Index
PTSD: posttraumatic stress disorder
RBD: REM sleep behavior disorder
RDI: respiratory disturbance index
REM: rapid eye movement
RERA: respiratory effort related arousal
RFA: radiofrequency ablation
RIP: respiratory inductive plethysmography
RLS: restless legs syndrome
RMMA: rhythmic masticatory motor activity
ROC: right outer canthus
ROS: reactive oxygen species
RR: risk ratio
RYGB: Roux-en-Y gastric bypass
SCID: Structured Clinical Interview for Diagnosis
SCN: suprachiasmatic nucleus
SDB: sleep-disordered breathing
SE%: sleep efficiency percentage
SEMs: small eye movements
SIDS: sudden infant death syndrome
SOL: sleep-onset latency
SOREM: sleep-onset REM
SOREMP: sleep-onset REM period
SSRI: selective serotonin reuptake inhibitor
SSS: Stanford Sleepiness Scale
SWS: slow wave sleep
TIB: total time in bed
TLR: Toll-like receptor
TMJ: temporomandibular joint
TRD: tongue-retaining device
TST: total sleep time
UARS: upper airway resistance syndrome
UPF: uvulopalatal flap
UPPP: uvulopalatopharyngoplasty
WASO: wake after sleep onset

Assessment and Pathophysiology

Approach and Evaluation of the Patient

Chapter

1

Beth A. Malow; Meir Kryger

Chapter Highlights

- This chapter emphasizes the clinical approach to the patient with disordered sleep, focusing on specific aspects of the history and physical examination.
- Patients who complain of disturbed sleep usually describe one or more of three types of problems: insomnia; abnormal movements, behaviors, or sensations during sleep or during nocturnal awakenings; or excessive daytime sleepiness.
- Taking a systematic history that includes medication use, family history, social history, and review of systems can provide important clues regarding the diagnosis.

Every clinician has patients in his or her practice who have sleep disorders. Because sleep breathing disorders are so common and impact several organ systems (for example, respiratory, cardiovascular, neurological endocrine), patients will present to different practitioners with differing complaints. The pulmonary specialist may be confronted with an obese patient with peripheral edema; the cardiologist may be evaluating a patient with newly diagnosed atrial fibrillation; the neurologist may be treating a patient with a recent stroke; the otolaryngologist may be asked whether surgery can be done for snoring that is disruptive to a bedpartner. Yet, some of the symptoms of sleep breathing disorders overlap with those of other sleep disorders. This section will focus on the approach to the patient with sleep disorders, so that the clinician can recognize which patients might have a sleep breathing disorder and which have another condition that explains their symptoms.

Patients who complain of disturbed sleep usually describe one or more of three types of problems: insomnia; abnormal movements, behaviors, or sensations during sleep or during nocturnal awakenings; and excessive daytime sleepiness. These sleep complaints are not mutually exclusive, and a given sleep disorder may be associated with more than one type. For example, patients with sleep apnea may complain of insomnia, excessive daytime sleepiness, choking or gasping during the night, or all three. Some patients, particularly those with sleep apnea, are frequently referred because a bed partner or family member has witnessed disruptive snoring or cessation of breathing.

CHIEF COMPLAINT AND HISTORY

Evaluation begins with the chief complaint, which provides a focus for delineating the patient's concerns and eliciting the history. It is often useful to ask why the patient is seeking help at the present time, particularly if the problem has been of long-standing. If the chief complaint is from the spouse or bed partner, it is important to determine whether the patient recognizes the problem, is unaware of it, or denies its existence. Many clinicians also obtain a brief patient profile during the interview that includes the patient's age, sex, occupational or academic status, marital status, and living arrangements. The profile often includes valuable information about how the sleep concern is affecting the patient's daily functioning (e.g., difficulty performing job responsibilities or participating in leisure activities with family). After the chief complaint is delineated, details concerning the sleep problem are sought, including its duration, the circumstances at its onset, the factors that lead to exacerbation or improvement, and any associated symptoms.

The patient's daily schedule is reviewed, including the usual bedtime and estimated time to sleep onset, the number and timing of awakenings, and the time of final awakening. Morning symptoms should be elicited, such as increased nasal congestion, dry mouth, or morning headaches. These symptoms may support a diagnosis of obstructive sleep apnea. Daytime symptoms, including during passive or repetitious activities (e.g., watching television or riding in a car), should be investigated to characterize the severity of sleepiness. A comprehensive sleep history also includes questions about the frequency and duration of daytime naps and the presence or absence of cataplexy, hypnic hallucinations, sleep paralysis, and automatic behavior.

Insomnia

Patients with insomnia usually complain that their nocturnal sleep is inadequate in some way. They may describe difficulty falling asleep, frequent awakening, or early morning awakening with inability to return to sleep. It is important to distinguish among these patterns of insomnia because they may have different causes. For example, awakenings from sleep because of obstructive sleep apnea may result in sleep maintenance insomnia but would not result in a patient's complaining of lying awake for hours not being able to fall asleep.

Excessive Sleepiness

Patients with daytime sleepiness typically complain of drowsiness that interferes with daytime activities, unavoidable napping, or both. Falling asleep while driving or at other particularly inappropriate or dangerous times is often the impetus that brings the patient to the clinician. Some of these patients complain that they need more sleep at night or that daytime drowsiness occurs regardless of how much sleep is obtained at night. Patients may also complain of difficulty with concentration or memory or increased irritability. Children may exhibit hyperactivity rather than sleepiness.

The differential diagnosis of excessive daytime sleepiness ranges from insufficient sleep to sufficient sleep that is disrupted by pathologic events, such as apneas, or neurologic disorders, such as narcolepsy. Inquiring about sleep routines and bedtimes and wake times is essential in excluding insufficient sleep as a cause of sleepiness. Asking patients who complain of sleepiness about other associated symptoms provides essential information. Loud snoring, gasping, snorting, and episodes of apnea suggest the diagnosis of obstructive sleep apnea syndrome (see Chapter 9). A history of episodic muscle weakness with buckling of the knees, laxity of the neck or jaw muscles, or complete loss of muscle tone associated with laughter, anger, or hearing or telling a joke suggests cataplexy and a diagnosis of narcolepsy. Questions assessing mood

are needed to identify patients with sleep disorders associated with depression. Circadian rhythm sleep disorders should be considered in patients with complaints of nocturnal insomnia and daytime sleepiness.

Nocturnal Movements, Behaviors, and Sensations

Information from collateral sources is needed for evaluation of episodic movements and behaviors during sleep. The bed partner should be asked to describe behaviors and vocalizations during the episodes, to relate episodes to sleep onset and time of night, and to note the degree of the patient's responsiveness during the episode. The patient's ability to recall the events is also significant. Episodes of inconsolable screaming and amnesia during the first third of the night suggest sleep terrors: episodes of dream-enactment behavior associated with dream recall that occur toward the end of the sleep cycle REM sleep behavior disorder. Epileptic seizures may occur at any time of the night and should be strongly considered if a history of stereotyped behavior or dystonic posturing is elicited.

MEDICATION USE AND MEDICAL HISTORY

Assessment of medication use, including nonprescription medications, herbal supplements, and illicit drugs, is critical because of the wide variety of medications that alter sleep, wakefulness, and sleep disorders.

The history of current or past medical, surgical, and psychiatric illnesses is important information. Seizure disorders, parkinsonism and dementia, arthritic conditions, asthma, ischemic heart disease, migraine or cluster headache, compressive neuropathies, and almost any painful illness can cause significant sleep disturbance. Anemia, renal disease, and pregnancy may cause or exacerbate restless legs syndrome or periodic limb movement disorder. Anxiety disorders, including panic disorder, and mood disorders are psychiatric disturbances that are often accompanied by insomnia, and some patients with depression complain of excessive daytime sleepiness.

FAMILY HISTORY

Specific inquiry should be made about the existence in family members of previously diagnosed sleep disorders or symptoms suggestive of narcolepsy, obstructive sleep apnea, periodic limb movements, enuresis, sleep terrors or sleepwalking, or insomnia. There is a strong genetic contribution to the development of narcolepsy, and genetic and familial influences sometimes have a role in the development and expression of obstructive sleep apnea and some of the parasomnias.

SOCIAL HISTORY

Assessment of psychosocial, occupational, and academic functioning as well as of satisfaction with personal relationships can yield valuable information about the impact of disordered sleep on the patient's life. Alcohol, caffeine, nicotine, and illicit drug use should be determined. Alcohol use or abuse may intensify snoring and obstructive sleep apnea, may be a contributor to insomnia, or may produce long-lasting changes in sleep patterns. Caffeine use produces significant sleep disturbance in susceptible persons, and nicotine dependency may lead to nocturnal awakenings.

REVIEW OF SYSTEMS

The review of systems may uncover symptoms of medical illnesses that can cause or contribute to sleep disorders (Box 1-1). Recent weight gain or increase in collar size increases the likelihood of obstructive sleep apnea. Particular attention should be paid to the cardiovascular and pulmonary systems because of their relation to breathing and oxygenation during sleep. Angina, orthopnea, paroxysmal nocturnal dyspnea, and wheezing may indicate that sleep disturbance is due to cardiac or pulmonary disease. Heartburn and reflux

---

Box 1-1   SAMPLE SLEEP REVIEW OF SYSTEMS

Sleep Habits
Bedtime on weekdays
Bedtime on weekends
Wake time on weekdays
Wake time on weekends
Time it takes to fall asleep
Awakenings during the night
Time it takes to fall back asleep

Morning Symptoms
Dry mouth
Refreshed
Morning headaches
Nasal congestion

Daytime Functioning
Sleepiness (specific situations when patient has fallen asleep)
Falling asleep while driving
Any accidents caused by sleepiness
Memory problems
Difficulty concentrating
Fatigue
Irritability
Naps (how many, how long, dreams?)

Bed Partner's Observations or What Patient Has Been Told
Loudness of snoring (mild, moderate, severe)
Witnessed apneas
Choking or gasping
Arousals

Sleep-Related Movements
Periodic leg movements
Leg cramps
Restless legs symptoms

Narcoleptic Symptoms
Cataplexy
Hallucinations
Sleep paralysis
Automatic behaviors
Disrupted sleep

Genitourinary System
Nocturia
Impaired sexual functioning

Other
Weight gain in recent years
Sleepwalking
Dream-enactment behavior

---

of gastric contents into the throat when the patient is recumbent may cause nocturnal choking episodes. Nocturia is a common cause of disturbed sleep, particularly in older men. Depression or anxiety can contribute to insomnia.

PHYSICAL EXAMINATION

Examination of the head and neck is particularly important in patients with suspected obstructive sleep apnea. Auscultation of the chest may reveal expiratory wheezes in patients with nocturnal asthma attacks. Thoracic abnormalities such as kyphoscoliosis may compromise ventilatory capacity, leading to hypoventilation and nocturnal breathing difficulties. Auscultation may reveal a prominent fourth heart sound originating from the enlarged right ventricle and murmurs related to pulmonary or tricuspid valve insufficiency. On abdominal examination, hepatomegaly may suggest that alcohol abuse is contributing to sleep disturbance or, in conjunction with other findings, that congestive heart failure is a factor.

Findings on mental status testing and neurologic examination may indicate the presence of a psychiatric or neurologic disease that causes or contributes to disturbed sleep. Impairment of short-term memory, judgment, language functions, and abstract reasoning suggests the presence of a dementing illness that may cause insomnia or nocturnal confusion. Assessment of mood may suggest the presence of mania or depression, either of which may be associated with insomnia. Delusional thoughts and agitation may indicate that acute psychosis is the cause of insomnia. Reduced alertness with slurred speech and nystagmus may be signs of hypnotic or sedative abuse. Impaired sensation and reduced or absent tendon reflexes may indicate peripheral neuropathy, sometimes accompanied by nocturnal paresthesias or burning pain. Elements of the physical examination relevant to the sleep patient are covered in greater detail in Chapter 3.

CLINICAL PEARL

A complete sleep and medical history often yields a specific cause of the patient's sleep complaint. For example, in patients complaining of excessive daytime sleepiness, the cause can often be pinpointed by close attention to the patient's (and bed partner's) account of nighttime symptoms, bedtime and wake time schedules, medications, and coexisting medical disorders.

SUMMARY

The evaluation of a patient with disordered sleep begins with the chief complaint, which can be classified as insomnia, daytime sleepiness, episodic nocturnal movements or behaviors, or a combination of these concerns. A thorough characterization of these concerns, coupled with a comprehensive sleep history that includes the daily schedule, bedtime routine, and morning and daytime symptoms, forms the foundation for diagnosis. As in other fields of medicine, it is essential to consider other medical and psychiatric conditions, medication use, family history, social history including the psychosocial situation, review of systems, and physical examination before formulating a differential diagnosis and performing diagnostic studies. This systematic approach allows accurate diagnosis and specific interventions for many treatable sleep disorders.

Cardinal Manifestations of Sleep Disorders

Bradley V. Vaughn; O'Neill F. D'Cruz

Chapter Highlights

- Sleep disorders include a wide range of conditions that impair health and quality of life. To identify patients afflicted with these disorders, to institute effective treatment, and to optimize patients' health and quality of life, early clinical recognition of the fundamental symptoms (insomnia, hypersomnia, and unusual sleep-related behaviors), as well as the more subtle signs of these conditions, is essential.

- Insomnia is a common symptom, and as a diagnostic entity it can be related to many contributing factors. Features that predispose to, precipitate, and perpetuate the insomnia can be identified in persons who suffer from chronic insomnias. Insomnia can have an intricate relationship with other medical and psychiatric disorders.

- Hypersomnia often is a presenting feature of other sleep disorders or may reflect lifestyle choices. The difficulty in diagnosis is in distinguishing sleepiness from fatigue, and in determining the underlying contributing features. The pattern of sleepiness, characteristics of the sleep period including

length, and response to these sleep periods give clear clues. Other manifestations, such as snoring, witnessed apnea, unrefreshing sleep, and morning headache, may indicate potential sleep-related breathing disorders or cataplexy, prompting an evaluation for narcolepsy.

- Unusual nocturnal sensations or events can provide a window into sleep issues. Features of restless legs syndrome, periodic limb movements in sleep, and parasomnias, such as sleepwalking, sleep terrors, and dream enactment, require detailed description of the sleep-related behaviors to help differentiate among potential causes. These events may indicate other underlying sleep disorders and brain disease.

- Sleep issues also may manifest as systemic problems. Findings of hypertension, unexplained weight gain, or mood or cognitive issues may be important flags signaling a need to inquire about underlying sleep issues. In addition, sleep issues may be early signs of brain disease.

Sleep is essential to health, restoring properties that promote wakefulness and a sense of well-being. Sleep disturbance, whether caused by a sleep breathing disorder, or one of the many other sleep disorders, can result in a wide range of systemic and neuropsychological symptoms. Sleep disruption due to intrusion of components of the sleep state into periods of wakefulness may manifest as hypersomnia. Similarly, intrusion of components of wakefulness into the sleep period may manifest as insomnia. Sleep disruption also has consequences for societal and public health by impairing work performance and psychosocial interactions. As the connection of sleep to health is increasingly appreciated, sleep disruption is now recognized to exacerbate symptoms of other diseases. These pathologic effects may manifest as worsening of a preexisting disorder or as impairment of the patient's ability to cope with its symptoms. The challenge for physicians is to recognize these manifestations and appropriately delineate them as being related to dysfunction of sleep.

Most patients referred to sleep centers present with one or a combination of three classic complaints: excessive sleepiness, difficulty attaining or sustaining sleep, or unusual events associated with sleep. These symptoms can be easily

recognized as related to sleep and are not mutually exclusive in nature. Patients may note more than one problem, such as difficulty sleeping at night and excessive sleepiness during the day. Others may complain of unusual events at night with daytime sleepiness or inability to sleep. Each of these symptoms conveys clues to the underlying pathologic process (Figures 2-1 to 2-3). This chapter reviews the cardinal manifestations of sleep disorders and describes some of the key features that guide the clinician to pursue further diagnostic evaluations.

INSOMNIA

The diagnosis of insomnia is dependent on the complaint of difficulty initiating or maintaining sleep combined with daytime sequelae. This combination of poor nighttime sleep with an adverse effect on daytime activities is important to establishment of the complaint as insomnia. The daytime manifestations of insomnia may take the form of excessive fatigue, impairment of performance, or emotional change. Individual sleep need may vary significantly. Some people may feel fine and note no impairment of performance with 5 hours

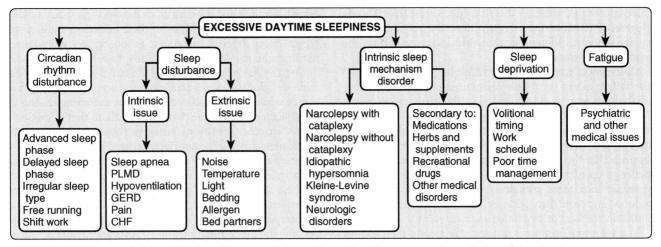

Figure 2-1 Diagnostic flow chart to approach excessive daytime sleepiness. CHF, Congestive heart failure; GERD, gastroesophageal reflux disease; PLMD, periodic limb movement disorder.

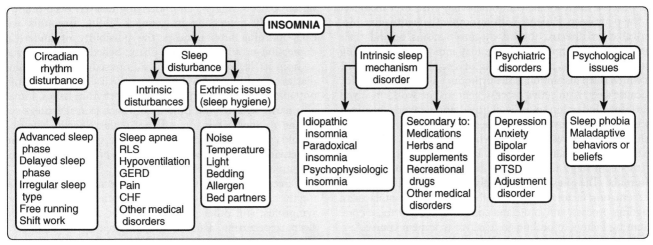

Figure 2-2 Diagnostic flow chart to approach insomnia. CHF, Congestive heart failure; GERD, gastroesophageal reflux disease; PTSD, posttraumatic stress disorder; RLS, restless legs syndrome.

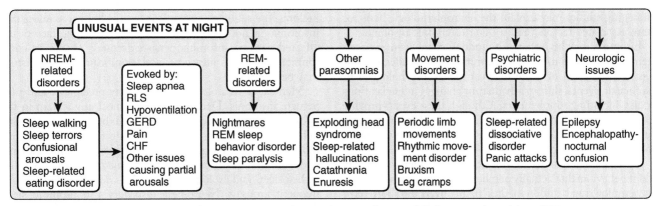

Figure 2-3 Diagnostic flow chart to approach unusual nocturnal events. CHF, Congestive heart failure; GERD, gastroesophageal reflux disease; RLS, restless legs syndrome.

of sleep per night, whereas others may need more than 9 hours to preserve daytime functioning. Thus the requirement of daytime sequelae differentiates individual sleep need from the complaint of insomnia.

Most people have an occasional night fraught with difficulty falling asleep or trouble maintaining sleep. These occasional nights may be closely linked to the surrounding events of the day, psychological challenges, or sudden changes in environment or onset or exacerbation of a medical condition. Surveys have shown that approximately one third of people complain that their sleep is disrupted on occasion and that a smaller group, of approximately 1 in 10, have a more persistent insomnia.[1] For these patients, lack of "good-quality" sleep produces a greater disruption of life and may lead to more significant medical or psychological symptoms.

As a symptom, insomnia is directly related to the patient's perception of poor sleep. Patients with insomnia believe that the sleep disruption produces their excessive sleepiness, fatigue, lack of concentration, muscle aches, and depression, and that a good night's sleep would reverse these symptoms. Patients with insomnia frequently describe themselves as tense, anxious, nervous, tired, irritable, unable to relax, obsessively worried, and depressed. Many of these traits may predate the onset of the insomnia, but others may arise after the onset of the poor sleep. Patients with insomnia frequently give historical clues directed toward the mechanisms behind their insomnia. The symptom complex may indicate an underlying disorder related to primary failure of sleep mechanics or one in which sleep disruption is the byproduct of another disorder. Because sleep is an active process, neuronal networks involved with sleep induction must be engaged and networks involved in wakefulness must be diminished for sleep to occur. Rarely is just one factor responsible for chronic insomnia (defined as lasting longer than 3 months). In most patients, multiple factors contribute to the risk of developing and maintaining insomnia. The presence of predisposing, precipitating, and perpetuating factors emphasizes the nature of insomnia as an ongoing process, and clinicians need to search for these contributing factors to outline an effective treatment course.

As indicated by epidemiologic studies, insomnia appears to be more common in women, older persons, and those with psychiatric or chronic medical illness. Insomnia also is more common in persons of lower socioeconomic status and with less education. Behavioral traits such as obsessive-compulsive nature, frequent rumination, and poor coping strategies and a "hyperalert" baseline state are correlated with greater risk for insomnia. So-called hyperarousal documented on recent neuroimaging studies may explain the neurophysiologic basis for these associated factors predisposing to chronic insomnia.[1]

Insomnia may be initiated by sudden changes in environment or challenges to the body or mind. These challenges may come in the form of acute medical illness, psychological or psychiatric events, shift in schedule, or changes in medications or diet, including supplements. Although these events provide good clues to preventing further recurrence of insomnia, initiating events may play little role in the patient's current, ongoing process..

Many patients, in attempting to improve their sleep, may adopt behaviors that actually perpetuate the insomnia. Patients may employ rituals and "remedies" that convert the short-term insomnia into a chronic form. During this evolution, the patient may institute changes in sleep schedule, resort to

certain somnogenic substances, or develop secondary medical or psychological issues. Many of these behaviors conflict with typical sleep hygiene practices, producing an environment detrimental to sleep. Such maladaptive habits may occur during the day or night and include issues such as heavy caffeine or alcohol use, watching television or playing video games while in bed, and even eating or exercising during the usual sleep period. Some patients may claim that television or radio distracts them from intrusive thoughts. In others, the development of sleep associations may be a mechanism to counterbalance negative experiences. A subgroup of patients actually fear going to bed or experience performance anxiety over the oncoming sleep period. This expectation of poor sleep promotes apprehension toward sleep and may perpetuate counterproductive sleep rituals. These maladaptive behaviors become the predominant feature of psychophysiologic insomnia. Many patients with these types of negative associations temporarily improve once placed in a new environment.

The timing of the insomnia during the sleep period also may be helpful in the evaluation. Circadian rhythm sleep-wake disorders can masquerade as complaints of insomnia or excessive sleepiness, and patients with insomnia may develop dysfunction of their circadian rhythm. Difficulty with the onset of sleep suggests an underlying delayed sleep phase or occasionally depression in younger adults. Insomnia with early-morning arousal raises the possibility of underlying depression or advanced sleep phase. Schedule changes, such as from jet lag or shift work, are important clues, and sleep diaries of bedtime and wake time can be useful in determining potential links to schedule or circadian rhythm issues. Timing also may correlate with other issues such as restless legs syndrome or medication or caffeine intake. Specific questions should explore the patient's daily routine, including the timing of activities that may be stimulating, such as exercise or work or gaming on a computer.

Perception of good sleep is an important factor in evaluating the complaint of insomnia. Some patients exaggerate their symptoms; still other patients may not even recognize that sleep is occurring. Paradoxical insomnia is one subtype of chronic insomnia in which people do not recognize that they have slept despite the recording of normal physiologic parameters of sleep. Other patients may endorse unrealistic expectations or unobtainable goals. Patients may assume that sleep should not be interrupted by any arousals or that it is essential to sleep for a set number of hours. These beliefs can be easily addressed with appropriate education about these issues.

For some people, insomnia may start in childhood and be lifelong. The subtype of chronic insomnia known as idiopathic insomnia is not associated with clear inciting factors. In affected persons, insomnia persists despite a change in environment or other measures, and significant family history may be identified.

Medical or neurologic disorders may precipitate and perpetuate insomnia. Derangement of almost any system in the body can disrupt sleep. Patients with heart, liver, or renal failure or disturbances of the gastrointestinal system or pulmonary disease commonly complain of insomnia. Patients with fulminant rash or significant burns frequently note disturbed sleep, and urologic issues such as nocturia may provoke frequent arousals. Neurologic disorders also promote sleep disruption. Neuromuscular disorders, for example, may be associated with discomfort or inadequate ventilation at night that provokes insomnia. Some patients who suffered a stroke have noted insomnia or sleep disruption after the vascular event. Paralysis from central or peripheral nervous system disorders can result in nighttime discomfort from inability to move. Patients with Parkinson disease may exhibit akinesis, tremor, or medication effects, and patients with dementia may have circadian rhythm abnormalities that promote awakenings at night.

Pain can disturb sleep and promotes insomnia. Musculoskeletal discomfort may become worse with periods of rest. Arthritis and other rheumatologic disorders frequently can disrupt sleep with increasing nighttime pain and stiffness. Pain from headaches, such as cluster headache, and even pain related to increased intracranial pressure or brain mass lesions can become more intense during sleep, and symptoms from entrapment neuropathies, such as carpal tunnel syndrome, typically are worse at night. Restless legs syndrome produces a classic urge to move that is worse in the evening.

Nearly all of the psychiatric illnesses have some link to poor sleep. Patients with depression or anxiety disorders may endure insomnia for years before presentation of the affective component. Although the cause and effect are still in debate, the association is clear. Insomnia may herald the onset of psychosis or mania.

The clinician may uncover few physical findings in patients with insomnia. Anxious or hyperalert persons may demonstrate mild tachycardia or rapid respiratory rate; cold hands may be an associated feature. These patients may easily startle or be distracted during the interview. The clinician should look carefully for signs of obstructive sleep apnea, narrow airway, and obesity because these too can be manifested as insomnia. Signs of Cushing syndrome (round face and buffalo hump) or hyperthyroidism (tachycardia and excessive sweating) are important clues to an endocrine disorder. Each patient with a complaint of insomnia should undergo a complete neurologic examination to look for potential neurologic lesions impairing sleep. This examination should include an assessment of cognition, mood, and affect. Insomnia or interrupted sleep can occur in many neurologic disease states, including several forms of dementia. The Mini Mental State Examination is a tool that helps assess cognitive abilities, with findings monitored for follow-up over time.[2] Clinicians also can use the Minnesota Multiphasic Personality Inventory to identify personality and affect issues, and the Hamilton Anxiety and Depression Scales may be helpful tools in clinical follow-up for persons so affected.

EXCESSIVE DAYTIME SLEEPINESS

Sleepiness is a common symptom noted by 5% to 20% of people.[3,4] Most people can relate some instances of falling asleep when they intended to be awake. Sleepiness is a normal feeling on approaching a typical sleep period or after prolonged wakefulness. Excessive sleepiness may manifest as sleep in an inappropriate setting or as episodes of unintentional sleep. Excessive sleepiness can occur in various degrees of severity. In mild sleepiness, the affected person may fall asleep while reading a book or while sitting quietly. This degree of sleepiness may produce only limited impairment in the person's perceived quality of life. Greater degrees of sleepiness may be associated with bouts of irresistible sleep or sleep attacks intruding on such activities as driving,

participating in a conversation, or eating meals. This degree of sleepiness may place the patient at significant risk for accidents and have a major impact on the person's health and sense of well-being.

As with other subjective symptoms, the person's perception of sleepiness influences the nature of the complaint. Some patients may overreport the degree of sleepiness and note this feeling even during periods of normal wakefulness. Others may underreport and not recognize periods of daytime sleepiness. For some people in the latter group, sleepiness may be described as periods of lapse of attention or diminished cognitive abilities, such as missing an exit on the highway or brief delay in performing a task. Perception of sleepiness also is reduced with continued sleep deprivation. People who are chronically sleep-deprived become accustomed to their impairment and are less likely to recognize their degree of sleepiness.

Clinicians should always question their hypersomnic patients for clues of potential sleep debt, dyssomnia, or medical or psychiatric causes. Sleep deprivation is common in today's society, and patients should be queried about their schedule during the week and weekends. Information elicited about sleep habits and environment may disclose important factors contributing to the sleepiness.

Excessive sleepiness may result from a wide range of medical disorders and medication. Patients with heart, kidney, or liver failure and rheumatologic or endocrinologic disorders such as hypothyroidism and diabetes may note sleepiness and fatigue. Similarly, a wide range of medications may cause daytime sleepiness even when taken at night. Neurologic disorders, such as strokes, tumors, demyelinating diseases, and head trauma, can be associated with excessive sleepiness. Sleepiness frequently is the cardinal symptom of many sleep disorders. Patients with sleep apnea, narcolepsy, idiopathic hypersomnia, or even parasomnias may identify excessive daytime sleepiness as their main complaint. Historical features of snoring, observed apneas, morning headaches, cataplexy, sleep paralysis, hypnagogic hallucinations, and confusion on arousals suggest contributions of a specific sleep disorder. Persons with idiopathic hypersomnolence experience unrelenting daytime sleepiness despite prolonged periods of sleep, which differentiates this disorder from sleep deprivation. Many adults with idiopathic hypersomnia find naps are not refreshing, whereas patients with narcolepsy (type 1 and type 2) note that brief naps actually improve their daytime sleepiness.

Physical findings are few in patients with sleepiness. Frequent pauses, slowed responses, drooping eyelids, and repetitive yawning support the complaint of sleepiness. Patients may be asleep when the clinician enters the examination room, and some patients may show signs of chronic sleepiness, such as dark circles under the eyes. The neurologic examination may yield findings of inattentiveness or even brief "microsleeps."

Sleepiness can be quantified subjectively by questionnaires or by objective assessments such as a multiple sleep latency test. The Epworth Sleepiness Scale is one example of a quantifiable subjective measure of sleepiness and has been translated into several languages (Table 2-1).[5] For scoring on this scale, the patient is asked to rate on a scale of 0 to 3 (0, no chance; 3, high likelihood) the chance of dozing in a series of eight situations. This score has a modest correlation with physiologic measures of sleep but has a better correlation with the respiratory disturbance index in patients with obstructive sleep apnea (Table 2-2).

Two quantitative tests are available to measure ability to fall asleep and to stay awake: the Multiple Sleep Latency Test (MSLT) and the Maintenance of Wakefulness Test. The

MSLT quantifies objective sleepiness on the basis of the time to onset of physiologic changes associated with sleep across five trials separated by 2 hours each across the typical wake period. Sleep is determined by the loss of the posterior dominant rhythm on the electroencephalogram or, in the absence of posterior dominant rhythm, slow eye movements, vertex sharp waves, and slowing of the background electroencephalographic activity. The MSLT uses these physiologic markers to quantify the time to sleep. Unfortunately, the MSLT is not well correlated with daytime function, and significant overlap has been documented between persons deemed "normal" and those deemed to have sleep disruption. Although the MSLT can "quantify" the degree of sleepiness on a particular day, the test is validated only for the diagnosis of narcolepsy (type 1 and type 2). The Maintenance of Wakefulness Test quantifies the propensity to stay awake during four attempts in a dimly lit room. This test has not been extensively tested in relationship to daytime function.

Table 2-1   The Epworth Sleepiness Scale

Name: _____
Today's date: _____ **Your age (years):** _____
Your sex (male = M; female = F): _____
How likely are you to doze off or fall asleep in the following situations, in contrast with feeling just tired? This refers to your usual way of life in recent times. Even if you have not done some of these things recently, try to work out how they would have affected you. Use the following scale to choose the most appropriate number for each situation:

   0 = would never doze
   1 = slight chance of dozing
   2 = moderate chance of dozing
   3 = high chance of dozing

Situation*	Chance of Dozing
Sitting and reading	_____
Watching TV	_____
Sitting, inactive in a public place (e.g., a theater or a meeting)	_____
As a passenger in a car for an hour without a break	_____
Lying down to rest in the afternoon when circumstances permit	_____
Sitting and talking to someone	_____
Sitting quietly after a lunch without alcohol	_____
In a car, while stopped for a few minutes in traffic	_____
Thank you for your cooperation.	

*The numbers for the eight situations are added together to give a global score between 0 and 24.
From Johns MW. A new method for measuring daytime sleepiness: the Epworth Sleepiness Scale. *Sleep* 1991;14:540–5.

FATIGUE

The complaint of fatigue is a complex symptom typically related to the perception of lack of energy. Many patients with excessive daytime sleepiness note fatigue or decreased energy. Patients may be aware of the lack of energy but not perceive the degree of sleepiness, or may confuse the symptom of fatigue with excessive sleepiness. Although frequently noted in combination, fatigue is distinct from excessive sleepiness. Patients with fatigue alone may not have an increased ability to fall asleep but believe that a good night's sleep would correct their lack of energy. Distinguishing sleepiness from fatigue can be difficult even for the most astute clinician. Detailed questioning regarding ability to fall asleep can be helpful. Patients with insomnia also frequently complain of fatigue related to disrupted sleep, as may patients with immunologic, endocrinologic, or organ failure. Similarly, patients with depression frequently have associated fatigue without sleepiness.

SNORING

Snoring is the sound created by turbulent airflow vibrating upper airway soft tissue. Usually more prominent during inspiration, snoring occurs in approximately 32% of adults and

Table 2-2   Sleep-Related Conditions and Sleepiness: Epworth Sleepiness Scale Score in Experimental Subjects

Condition/Diagnosis	Total No. of Subjects (Males/Females)	Age (Years): Mean ± SD	Epworth Sleepiness Scale Score Mean ± SD	Range
Healthy control subjects	30 (14/16)	36.4 ± 9.9	5.9 ± 2.2	2–10
Primary snoring	32 (29/3)	45.7 ± 10.7	6.5 ± 3.0	0–11
Obstructive sleep apnea syndrome	55 (53/2)	48.4 ± 10.7	11.7 ± 4.6	4–23
Narcolepsy	13 (8/5)	46.6 ± 12.0	17.5 ± 3.5	13–23
Idiopathic hypersomnia	14 (8/6)	41.4 ± 14.0	17.9 ± 3.1	12–24
Insomnia	16 (6/12)	40.3 ± 14.6	2.2 ± 2.0	0–6
Periodic limb movement disorder	18 (16/2)	52.5 ± 10.3	9.2 ± 4.0	2–16

SD, Standard deviation.
From Johns MW. A new method for measuring daytime sleepiness: the Epworth Sleepiness Scale. *Sleep* 1991;14:540–5.

in more than 7% of children.[6,7] Many adults have little knowledge or recognition of their snoring habits, and accounts from bed partners may be more helpful for the clinician.

Snoring usually is worse with the patient in the supine position, after sleep deprivation or alcohol ingestion. Loud snoring may not disturb sound sleepers, but some patients may report complaints from family members and even neighbors. Snoring may continue for decades. Persistent loud snoring is a classic symptom of obstructive sleep apnea syndrome, but the absence of snoring does not exclude the diagnosis of apnea. In some cases, the airway dynamics are not conducive to snoring. This is especially true in patients who have had upper airway surgical procedures that eliminated flaccid tissue. Other patients, such as those with neuromuscular disorders, may not generate enough force to produce turbulent airflow.

Snoring, for many people, produces little disruption in their lives, but snoring may have implications for overall health. People who snore are at greater risk for vascular disease. Witnesses may describe the snoring occurring in bursts or associated with snorts, gasps, choking, body jerks, and movements. Patients may recall being awoken by their own gasps and relate symptoms of gastroesophageal reflux. These associated symptoms raise the clinical suspicion of obstructive sleep apnea.

SLEEP APNEA

Apnea is the absence of ventilation. In the sleep laboratory, an apneic event is defined as the cessation of breathing for more than 10 seconds and usually is associated with oxygen desaturation and arousal.[8] Although snoring is very common, witnessed apneic events and nocturnal gasping or choking are the most reliable subjective indicators of sleep apnea.[9] Some patients may experience hundreds of events in a single night and are unable to obtain good-quality sleep because of the frequent arousals. These patients typically are unaware of the arousals, but some may report being aware of occasional awakening with a gasp or snort. Sleep apnea is classified in two major forms: obstructive and central.

Obstructive apnea is the most common form of sleep apnea. These apneas are due to obstruction in the upper airway and more commonly are noted during stage N1 or N2 or rapid eye movement (REM) sleep. Snoring is a frequent associated complaint, but a wide variety of symptoms may be present. Some questionnaires, such as the Sleep Apnea section of the Sleep Disorder Questionnaire, Berlin Questionnaire, or the STOPBANG, a combination of items regarding snoring, witnessed apneas, body habitus, and associated disorders such as hypertension[10,11] (Table 2-3), provide a summary score that correlates with presence of obstructive sleep apnea, but the questionnaires have been tested in selected populations only. Thus the questionnaires themselves serve as rough guides and do not confirm the diagnosis of sleep apnea. Astute clinicians should not rule out the presence of apnea on the basis of a low score on a questionnaire. The physical examination may show structural evidence for airway obstruction. Many patients are obese, with a thick neck or crowded upper airway, yet some have a normal body habitus. Common structural abnormalities, such as a narrow nasal passage, long soft palate, large tonsils, or retroflexed mandible leading to a small airway, contribute to airway obstruction. Sleep apnea is associated

Table 2-3 Key Features of the Berlin Questionnaire

Height _____	Age _____
Weight _____	Gender _____
Has your weight changed in the last 5 years?	Increased Decreased No change
Do you snore?	Yes No Do not know
Your snoring is:	Slightly louder than breathing As loud as talking Louder than talking Very loud
How often do you snore?	Nearly every day 3 to 4 times per week 1 to 2 times per week 1 to 2 times per month Never or almost never
Has your snoring bothered other people?	Yes No
Has anyone noticed that you quit breathing during your sleep?	Almost every day 3 to 4 times per week 1 to 2 times per week 1 to 2 times per month Never or almost never
Are you tired or fatigued after your sleep?	Nearly every day 3 to 4 times per week 1 to 2 times per week 1 to 2 times per month Never or almost never
During your wake time, do you feel tired, fatigued, or not up to par?	Nearly every day 3 to 4 times per week 1 to 2 times per week 1 to 2 times per month Never or almost never

Have you ever fallen asleep while driving?	Yes
	No
	If so, how often does it occur?
	    Nearly every day
	    3 to 4 times per week
	    1 to 2 times per week
	    1 to 2 times per month
	    Never or almost never

Do you have high blood pressure?	Yes No Do not know

Modified from Reprinting of the Berlin questionnaire. *Sleep Breath* 2000;4(4): 187–92, with the permission of Kingman P. Strohl.

with significant health risks and lowers the quality of life of both patient and bed partner. Mounting evidence from multiple studies such as the Sleep Heart Health Study indicates that hypopneas with oxygen desaturation correlate with greater risk of vascular disease.[12] These are discussed in greater detail in Chapters 25 to 27.

Central apnea is the absence of ventilation due to an absence of contraction of the lower respiratory musculature. Affected patients experience pauses in respiration, also associated with oxygen desaturation and arousals. Central apneas can be caused by narcotics or a neurologic abnormality in the brainstem or other areas involved in regulation of respiration. Cheyne-Stokes breathing can manifest features of both central and obstructive apnea. The classic pattern of crescendo-decrescendo breathing with a central apnea can be seen in persons with heart failure, neurologic lesions, and metabolic or toxic encephalopathies. This pattern may be present only in sleep and may signal underlying disease. Apneic episodes may follow other neurologic events, such as nocturnal seizures, and are more prevalent after acute strokes and seizures. Central apnea is reviewed in Chapters 12 and 15.

CATAPLEXY

Cataplexy is the abrupt loss of muscle tone triggered by strong emotional stimuli or physical exercise.[13] Patients are aware of their surroundings and have clear memory for the complete events. Events can be triggered by a joke, surprise, anger, fear, or enthusiastic athletic endeavors. Individual experiences range in intensity from a mild feeling of weakness to severe weakness precipitating a fall. Cataplectic attacks arise over several seconds and may start with brief waves of loss of tone that may appear like jerks initially. In most cases, symptoms initially affect the face and neck and then progress to involve the rest of the body. Patients may describe more subtle events as a feeling of slowness to respond or slurring or speech. The attacks generally are brief, lasting less than a few minutes. Patients then regain muscle control and exhibit no postictal confusion or memory deficits. More prolonged attacks may be ended with the patient's entering sleep and then awakening. Examination of the patient during the cataplectic attack will demonstrate paralysis with diffuse hypotonia, absence of deep tendon reflexes, diminished corneal reflexes, preservation of pupillary responses, and in many instances, phasic muscle twitching. Phasic muscle twitching can occur as single jerks or repetitive muscle twitching and most frequently is seen in the face, sometimes being confused with seizure activity.

The combination of excessive daytime sleepiness and cataplexy is nearly always related to narcolepsy type 1. Cataplexy can rarely be seen as an isolated symptom suggestive of an underlying neurologic lesion in the brainstem. Maintenance of consciousness and memory helps differentiate these events from most seizures and syncope. The historical feature of clear emotional triggers differentiates cataplexy from vertebral basilar insufficiency and the group of neuromuscular disorders known to produce periodic paralysis. Cataplexy also is differentiated from myasthenia gravis by the abrupt onset and absence of muscle fatigue with repetitive stimulation that is typical of myasthenia gravis.

SLEEP PARALYSIS

Sleep paralysis is an inability to move during the transition into or out of sleep. The association with intentional sleep distinguishes these events from cataplexy. Patients may describe complete awareness of their surroundings or feeling partially asleep with awareness but being unable to move even the fingers or to vocalize. Patients may try to scream but produce only a whisper. Some affected persons may describe a feeling of suffocation, with resumption of breathing only

when the event has passed. Patients frequently describe a strong feeling of impending doom, being chased, or having to escape imminent danger. On occasion, patients may note the feeling that someone else is in the bedroom. Auditory and tactile hallucinations may accompany the events, and patients may recount dramatic stories. These events can be emotionally profound and leave a lasting memory that patients vividly recall years later. Most sleep paralysis episodes last a few minutes and usually end after the patient is touched or is alerted. If the event is allowed to persist, the patient usually reenters sleep and awakens later. These events are experienced by many people in association with severe sleep deprivation, schedule disruption, or ingestion of alcohol and may be more frequent in patients with narcolepsy.

HYPNAGOGIC AND HYPNOPOMPIC HALLUCINATIONS

Hallucinations can occur with sleep onset (hypnagogic) or at the end of sleep (hypnopompic). Such hallucinations may include visual, auditory, or tactile components and may last seconds to minutes. The events occur at the transition between wake and sleep and incorporate some dream-like features. They can be relatively pleasant or very terrifying and difficult to distinguish from reality. Patients may note a feeling of weightlessness, falling, or flying or describe an out-of-body experience; the episode may sometimes terminate with a sudden jerk (hypnic jerk). Visual hallucinations may be described as poorly formed colors and shapes or well-formed images of people and animals. The events are terminated once the patient awakens.

Exploding head syndrome is characterized by the subjective experience of a loud, painless explosion that occurs near sleep onset. This parasomnia is benign and may be associated with a hallucinatory flash of light.

In the face of excessive daytime sleepiness, patients with hypnagogic hallucinations should be evaluated for narcolepsy. These events may be repetitive but usually are not stereotypical. This lack of stereotypical features distinguishes these events from seizures. Affected patients may experience these events after sleep deprivation or a change in the sleep schedule. Alcohol ingestion or withdrawal of REM suppressants may also provoke these events. The relationship of sleep to these hallucinations distinguishes them from hallucinations of psychosis and dementia. Hypnagogic hallucinations are shorter in duration than peduncular hallucinations. Some people with dementia experience hallucinations at night. These types of hallucinations are associated with cognitive impairment during the day and most commonly are seen in patients with Lewy body dementia but can occur with other forms of dementia. Small people or animals predominate in these hallucinations, and many patients experience these events while awake.

AUTOMATIC BEHAVIOR

Automatic behavior consists of purposeful but inappropriate activities that occur with the patient partially asleep. Patients relay stories of putting milk containers in the microwave oven, cereal bowls in the dryer, or even missing an exit on the highway. Sleep-deprived soldiers have been reported to continue marching in the wrong direction. Patients appear drowsy or groggy during the event and usually are partially or totally amnestic for the actual happenings. Events may last minutes to up to an hour. Automatic behavior and "sleep inertia," the persistence of profound sleepiness into the awake state, are more common in persons with idiopathic hypersomnolence but also are common in patients with a delayed sleep phase.

These events are distinguished from seizures by the lack of stereotypical behavior. Automatisms associated with seizures usually are stereotypical and repetitive, such as picking, rubbing, or lip smacking. Patients with sleep-related automatic behavior appear sleepy but can be alerted and answer questions appropriately, in contrast with those with postictal confusion and metabolic or toxic encephalopathy. The quick return of orientation with lack of bewilderment and anxiety also differentiates this entity from transient global amnesia.

EXCESSIVE MOVEMENT IN SLEEP OR PARASOMNIA

Patients and their bed partners may complain of frequent movement during the sleep period. This complaint may be more concerning to the bed partner than to the patient. Excessive sleep movement also is a common complaint among patients who complain of insomnia and in persons with sleep apnea. Some patients may complain of being active sleepers and describe a corresponding high level of mental activity or an inability to turn off their mind. These patients need an evaluation focusing on features of insomnia. Those who are physically active need evaluation for the movements or a parasomnia.

Parasomnia refers to undesirable physical or behavioral phenomena that occur predominantly during sleep. They include disorders of arousals, such as sleepwalking and night terrors; sleep-wake transition disorders, such as bruxism or rhythmic movement disorder (e.g., head banging); and REM parasomnias, such as REM sleep behavior disorder. These behavioral events may mimic epileptic seizures or other psychiatric events, and a clear description from a keen observer is very helpful in leading to the correct diagnosis.

Key features of age at onset, time of night of the events, memory for the events, and family history are important in determining the etiology of parasomnias. Stereotypical behavior—recurrence of the same behavior with each event—also can help in categorizing the events. Events such as periodic limb movements, rhythmic movement disorder, and epileptic seizures are associated with stereotypical behavior, whereas sleeptalking, sleepwalking, night terrors, and dream enactment incur different behavior with each event. Although historical features can be useful in distinguishing among these disorders, most patients require polysomnographic recording to delineate the cause.

Sleeptalking

Sleeptalking is a relatively frequent event, ranging from occasional utterances to coherent conversation during sleep. This usually occurs in the lighter stages of NREM sleep but can occur in REM ("stage R") sleep. Patients have no memory for such events, during which they may convey information that may have little resemblance to the truth. Many people talk in

their sleep, and this is considered a normal variant. In the absence of other sleep disturbances, sleeptalking is of little medical concern.

Sleepwalking

Sleepwalking events usually are part of the disorders of arousal, indicating incomplete arousal typically from slow wave sleep (stage N3) occurring during the first half of the sleep period. The events can consist of minor behaviors and movement or elaborate behaviors including dressing, unlocking locks, minor housekeeping or work tasks, and even driving. Patients usually have little or no memory of the event. They typically can recall various associated feelings or impressions, however, and some imagery is more common in adults. Affected patients do not exhibit significant tachycardia, sweating, or manifestations of fear. The lack of screaming and autonomic features differentiates sleepwalking from sleep terrors. Both children and adults with a history of recent sleepwalking should be questioned regarding signs of other sleep disorders. Any disorder evoking arousals may increase the likelihood of these events, so a careful assessment to uncover symptoms of other sleep disorders is essential. Patients typically exhibit normal neurologic examination findings during wakefulness.

Sleep Terrors

Sleep terrors are a more intense form of disorder of arousal with a predominance of autonomic expression. Witnesses rarely forget the patient's sudden arousal accompanied by a piercing scream or cry, autonomic output, and behavioral manifestation of intense fear, but the patient has little to no memory of the event. The onset of the episode is abrupt, accompanied by tachycardia, tachypnea, flushing, diaphoresis, and mydriasis. The affected patient is confused and disoriented, and attempts to intercede may result in prolongation of the event and potential harm to the person trying to wake the patient. Patients can become violent, resulting in injury to the patient and bed partners. Less than 1% of adults may experience these events.[14] They usually occur in the first third of the night, and the events are nonstereotypical. Diurnal neurologic examination typically yields normal findings, and as with sleepwalking, a careful assessment for the presence of other sleep disorders is indicated.

Confusional Arousals

Confusional arousals can occur during any arousal from NREM sleep. These events are characterized by disorientation, slowed speech and mentation, or inappropriate behavior. Affected patients have memory impairment for the event, and the events can be induced with forced arousal. These events usually become less frequent with age, but rate of occurrence may remain stable in adulthood.

Patients may exhibit other complex sleep-related behaviors. In a well-characterized variant of such behavior, eating is the sleep-related event, as seen in sleep-related eating disorder. Affected persons consume quantities of high-calorie, sometimes bizarre foods and have no or little memory of the episode. Morning anorexia and unexplained weight gain are typical. Another reported complex sleep behavior consists of engaging in multiple episodes of sexual intercourse during sleep. Again, the affected person relates no memory of the event.

Sleep-Related Groaning (Catathrenia)

Rarely, patients or families may present because of repetitive nocturnal groaning. Bed partners usually express concern because the patients voice long expiratory groans that sound mournful. Patients usually have no recollection of the sound or feeling distressed but may have morning hoarseness. No other detectable abnormalities are found on physical examination. These groaning events have been compared with central apneas, and the disorder is now classified under sleep-related breathing disorders.[15]

Dream Enactment

REM sleep ("stage R") is characterized by diffuse muscle atonia. Normally, only brief phasic muscle activity is noted during REM sleep, but pathologic dream enactment behavior can include punching, kicking, leaping, running, talking, yelling, and any behavior that could occur during a dream. Bed partners frequently are injured, and patients may go to great lengths to protect themselves and bed partners. This dream enactment commonly is seen as part of REM sleep behavior disorder (RBD). Patients usually have a vivid recall of the actual dreams that correlates with the witnessed behavior, and many dreams involve fleeing or defending themes. Dream recall is not uniformly noted, and patients may not be willing to talk about the dream that led them to seek medical attention. These events occur more commonly in the latter half of the night but can occur any time on entry into REM sleep. Patients may experience multiple events during a single night. In most cases, the dream enactment behavior begins in late adulthood, but children with symptoms of RBD have been described. RBD can be induced by medication, and tricyclic antidepressants, monoamine oxidase inhibitors, and serotonin reuptake inhibitors all have been implicated in causing RBD-like behavior. Acute forms of RBD also can occur during alcohol withdrawal and potentially benzodiazepine withdrawal. In the more chronic form of RBD, behaviors may occurr for years before the patient presents for medical evaluation. RBD has been linked to alpha-synucleinopathies. This group of disorders includes Parkinson disease, multiple system atrophy, and Lewy body dementia. Patients need a complete neurologic evaluation to look for signs of degenerative disorders. Other identifiable neurologic disorders, such as strokes, posterior fossa tumors, and demyelination, have been reported in association with RBD.[16]

Nightmares

Nightmares or recurrent disturbing dream mentation can be a presenting symptom of sleep disturbance. The hallmark of nightmares is emotionally intense dreaming associated with fear, anxiety, anger, sadness, or other negative emotions. Affected persons awaken from stage R or light NREM sleep to full alertness and usually recall the event immediately. Nightmares most commonly are associated with a psychologically disturbing event but may also be a result of medications, such as antihypertensives, antidepressants, or dopamine agonists. Nightmares can occur in patients with narcolepsy as well as in patients with sleep apnea.

Sleep-Related Rhythmic Movement Disorder

Rhythmic movement disorder can be manifested as a variety of distracting behaviors that occur before sleep onset. The movements are stereotypical, usually involving large muscles, and are sustained into light sleep. Movements and related behaviors may include head banging, body rocking, leg rolling, humming, and chanting and frequently are more concerning to the bed partner and family than to the patient. Many patients are relatively unaware of the movement, and others may describe such movement as inducing a calming effect or as a compulsion before sleep. This behavior frequently is seen in infants and young children, and the prevalence diminishes with age. It is more commonly seen in persons with mental challenges or autism and is more prevalent in males. Emotional stress may provoke it. Patients can be easily alerted during the events, which helps differentiate these events from seizures.

Sleep-Related Bruxism

Sleep bruxism also can occur as a rhythmic or repetitive movement during sleep.[17] Grinding or clenching of the teeth during sleep may produce bizarre sounds, and patients rarely may even vocalize with the episodes. Patients may exhibit abnormal wear of the teeth and complain of jaw pain, headache, facial pain, or tooth pain. They may experience hundreds of events per night, and the events increase with emotional stress. Some studies suggest that as many as 85% of the population grinds the teeth to some degree during the day or night. These events often occur in children, and persistence of symptoms occasionally is associated with a familial tendency.

RESTLESS LEGS SYNDROME AND PERIODIC MOVEMENTS OF SLEEP

Patients may complain of an unpleasant crawling, deep aching sensation in the legs or arms that is relieved in some measure by motion of the extremities. Diagnostic criteria focus on four main symptoms: the sensation or urge to move the limbs, worsening of symptoms with rest, improvement with movement, and higher frequency in the evening.[18] In addition, the patient must note a symptom of concern, distress, sleep disturbance, or some impairment related to the sensations. Patients with restless legs syndrome may relay that the discomfort can be debilitating at times, and some people are driven to pursue extreme measures to decrease the symptoms. Most patients experience the symptoms while sitting or lying down and may complain of the need to walk or to have continuous movement of their legs. These symptoms can lead to the affected person's walking until the early morning hours or trying to sleep despite the continuous leg motion. Other afflicted persons may use a combination of medication and alcohol to reduce the symptoms. Some patients note that their legs move or dance on their own, indicating periodic limb movements in wakefulness. Restless legs syndrome usually occurs along with periodic movements of sleep.

Periodic movements of sleep are repetitive stereotypical movements, typically of the lower extremities, that occur during sleep; in the legs, they consist of the extension of the great toe with dorsiflexion of the ankle and flexion of the knee and hip. The patient or a bed partner may complain of kicking or arm movements at night. These movements may occur as periodic events or appear random. Movements also can occur in the arms and axial muscles. The individual movements are relatively brief, lasting 0.5 to 5.0 seconds, and occur at 5- to

90-second intervals. Although a majority of people with restless legs also experience periodic limb movements of sleep, only a minority of patients with periodic movements of sleep will experience excessive daytime sleepiness or insomnia. Patients may be unaware of the movements, but bed partners usually are unable to ignore them. Similar factors that provoke periodic limb movements increase the likelihood of restless legs syndrome. Periodic movements of sleep have been associated with uremia, peripheral vascular disease, anemia, arthritis, peripheral neuropathy, spinal cord lesions, antidepressants, antiemetics, and caffeine use.

MORNING HEADACHE

Morning headache is a common symptom.[19] Almost three fourths of the population has occasional headache; this symptom is relatively nonspecific. Morning headache is more specifically linked to sleep dysfunction but also may indicate elevated blood pressure at night. Characteristics of the headache, such as location, quality, and nature of pain, and potential associations can aid in determining the etiology. Approximately one half of the patients with obstructive sleep apnea and hypoventilation note morning headache, typically dull and generalized in nature, which usually clears within an hour of waking. Patients with chronic obstructive pulmonary disease, obstructive sleep apnea and the obesity hypoventilation syndrome may develop morning headache from the increase in carbon dioxide, low oxygen saturation, or vascular changes. Patients with sinus disorders, muscle contraction headache, post–alcohol intake, and withdrawal from medication (rebound headaches) may have distinct patterns. Cluster headaches are noted to occur in REM sleep. Hypnic headaches, or "alarm clock headaches," so called because of their regularity, are throbbing or sharp pains lasting 15 to 60 minutes that awaken the patient typically between 1 A.M. and 3 A.M. Headaches that routinely awaken patients from sleep should be further evaluated, potentially including head imaging. Patients with brain tumors frequently note worsening of headache at night.

SYSTEMIC FEATURES

Recognition of the connection of good sleep to good health continues to expand the current understanding of the importance of sleep. Sleep plays a role in endocrine regulation, weight maintenance, and metabolism and has been hypothesized to improve neuronal network proficiency and function. Therefore sleep disorders may influence both regulatory processes and compensatory mechanisms.

Sleep disorders may influence systemic disorders by three general mechanisms: (1) they may directly cause the primary physiologic changes that result in systemic disease; (2) they may exacerbate a preexisting disorder by altering a normal compensatory mechanism; or (3) they may be the hallmark symptom of the systemic disease, sharing a common pathophysiologic mechanism. Sleep disorders may result in systemic manifestations, as noted in sleep-related breathing disorders. Sleep-related disordered breathing can result in a variety of vascular and autonomic changes that increase the likelihood of hypertension and other vascular disorders.

In patients with high-risk disorders, including those with hypertension, vascular disease, heart disease, diabetes mellitus, and obesity, the clinical assessment should include specific evaluation for symptoms of sleep dysfunction that may indicate sleep disorders acting as a cofactor. Sleep disorders (e.g., obstructive sleep apnea or hypoventilation) may exacerbate underlying conditions such as hypertension, diabetes mellitus, congestive heart failure, epilepsy, and depression. Thus the clinician must pay attention to aggravation of symptoms of medical, neurologic, or psychiatric dysfunction as a clue to disordered sleep. The interplay of sleep and brain function makes symptoms of neurologic and psychiatric disease natural manifestations of sleep dysfunction. This association has been documented in persons with epilepsy as well as in those with symptoms of depression and anxiety. Patients may not be aware of the connection of sleep to their other medical problems or may not place emphasis on their sleep symptoms. Therefore the clinician needs to consider the potential of sleep disturbance as an aggravating factor and to recognize the relationship of systemic findings to sleep disruption. Patients also may present with a systemic illness that may share a common pathophysiologic mechanism with a sleep disorder. In persons with anemia and restless legs, iron deficiency may be the common link, so appropriate treatment of the underlying cause may address the symptoms of both. Finally, the sleep symptom may be the hallmark of another process, as observed with REM sleep behavior disorder preceding the development of other neurologic disorders such as Parkinson disease. Although these symptoms may not be considered the typical cardinal manifestations of sleep disorders, their clinical identification does represent an important aspect of diagnosis and may constitute an appropriate entry point for patients into the medical system. Recognition of the systemic manifestations of sleep disorders is an important step in understanding the full relationship of sleep to the body.

PEDIATRIC CARDINAL MANIFESTATIONS

Symptoms of sleep disorders in children can be strikingly different from those in adults and are likely to be overlooked or misinterpreted.[20] Moreover, disruption of family dynamics, psychosocial factors that influence the family unit, and temperamental differences between parent-child pairs may be reported as childhood sleep disorders. Sleep-onset associations, cultural norms, and parental expectations can influence the perception of sleep problems in infants and toddlers. Children can present with a range of physical and behavioral manifestations. In young children, sleep disturbances may manifest as poor growth, learning difficulties, persistent fussiness, inconsolability, or increased oppositional behavior. School-aged children may exhibit suboptimal academic performance, inattention or hyperactivity, or daydreaming behavior in sedentary settings. Adolescents typically fall asleep in class and may present with affective symptoms that need to be differentiated from primary psychiatric disorders. In children with symptoms of RLS (often reported as "growing pains"), a strong family history often is present, suggesting a hereditary predisposition with age-dependent expression. In all pediatric age groups, unrefreshing nocturnal sleep often is a clue to sleep disturbance. Although many of these symptoms are nonspecific, the clinician must be aware of the potential role of sleep dysfunction in the genesis of the symptoms.

CLINICAL PEARL

Patients may present with initial complaints that may seem unrelated to sleep, such as morning headache, "fogginess" during the day, or elevated blood pressure. The patient initially may not have any concerns about his or her sleep or may not even be aware of sleep symptoms. Clarifying functional questions (e.g., asking patients to describe how they feel during certain activities such as on getting up in the morning or after lunch) may give additional clues. Also, family members may be aware of sleep issues before the patient notices a problem, thus lending insight into the impact of sleep on the clinical picture.

SUMMARY

Sleep provides the benchmark for many aspects of daily life. The restorative powers of sleep improve baseline status in wakefulness and maximize the ability to attain higher levels of functioning, whereas poor sleep has a negative impact on health, sense of well-being, and performance. Obvious manifestations of poor sleep, such as daytime sleepiness, insomnia, and sleep-related events, are the hallmark signs indicating the need for further investigation. A proper understanding of the intricate relationship of sleep and health must go beyond the most apparent manifestations of sleepiness. The astute clinician should be alert to less obvious and discrete signs. Predominance of negative over positive memories, trouble with creative solutions, obesity, and poor healing all may suggest sleep disruption. In both research and clinical practice, it is essential to continue to search for more clues that delineate the connection of sleep to health. The insights thus obtained can be expected to expand the clinical recognition of these cardinal manifestations of sleep disorders. Identification of persons who need further evaluation and application of appropriate therapies, will lead to optimal management of individual patients and also address the societal and public health issues associated with these disorders.

Selected Readings

Alibhai FJ, Tsimakouridze EV, Reitz CJ, et al. Consequences of circadian and sleep disturbances for the cardiovascular system. *Can J Cardiol* 2015;**31**: 860–72.

American Academy of Sleep Medicine. *International classification of sleep disorders*. 3rd ed. Darien (Ill.): American Academy of Sleep Medicine; 2014.

Bauters F, Rietzschel ER, Hertegonne KB, Chirinos JA. The link between obstructive sleep apnea and cardiovascular disease. *Curr Atheroscler Rep* 2016;**18**(1):1. doi:10.1007/s11883-015-0556-z.

Baumann CR, Mignot E, Lammers GJ, et al. Challenges in diagnosing narcolepsy without cataplexy: a consensus statement. *Sleep* 2014;**37**: 1035–42.

Boeve BF, Silber MH, Ferman TJ, et al. Clinicopathologic correlations in 172 cases of rapid eye movement sleep behavior disorder with or without a coexisting neurologic disorder. *Sleep Med* 2013;**14**:754–62.

Buysse DJ. Insomnia. *JAMA* 2013;**309**:706–16.

Chung F, Abdullah HR, Liao P. STOP-Bang Questionnaire: A Practical Approach to Screen for Obstructive Sleep Apnea. *Chest* 2016;**149**(3): 631–8.

Hoban TF. Sleep disorders in children. *Ann N Y Acad Sci* 2010;**1184**:1–14.

Howell MJ. Parasomnias: an updated review. *Neurother* 2012;**9**:753–75.

Leschziner G, Gringras P. Restless legs syndrome. *BMJ* 2012;**344**:e3056.

Mannarino MR, Di Filippo F, Pirro M. Obstructive sleep apnea syndrome. *Eur J Intern Med* 2012;**23**:586–93.

Scammell TE. Narcolepsy. *N Engl J Med* 2015;**373**(27):2654–62.

Zeitzer JM. Control of sleep and wakefulness in health and disease. *Prog Mol Biol Transl Sci* 2013;**119**:137–54.

A complete reference list can be found online at ExpertConsult.com.

Physical Examination in Sleep Medicine

Alon Y. Avidan; Meir Kryger

Chapter Highlights

- Because many patients who present with sleep disorders have sleep-disordered breathing, assessment of vital signs (heart rate, blood pressure, pulse rate), along with height and weight to calculate the body mass index (BMI), is key.

- Head and neck physical examination is critical for evaluation of any directly visualized anatomic factors that could hinder airflow at the level of the upper airway. This chapter reviews the Mallampati and Friedman classification systems used to assess upper airway patency.

- In addition to increased BMI, other factors that predispose to sleep apnea include increased neck circumference, macroglossia, retrognathia, tonsillar adenoid hypertrophy, overjet, and decreased cricomental space. This chapter provides some specific examples of how these factors are measured and contribute to sleep apnea.

- Specific phenotypes that contribute to sleep-disordered breathing include systemic diseases such as systemic amyloidosis and mucopolysaccharidosis, which lead to abnormal upper airway tissue infiltration and airway restriction.

- Craniofacial disorders related to Down syndrome, acromegaly, and primary mandibular deficiency result in abnormal reduction of upper airway size and contribute directly to obstructive sleep apnea.

- Facial and body habitus phenotype in specific endocrinopathies such Graves disease, Cushing disease, and polycystic ovarian syndrome can predispose patients to both sleep apnea and insomnia and should prompt the clinician to review for these complaints in the appropriate patients.

- Patients with neurologic disorders have significant sleep comorbidities. For example, those with neuromuscular disorders and motor neuron disease are especially vulnerable to nocturnal hypoventilation. Specific neurologic signs such as bulbar weakness, Gower maneuver from sitting to standing, and hypophonia are critical and should prompt the clinician to ask about breathing patterns, sleepiness, and nighttime sleep disruption.

- Patients with parasomnias and nocturnal seizures may present with unexplained bruises, ecchymosis, and nonspecific injuries the next day.

- Symptoms of rapid eye movement sleep behavior disorder often precede the onset of Parkinson disease. Patients with Parkinson disease present with neurologic examination findings of bradykinesia, cogwheel rigidity, masked facies, and resting tremor.

- Patients with bruxism, when severe, often demonstrate dental consequences, including teeth fractures and masseter muscle hypertrophy.

- Patients with narcolepsy often lack characteristic features on physical examination. However, cataplectic facies is a physical finding that was recently used to describe facial weakness and grimaces among patients with cataplexy in the setting of narcolepsy type 1.

The physical examination of the patient presenting with sleep complaints provides important supporting information for the diagnosis of a sleep disorder. In this chapter, the examination findings characteristic of the major categories of sleep disorders are described and illustrated. These include findings observed in obstructive sleep apnea (OSA), central sleep apnea, hypoventilation syndromes, narcolepsy, Willis-Ekbom disease (WED), parasomnias, and bruxism.

After obtaining the narrative medical history, the sleep care provider performs the physical examination, a key and necessary element in evaluating patients with sleep disorders. Patients may have more than one sleep disorder. The examination may provide important clues that lead to elucidation of the etiology and pathophysiology of the sleep disorder. These will help guide the clinician in determining what diagnostic tests will be ordered, what comorbidities require management, and ultimately what therapy will be employed. The physical examination is a critical component of monitoring outcome of treatment of many sleep disorders.

SLEEP APNEA

OSA is associated with multiple anatomic and physical risk factors. Some of these require elaborate measurements of nasopharyngeal anatomy using fiberoptic visualization or cephalometric radiographic techniques, whereas others measure changes in response to maneuvers. The most commonly used signs are static, anthropometric measurements from simple examination of oropharyngeal and craniofacial structure.[1] However, at the time of the initial evaluation of the sleep apnea patient, the main ones are obesity, as reflected by elevated body mass index (BMI), and increased neck circumference.[2]

Figure 3-1 summarizes the key anatomic changes that result from increasing age and BMI. The airways become restricted, and the soft palate, which becomes longer and thicker, is now closer to the posterior and lateral pharyngeal walls, restricting the retropalatal space even further.[2] Increased adipose volume in the floor of the mouth displaces the tongue superiorly and posteriorly, thus decreasing the retroglossal airway space. Chronic allergic rhinitis expands the turbinate tissue, leading to diminished intranasal airway space (see Figure 3-1). The spread of adipose volume in the

submental triangle and in the supraplatysmal regions produces the so-called double-chin appearance with a full neck phenotype.[2]

Anthropometric Measurements in Patients with Suspected Sleep Apnea

Obesity, as measurement of BMI, is strongly associated with OSA. However, recent data indicate that general body adiposity and regional adiposity are also important risk factors in the evolution of OSA. Besides BMI, other anthropometric obesity indexes, such as increased waist circumference and neck circumference, are significant risk factors for the evolution of OSA.[3]

Body Mass Index Calculations

The following BMI criteria are used to quantitate weight phenotype[4]: Patients with a BMI below 18.5 are considered underweight, those between 18.5 and 24.9 are classified as normal weight, those between 25.0 and 29.9 are classified a overweight, and those with a BMI higher than 30.0 are obese (Table 3-1).

Figure 3-2 illustrates the obesity phenotype in two brothers. Visceral fat accumulation, as depicted in Figures 3-3 and 3-4, is an important risk indicator for sleep apnea, particularly in male patients.[1,2,4] Expansion of regional fat deposition is believed to compromise airway space, whereas visceral or

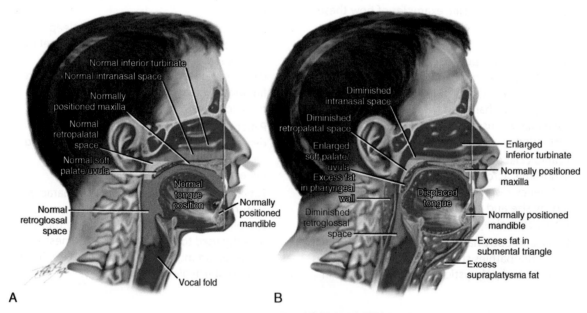

Figure 3-1 Normal and abnormal airway anatomy. **A,** This illustrated midline sagittal cross-section of the head and neck depicts the normal upper airway and maxillofacial spaces and anatomy of a healthy, normal-weight 20-year-old man. The patient has a normal upper and lower facial skeleton and normal soft tissue indicators (soft palate, tongue, tonsils, and adenoids), without any compromise of the intranasal cavity. **B,** With increasing age and weight gain, the same individual, three decades later has an elevated body mass index. Although the anatomy of the upper and lower facial skeleton remains fixed without any changes, fatty tissue consisting of adipose cells has expanded and infiltrated the crevices and space in the upper airway. Particularly compromised are the retropharyngeal and the lateral pharyngeal tissues, the soft palate, and the floor of the mouth, culminating in restricted airflow. At age 20 years, the patient had normal upper airway space (the intranasal, retropalatal, and the retroglossal sites were all well visualized and with appropriate space for air flow to proceed smoothly and unimpeded. At age 50 years, he has developed obstructive sleep apnea: The normal airspace (*green*) is severely compromised because of restriction of the upper airway, intranasal space, and retropalatal and the retroglossal spaces. A *perfect storm* indeed. (From Posnick JC. Obstructive sleep apnea: evaluation and treatment. In: Posnick JC, editor. *Orthognathic surgery: principles and practice*. Philadelphia: Elsevier; 2014. p. 992–1058.)

abdominal obesity reduces lung volume and therefore caudal traction on the pharynx.[5]

Neck circumference at the superior border of the cricothyroid membrane can be measured to evaluate excessive adiposity in the upper body. This measurement is performed with the patient in the upright position (Figure 3-5). Recent data suggest that in adults with metabolic syndrome, measurement of neck circumference is associated with OSA and should be considered in the definition of metabolic syndrome (Figure 3-6).[6] In pediatric and adolescent patients, neck circumference percentile, particularly that greater than the 95th percentile for age and sex, may be an additional screening tool for OSA.[7] In adults, having a large neck circumference in the context of OSA can predict difficult intubations in the anesthesia setting[8] and has been documented in several metabolic derangements, as in the patients presented in Figure 3-7.[9]

However, many patients with OSA are not obese but may exhibit reduced oropharyngeal airspace, retrognathia, or micrognathia, which put patients are risk for OSA (Figure 3-8). In contrast, central sleep apnea usually presents with abnormalities reflective of impaired respiratory effort, including the manifestations of heart failure, central nervous system (CNS) disease, or neuromuscular disease. Hypoventilation may be secondary to obesity but may also reflect pulmonary disease or neuromuscular and chest wall disorders. We review the manifestations of sleep apnea on the basis of anatomic site.

Overall Inspection

As noted in the previous section, sleep apnea often presents in association with obesity, which increases the prevalence 10-fold (20% to 40%).[10] Obesity and, in particular, the central type of obesity (see Figure 3-4) are significant risk factors for OSA.[11] They impose increased pharyngeal collapsibility through mechanical compression of the pharyngeal soft

Table 3-1	Body Mass Index Calculations
Measurement Units	**Formula and Calculation**
Kilograms and meters (or centimeters)	Formula: Weight (kg)/height (m²) Using the metric system, the formula for body mass index (BMI) is weight (expressed in kilograms) divided by height in meters squared. Because height is commonly measured in centimeters, divide height in centimeters by 100 to obtain height in meters For example: Weight = 68 kg, height = 165 cm (1.65 m) Calculation: $68 \div 1.65^2 = 24.98$
Pounds and inches	Formula: weight (lb)/height (in²) × 703 Calculate BMI by dividing weight in pounds (lb) by height in inches squared (in²) and multiplying by a conversion factor of 703 Example: Weight = 150 lb, height = 5'5" (65") Calculation: $[150 \div 65^2] \times 703 = 24.96$

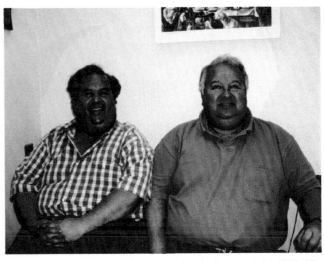

Figure 3-2 Obesity is strongly associated by body mass index (BMI). The example depicts two brothers with sleep apnea with elevated BMI, in the morbidly obese range. (From Kryger MH. *Atlas of clinical sleep medicine.* 2nd ed. Philadelphia: Saunders; 2014: Fig. 13.1-3, A.)

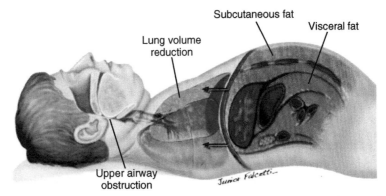

Figure 3-3 The contribution of obesity to obstructive sleep apnea. The illustration depicts the principle anatomic factors that place obese patients at significant risk for obstructive sleep apnea. (From Drager L, Togeiro SM, Polotsky VY, Lorenzi-Filho G. Obstructive sleep apnea: a cardiometabolic risk in obesity and the metabolic syndrome. *J Am Coll Cardiol* 2013;62[7]:569–576.)

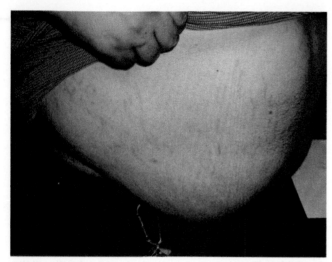

Figure 3-4 Central obesity in obstructive sleep apnea. (From Kryger MH. *Atlas of clinical sleep medicine.* 2nd ed. Philadelphia: Saunders; 2014: Fig. 13.1-42.)

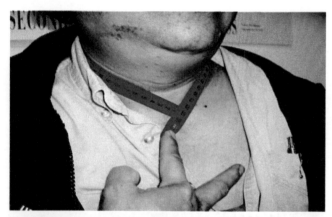

Figure 3-5 Measuring neck collar size. Neck circumference (NC) values of 17 inches or greater in men and 16 inches or greater in women are strongly correlated with the risk for obstructive sleep apnea. (From Kryger MH. *Atlas of clinical sleep medicine.* 2nd ed. Philadelphia: Saunders; 2014: Fig. 13.1-40.)

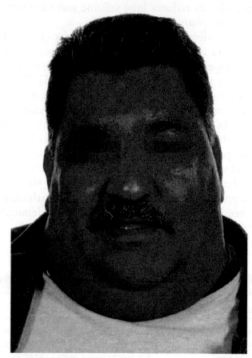

Figure 3-6 The typical facial features of a patient with obstructive sleep apnea. Notice the width of the neck. (From Venn PJH. Obstructive sleep apnoea and anaesthesia. *Anaesth Intens Care Med* 2014;12:313–8.)

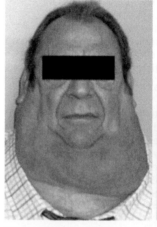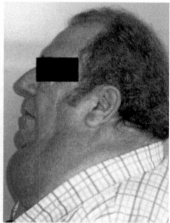

Figure 3-7 Significantly large neck size due to symmetrical accumulation of adipose tissue in a patient with multiple symmetrical lipomatosis, a conditions characterized by a diffuse, symmetrical accumulation of adipose tissue, primarily around the neck. (From Esteban Julvez L, Perello Aragones S, Aguilar Bargallo X. Sleep apnea-hypopnea syndrome and multiple symmetrical lipomatosis. *Arch Bronconeumol* 2013;49:86–7.)

tissues and decreased lung volume through CNS-acting signaling proteins (adipokines) that may alter airway neuromuscular control.[11,12] OSA may independently predispose individuals to worsening obesity as a result of sleep deprivation, hypersomnia, and disrupted metabolism.[13]

Sleep apnea is also associated with endocrinopathies such as hypothyroidism[14,15] and acromegaly.[16] Hypothyroidism is a known cause of secondary OSA; oropharyngeal airway myopathy, edema, and obesity predispose patients to upper airway collapse and obstruction. Acromegaly as depicted in Figure 3-9 results from excessive growth hormone, resulting in enlarged growth of the craniofacial bones, enlargement of the tongue (macroglossia as shown in Figure 3-10), and thickening and enlargement of the laryngeal region; all of these factors can contribute to upper airway obstruction.[17] Goiter, which is associated with acromegaly and hypothyroidism as well as a euthyroid state,[18] can contribute to OSA (Figure 3-11). Patients with Down syndrome (Figure 3-12) regularly experience snoring and obstructive apneas, two common manifestations of upper airway obstruction in this condition, which independently predict neurocognitive impairment.[19] Recent data show significant prevalence of OSA in Down

syndrome patients, conferred through several factors, including craniofacial anatomy, high BMI, adenotonsillar hypertrophy, and muscle hypotonia.[20]

Metabolic derangement such as deposition disorders, including mucopolysaccharidosis (Figure 3-13) and amyloidosis (Figure 3-14),[21] are strongly correlated to OSA. In fact, in patients with mucopolysaccharidosis the prevalence of OSA syndrome can be as high as 70%.[22]

Specific endocrinopathies, in particular polycystic ovarian syndrome, are extremely common among women of reproductive age but often go undiagnosed.[23] Polycystic ovarian

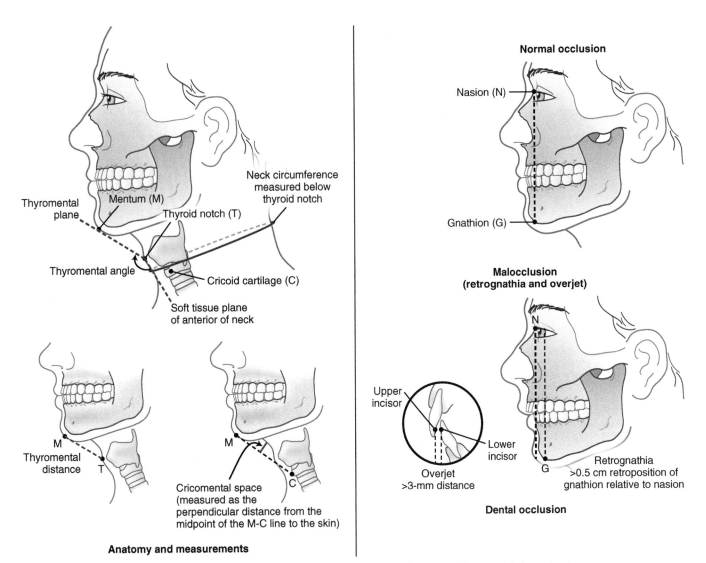

Anatomy and measurements

Figure 3-8 Anatomy and surface measurements in the assessment of a patient with suspected obstructive sleep apnea (OSA). Retrognathia, overjet, and reduced cricomental space are key craniofacial properties that are predictive of OSA. (From Myers KA, Mrkobrada M, Simel DL. Does this patient have obstructive sleep apnea? The rational clinical examination systematic review. *JAMA* 2013;310:731–41.)

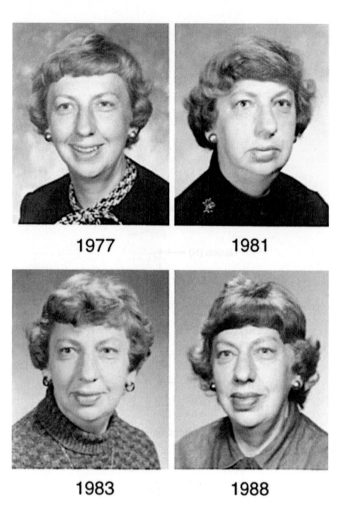

1977   1981

1983   1988

Figure 3-9 Progressive change in facial features in a patient with acromegaly. The onset of physical changes is sometime insidious, and patients may not present with specific complaints relating directly to these distinguishing signs of acromegaly. However, patients may be more likely to present with symptoms referred to other conditions such as diabetes, hypertension, and obstructive sleep apnea. At the advanced stages of the condition, patients exhibit more dramatic physical characteristics, such as enlarged hands, feet, lips, and tongue; prominent supraorbital ridges; and lower jaw protrusion. (From Molitch ME. Clinical manifestations of acromegaly. *Endocrinol Metab Clin North Am* 1992;21[3]:597–614.)

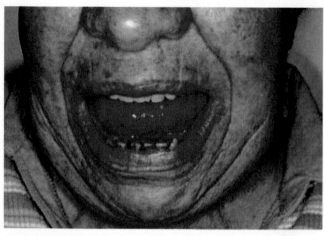

Figure 3-10 Patient with acromegaly showing the coarse facial features, macroglossia, and interdental separation typically seen in this condition, which lead to airway restriction and contribute to the development of obstructive sleep apnea. (From Burke G. Endocrine disease. In: Sprout C, Burke G, McGurk M, editors. *Essential human disease for dentists*. Edinburgh: Churchill Livingstone; 2006. p. 99–119.)

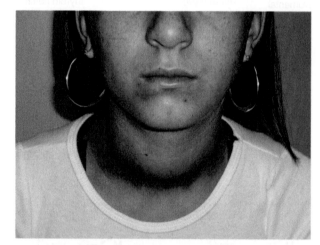

Figure 3-11 Goiter. (From Kryger MH. *Atlas of clinical sleep medicine*. 2nd ed. Philadelphia: Saunders; 2014: Fig. 15.1-8, B.)

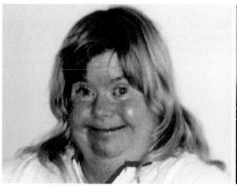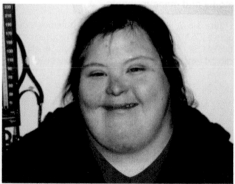

Figure 3-12 Two patients with the characteristic phenotype of Down syndrome. Contributing factors to obstructive sleep apnea in Down syndrome include alteration in craniofacial anatomy, macroglossia, adenotonsillar hypertrophy, and muscle hypotonia. (Courtesy Dr. Meir H. Kryger.)

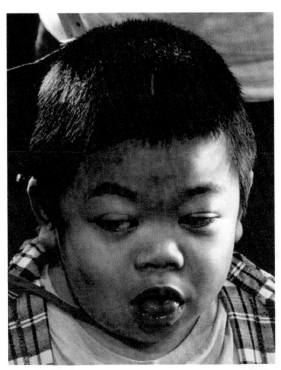

Figure 3-13 Hunter syndrome (mucopolysaccharidosis type II) depicting significant macroglossia, a risk factor for OSA. In this 8-year-old boy with Hunter syndrome, infiltration of the macroglossia can be seen. Other features include macrocephaly, coarse hair, abnormally short neck, hairy face, puffy eyelids, depressed nasal bridge, upturned nose, full lips, and thick skin texture. (From Chou W-C, Weng C-Y, Lin S-P, Chu S-Y. Postenzyme replacement therapy era for type 2 mucopolysaccharidosis. *Tzu Chi Med J* 2013;25:128–9.)

syndrome is associated with metabolic syndrome and carries a greatly increased risk for obesity with metabolic syndrome, OSA, impaired glucose tolerance, type 2 diabetes mellitus, and cardiovascular disease (Figure 3-15).[23]

Craniofacial Factors

As summarized in Figure 3-8, cephalometric measurements reveal that subjects with OSA have significant changes in the size and position of the soft palate and uvula, volume and position of the tongue, hyoid position, and mandibulomaxillary protrusion compared with controls. Mandibular retrognathia (Figure 3-16) and micrognathia (Figure 3-17), which cause the tongue to rest in a more superior and posterior position, impinging on the upper airway, can be detected on examination, especially by observing the patient from the side. As seen in Figure 3-17, *B*, the cricomentalis space defined by the distance between the neck and the bisection of a line from the chin to the cricoid membrane, when the head is in a neutral position, is extremely limited.[24] A scalloped tongue (Figure 3-18) may accompany micrognathia. Men with retrognathia or micrognathia may grow a beard to compensate for this anatomic variant. Crowded teeth (Figure 3-19) and overjet (Figure 3-20), with the mandibular teeth excessively posterior to the maxillary teeth (Figure 3-20, *B*), often accompany retrognathia or micrognathia. Figure 3-21 depicts the global consequences of primary mandibular insufficiency on the patency of the upper airways, leading to compromised retronasal, retropalatal, and retroglossal spaces.[2] Commonly encountered craniofacial features predisposing to sleep apnea consist of mandibular deficiency syndrome, an inferiorly placed hyoid bone relative to the mandibular plane, narrowing of the posterior airspace, and elongation of the soft

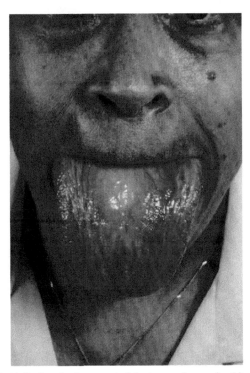

Figure 3-14 Profound enlargement of the tongue (macroglossia) as a result of amyloid infiltration. The patient had severe obstructive sleep apnea. The tongue fills the oral cavity completely, contributing to profound hypopharyngeal and oropharyngeal airway blockade. (From Hoffman R, Benz EJ, Silberstein LE, et al. *Hematology: diagnosis and treatment*. Philadelphia: Elsevier Science; 2013. p. 1352, Figure 87-3.)

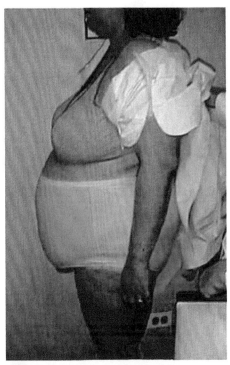

Figure 3-15 A 31-year-old woman with polycystic ovary syndrome. Shown here is the particular phenotype of increased central fat distribution among these patients. (From Magnotti M, Futterweit W. Obesity and the polycystic ovary syndrome. *Med Clin North Am* 2007;91:1151–68, ix-x.)

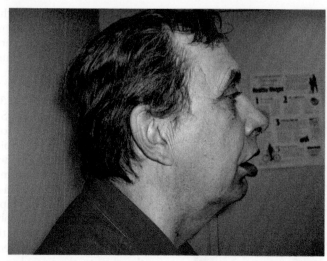

Figure 3-16 Mandibular retrognathia contributing to obstructive sleep apnea. (From Kryger MH. *Atlas of clinical sleep medicine*. 2nd ed. Philadelphia: Saunders; 2014: Fig. 13.1-16.)

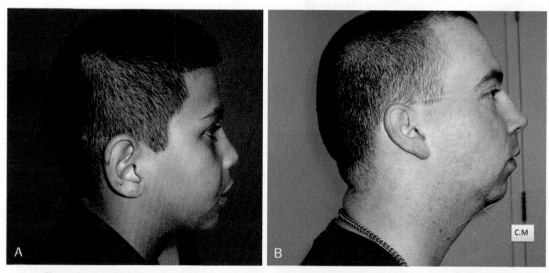

Figure 3-17 A child **(A)** and an adult **(B)** with significant mandibular micrognathia contributing to obstructive sleep apnea. The cricomentalis (C–M) space (as delineated by the *dotted line*) is severely reduced in the adult with mandibular micrognathia. (From Kryger MH. *Atlas of clinical sleep medicine*. 2nd ed. Philadelphia: Saunders; 2014: Fig. 13.1-12, A.)

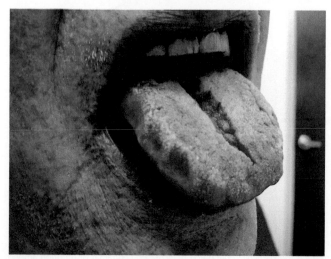

Figure 3-18 Scalloped tongue in a patient with obstructive sleep apnea and micrognathia. The scalloping and furrow result from the tongue's pressing against teeth (especially on the right side). In addition, the tongue is atrophied, raising the possibility of iron or vitamin B_{12} deficiency. (Courtesy Dr. Meir H. Kryger.)

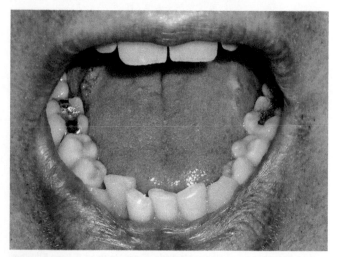

Figure 3-19 Crowded teeth indicate a small mandible, contributing to obstructive sleep apnea. (From Kryger MH. *Atlas of clinical sleep medicine*. 2nd ed. Philadelphia: Saunders; 2014: Fig. 13.1-12.)

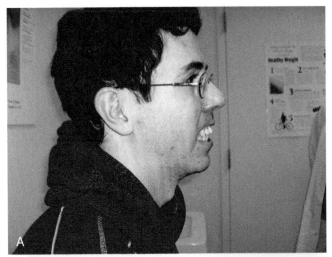

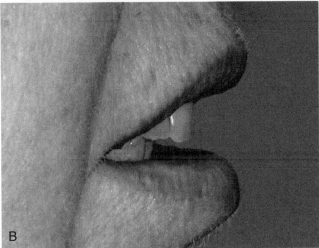

Figure 3-20 Overjet contributing to obstructive sleep apnea. (From Kryger MH. *Atlas of clinical sleep medicine*. 2nd ed. Philadelphia: Saunders; 2014: Fig. 13.1-14.)

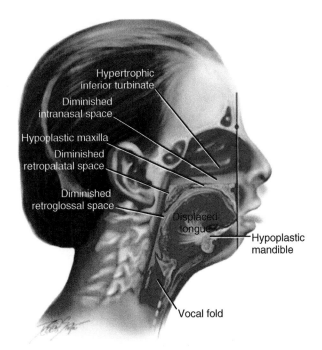

Figure 3-21 An illustration of a sagittal cross-sectional head and neck view from a 16-year-old patient with primary mandibular deficiency and overjet malocclusion predisposing to obstructive sleep apnea. (From Posnick JC. Obstructive sleep apnea: evaluation and treatment. In: Posnick JC, editor. *Orthognathic surgery: principles and practice*. Philadelphia: Elsevier; 2014. p. 992–1058.)

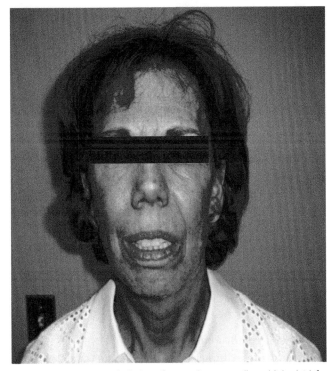

Figure 3-22 A patient with the long face syndrome, a well-established risk for obstructive sleep apnea, that is conferred through an increase of anterior facial height generally associated with retrognathia. (Courtesy Dr. Meir H. Kryger.)

palate.[25] In addition, marfanoid habitus, including the long face phenotype (Figure 3-22), leads to upper airway restriction, thereby predisposing to OSA.[26] Indeed when the well-established role of obesity in the development of OSA is taken into account, a model of OSA emerges in which the degree of craniofacial abnormalities determines the extent of obesity required to produce OSA in a given individual.

Racial differences in cephalometric properties probably play a major role in conferring risk for OSA in the absence of obesity. For example, in Chinese patients with OSA, a more retropositioned mandible was associated with more severe OSA, after controlling for obesity.[27] In Japanese patients with OSA, micrognathia was a major risk factor.[28] Children and adults with Down syndrome (see Figure 3-12) frequently have sleep apnea most likely related to a combination of craniofacial abnormality and macroglossia.

Patients with OSA have an increased pharyngeal narrowing ratio, which is defined as a ratio between the airway cross section at the hard palate level and the narrowest cross section from the hard palate to the epiglottis.[29]

Nasal Factors

Examination of the nasal airway should focus on anatomic abnormalities that may contribute to nasal obstruction. These

may be congenital, traumatic, infectious, or neoplastic in etiology (Figure 3-23).

Neck Circumference

Increased neck circumference (see Figure 3-6) is an important risk factor for OSA. Patients with a neck circumference

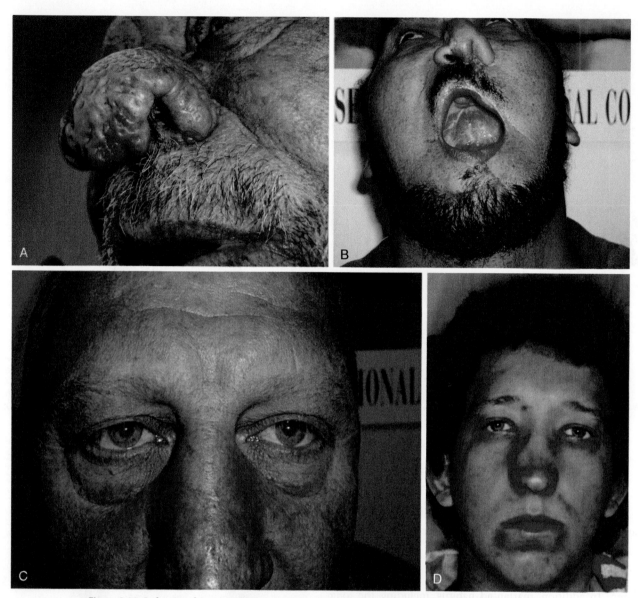

Figure 3-23 Deformity of the nose can be a very important contributor to sleep disordered breathing. **A,** Rhino-phyma ("bulbous nose" or "phymatous rosacea") is a nodular hypertrophy characterized by progressive thickening of the nose and leading to compromise of the nasal orifice airflow. **B,** Gun shot wound leading to significant facial injury and nasal collapse, requiring maxillomandibular reconstruction and plastic surgery. **C,** Nasal deviations due to remote broken nose caused by boxing. **D,** Nasal deformity due to the presence of nasal polyps. (**A, B,** and **C,** Courtesy Dr. Meir H. Kryger. **D,** From McGurk M. ENT disorders. In: Sprout C, Burke G, McGurk M, editors. *Essential human disease for dentists.* Edinburgh: Churchill Livingstone; 2006. p. 195–204.)

greater than 48 cm (19.2 inches) have a 20-fold increased risk for OSA.[30]

Examination of the Pharynx

There are two well-established classifications to determine the relation of the tongue to the pharynx. The Mallampati classification was first described as a method for anesthesiologists to predict difficult tracheal intubation (Figure 3-24).[31] The Friedman classification identifies prognostic indicators for successful surgery for sleep-disordered breathing, combining palate position with tonsillar size.[32] The Mallampati classification can be seen in Table 3-2 and Figures 3-25 through 3-28. The Friedman classification is illustrated in Figure 3-29.

Table 3-2	Mallampati Classification
Class I	Soft palate, fauces, uvula, and posterior and anterior pillars are visible (Figure 3-25).
Class II	Soft palate, fauces, and uvula are visible (Figure 3-26).
Class III	Soft palate, fauces, and only base of uvula are visible (Figure 3-27).
Class IV	Soft palate is not visible (Figure 3-28).

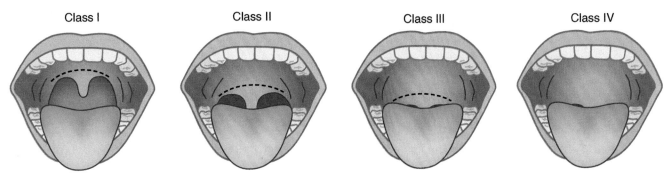

Class I	Class II	Class III	Class IV

Figure 3-24 The Mallampati classification system is visualized with the tongue protruded, but without the patient phonating. A *modified* form of the Mallampati system is measured with the tongue remaining on the floor of the mouth. The system was initially developed to predict ease of intubation but was later adopted by sleep medicine to help forecast the severity of obstructive sleep apnea in the ambulatory setting. It can also be used to help predict the appropriateness of upper airway surgery in certain patients by delineating the relationship of the various upper airway structures and noting the tongue size in relation to the uvula, tonsils, soft palate, and oropharyngeal wall. The standard for tongue size measurement involved the patient holding his or her head in a neutral position, opening the mouth as wide as possible, and sticking out the tongue. Class I is characterized by direct visualization of the soft palate, uvula, palatine tonsils, and pillars. However, as these structures become obscured, so does the Mallampati class, until only the hard palate is visible (class IV). (From Townsend CM Jr, Beauchamp RD, Evers BM, et al. *Sabiston textbook of surgery*. 19th ed. Philadelphia: Elsevier; 2012.)

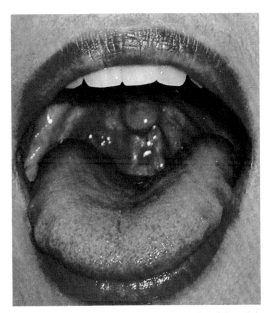

Figure 3-25 Mallampati class I. (From Kryger MH. *Atlas of clinical sleep medicine*. 2nd ed. Philadelphia: Saunders; 2014: Fig. 13.1-28.)

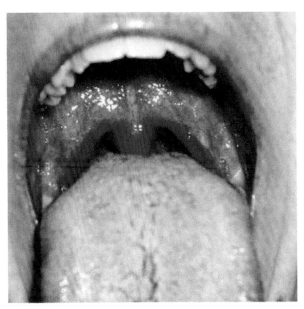

Figure 3-26 Mallampati class II. (From Kryger MH. *Atlas of clinical sleep medicine*. 2nd ed. Philadelphia: Saunders; 2014: Fig. 13.1-29, A.)

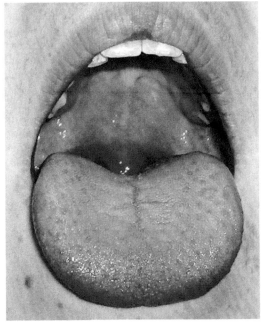

Figure 3-27 Mallampati class III. (From Kryger MH. *Atlas of clinical sleep medicine*. 2nd ed. Philadelphia: Saunders; 2014: Fig. 13.1-30, A.)

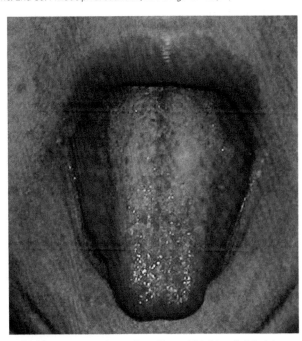

Figure 3-28 Mallampati class IV. (From Kryger MH. *Atlas of clinical sleep medicine*. 2nd ed. Philadelphia: Saunders; 2014: Fig. 13.1-31.)

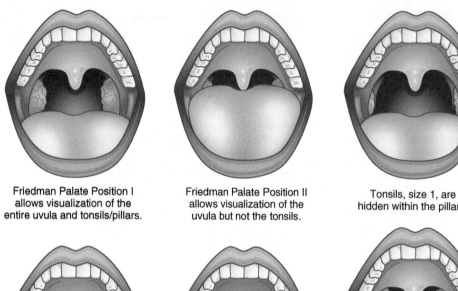

Friedman Palate Position I allows visualization of the entire uvula and tonsils/pillars.

Friedman Palate Position II allows visualization of the uvula but not the tonsils.

Tonsils, size 1, are hidden within the pillars.

Tonsils, size 2, extend to the pillars.

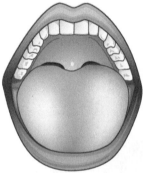
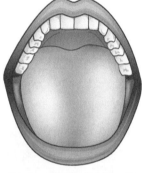
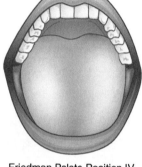
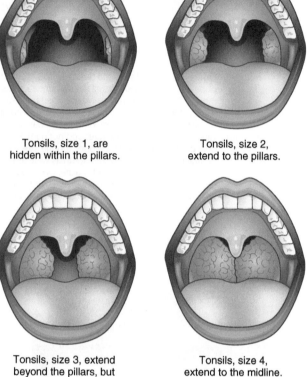

Friedman Palate Position III allows visualization of the soft palate but not the uvula.

Friedman Palate Position IV allows visualization of the hard palate only.

Tonsils, size 3, extend beyond the pillars, but not to the midline.

Tonsils, size 4, extend to the midline.

Figure 3-30 Tonsil size grading. (From Friedman M, Ibrahim H, Bass L. Clinical staging for sleep-disordered breathing. *Otolaryngol Head Neck Surg* 2002;127:13–21.)

Figure 3-29 Friedman classification. This grading is based on the tongue in a natural position inside the mouth (I). Palate grade I allows the observer to visualize the entire uvula and tonsils or pillars. Palate grade II allows visualization of the uvula but not the tonsils. Palate grade III allows visualization of the soft palate but not the uvula. Palate grade IV allows visualization of the hard palate only. (From Friedman M, Ibrahim H, Bass L. Clinical staging for sleep-disordered breathing. *Otolaryngol Head Neck Surg* 2002;127:13–21.)

Examination of the Tonsils

Enlarged tonsils and adenoids are a major cause of airway obstruction and sleep apnea in children, but a minority of adults may also have enlargement of these structures contributing to airway obstruction.[33] Adenoids cannot be visualized in a routine physical examination, and the examination of tonsils may require use of a tongue blade. Tonsillar size is graded on a scale of 1 to 4 (Figure 3-30). Children with marked adenotonsillar hypertrophy and nasal obstruction have been noted to have a peculiar "dull" expression (i.e., "adenoid facies"), as shown in Figure 3-31, *A* and *B*. Children with chronic sinus allergies may present with an "allergic salute" sign (see Figure 3-31, *C*).

Neurologic Examination

The neurologic examination may hold important clues to the presence of obstructive or central sleep apnea and hypoventilation syndromes. Features of neuromuscular disease evident on physical examination may indicate these syndromes. For example, progressive muscle atrophy and fasciculations of the hand (Figure 3-32) or tongue may indicate amyotrophic lateral sclerosis. In amyotrophic lateral sclerosis, phrenic nerve dysfunction is common and results in diaphragmatic paralysis, with prominent hypoventilation during rapid eye movement (REM) sleep. In addition, coexisting OSA may occur in amyotrophic lateral sclerosis with bulbar involvement. Weakness of thoracoabdominal or respiratory accessory muscles, often with accompanying kyphoscoliosis, may be observed in poliomyelitis. Postpolio syndrome, muscular dystrophies, myasthenia gravis, and metabolic myopathies may also manifest with weakness of the chest wall musculature[34] and diaphragm weakness. Myasthenia gravis (Figure 3-33) may also involve facial structures, resulting in OSA. Craniofacial abnormalities may occur in myotonic dystrophy (Figure 3-34) or muscular dystrophy; macroglossia may also occur (e.g., Duchenne muscular dystrophy).[35]

Figure 3-35 depicts a patient with facial weakness in the setting of progressive muscular dystrophy. Figure 3-36 shows a patient with myotonic dystrophy with tightness of the muscles (called myotonia), leading to difficulty relaxing certain muscles after using them, such as being able to release grip in a handshake or on a doorknob, or as in the example provided. Figure 3-37 depicts the classic Gower maneuver in Becker muscular dystrophy. Defects in upper airway neuromuscular control in many of the patients with dystrophinopathies play a critical role in sleep apnea pathogenesis, and the sleep care provider must maintain a vigil eye on sleep disturbances in this group of patients.[36]

Finally, obesity (e.g., from steroid use, as in Figure 3-38, or inactivity) may also contribute to sleep apnea in neuromuscular disease.

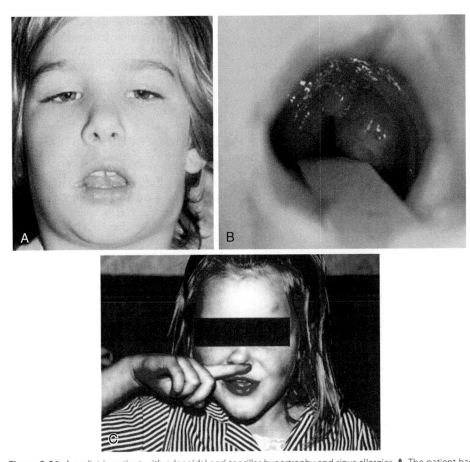

Figure 3-31 A pediatric patient with adenoidal and tonsillar hypertrophy and sinus allergies. **A,** The patient has a "dull expression" of a child with marked adenotonsillar hypertrophy and nasal obstruction (i.e., "adenoid facies"). He must keep his mouth open to breathe and shows signs of fatigue as a result of the result of sleep disruption as a consequence of obstructive sleep apnea. **B,** A severely crowded oropharynx due to tonsillar hypertrophy. **C,** Allergic salute in a patient with chronic allergic rhinitis. (**A** and **B,** From Landsman IS, Werkhaven JA, Motoyama EK. Anesthesia for pediatric otorhinolaryngologic surgery. In: Davis PJ, Cladis FP, Motoyama EK, editors. *Smith's anesthesia for infants and children*. Philadelphia: Mosby; 2011. p. 786–820. **C,** From Scadding GK, Church MK, Borish L. Allergic rhinitis and rhinosinusitis. *Allergy* 2012;203–226.)

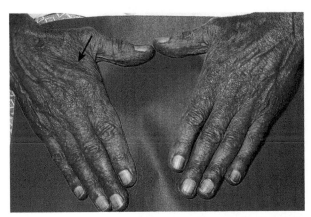

Figure 3-32 Hand atrophy (*arrow*) in amyotrophic lateral sclerosis. (From Goldman L, Ausiello DA, editors. *Cecil medicine*. 23rd ed. Philadelphia: Elsevier; 2008.)

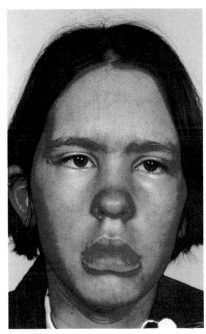

Figure 3-33 Facial muscle weakness in myasthenia gravis. (From Goldman L, Ausiello DA, editors. *Cecil medicine*. 23rd ed. Philadelphia: Elsevier; 2008.)

Cardiopulmonary Examination

The presence of congestive heart failure (see Chapter 28) indicates a high likelihood of central sleep apnea. Peripheral edema (Figure 3-39) is a common finding in patients with obesity-hypoventilation syndrome (as a manifestation of cor

pulmonale) and in some patients with OSA who also have left ventricular cardiac failure. Resolution of peripheral edema with treatment correlates with clinical improvement. Chronic obstructive pulmonary disease (see Chapter 29) and asthma (see Chapter 29) are also seen in association with OSA. In patients with cardiopulmonary insufficiency, clubbing of digits and nails may be a cardinal sign (Figure 3-40).

CENTRAL NERVOUS SYSTEM HYPERSOMNIA

Narcolepsy

Physical findings in patients with narcolepsy are nonspecific and may be subtle, infrequent, and absent during the clinic visit. During cataplectic spells, patients present with muscle atonia, absence of deep tendon reflexes, and decrease in the H-reflex.[37] Cataplexy attacks may range from partial episodes characterized by sagging of the jaw and mild dropping of the head and shoulders, to generalized spells leading to loss of muscle tone with unbuckling of the knee. However, it is rare to encounter cataplexy during the actual clinic visit or physical examination, which makes it difficult to describe during routine clinic visits. In general, patients with narcolepsy tend to be obese, with increased predilection to type 2 diabetes mellitus, and have a lower basal metabolism compared with controls.[38,39] Children with obesity and precocious puberty should be screened for narcolepsy and cataplexy.[40]

Narcolepsy related to medical conditions (symptomatic narcolepsy) is seen in disorders such as CNS tumors, head trauma, multiple sclerosis, neurosarcoidosis, acute disseminated encephalomyelitis, CNS vascular disorders, encephalitis, and neurodegeneration.[41] An abnormal neurologic examination can be an important sign that hypersomnia may be due

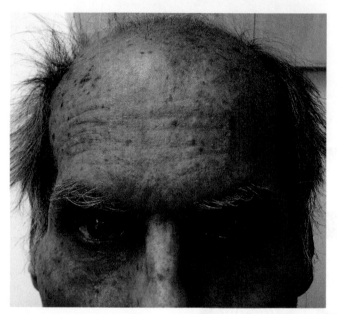

Figure 3-34 Myotonic muscular dystrophy (DM1). Findings in a patient with myotonic muscular dystrophy include wasting of the temporal muscles (shown) and male-pattern baldness that began at an early age. These patients may also have weakness of other facial muscles and micrognathia. (Courtesy Dr. Meir H. Kryger.)

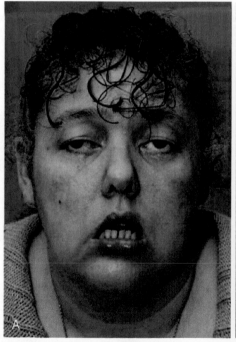
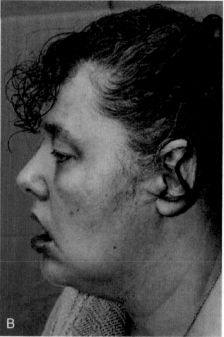

Figure 3-35 A and **B,** Bilateral facial weakness due to progressive muscular dystrophy. The patient exhibits the classic signs, including bilateral ptosis. Facial weakness involves the orbicularis oculi, orbicularis oris, and zygomaticus muscle, producing the characteristic myopathic facial. Weakness of muscles of the thoracic region often leads to respiratory insufficiency, and many patients also present with bulbar symptoms (dysarthria, dysphagia). (From Laina V, Orlando A. Bilateral facial palsy and oral incompetence due to muscular dystrophy treated with a palmaris longus tendon graft. *J Plast Reconstr Aesthet Surg* 2009;62[11]:e479–81.)

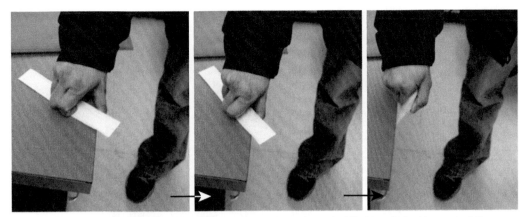

Figure 3-36 Muscular dystrophy. An attempt at grasp by the patient with difficulties relaxing his muscles following the grasp. (Courtesy Dr. Meir H. Kryger.)

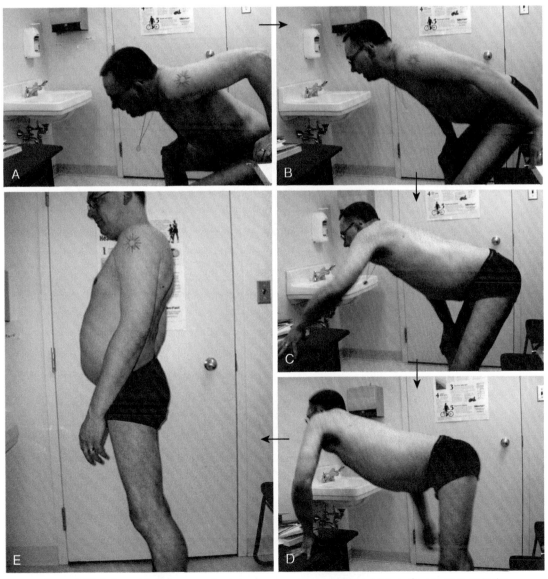

Figure 3-37 Patient with Becker muscular dystrophy caused by an in-frame deletion of exons 45 to 47 in the dystrophin gene. The patient is using the Gower maneuver to rise from sitting to standing position: While sitting **(A),** he uses the force of his hands to stand **(B, C, D)**. In **E,** using his thighs, he pushed himself upright, leading to the characteristic hyperlordosis posture. (Courtesy Dr. Meir H. Kryger.)

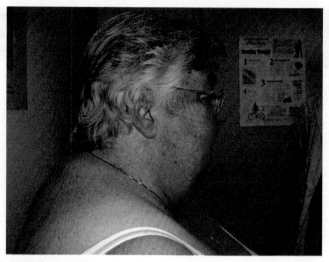

Figure 3-38 "Buffalo hump" in a patient with chronic steroid use. (Courtesy Dr. Meir H. Kryger.)

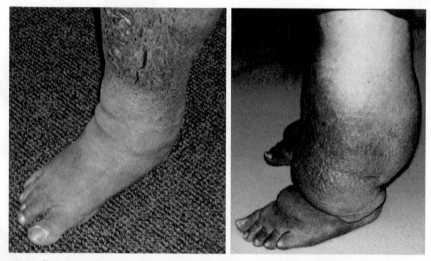

Figure 3-39 Chronic peripheral edema is a common finding in patients with obesity-hypoventilation syndrome. (Courtesy Dr. Meir H. Kryger.)

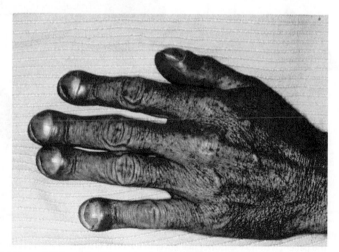

Figure 3-40 Clubbing of digits and nails may be associated with cardiopulmonary insufficiency. (Courtesy Dr. Meir H. Kryger.)

to a CNS etiology. In lesions of the diencephalon due to inflammatory changes such as neurosarcoidosis, one finds additional physical findings associated with panhypopituitarism such as orthostatic hypotension, temperature fluctuations, and other finding of autonomic dysregulation.

Patients with narcolepsy type 1 who experience cataplexy are sometimes observed to have a state of peculiar semipermanent ptosis and jaw weakness, on which partial and complete cataplectic attacks were superimposed cataplectic facies,[42,43] as depicted in Figure 3-41.

PARASOMNIAS

Nocturnal Eating Disorder and Sleep-Related Eating Disorder

In nocturnal eating disorder, patients often manifest compulsive food-searching behaviors and a return to sleep after food ingestion. Body mass index was abnormally high in 6 of 10 patients after careful exclusion of both anorexia nervosa and bulimia.[44] Sleep-related eating disorder, which also occurs in the setting of WED, is characterized by recurrent episodes of eating after an arousal from nighttime sleep with or without amnesia[45] and may also result in obesity.

REM Sleep Behavior Disorder

Patients with idiopathic REM sleep behavior disorder (RBD) can develop dramatic and aggressive dream enactment events sometimes leading to serious injury. Figure 3-42 depicts a patient who presented at the author's sleep clinic together with his wife who complained that he was dreaming about golfing, was in an argument, and fell to the floor. In the process he hit his neck on the corner of the bedside table and bruised his ear and cheek on bedside table. Although the condition is unlikely to produce severe injury to the patient, the bed partner paradoxically ends up suffering severe sleep interruptions, is more likely to experience sleepiness, and is at risk for injury. Patients with RBD are frequently at risk for development of α-synucleinopathies such as Parkinson disease, and most present with hyposmia (impaired smell), which is a potential preclinical nonmotor sign of the disease.[46] Odor identification was also found impaired in Japanese patients with idiopathic RBD and Parkinson disease.[47]

Cardinal features of Parkinson disease are shown in Figure 3-43. Patients with multiple system atrophy may present with inspiratory stridor, which along with RBD may serve as a clue to the disease in a patient with autonomic failure.[48]

SLEEP-RELATED MOVEMENT DISORDERS

Willis-Ekbom Disease

The prevalence of WED, also known as restless legs syndrome, in patients with type 2 diabetes is 17.7%,[49] and the prevalence may be higher in patients with hereditary neuropathy.[50] WED occurs in about one third of patients with polyneuropathy,[51] with preferential involvement of small sensory fibers. Electrophysiologic studies demonstrate that axonal neuropathy is common in WED, which further necessitates comprehensive peripheral nerve evaluations in these patients.[52]

Reduced iron stores can also cause WED. With iron deficiency, examination of the pharynx may reveal inflammation (redness) or loss or atrophy of the lingual mucosa, indicating

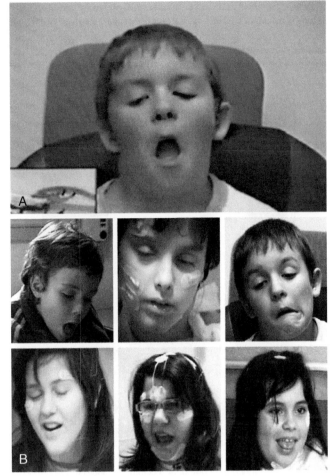

Figure 3-41 A, Patients with cataplexy are shown responding to the trigger stimulus (a cartoon). The facial weakness is also present during normal activity without stimulus. **B,** The patient experiences facial muscle weakness, as noted by bilateral, facial grimaces while attempting to keep the eyes open. Facial slackening and tongue protrusion with the mouth opened and a quasi "drunken or droopy look" phenotype, characterize the "cataplectic facies." (From Leonardo S, Pasquale M, Emmanuel M, et al. Cataplexy features in childhood narcolepsy. *Mov Disord* 2008;23:858–65.)

glossitis (Figure 3-44). The patient may complain of a sore or tender tongue.

On neurologic examination, symptoms include sensory loss, often described by patients as a sense of numbness or tingling. In the generalized polyneuropathies, symptoms frequently begin in the most distal aspect of the longest sensory fibers, which produce disturbances in sensation in the toes and feet. In addition to sensory loss, patients frequently complain of paresthesias and dysesthesias, often characterized by numbness, tingling, prickling, and pins-and-needles sensations. The sensory examination will often disclose a distal to proximal loss of the various sensory modalities. In certain polyneuropathies, pain predominates in the clinical picture, and the sensory examination tends to disclose deficits predominantly of pain and thermal sensation. When significant proprioceptive deafferentation occurs, patients may present with altered joint position sense that can manifest as an ataxia or tremor of the affected limbs and an imbalance of gait and station.

Pain may be a significant symptom for many patients with WED in which the etiology is related to a polyneuropathy. It may be described as a dull aching sensation, an intense burning sensation, or, occasionally, intermittent lancinating pulses of pain. On occasion, patients notice that their skin is hypersensitive to tactile stimulation, such as from the touch of bed sheets or clothing or standing on the feet. Some patients note

an exaggerated painful sensation resulting from any stimulus to the affected area, a form of pain termed allodynia. Various limb deformities and trophic changes may be observed in chronic polyneuropathies. Pes cavus, characterized by high arches and hammertoes, and the clawfoot deformity are typical foot deformities in hereditary polyneuropathies with childhood onset. These deformities are due to progressive weakness and atrophy of intrinsic foot muscles. A similar clawlike deformity may be observed in the hand. Autonomic involvement of a limb may cause the affected area to appear warm, red, and swollen at times and pale and cold at other times owing to dysregulation of small vessels due to autonomic denervation. Various trophic changes, including tight, shiny skin, may occur. In patients who have had severe sensory

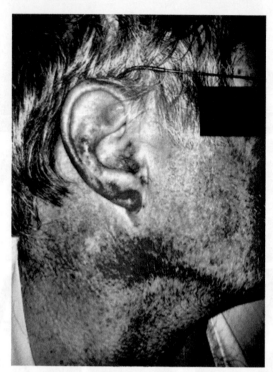

Figure 3-42 A patient with aggressive dream enactment behavior who experienced severe injury during one of his nocturnal episodes in the setting of REM sleep behavior disorder. (Copyright Alon Y. Avidan, MD, MPH.)

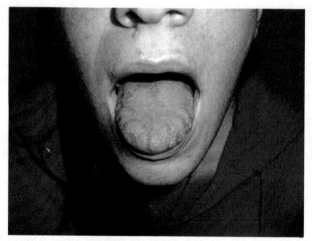

Figure 3-44 Tongue glossitis in iron deficiency. (Courtesy Dr. Meir H. Kryger.)

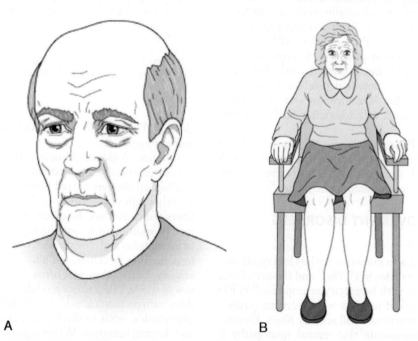

A   B

Figure 3-43 A, Patients with Parkinson disease (PD) blink less frequently and make fewer facial expressions, with less frequent head movements ("masked facies"). **B,** Patients with PD rarely participate in normal gestures or repositioning movements. They are observed to sit motionless with their legs uncrossed and their feet flat. The upper extremities remain motionless on the chair or in their lap. (From Kaufman DM: Involuntary movement disorders. In: Kaufman DM, editor. *Clinical neurology for psychiatrists.* 6th ed. Philadelphia: Elsevier; 2007. p. 401–64.)

loss in the limbs, the affected areas may be subject to incidental traumas, including burns, pressure sores, and other injuries that are not perceived by the patient, in whom repeated injuries and traumas may result in chronic infections and, when severe, lead to osteomyelitis. A clinical evaluation of peripheral neuropathy is provided by Kelly.[53,54]

Bruxism

Bruxism represents a stereotyped movement disorder clinically characterized by grinding or clenching of the teeth during sleep. The sounds made by friction of the teeth are usually perceived by a bed partner as very unpleasant.[55] The condition is typically brought to the attention of the medical or dental practitioner in efforts to eliminate the disturbing sounds. Bruxism can lead to abnormal wear of the teeth (Figure 3-45), periodontal tissue damage, or jaw pain. Other symptoms include facial muscle and tooth pain and headache. Bruxism induces dental damage with abnormal wear to the teeth and damage to the structures surrounding the teeth. Chronically, over time and when untreated, this leads to recession and inflammation of the gums, alveolar bone resorption, muscles of mastication hypertrophy (Figure 3-46), and temporomandibular joint disorders, often associated with facial pain. Additional physical findings include tenderness of the muscles of mastication (masseter, temporalis, pterygoid, sternocleidal), temporomandibular disorders, tongue indentation, subjective appreciation of a tense personality, and hypervigilant patient.[56]

Case reports in patients with bruxism demonstrate bilateral enlargement in the region of the mandibular angle, corresponding with the masseter hypertrophy (see Figure 3-46).[57] Children with bruxism have a significantly longer and higher palate in the sagittal plane and bigger dental arches compared with normal children.[58] Psychiatric patients have a higher prevalence of bruxism and signs of temporomandibular disorders, possibly related to neuroleptic-induced phenomenon.[59]

Insomnia

Insomnia, especially comorbid in type, is often seen in the context of endocrinopathies, mood disorders, anxiety disorders (Figure 3-47), rheumatologic conditions, pain, and a long

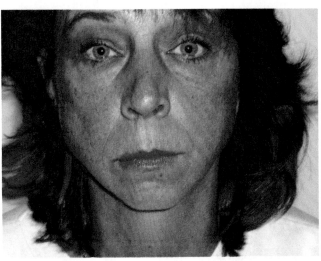

Figure 3-46 Hypertrophic masseter in bruxism. The masseter muscle bulk is markedly increased over the mandibular angle region. (Courtesy Dr. Meir H. Kryger.)

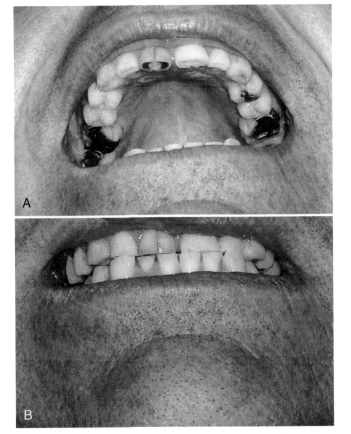

Figure 3-45 Bruxism with abnormal wear of the teeth.

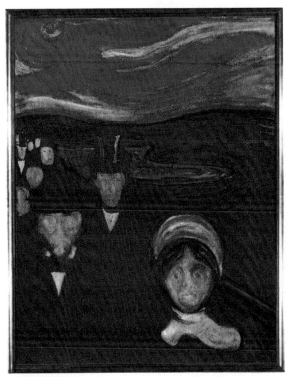

Figure 3-47 The painting of anxiety, a common comorbidity in chronic insomnia. (From Gross M. Shining new light on the brain. *Curr Biol* 2011;21[20]:R831–3.)

list of other medical, psychiatric, and primary sleep disorders. Patients with Graves disease (Figure 3-48), an autoimmune disorder and a common cause of hyperthyroidism, is characterized by the presence of autoantibodies that bind and stimulate the thyroid-stimulating hormone receptor, resulting in hyperfunction of the thyroid. Graves disease is characterized by a phenotype of heat intolerance, involuntary weight loss, thyromegaly, tremor, and hyperactivity manifesting as restless sleep and insomnia.[60] Finally, floppy eyelid syndrome (Figure 3-49) is sometimes confused with tiredness, a thyroid disorder,

or a neuromuscular disorder and is characterized by flaccid and easily everted upper lids, occurring spontaneously or with minimal manipulation.[61] It is can seen in middle-aged men who are overweight and has been associated with OSA.

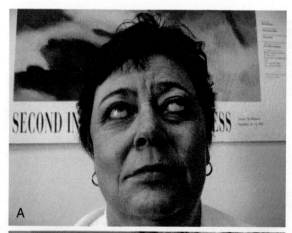
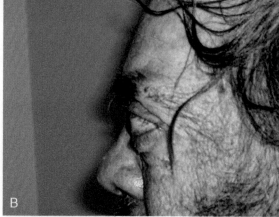

Figure 3-48 Proptosis seen in the setting of Graves disease. **A,** Eye signs in Graves disease. **B,** Severe proptosis in Graves disease. (**A** and **B,** Courtesy Dr. Meir H. Kryger.)

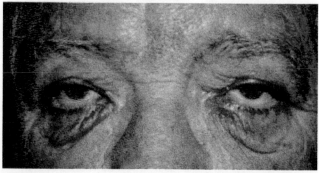

Figure 3-49 Bilateral upper lid ptosis in a patient with floppy eyelid syndrome. (From Leibovitch I, Selva D. Floppy eyelid syndrome: clinical features and the association with obstructive sleep apnea. *Sleep Med* 2006;7[2]: 117–122.)

CLINICAL PEARLS

- Overall inspection of the patient, coupled with observation of craniofacial, nasal, and pharyngeal factors, allows detection of key risk factors for sleep apnea.
- Examination of patients with insomnia should focus on the potential associated comorbidities, including hypothyroidism and rheumatologic disorders.
- Patients with motor disorders of sleep and parasomnias also have clinical findings conferred by the underlying medical, neurologic, and associated psychiatric comorbidities. For example, anosmia, orthostatic fluctuations in the setting of dream enactment behavior, and loss of electromyographic tone on polysomnogram may be predictive of an evolving α-synucleinopathy.
- Clues to the presence of abnormal nocturnal events such as parasomnias or nocturnal seizures may include unexplained bruising, lacerations in the former, and tongue laceration in the latter. However, even tongue biting, which is believed to be a clinical sign of epilepsy, can occur in syncope and nonepileptic seizures. These difficulties highlight the importance of a well-tailored approach in which the clinical history, physical examination, and supportive laboratory and polysomnographic data are used to arrive the most plausible clinical diagnosis.

SUMMARY

The physical examination of any patient with sleep disorders is the cornerstone for making critical decisions about the possible clinical diagnosis, determining the need for formal polysomnography, and ensuring that treatment is successful. Given that medial trainees often do not receive formalized sleep medicine education in medical school, appreciating the fundamental phenotypical patterns responsible for sleep-disordered breathing is critical. A basic appreciation of the abnormal neurologic examination is important for nonneurologists who may encounter patients with parasomnias and motor and movement disorders of sleep. Finally, no clinical examination of a sleepy patient should conclude without a comprehensive review of the patient's medical, endocrine, metabolic, genetic, and disease background, given that may phenotypes contribute directly to disruptive sleep.

Selected Readings

Friedman M. *Sleep apnea and snoring: surgical and non-surgical therapy.* Philadelphia: Elsevier Science; 2008.

Kryger MH, Avidan AY, Berry R. *Atlas of clinical sleep medicine.* 2nd ed. Philadelphia: Saunders; 2014.

Myers KA, Mrkobrada M, Simel DL. Does this patient have obstructive sleep apnea? The rational clinical examination systematic review. *JAMA* 2013;**310**:731–41.

Posnick JC. *Orthognathic surgery: principles and practice.* Philadelphia: Elsevier Science; 2014.

Wilhelm CP, deShazo RD, Tamanna S, et al. The nose, upper airway, and obstructive sleep apnea. *Ann Allergy Asthma Immunol* 2015;**115**(2): 96–102.

A complete reference list can be found online at ExpertConsult.com.

Use of Clinical Tools and Tests in Sleep Medicine

Cathy A. Goldstein; Ronald D. Chervin

Chapter Highlights

- A clinician confronted with a sleep-related complaint combines symptoms, signs, and test results to make a diagnostic assessment.
- Information about test performance characteristics, such as sensitivity, specificity, and predictive value, can be used more formally to decide on optimal approaches.

- In addition to the history and physical examination, tools and tests used in the evaluation of a patient with sleep-related symptoms may include questionnaires, sleep diaries or logs, actigraphy, nocturnal polysomnography, an out-of-center sleep test, or a multiple sleep latency test.

This chapter focuses on the comparative value of different approaches to clinical assessment of sleep-related problems. It is important to remember that the patient being evaluated for sleep complaints may have more than one sleep disorder. This chapter therefore highlights the clinical reasoning process by which a clinician challenged with a sleep complaint can combine information from different sources, appropriately weigh available evidence, and arrive at sound diagnoses and treatment plans. Here we review the value of tests in evaluations of suspected obstructive sleep-disordered breathing, hypersomnolence, insomnia, suspected circadian rhythm sleep-wake disorders, restless legs syndrome (RLS), and suspected parasomnias. A selection of evidence-based practice parameters and reviews produced by the American Academy of Sleep Medicine (AASM) can be accessed at http://aasmnet.org/practiceguidelines.aspx (Table 4-1) to supplement overviews presented in this chapter.

EVALUATION FOR SLEEP-RELATED BREATHING DISORDERS

History and Questionnaires

Sleep-related breathing disorders are by far the most common disorders diagnosed at sleep centers, and obstructive sleep apnea (OSA) alone accounts for nearly 70% of all patients evaluated.[1]

Subjective clinical impressions of OSA tend to have inadequate sensitivity (probability of a positive test result or assessment given that the disorder is present) and specificity (probability of a negative test result given that the disorder is absent).[2] Combinations of some signs and symptoms can have sensitivity above 0.90, but specificity is usually poor. Performance of these models in clinical practice can be worse than originally reported.[3] However, sensitivity and specificity data suggest that the negative predictive value (NPV) of some symptom combinations may be good, whereas the positive predictive value (PPV) is probably poor, especially when the prevalence of OSA in the tested population is not high.[4] Accordingly, patients without a history suggestive of OSA usually do not receive further testing for it. Among patients referred for suspected OSA, models based on historical information may accurately classify a minority as apnea free without further tests.[5] In practice, patients who do have symptoms of OSA generally are tested.

Although, in general, the PPV of symptoms alone is not high, a minority of patients have a clinical presentation so convincing as to be essentially diagnostic. However, the *International Classification of Sleep Disorders*, third edition (ICSD3), requires minimal objective criteria, in addition to symptoms, to establish a diagnosis of OSA.[6] Tests in such cases may also serve to define the severity of OSA. In a patient with a history strongly suggestive of OSA, the diagnosis must still be suspected when it is not confirmed by a single polysomnogram (PSG) and especially when it is not confirmed by a more abbreviated home sleep test.[7]

The diagnostic values of specific symptoms are difficult to judge on the basis of studies with significant methodologic differences. For example, among patients referred specifically for possible OSA, the symptom of excessive daytime sleepiness may[8] or may not[9] be useful in making the diagnosis, and a history of hypertension may be better than a report of snoring as an indication that OSA is present.[10] Among patients referred to a sleep center, snoring has high sensitivity (80% to 90%) and low specificity (20% to 50%) for the diagnosis of OSA, whereas nocturnal choking or gasping is less sensitive (52%) and more specific (84%).[2] In patients referred for suspected sleep-disordered breathing, the presence of nocturnal choking or gasping yields a PPV for OSA of 35%, which is greater than the PPV for morning headache, reported apnea, excessive daytime sleepiness, or snoring.[2] In contrast, in the community, the symptom with the highest predictive value for OSA is habitual snoring, although excessive daytime sleepiness and observed apneas are also useful.[11]

Physical Examination

In the community, among variables related to body weight, neck circumference and body mass index (BMI) correlate well with the presence and severity of OSA.[12] Among patients referred for possible OSA, these variables still may be useful, but their predictive value is not large except in extreme

Type	Published (mo/yr)	Subject Matter	Paper Title
Table 4-1			**Practice Guidelines for the Use of Tools and Tests in Sleep Medicine from the American Academy of Sleep Medicine (AASM)**
P	1/2008	Sleep-related breathing disorders	Practice Parameters for the Use of Autotitrating Continuous Positive Airway Pressure Devices for Titrating Pressures and Treating Adult Patients with Obstructive Sleep Apnea Syndrome: An Update for 2007
CG	6/2009	Sleep-related breathing disorders	Clinical Guideline for the Evaluation, Management, and Long-term Care of Obstructive Sleep Apnea in Adults
CG	2/2008	Sleep-related breathing disorders	Clinical Guidelines for the Manual Titration of Positive Airway Pressure in Patients with Obstructive Sleep Apnea
P	11/2007	Circadian rhythm sleep disorders	Practice Parameters for the Clinical Evaluation and Treatment of Circadian Rhythm Sleep Disorders
R	11/2007	Circadian rhythm sleep disorders	Circadian Rhythm Sleep Disorders: Part I, Basic Principles, Shift Work, and Jet Lag Disorders
R	11/2007	Circadian rhythm sleep disorders	Circadian Rhythm Sleep Disorders: Part II, Advanced Sleep Phase Disorder, Delayed Sleep Phase Disorder, Free-Running Disorder, and Irregular Sleep-Wake Rhythm
CG	10/2008	Insomnia	Clinical Guideline for the Evaluation and Management of Chronic Insomnia in Adults
P	11/2012	Pediatrics	Practice Parameters for the Non-Respiratory Indications for Polysomnography and Multiple Sleep Latency Testing for Children
P	3/2011	Pediatrics	Practice Parameters for the Respiratory Indications for Polysomnography in Children
R	11/2012	Pediatrics	Non-Respiratory Indications for Polysomnography and Related Procedures in Children: An Evidence-Based Review
R	3/2011	Pediatrics	Executive Summary of Respiratory Indications for Polysomnography in Children: An Evidence-Based Review
P	4/2007	Diagnostics	Practice Parameters for the Use of Actigraphy in the Assessment of Sleep and Sleep Disorders: An Update for 2007
P	4/2005	Diagnostics	Practice Parameters for the Indications for Polysomnography and Related Procedures: An Update for 2005
P	1/2005	Diagnostics	Practice Parameters for Clinical Use of the Multiple Sleep Latency Test and the Maintenance of Wakefulness Test
P	9/2003	Diagnostics	Practice Parameters for Using Polysomnography to Evaluate Insomnia: An Update
R	10/2011	Diagnostics	Obstructive Sleep Apnea Devices for Out-Of-Center (OOC) Testing: Technology Evaluation
R	1/2005	Diagnostics	A Review by the MSLT and MWT Task Force of the Standards of Practice Committee of the American Academy of Sleep Medicine: The Clinical Use of the MSLT and MWT
CG	12/2007	Diagnostics	Clinical Guidelines for the Use of Unattended Portable Monitors in the Diagnosis of Obstructive Sleep Apnea in Adult Patients

MSLT, Multiple Sleep Latency Test; MWT, Maintenance of Wakefulness Test.
Practice guidelines are written by the Standards of Practice Committee of the AASM. Practice Parameters (P), Systematic Reviews (R), Clinical Guidelines (CG), and Best Practice Guides (BPG) are generally available at http://aasmnet.org/practiceguidelines.aspx.

ranges.[9,13,14] Patients with OSA who are not obese often have pharyngeal crowding, obstructed nasal passages, or other craniofacial abnormalities associated with narrowing of the upper airway.[15] The predictive value of such findings may differ somewhat between men and women.[16] The Mallampati score, which reflects oropharyngeal crowding on a 4-point scale, was found to predict OSA.[17] Each 1-point increase in the score was associated with an odds ratio of 2.5 (95% confidence interval [CI] [1.2, 5.0]) for OSA and predicted a 5-point higher apnea-hypopnea index (coefficient = 5.3 [0.2 to 10]), independent of many other physical findings and symptoms.

Physical findings can also be combined into predictive quantitative models to aid in the diagnosis of OSA. Models based on measures that can be obtained during the physical examination, such as BMI, neck circumference, craniofacial measurements, pharyngeal scores, and tonsil size, demonstrate excellent PPV (90% to 100%) but less strong NPV (49% to 89%).[18-20] Other physical findings may also have value in the diagnosis of OSA. High blood pressure increases the chance that OSA will be present, especially among persons who are less obese.[21] Signs of neuropathy or neuromuscular disease also may increase the likelihood of OSA.

Table 4-2   Value of Specific Questionnaire Instruments that Combine Symptoms and Physical Findings to Diagnose Obstructive Sleep Apnea

Instrument	Study	Subjects	Gold Standard	Sensitivity	Specificity	Predictive Value
Berlin Questionnaire	Subramanian et al., 2011[154]	Referral based	PSG RDI ≥15	0.93	0.14	
			PSG RDI ≥5	0.92	0.18	
	Hrubos-Strøm et al., 2011[155]	Population based	PSG AHI ≥15	0.43	0.80	PPV = 0.34, NPV = 0.86
			PSG AHI ≥5	0.37	0.84	PPV = 0.61, NPV = 0.66
	Sun et al., 2011[156]	Referral based	PSG AHI ≥15	0.97	0.48	
	Kang et al., 2013[157]	Population based	PSG AHI ≥5	0.69	0.83	
	Cowan et al., 2014[158]	Referral based	Home PG AHI ≥15	0.94	0.08	PPV = 0.44, NPV = 0.67
			Home PG AHI ≥5	0.93	0.06	PPV = 0.75, NPV = 0.22
STOP-BANG	Chung et al., 2008[159]	Preoperative population	PSG AHI ≥15	0.93	0.43	PPV = 0.52, NPV = 0.90
			PSG AHI ≥5	0.84	0.56	PPV = 0.81, NPV = 0.61
	Ong et al., 2010[160]	Referral based	PSG AHI ≥15	0.91	0.40	PPV = 0.61, NPV = 0.82
			PSG AHI ≥5	0.85	0.53	PPV = 0.84, NPV = 0.53
	Cowan et al., 2014[158]	Referral based	Home PG AHI ≥15	1.0	0.21	PPV = 0.5, NPV = 1.0
			Home PG AHI ≥5	0.95	0.3	PPV = 0.81, NPV = 0.64
NAMES	Subramanian et al., 2011[154]	Referral based	PSG RDI ≥15	0.91	0.23	PPV = 0.62, NPV = 0.63
			PSG RDI ≥5	0.88	0.29	
NAMES2	Subramanian et al., 2011[154]	Referral based	PSG RDI ≥15	0.92	0.34	
			PSG RDI ≥5	0.85	0.42	
Snoring Severity Scale with BMI	Morris et al., 2008[161]	Referral based	PSG RDI ≥15	0.97	0.40	PPV = 0.82, NPV = 0.84

AHI, Apnea-hypopnea index (number of apneas or hypopneas per hour of sleep); BMI, body mass index; RDI, respiratory disturbance index (number of apneas, hypopneas, or respiratory effort related arousals per hour of sleep); NPV, negative predictive value; PPV, positive predictive value; PSG, polysomnography; SDB, sleep-disordered breathing.
The NAMES instrument assesses neck circumference, airway classification, comorbidities, Epworth scale, and snoring. The NAMES2 instrument contains the same variables in NAMES with the addition of BMI and gender. The STOP-BANG instrument assesses snoring, tiredness, observed apneas, blood pressure, BMI, age, neck circumference, and gender. The Snoring Severity Scale (SSS) assesses snoring loudness, frequency, and duration.

Instruments that use a combination of symptoms, comorbidities, and physical findings to assess risk for OSA include the Berlin Questionnaire, STOP-BANG, NAMES, NAMES2, and the Snoring Severity Scale combined with BMI. Table 4-2 shows sensitivity, specificity, and predictive values for these tools. Of these tools, the Berlin Questionnaire and the STOP-BANG instrument (Figure 4-1) are most frequently encountered in clinical practice.

Nocturnal Polysomnography

A nocturnal, laboratory-based PSG is commonly used to objectively test for OSA. The PSG often is considered a gold standard for OSA diagnosis, assessment of severity, and identification of some other sleep disorders that can accompany OSA. The PSG allows direct monitoring and quantification of respiratory events and physiologic consequences—such as hypoxemia, arousals, and awakenings—that are suspected to cause daytime symptoms. A single-night PSG is usually sufficient to diagnose or to exclude OSA. However, the test is not infallible. Accuracy may be reduced by variability in biologic severity, laboratory equipment, human scoring, or scoring protocols. Night-to-night variability may be particularly high in subjects with low but clinically significant rates of apneas and hypopneas during sleep. A repeat PSG may confirm OSA in 20% to 50% of individuals who have symptoms suggestive of OSA but initial PSG negative for OSA.[22,23]

SNORING?
Do you **snore loudly** (louder than talking or loud   Yes   No
enough to be heard through closed doors)?

TIRED?
Do you often feel **tired, fatigued, or sleepy** during   Yes   No
the daytime?

OBSERVED?
Has anyone **observed** you **stop breathing**   Yes   No
during your sleep?

PRESSURE?
Do you have or are you being treated for **high**   Yes   No
blood pressure?

BODY MASS INDEX more than 35 kg/m^2?   Yes   No

AGE older than 50 years?   Yes   No

NECK circumference?
Neck circumference greater than 40 cm?   Yes   No

Gender=male?   Yes   No

Figure 4-1 The STOP-BANG questionnaire. Low risk for OSA: yes to 0 to 2 questions. High risk for OSA: yes to 3 or more questions. (From Chung F, Yegneswaran B, Liao P, et al. STOP questionnaire: a tool to screen patients for obstructive sleep apnea. *Anesthesiology* 2008;108[5]:812–21, with permission.)

Publication by the AASM in 2007 (since updated twice) of new sleep scoring guidelines also included recommendations for polysomnographic equipment; scoring of abnormal respiratory events, electrocardiographic findings, movements, and arousals during sleep; and modifications necessary for children.[24] These guidelines serve to improve uniformity of procedures between laboratories.

Arguably, the change in the updated manual with the highest potential to influence clinical practice is the modification to the scoring rules for hypopneas. The scoring manual recommends that the technician scores a hypopnea when the nasal pressure transducer signal (or positive airway pressure flow during a titration study) drops by at least 30% from the preevent baseline, the duration of this amplitude reduction is at least 10 seconds, and the event results in either an arousal or oxygen desaturation of at least 3%.[25] The recommended hypopnea definition aims to increase the sensitivity of PSG to detect OSA in patients with sleep fragmentation and daytime impairment but without significant oxygen desaturations.[25] The scoring manual also defines an acceptable rule as an alternative method to score hypopneas that requires an oxygen desaturation of 4%.[25]

The distinction between the recommended rule and acceptable rule for scoring hypopneas is important from a diagnostic standpoint. For example, PSGs were rescored in a group of lean patients with known OSA based on use of a scoring rule that did not require oxygen desaturation to score hypopneas.[26] The PSGs were rescored with a hypopnea definition that required a 4% oxygen desaturation but not necessarily an arousal. This change resulted in a reduction of the apnea-hypopnea index (AHI) and classified 40% of these symptomatic patients as negative for OSA.[26] These findings highlight the potential benefits of the recommended hypopnea definition set forth in the 2012 scoring manual.

Most laboratories report an AHI that represents the sum total of apneas and hypopneas per hour of sleep. Additionally, the respiratory disturbance index (RDI) calculates the sum total of apneas, hypopneas, and respiratory effort related arousals (RERAs) per hour of sleep. Nasal or esophageal pressure monitoring allows for the scoring of RERAs. Although additional data are still needed, the importance of scoring RERAs is likely to depend in part on which hypopnea definition is used. With the less sensitive definition that focuses on 4% desaturations and ignores arousals, scoring RERAs makes a much larger difference in the computed total rate of respiratory events and may frequently make the difference between diagnosis and failure to diagnose OSA. If the more sensitive definition for hypopneas is used that includes arousal but does not require oxygen desaturation, fewer additional events are detected when RERAs are scored; RERAs then have less impact on the total rates of apneic events and therefore less clinical impact.

As a result of these challenges and the imperfect reliability of PSGs, interpretation of PSG reports remains more complicated and may not be definitive, particularly in borderline cases. The patient's clinical presentation should be considered when interpreting the PSG to help mitigate underdiagnosis and overdiagnosis. Although many clinicians believe that an AHI above 5 indicates OSA, the PSG finding of an AHI greater than 5 may not be associated with symptoms. For example, a large population-based epidemiologic study found that only 22.6% of women and 15.5% of men who met this criterion clearly complained of daytime hypersomnolence.[12] Conversely, some patients with an AHI less than 5 may still have OSA that merits treatment to improve symptoms and morbidity.[27,28]

Further research is needed to define and to improve the ability of PSGs to measure those aspects of sleep-disordered breathing that most affect health and daytime sleepiness. The AHI and minimum oxygen saturation do not correlate strongly with daytime sleepiness,[29] although the AHI may correlate better with cardiovascular morbidity.[22] Esophageal pressure monitoring is the gold standard to assess respiratory effort and may identify increased respiratory effort and RERAs in patients without significant apneas and hypopneas.[30,31] However, criteria for abnormal esophageal pressure recordings, as defined by association with poor outcomes, remain to be studied more definitively. Nasal pressure monitoring may provide a well-tolerated alternative; however, despite increased sensitivity, studies have yet to demonstrate improved prediction of outcomes, and initial comparisons to thermistor results show correlations high enough (e.g., 0.90 or higher)[32,33] to suggest redundancy of information. Other polysomnographic measures that may (or may not) prove to enhance the ability of PSGs to predict outcomes of sleep-disordered breathing include end-tidal or transcutaneous carbon dioxide monitoring,[34] pulse transit time,[35] peripheral arterial tonometry,[36] scoring of arousals,[37,38] and analysis of respiratory cycle–related electroencephalographic changes.[38,39]

In short, the PSG is the single most useful and definitive test in the diagnosis of sleep-related breathing disorders, but the information it provides cannot be reliably interpreted by persons without experience in sleep medicine, summarized by any single number, or applied to patient care without careful use of additional clinical data. Failure to recognize these limitations, by health care policy makers or clinicians, could trigger unnecessary intervention or deprive a patient of effective treatment.

Modified Forms of the Polysomnogram

In comparison to the standard PSG, daytime and split-night studies may reduce costs and expedite evaluation. Studies of daytime PSGs have sometimes found a high NPV, with lower PPV, but inconsistent results and the lack of sufficient data explain why daytime PSGs have not generally been recommended.[4] A successful split-night study may save a patient from a second night in the sleep laboratory. Studies of diagnostic accuracy and treatment outcomes appear promising.[40] Concordance is high between AHI measured in the first 2 hours of PSG recording and AHI measured in a full-night PSG (concordance correlation coefficient = 0.93).[41] Although the traditional gold standard has been separate, full-night studies for diagnostic assessment and then positive airway pressure titration, split-night studies may be adequate alternatives in most cases.[42,43]

Home Sleep Tests

Many different devices exist to assess OSA at home, although most do not record sleep. These "portable" recordings usually are less costly than laboratory-based PSGs, and patients often prefer home studies to laboratory studies. However, the diagnostic value of unattended portable monitoring is often reduced by the inability to make behavioral observations, standardize recording conditions, address technical problems, make interventions during the night, or monitor variables equivalent to those recorded in the laboratory setting. Home sleep tests that do not monitor signals necessary to identify sleep stages or leg movements only evaluate for sleep apnea. Additionally, scored respiratory events may not have occurred during sleep and thus may result in inaccurate sleep apnea severity.

A Portable Monitoring Task Force of the AASM recommended home studies only after a comprehensive sleep evaluation by a clinician board-eligible or certified in sleep medicine, and then interpreted by someone with the same level of specialty training.[7] This recommendation is based on the fact that studies demonstrating effectiveness of home sleep tests were conducted in the context of thorough clinical evaluations by sleep specialists. Further, home studies have significant limitations and therefore must be interpreted by specialists aware of these constraints. Under these conditions, home studies can be used as an alternative to laboratory-based PSGs when clinical judgment suggests that pretest probability of moderate to severe OSA is high. Home studies should generally not be used when the patient is a child or older person, has significant health comorbidities (e.g., severe pulmonary disease, neuromuscular disease, or congestive heart failure), or in whom other additional sleep disorders are suspected.[7] Home studies may be indicated for patients who do not have access to laboratory-based PSG, cannot tolerate the procedure, or need follow-up assessment of response to non–positive airway pressure treatments of OSA.

Published guidelines for home studies recommend that at minimum they monitor airflow, respiratory effort, and blood oxygenation and that the equipment should be applied by a sleep technologist or health care practitioner with appropriate training.[7] Home studies can underestimate sleep-disordered breathing. Many home studies do not monitor an electroencephalogram (EEG) and as such do not allow for hypopneas to be scored when they terminate in cortical arousal but do not result in oxygen desaturation. Additionally, the AHI on a home study that does not monitor sleep is calculated with total recording time (as opposed to total sleep time) as the denominator.[42] Therefore, if a home study in an appropriately selected individual does not demonstrate OSA, a more definitive laboratory-based sleep study should be considered. A suggested algorithm for use of home studies is shown in Figure 4-2.

In carefully selected patients, portable recording devices are effective tools to diagnose OSA. A meta-analysis of level 3 portable monitoring devices demonstrated sensitivity from 0.79 to 0.97 and specificity from 0.60 to 0.93 for OSA, depending on AHI cutoffs.[44] However, these validation studies, generally performed in a controlled laboratory setting, do not take into account the potential for technical failure of portable devices in an ambulatory environment. Despite these limitations, initial investigations demonstrate similar outcomes in patients randomized to home sleep tests versus attended PSG.[45,46] Portable devices that have low costs, high sensitivities, and high specificities have the potential to be cost-effective in comparison to PSGs. However, cost-effectiveness analyses thus far suggest that full-night PSG is superior to portable tests for OSA[47,48] (discussed under Beyond Sensitivity, Specificity, and Predictive Value in this chapter). In some situations, home studies could increase costs, delay confirmatory laboratory testing, encourage

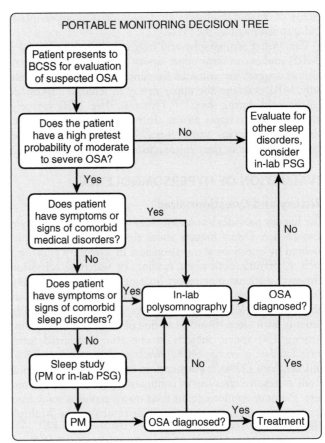

Figure 4-2 Recommended use of home studies. BCSS, Board-certified sleep specialist; OSA, obstructive sleep apnea; PM, portable monitoring; PSG, polysomnography. (From Collop NA, Anderson WM, Boehlecke B, et al. Clinical guidelines for the use of unattended portable monitors in the diagnosis of obstructive sleep apnea in adult patients. Portable Monitoring Task Force of the American Academy of Sleep Medicine. *J Clin Sleep Med* 2007;3:737–47, with permission.)

treatment of patients with false-positive results, or allow development of medical morbidity from undiagnosed and therefore untreated OSA.

Studies of Airway Morphology

Although imaging of the upper airway for research purposes has led to a better understanding of OSA pathophysiology, such studies are not routinely performed in diagnostic evaluations of patients, in part because findings that predict OSA or its severity with sufficient accuracy to allow use in management of individual patients have not been identified. However, cephalometric radiography and pharyngoscopy may be useful in preoperative identification of sites of obstruction and in selection of appropriate surgical procedures. The diagnostic value of cephalometrics may be limited in part because only sagittal plane dimensions are provided while coronal plane dimensions or volume may be more pertinent to OSA.[49] Pharyngoscopy allows three-dimensional anatomic characterization, but whether airway collapse with Müller's maneuver predicts response to uvulopalatopharyngoplasty is debated. Pharyngoscopy may be particularly valuable if it is performed during supine sleep.[50] Techniques for quantitative computer-assisted video endoscopic airway analysis are also being developed and have shown, for example, correlation between the extent of anatomic change after uvulopalatopharyngoplasty and improvement in the AHI.[51]

Computed tomography and magnetic resonance imaging (MRI) studies can show upper airway morphology,[49] and some authors suggest the potential for clinical usefulness.[52] Specifically, MRI evaluates the upper airway in multiple planes and can be used during sleep.[53-55] Dynamic sleep MRI protocols may characterize upper airway obstruction better than single-plane images during wakefulness.[53-55] However, the value of these techniques in the clinical setting is not well defined.

EVALUATION OF HYPERSOMNOLENCE

History and Questionnaires

The history provides important clues to the severity of hypersomnolence. Direct inquiry about sleepiness can be supplemented by questions about sleepiness in sedentary situations, such as driving, desk work, reading, or watching television. However, patients may report little of the excessive daytime sleepiness suggested by family members, clinical signs, or objective tests. Words other than *sleepiness* are often used by patients with sleep disorders to describe the chief complaint. Among 190 apneic subjects in one study, preferred terms included *lack of energy* (40%), *tiredness* (20%), *fatigue* (18%), and *sleepiness* (22%).[56] Furthermore, each of these symptoms tends to resolve after use of continuous positive airway pressure. Patients' opinions about their own sleepiness sometimes show no significant association with results of the Multiple Sleep Latency Test (MSLT).[57]

Questionnaires such as the Epworth Sleepiness Scale[58] and the Stanford Sleepiness Scale[59] provide a more formal and perhaps reliable measure of excessive daytime sleepiness. The impact of sleepiness on activities of daily living can be assessed with the Functional Outcomes of Sleep Questionnaire.[60] Epworth results correlate reasonably well with patients' self-ratings for overall sleepiness but not well with MSLT results.[61] Although the Epworth Sleepiness Scale and the Stanford Sleepiness Scale can have clinical utility, for example, in monitoring response to treatment over time, they do not substitute for well-validated objective measures of sleepiness. Unfortunately, the ability of subjective tests of sleepiness to predict future health outcomes remains largely unknown.

In addition to the severity of EDS, it is critical to assess napping patterns and other symptoms associated with hypersomnolence to determine its etiology. For example, cataplexy is the essential feature that distinguishes narcolepsy type 1 from narcolepsy type 2 and other disorders of sleepiness.[6] Cataplexy must be derived from patient report because it is rarely observed during the clinical evaluation for hypersomnolence. Sleep paralysis and hypnagogic and hypnopompic hallucinations are reported in about 50% of patients with narcolepsy; however, these symptoms are often present in individuals without the disease and thus are not specific.[62] Inquiry about nap duration and quality is also useful because patients with narcolepsy, in contrast to other sleep disorders, may experience a greater (although transient) alerting affect from short naps.[63] In contrast, more than two thirds of patients with idiopathic hypersomnia report that naps are nonrestorative.[64-66]

Physical Examination

Although the alerting effect of an examination obscures physical signs of sleepiness in most patients, overt signs of sleepiness—such as the inability to stay awake or to keep eyes open in the examination room—have high PPV and may obviate the need for additional tests. The examination may also help distinguish severe sleepiness from stupor due to neurologic impairment or drugs.

Sleep Logs and Actigraphy

The evaluation of hypersomnolence includes assessment of sleep duration and timing to rule out insufficient sleep syndrome or circadian rhythm sleep-wake disorders. The clinician should ask about sleep schedules at the time of clinical evaluation. Unfortunately, singular point estimates of sleep duration and timing demonstrate poor agreement with longitudinal measures.[67-69] Therefore tools such as sleep logs and actigraphy are valuable to track sleep patterns over days to weeks. Historically, sleep logs have been used to ensure adequate sleep duration before objective assessment of hypersomnolence with MSLT despite the absence of data supporting this use.[70]

An actigram is a device worn on the nondominant wrist that uses accelerometry to detect movement to estimate sleep and wake. Agreement between actigraphy and PSG in the detection of sleep is approximately 90%, and this device is accepted as a valid method to evaluate sleep patterns.[71-73] Actigraphy and sleep logs recorded for 2 weeks before MSLT were compared in a group of patients who underwent evaluation for hypersomnolence. Sleep logs were found to overestimate average nightly sleep duration by 1.43 hours (±1.31 hours) compared with actigraphy.[67] In the subgroup of patients whose MSLT results objectively confirmed excessive daytime sleepiness, average nightly sleep duration was 4.53 ± 1.37 hours by actigraphy, which was 2.55 ± 1.41 hours shorter than that recorded on sleep logs.[67] This study may be difficult to generalize because it was conducted in a military population. However, in a subsequent study at a large academic institution, poor agreement was seen between actigraphy and sleep logs typically owing to increased total sleep time reported on sleep logs compared with actigraphy.[74] Actigraphy is highly sensitive but not specific for EEG-defined sleep and may overestimate true sleep. Therefore the finding that sleep duration reported on sleep logs exceeds sleep duration derived by actigraphy is troublesome when determining whether sleep duration is adequate before MSLT. The ICSD-3 recommends documentation of sleep duration for 7 days on a sleep log and, whenever possible, actigraphy in conjunction with the sleep log, before the MSLT.[6]

Nocturnal Polysomnography

Many patients referred to sleep centers for excessive daytime sleepiness have nocturnal sleep disorders, and PSG is often more notable for the manifestations of such disorders than for signs of excessive daytime sleepiness. The single polysomnographic variable that best reflects sleepiness, as measured by the mean sleep latency on the MSLT, is nocturnal sleep latency.[75] Polysomnographic measures of sleep pathology, such as the AHI and minimum oxygen saturation, show only low magnitudes of correlation with MSLT results.[76] However, a short latency to REM sleep on overnight PSG can provide a valuable clue to the presence of narcolepsy. Among patients referred to a sleep laboratory, REM onset latency less than 15 minutes on nocturnal PSG had poor sensitivity (approximately 40%) but excellent specificity (99.6%) for type 1 narcolepsy.[77] The ICSD-3 now allows a sleep-onset REM period, on overnight PSG, to account for one of the two REM periods necessary to diagnose narcolepsy with an MSLT.[6]

Multiple Sleep Latency Test

The mean sleep latency on the MSLT is the most commonly used objective measure in the assessment of daytime sleepiness.[78] The MSLT may contribute to diagnosis but is usually not sufficient, alone, to establish a diagnosis. The mean sleep latency is most useful when it is clearly abnormally low. A patient with a mean sleep latency of 2 minutes on a properly performed MSLT is unlikely to be exaggerating a complaint of excessive daytime sleepiness, to suffer from fatigue rather than sleepiness, or to be free of any sleep disorder. The MSLT can help determine the clinical significance of a sleep disorder or assess response to treatment.

As a general guideline, mean sleep latencies shorter than 8 minutes on a properly conducted MSLT are considered abnormal,[78] and latencies shorter than 5 minutes often indicate severe excessive daytime sleepiness. However, proper interpretation of MSLT results requires integration of other factors and especially knowledge of the limitations of this test. Results may be misleading if they are affected by youth (different criteria apply for children), noise, anxiety, or atypical sleep on the previous night. Use of medications such as stimulants or antidepressants, their recent discontinuance, or inability to be weaned off them at least 10 days before testing can complicate interpretation of an MSLT. Sleep apnea and other sleep disorders may make sleep onset more difficult and thereby interfere with the test. In general, the NPV of a long mean sleep latency is less than the PPV of a particularly short mean sleep latency. When an MSLT is normal, clinicians must carefully consider other possible explanations before telling a subjectively sleepy patient that there is no objective evidence of excessive daytime sleepiness. Formal prospective studies of "real-life" outcomes associated with different mean sleep latencies are still needed, but until such data are available, clinicians should realize that MSLT results form a continuum without strictly interpretable cutoffs. Community-based samples of adults show mean sleep latencies of 8 minutes or less in well more than 20% of subjects.[79] High test-retest reliability among normal subjects[80] does not necessarily generalize to patients.[81] In fact, 40% of central hypersomnia patients had mean sleep latencies that crossed to the other side of the 8-minute threshold when MSLTs conducted about 4 years apart were compared.[82] Interrater reliability can be excellent but adds another source of potential variation in test results.[83]

Nocturnal Polysomnography and MSLT in the Diagnosis of Narcolepsy

The diagnostic criteria for narcolepsy—two or more sleep-onset REM periods (SOREMPs) and short mean sleep latency—were once thought to have high sensitivity and specificity. Original case series suggested that all narcoleptic subjects and virtually no normal controls had two or more SOREMPs[84]; the PPV of two or more SOREMPs for the diagnosis of narcolepsy was 98%, and the NPV was 89%.[85] Subsequent studies did not find the SOREMP criteria to provide such diagnostic accuracy, partly because the most common reasons for sleep laboratory referral evolved. Two or more SOREMPs were found in 25% of 187 sleep apneic subjects,[86] 17% of 139 normal subjects,[87] and 83% of 200 narcoleptic subjects who had cataplexy.[88] Among 2083 patients

evaluated with MSLTs at one sleep center, the PPV of two or more SOREMPs was 57% and the NPV was 98%.[89] Thus the presence of SOREMPs must be interpreted in conjunction with other clinical and polysomnographic findings. The criterion of two or more SOREMPs cannot be used to diagnose narcolepsy when the patient has untreated OSA. Furthermore, the number of SOREMPs can change enough to alter the diagnosis (idiopathic hypersomnia versus narcolepsy without cataplexy) in up to 30% of patients on repeated MSLT.[82] As an alternative to the MSLT, cerebrospinal fluid hypocretin-1 levels can be used to confirm type 1 narcolepsy. These levels are low (≤110 pg/mL or <one third of the mean for controls) in more than 90% of affected patients but almost never among patients without this diagnosis.[6]

Variations of the Multiple Sleep Latency Test and Other Physiologic Tests

Results of the Maintenance of Wakefulness Test (MWT) can differ markedly from those of the MSLT,[90] but whether the MWT results are more predictive of adverse effects of sleepiness in daily life remains unknown. Results of both the MWT and MSLT can be influenced by the patient's motivation.[91] The MWT results correlate with measures of sleep apnea severity to about the same extent as MSLT results do[92] but may better reflect improvement with treatment.[90] Shorter sleep latencies on MWTs correlate with increased errors on driving simulation tests.[93,94] However, until MWT and MSLT results are shown to differ in a clinically meaningful way, the MSLT continues to offer advantages of more published experience, familiarity among clinicians, and relevance to the diagnosis of narcolepsy. The Federal Aviation Administration and other agencies may at times request or require an MWT, but given the dearth of proven real-life predictive value, the role of this test or the MSLT in predicting workplace safety remains controversial.[95,96]

MSLT modifications, for which limited validity data exist, include addition of performance tasks[97,98]; analysis of sleep stages during naps[99]; focus on the percentage of time spent awake[100]; definition of sleep onset by failure to respond to a repeated signal[101]; and use of survival analysis to better account for failure to sleep on some naps.[102] In the clinical setting, none of these modifications have been adopted; neither have a range of other physiologic tests, including pupillometry and brainstem auditory evoked potentials. A variety of performance-based tests are used, usually in research settings, to assess variables related to sleepiness. Examples are the Psychomotor Vigilance Task[103] and the Steer Clear driving simulation test.[104]

Another available method to assess hypersomnia is the 24-hour PSG. About 40% of patients with idiopathic hypersomnia demonstrate mean sleep latencies greater than 8 minutes on the MSLT despite severe subjective sleepiness.[65,105,106] This finding is more common in patients with long nocturnal sleep durations. In these individuals, prolonged PSG reveals a total sleep duration near 700 minutes over 24 hours.[105] Therefore a 24-hour PSG that documents total sleep time of at least 660 minutes can be used to diagnose idiopathic hypersomnia in patients with symptoms consistent with the disorder but mean sleep latency greater than 8 minutes.[6] The ICSD-3 also allows actigraphy for this purpose; however, it has not been validated in this particular setting.[6]

EVALUATION OF INSOMNIA

History and Questionnaires

Like excessive daytime sleepiness, the complaint of inadequate, insufficient, or nonrestorative sleep can have many different causes. However, causes of insomnia are often diagnosed by history alone.[107,108] In part because the gold standard is not a physiologic test, few data are available with which to assess the relative value of individual symptoms. Predictive values for some symptoms are likely to be high because symptoms define the disorders. When a history does not reveal a cause of the insomnia, PSG may be useful (discussed under Nocturnal Polysomnography in this section). Psychometric tests can reveal cognitive differences between insomniac subjects and normal controls,[109] but these tests are not commonly used for diagnostic purposes in the clinical sleep medicine setting.

The Insomnia Severity Index is a seven-item self-report instrument that is typically used in insomnia research.[110] However, this tool may also be beneficial in the clinical setting. A score of 10 or higher on the Insomnia Severity Index identified insomnia with a sensitivity of 86% and a specificity of 88% in a community sample.[111]

Sleep Logs and Actigraphy

Sleep logs are an important tool in the evaluation of insomnia.[112] Patients record sleep-onset latency (SOL) and wake after sleep onset (WASO) on sleep logs, and investigators have tested the ability of different cutoffs of these quantitative parameters to predict insomnia. In one study, SOL or WASO of 31 minutes or longer identified insomnia with a sensitivity of 64% and specificity of 77% in subjects with insomnia at least 3 times per week for 6 months.[113] A subsequent investigation that also used sleep logs found that SOL or WASO of 20 minutes or more alone identified insomnia with a sensitivity of 94% and specificity of 80%.[114] Logs are not necessary to establish the presence of insomnia but can help define severity and facilitate identification of causes such as inadequate sleep hygiene or circadian rhythm sleep-wake disorders.

Actigraphy should be used with caution in patients with insomnia. The ability of actigraphy to measure sleep parameters (e.g., total sleep time or WASO) deteriorates as sleep efficiency decreases, which limits utility in patients with insomnia. Among patients with insomnia, in an epoch-by-epoch analysis that compared actigraphy with PSG, the accuracy, sensitivity, and specificity of actigraphy were 0.83, 0.95, and 0.35, respectively.[73] SOL is consistently underestimated by actigraphy in patients with insomnia.[115] Actigraphy is an effective tool to assess sleep-wake patterns when insomnia symptoms are thought to be secondary to a circadian rhythm sleep-wake disorder. However, because of the limitations described previously, actigraphy is not used routinely to confirm a diagnosis of insomnia.[108]

Nocturnal Polysomnography

PSG is not indicated for routine evaluation of insomnia; although when a patient's history and physical examination suggest that insomnia may be due to sleep-disordered breathing, periodic limb movement disorder, paradoxical insomnia, or uncertain causes, it can be an important aid to diagnosis.[116] Additionally, PSG may be indicated if insomnia fails to respond to treatment or in patients who have precipitous

arousals with violent or injurious behavior.[108] Of note, injudicious use of PSG can sometimes enhance patient's conviction that insomnia is due to physical rather than behavioral causes or lead to diagnoses that eventually prove irrelevant to the main complaint.

EVALUATION OF SUSPECTED CIRCADIAN RHYTHM SLEEP-WAKE DISORDERS

History and Questionnaires

Discrepancies between the desired time for sleep and wake and the circadian propensity for sleep and wake may present as insomnia or hypersomnolence. Approximately 7% to 16% of patients who present to sleep disorders clinics with symptoms of insomnia are ultimately diagnosed with delayed sleep-wake phase disorder.[117,118] To distinguish circadian rhythm sleep-wake disorders from other causes of insomnia and hypersomnolence, examples of useful questions may include, "What time of day do you feel most alert?" and "When do you perform the best?" Comparison of regular sleep schedules to schedules on days free from work or school can reveal discrepancies that help to identify a circadian rhythm disorder.

Questionnaires such as the Horne-Ostberg Morningness-Eveningness Questionnaire (MEQ) and the Munich Chronotype Questionnaire (MCTQ) evaluate circadian preference, also known as chronotype.[119,120] The MEQ is the most widely used instrument to assess chronotype. It is a 19-item self-assessment tool that evaluates personal preference for the timing of sleep and other behaviors.[119] The MCTQ is also self-completed but assesses the actual (opposed to preferred) timing of sleep on work or school days versus free days.[120] The midpoint of sleep on free days and self-rated chronotype derived from the MCTQ both correlate highly with chronotype based on MEQ score ($r = -0.7$ and -0.8, respectively).[120,121] In addition to correlating with each other, the MEQ and MCTQ correlate with objective markers of circadian phase. The MEQ scores correlate with salivary dim-light melatonin onset (DLMO) ($r = -0.4$ to -0.5) and peak serum melatonin ($r = -0.4$).[122-124] The midpoint of sleep on free days derived from the MCTQ correlates with DLMO ($r = 0.5$).[124] The MEQ has also been validated against core body temperature and cortisol secretion.[119,125,126]

Sleep Logs and Actigraphy

The AASM recommends the use of sleep logs and, whenever possible, actigraphy for 7 to 14 days to evaluate suspected circadian rhythm sleep-wake disorders. Actigraphy has been validated in patients with circadian rhythm sleep-wake disorders.[72] Inclusion of ad libitum sleep-wake times (e.g., days off from school or work) is essential when sleep is tracked with actigraphy or sleep logs and will provide a more accurate estimate of true, endogenous circadian phase.[122,127,128] Vacation times may be particularly revealing; in fact sleep-wake times of individuals on an unrestricted sleep-wake schedule demonstrate higher correlation ($r = 0.77$) with DLMO than sleep-wake times of those on a fixed schedule ($r = 0.40$).[127]

Nocturnal Polysomnography

PSG is not necessary to diagnose circadian rhythm sleep-wake disorders, although it may be performed to rule out other comorbid sleep conditions. A PSG conducted at conventional times may demonstrate a delay of sleep onset or early morning awakening in patients with delayed or advanced sleep-wake phase disorders, respectively.[129-131]

Multiple Sleep Latency Test

The MSLT is not used to diagnose circadian rhythm sleep-wake disorders; however, if obtained, mean sleep latency may be reduced in circadian rhythm sleep-wake disorders in the setting of sleep loss and excessive daytime sleepiness. Notably, in a large epidemiologic study, shift workers (night or rotating) were almost eight times more likely to have a mean sleep latency of less than 8 minutes combined with at least two SOREMPs on MSLT.[132] Additionally, adolescents with a delay in circadian phase can demonstrate SOREMPs during the MSLT (particularly during the first nap) when they wake according to their school schedule.[133]

Objective Markers of Circadian Phase

The *International Classification of Sleep Disorders*, third edition notes that endogenous markers of circadian phase can confirm the diagnosis of certain circadian rhythm sleep-wake disorders.[6] The salivary (DLMO) or urinary (6-sulfatoxymelatonin, aMT6s) melatonin assays are the most commonly used objective markers of circadian phase. These measures objectively document a stable advance, stable delay, or progressive delay of circadian phase in advanced sleep-wake phase disorder, delayed sleep-wake phase disorder, and non–24-hour sleep-wake rhythm disorder, respectively.[6] Although melatonin assays are infrequently used in clinical practice, at-home DLMO assays correlate well with in-lab DLMO assessments ($r = 0.85$ when a fixed threshold of 3 pg/mL is used).[134] Salivary melatonin assays can capture the onset of melatonin secretion but are not practical to determine the secretion profile overnight in the ambulatory setting. Alternatively, urinary aMT6s can be collected at 8-hour intervals; therefore the first morning void allows for calculation of overnight aMT6s secretion in the home setting.[135] Further investigation is required to determine whether ambulatory measurement of circadian phase markers is reliable and feasible.

EVALUATION OF RESTLESS LEGS SYNDROME

History and Questionnaires

The diagnosis of RLS is made by a clinical history of an urge to move the limbs that is worse at rest, improved with movement, and worse in the evening or night.[6] These four criteria have a PPV of 76% when expert interview is used as a gold standard.[136] Differentiating RLS carefully from leg cramps or positional discomfort improves the specificity of the four criteria from 84% to 94%.[6,136]

Several instruments exist to assist in the evaluation of RLS or its severity, including the International Restless Legs Scale (IRLS), RLS-6, and Johns Hopkins Severity Scale. The IRLS scale is a 10-item questionnaire that assesses the severity of RLS symptoms.[137] This scale has good internal consistency, interexaminer reliability, and test-retest reliability,[137] and a 6-point decrease is considered to be a clinically relevant improvement.[138] Although these scales are used mostly in research, they may be beneficial in the clinic setting to quantify symptom severity; determine the impact of RLS symptoms on patient quality of life, mood, and sleep; measure the progression of RLS symptoms; and evaluate therapeutic response.[139]

Physical Examination

A full neurologic examination is indicated to evaluate for RLS because this condition may arise in the context of other neurologic diseases, such as neuropathy, multiple sclerosis, or Parkinson disease. Assessment of affect and mood to help identify psychiatric disorders is important because mental health morbidity frequently coexists with RLS.

Laboratory Tests

Evaluation of a patient with RLS should include serum iron and ferritin levels. More than one third of individuals with RLS have low serum iron levels, and greater than two thirds have ferritin values of 50 ng/mL or less. Depression, fatigue, and increased severity of symptoms are associated with low serum iron levels in RLS patients.[140] Ferritin levels are inversely related to RLS severity.[141,142] Iron supplementation may reduce symptoms in RLS, although findings are inconsistent.[143] Therefore evaluation of serum iron and ferritin is an integral part of the evaluation of RLS for both diagnosis and treatment.

Nocturnal Polysomnography

PSG is not routinely indicated in the evaluation of RLS and should be performed only if the clinician suspects a comorbid sleep disorder such as OSA. Periodic limb movements during sleep are found in up to 90% of patients with RLS. However, periodic limb movements during sleep are nonspecific because they also occur in approximately 25% of individuals without RLS.[144,145]

EVALUATION FOR SUSPECTED PARASOMNIAS

History and Questionnaires

With the notable exception of REM sleep behavior disorder (RBD), parasomnias often can be diagnosed by history alone.[6] Information obtained from a bed partner may contribute more than that obtained from the patient.

Physical Examination

The physical examination of patients evaluated for parasomnias can be useful, but its value is not well quantified. Some signs may suggest sleep apnea as an underlying trigger for confusional arousals, sleepwalking, sleep terrors, RBD, or nocturnal enuresis. Worn occlusive surfaces of molars can provide key evidence of sleep bruxism. The urogenital examination is important in patients thought to have sleep enuresis. A neurologic examination may suggest a primary cause of sleep enuresis or RBD. Similarly, appropriate laboratory findings may be helpful in some cases; for example, a urinalysis may reveal the cause of sleep enuresis.

Nocturnal Polysomnography

Few studies have examined the predictive value of PSG for parasomnia diagnoses. When the behavior in question occurs during the PSG, the diagnostic value of the test is likely to be high, especially if appropriate additional recording devices, such as extra EEG leads, extra surface electromyogram (EMG) leads, or video monitoring, are used.[146] Additional EEG leads used during PSG, combined with clinical history, may effectively differentiate sleep-related epilepsy from parasomnias.

However, EEG does not reliably diagnose nocturnal frontal lobe epilepsy (NFLE) because more than 60% of patients with

NFLE fail to demonstrate a definite ictal rhythm.[147] Therefore semiology of the events is the key to diagnosis. Derry and colleagues created a rigorous decision tree algorithm based on 120 nocturnal events recorded on video PSG to distinguish NREM disorders of arousal from NFLE.[147] The algorithm included the following characteristics suggestive of NFLE as opposed to parasomnia: complete arousal after the ictus, discrete offset of the behavior, presence of versive head turning or posturing, and persistence of recumbent posture. This decision tree algorithm classified 94% of events correctly. Unfortunately, PSG often fails to document the behavior—especially in cases of suspected RBD, sleepwalking, night terrors, and epilepsy—either because the behavior does not occur on most nights or perhaps because the sleep laboratory is not an environment familiar to the patient. For evaluation of parasomnias, the NPV of a completely normal study is less clear than the PPV of an abnormal study. In one series of 122 patients with suspected parasomnias, one or two nights of PSG with video monitoring contributed useful diagnostic information in more than 50% of cases.[146]

Even in the absence of abnormal behaviors on the night of the PSG, other findings can be valuable. Examples include excessive limb twitching during REM sleep characteristic of RBD and interictal spike and wave complexes that may represent an interictal expression of epilepsy. REM sleep without atonia (RSWA) is the PSG hallmark of RBD and is required to confirm the diagnosis.[6] RSWA may be quantified manually by the eye or by automated computer programs. When scored manually, RSWA is defined by the AASM manual for the scoring of sleep and associated events as either excessive phasic or tonic elevation in EMG tone.[28] Multiple computer algorithms exist to automatically score RSWA, including the REM atonia index and supra-threshold REM EMG activity metric.[148] A supra-threshold REM EMG activity metric cutoff of 15 or higher is able to detect RBD with 100% sensitivity and 71% specificity.[149]

At this time, manual scoring remains the gold standard to detect RSWA.[148] However, the AASM manual does not specify a minimum number or proportion of epochs that must contain RSWA to meet the PSG criteria to confirm suspected RBD.[28] To address this, different cut points have been investigated. When using the submentalis muscle alone, the presence of RSWA (phasic) in 15% of 2-second REM mini-epochs will correctly classify 84% of patients.[150] The Sleep Innsbrook Barcelona group has extensively tested different methods to quantify EMG tone in stage REM sleep and recommends recording EMG in both the submentalis muscle and the bilateral flexor digitorum superficialis muscles to score RSWA.[151] Use of this montage with specificity set at 100% (no false-positive RBD diagnoses permitted) yields a cut point of 32% of 3-second REM mini-epochs to diagnose RBD (area under the receiving operator characteristic curve = 0.998).[151] Upper limb as opposed to lower limb EMG more reliably distinguishes patients with RBD from those without RBD.[148]

BEYOND SENSITIVITY, SPECIFICITY, AND PREDICTIVE VALUE: DECISION AND COST-EFFECTIVENESS ANALYSES

Data on sensitivity, specificity, pretest probability, and utility of outcomes can be used to construct a decision analysis. A clinical decision analysis typically models a choice between diagnostic and therapeutic alternatives. Logical rules are used to weigh information and to make the best decision for an individual patient.[152] Decision analysis may be useful, for example, when one procedure has a high probability of a small benefit but an alternative has a low probability of a large benefit.

Beyond utility, economic data on a procedure can include cost studies, cost-effectiveness analyses that compare different methods to achieve the same end, cost-utility analyses that compare costs per common unit of utility (often quality-adjusted life years), and cost-benefit analyses that compare monetary costs with monetary gains.[153] Such studies require quantitative information on costs and outcomes, data that are not abundant for sleep disorders.[95,96] Despite uncertainty of some important data points, cost-utility models have focused on the decision of whether to diagnose OSA with the aid of a full-night PSG, split-night PSG, portable cardiorespiratory monitoring, or no ancillary test.[47,48] The full-night PSG costs less and results in more quality-adjusted life-years than split-night PSG or unattended portable monitoring over the course of an individual's lifetime.[48] Despite the increased upfront cost of full-night PSG, these results reflect the high utility of an accurate OSA diagnosis and the expense of diagnostic mistakes. These findings highlight the importance of performing decision and cost-utility analyses before conclusions are made about relative values of diagnostic tests.

CLINICAL PEARL

Evaluation of common sleep complaints is based on symptoms, signs, and test results, combined with an understanding of the diagnostic value that each type of data contributes.

SUMMARY

Clinical tools and tests must be used carefully in the evaluation of suspected sleep disorders. All patients with sleep-related complaints should undergo a history and physical examination. Evaluations for obstructive sleep-disordered breathing start with a history and physical examination, which generate valuable information. Symptom-based questionnaires alone usually show inadequate specificity. Laboratory-based nocturnal polysomnography is a gold standard but not infallible. Final diagnostic decisions should be based on integration of multiple clinical and objective data points rather than on any specific cutoff for one specific variable, such as the apnea-hypopnea index. Evaluation for hypersomnolence also relies on historical symptoms collected during an interview or by use of a questionnaire. Objective testing with an MSLT is particularly useful when a shortened mean sleep latency confirms excessive daytime sleepiness or a shortened latency in addition to sleep-onset REM periods confirm narcolepsy. Results must be interpreted carefully, especially when they are normal, because of potential confounds. Evaluation for insomnia often relies solely on historical information. Sleep logs can be helpful, but polysomnography is indicated only when other occult sleep disorders may underlie the insomnia. Questionnaires to determine chronotype and actigraphy are valuable tools when symptoms suggest a circadian rhythm sleep-wake disorder. RLS is a diagnosis based on clinical history, but serum iron studies provide valuable information with repercussions for treatment. Evaluation for a parasomnia starts with a thorough history, obtained whenever possible from a bed partner in addition to the patient. Polysomnography may confirm a diagnosis or distinguish between several possibilities.

Selected Readings

Andlauer O, Moore H, Jouhier L, et al. Nocturnal rapid eye movement sleep latency for identifying patients with narcolepsy/hypocretin deficiency. *JAMA Neurol* 2013;**70**(7):891–902.

Aurora RN, Collop NA, Jacobowitz O, et al. Quality measures for the care of adult patients with obstructive sleep apnea. *J Clin Sleep Med* 2015;**11**(3):357–83.

Berry RB, Budhiraja R, Gottlieb DJ, et al. Rules for scoring respiratory events in sleep: update of the 2007 AASM Manual for the Scoring of Sleep and Associated Events. Deliberations of the Sleep Apnea Definitions Task Force of the American Academy of Sleep Medicine. *J Clin Sleep Med* 2012;**8**(5):597–619.

Chung F, Abdullah HR, Liao P. STOP-Bang Questionnaire: A Practical Approach to Screen for Obstructive Sleep Apnea. *Chest* 2016;**149**(3):631–8.

Collop NA, Anderson WM, Boehlecke B, et al. Clinical guidelines for the use of unattended portable monitors in the diagnosis of obstructive sleep apnea in adult patients. Portable Monitoring Task Force of the American Academy of Sleep Medicine. *J Clin Sleep Med* 2007;**3**:737–47.

Epstein LJ, Kristo D, Strollo PJ Jr, et al. Clinical guideline for the evaluation, management and long-term care of obstructive sleep apnea in adults. *J Clin Sleep Med* 2009;**5**(3):263–76.

Frauscher B, Ehrann L, Högl B. Defining muscle activities for assessment of rapid eye movement sleep behavior disorder: from a qualitative to a quantitative diagnostic level. *Sleep Med* 2013;**14**(8):729–33.

Krahn LE, Hershner S, Loeding LD, et al. Quality measures for the care of patients with narcolepsy. *J Clin Sleep Med* 2015;**11**(3):335–55.

Littner MR, Kushida C, Wise M, et al. Practice parameters for clinical use of the multiple sleep latency test and the maintenance of wakefulness test. *Sleep* 2005;**28**:113–21.

Morgenthaler T, Alessi C, Friedman L, et al. Practice parameters for the use of actigraphy in the assessment of sleep and sleep disorders: an update for 2007. *Sleep* 2007;**30**(4):519–29.

Myers KA, Mrkobrada M, Simel DL. Does this patient have obstructive sleep apnea? The Rational Clinical Examination systematic review. *JAMA* 2013;**310**(7):731–41.

Pietzsch JB, Garner A, Cipriano LE, Linehan JH. An integrated health-economic analysis of diagnostic and therapeutic strategies in the treatment of moderate-to-severe obstructive sleep apnea. *Sleep* 2011;**34**(6):695–709.

Trotti LM, Goldstein CA, Harrod CG, et al. Quality measures for the care of adult patients with restless legs syndrome. *J Clin Sleep Med* 2015;**11**(3):293–310.

A complete reference list can be found online at ExpertConsult.com.

Monitoring Techniques for Evaluating Suspected Sleep-Disordered Breathing

Max Hirshkowitz; Meir Kryger

Chapter Highlights

- Polysomnography evolved from a research tool into a medical diagnostic procedure largely applied for diagnosing and treating sleep-related breathing disorders.
- Principal components of an evaluation for sleep-related breathing disorders are airflow measurement, respiratory effort assessment, and oxyhemoglobin desaturation recording. Appreciating the relationship between

sleep-disordered breathing events and sleep disruption also provides crucial information for patient care.

- Techniques are available to measure lung volume changes, blood pressure changes, and carbon dioxide; however, they are not routinely used for sleep-related breathing disorder evaluation in adults.

OVERVIEW

Soon after their discovery, sleep-related breathing disorders (SRBDs) became clinical polysomnography's dominant focus.[1] Polysomnography began as a laboratory research technique to study sleep, but with a few additional channels, it quickly found a new role as the "gold standard" modality for diagnosing obstructive sleep apnea. Penetration for assessing sleep-disordered breathing has been so complete that undoubtedly the vast majority of sleep studies performed tonight, or on any given night, will serve this function. Nonetheless, home sleep testing increasingly makes inroads as the technique to diagnose sleep-related breathing disorders.[2] With few exceptions, polysomnography and home testing devices use similar techniques. This chapter presents an overview of recording techniques and their application for evaluating breathing during sleep.

Abnormal breathing during sleep takes several different forms and arises from various underlying etiologies. It goes by many names, including sleep apnea, sleep apnea-hypopnea syndrome, sleep-disordered breathing (SBD), sleep-related breathing disorder (SRBD), periodic breathing, Cheyne-Stokes respiration (CSR), and hypoventilation (Box 5-1). However, obstructive forms of sleep apnea-hypopnea syndrome remain by far the most common SRBD. Detailed descriptions regarding SRBD-associated etiology, morbidity, and treatments appear elsewhere in this book.

The specific pathophysiologic events underlying SRBD include apnea episodes, hypopnea episodes, respiratory effort–related arousals, oxyhemoglobin desaturations, and snore arousals. As their names imply, *apnea* is cessation of breathing and *hypopnea* is shallow breathing. The face validity, that not breathing is undesirable for the health of the organism, seems obvious. However, the association between apnea and morbidity can be, but is not necessarily always, a matter of

cause and effect. Other pathophysiologic processes, especially those related to metabolic and cardiac diseases, can produce downstream effects on breathing.

Polysomnographic and home sleep testing criteria for designating a breathing event as an apneic spell have been consistently defined for decades. Cessation of breathing for 10 seconds or longer constitutes an apnea. Ten seconds was chosen because it approximates missing two breaths. The definition for hypopnea, by contrast, remains controversial. *Hypopnea* essentially means "shallow breath." The difficulty in defining hypopnea stems from several sources. The first involves measurement technique, the second from the fact that hypopneas are not intrinsically pathophysiologic, and finally from decades of usage without any standard.

Polysomnographic and home sleep testing airflow monitoring techniques mostly rely on surrogate and uncalibrated measurements (as detailed further on). Furthermore, airflow signal magnitude from thermistors, thermocouples, capnographs, and nasal pressure transducers correlates poorly with tidal volume. Consequently, operational definitions for hypopnea based on a percentage decrease of flow signal use arbitrary cutoff points (regarding which considerable disagreement continues).

Brief hypopneic intervals routinely occur during wakefulness without causing harm. For example, hypopnea accompanies speaking, and except in extraordinary circumstances, talking does not produce adverse health consequences. During sleep, however, a hypopnea may provoke significant oxyhemoglobin desaturation or a central nervous system (CNS) arousal. Thus, the consequence of the hypopnea (not the hypopnea itself) conceivably may be deemed pathophysiologic. Accordingly, prerequisites for designating sleep hypopnea as abnormal involve (1) accurately measuring physiologic consequences, (2) determining at what point these consequences reach significance, and (3) demonstrating their role in morbidity.

Box 5-1   SLEEP-RELATED BREATHING EVENTS, DISORDER CLASSIFICATIONS, AND PARAMETERS

- **Apnea** (A): The complete or near-complete cessation of breathing for 10 seconds or longer in an adult.
- **Oxyhemoglobin desaturation event** (ODE): A decrease in blood oxygen saturation. Usually, the magnitude must be 3% or greater to distinguish it from signal noise.
- **Hypopnea** (H): A reduction in (but not cessation of) ventilation. To be clinically significant, the hypopnea must be associated with an oxyhemoglobin desaturation event or a CNS arousal.
- **Desaturating hypopnea** (DH): A hypopnea with oxyhemoglobin desaturation of 4% or greater (also known as a "Medicare hypopnea").
- **Respiratory effort–related arousal** (RERA): A CNS arousal terminating obstructive breathing events that do not meet the criteria for apnea or hypopnea.
- **Obstructive apnea** or **hypopnea** episode (OA or OH): Breathing event caused by upper airway obstruction or reduced upper airway patency.
- **Central apnea** or **hypopnea** episode (CA or CH): Breathing event caused by absent or reduced respiratory effort (i.e., decreased output to inspiratory muscles from CNS respiratory control centers).
- **Mixed apnea** or **hypopnea** episode (MA or MH): Breathing event with both obstructive and central features. Many laboratories assign mixed events to the obstructive category.
- **Periodic breathing** (PB): A regularly repeating pattern in which normal or increased ventilation alternates with decreased or absent ventilation.
- **Central sleep apnea syndromes** (CSASs): These syndromes include primary central sleep apnea, Cheyne-Stokes breathing pattern, high-altitude periodic breathing, central sleep apnea due to medical conditions other than Cheyne-Stokes, and central sleep apnea due to drug or substance use/abuse.*
- **Obstructive sleep apnea syndromes** (OSASs): These syndromes include obstructive sleep apnea and obesity-hypoventilation syndrome (see Sleep-Related Hypoventilation Syndromes[†]). Primary snoring is a normal variant of an obstructive airway process.*

*Opiate and other sedatives are known to depress respiration by blunting respiratory drive.
[†]ICSD-2 diagnostic classification.
CNS, Central nervous system.

Unfortunately, measurement and morbidity determination issues have remained unresolved for many decades. Many operational definitions for hypopnea* have appeared in published clinical and research literature. Emergence of differing criteria for percentage airflow decrease and oxyhemoglobin decrease and inclusion versus exclusion of CNS arousal as part of the definition seriously complicated matters. Definitional criteria set forth in a standardization attempt sponsored by the American Academy of Sleep Medicine, often referred to as the "Chicago Criteria," were adopted for research but not for clinical use.[3]

Subsequently on April 1, 2002, like it or not, the Centers for Medicare and Medicaid Services (CMS) defined a

*At last count, this author (MH) is aware of more than 15 different definitions for hypopnea.

hypopnea as "an abnormal respiratory event lasting as least 10 s with at least a 30% reduction in thoracoabdominal movement or airflow as compared to baseline, and with at least 4% desaturation."[4] Eliminating CNS arousal from the hypopnea criteria and requiring 4% desaturation (rather than 3%) decreased the number of scorable hypopneic spells in many patients.[5,6]

On the face of it, respiratory-related and snore-related arousals certainly seem irrefutably abnormal (because they compromise sleep integrity); however, issues have arisen concerning detection reliability (and impossibility with use of many home sleep testing devices). Ignoring CNS arousal provoked by respiratory events seemed so ridiculously misguided to many clinicians that they began tabulating such events (even though they fell short of the 4% desaturation criteria). The designation *respiratory effort–related arousals* (RERAs) was commandeered from the Chicago Criteria even though it originally had quite different criteria.

In a major effort to standardize sleep medicine clinical practice, the AASM published *The AASM Manual for the Scoring of Sleep and Associated Events: Rules, Terminology and Technical Specifications* in 2007,[7] sometimes referred to as the *AASM Manual*. With regard to hypopnea, two definitional criteria were offered, neither of which agreed with the CMS criteria. Member centers were required to adopt and use the AASM criteria to maintain accreditation. One of the definitional criteria used a 3% oxyhemoglobin desaturation and the other included CNS arousal. These conflicting mandates and ambiguities placed American sleep specialists in an intellectual, clinical, and legal dilemma. Clinicians seeing even a single Medicare- or Medicaid-covered patient are required to use CMS criteria for all patients seen in their practice. Failure to comply with this regulation constitutes Medicare fraud. This CMS directive's intent is to prevent a two-tier medical system from developing. AASM issued clarifications of the rule in 2012, and ultimately, in 2013, AASM adopted CMS criteria[8] for scoring hypopnea.

Mitterling and colleagues examined scoring outcome using the different definitions.[9] Applying the 2012 scoring criteria produced higher apnea-plus-hypopnea indices compared with scoring based on the 2007 rules. These investigators used a sample of 100 healthy sleepers, ranging in age from 19 to 77 years.

Apnea and hypopnea episodes can be further categorized as obstructive, central, or mixed, depending on the presence or absence of respiratory effort during the entirety or some part of the breathing event. Beyond mere presence or absence, changes in the effort's magnitude can provide information concerning airway resistance. Increasing effort leading to a CNS arousal provides insight regarding pathophysiology. Therefore respiratory effort represents a crucial measure for evaluating patients with SRBD.

Sleep-disordered breathing severity can be based on a clinical dimension (e.g., sleepiness), event frequency (e.g., number of events per hour), or magnitude of the consequence (e.g., degree of oxyhemoglobin desaturation). Table 5-1 provides examples for dimensionally classifying severity of sleep-disordered breathing. General agreement is lacking on assignment of severity descriptors to indices of sleep-disordered breathing; however, two schemes are commonly used. In the first, "liberal" classification, an apnea-hypopnea index (AHI) between 5 and 15 is mild, between 15 and 30 is

Table 5-1	Clinical/Laboratory Features of Obstructive Sleep Apnea Syndrome by Severity		
Dimension	**Mild**	**Moderate**	**Severe**
Sleepiness or unintended sleep episodes	During activities requiring little attention (e.g., watching television)	During activities requiring some attention (e.g., business meeting)	During activities requiring active attention (e.g., driving)
PSG SRBD events: number per night	5–15	15–30	>30
PSG/HST SRBD events and oxyhemoglobin (SaO₂)	RDI or AHI 2–20 and/or SaO₂ nadir >85%	RDI or AHI 20–40 and/or SaO₂ Nadir 65%–85%	RDI or AHI >20 and/or SaO₂ nadir <65%

AHI, Apnea-hypopnea index; HST, home sleep test; PSG, polysomnography; RDI, respiratory disturbance index; SaO_2, arterial oxygen saturation; SRBD, sleep-related breathing disorder.

moderate, and greater than 30 is severe. In the second, "conservative" classification, an AHI between 10 and 20 is mild, between 20 and 50 is moderate, and greater than 50 is severe.[10]

MEASURING AIRFLOW

General Considerations

Most clinical techniques use qualitative surrogate measures to estimate airflow changes. Fully quantitative airflow determination requires pneumotachography or having the patient sleep in a "body box"; however, such techniques are unsuitable for routine clinical sleep studies. Although semiquantitative measures are attainable using calibrated inductance plethysmography, most clinical evaluations rely on qualitative nasal-oral thermography and nasal pressure. This approach provides adequate data and minimizes patient discomfort, reduces costs, and simplifies data acquisition. The AASM Manual recommends using a thermal sensor to identify apnea and a nasal pressure sensor to detect hypopnea.[7] However, other methods also provide reliable assessment. Airflow also can be measured qualitatively by detecting chemical differences between ambient and expired air (e.g., capnography). However, respiratory activity requires careful classification. Sometimes the patient's airway can be completely occluded during inspiration but release small puffs upon expiration (detectable by thermistor or CO_2 analyzer). Such events are erroneously categorized as hypopneas or even normal (unobstructed breathing). Figure 5-1 illustrates the problem.

Measuring Temperature

Exhaled air usually is warmer than ambient temperature. Air in the lungs is warmed by core body heat, thereby creating a temperature difference between air entering and exiting the respiratory system. Consequently, measuring temperature fluctuation at the nares and in front of the mouth provides a simple surrogate measure of airflow. Measurement is possible using several different technologies.

Thermistors are thermally sensitive variable resistors that produce voltage alterations when connected in a low-current (but constant-current) circuit. Low current minimizes the tendency for the thermistor to heat itself. Thermistors maximize sensing area while minimizing sensor size and mass. Small temperature changes can produce large resistance changes that can in turn be transduced with a bridge amplifier. Care must be taken to ensure that the thermistor remains below body temperature (i.e., it must not rest on the skin); otherwise, expired air will not be warmed, and no resistance

ERROR IN DETECTING APNEA

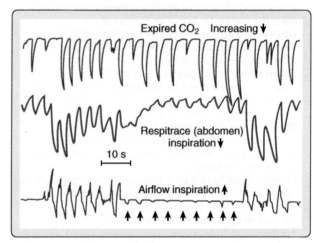

Figure 5-1 An example of the limitations of noninvasive airflow detection. Airflow is recorded simultaneously with a CO_2 analyzer and a pneumotachograph. During the obstructive apnea event, periods of expiratory airflow occur (recorded by the pneumotachograph and the CO_2 analyzer) in the absence of inspiratory flow (obvious in the pneumotachograph recording and unclear in the CO_2 recording). Without the information from the pneumotachograph, the recording from the CO_2 analyzer would be interpreted as evidence of uninterrupted inspiratory and expiratory airflow. *Top,* Airflow is detected with the CO_2 analyzer. *Middle,* Respiratory inductance plethysmograph (RIP) ("Respitrace"). *Bottom,* Airflow measured with a pneumotachograph. With each apnea-related expiratory deflection documented by the pneumotachograph (*arrows, bottom*), there is a sustained shift in the baseline of the RIP tracing. This correlation suggests an incremental decrease in functional residual capacity resulting from absence of inspirations with continued small expiratory puffs. If only the top two tracings were available, this pattern would have been mistakenly called hypoventilation or hypopnea, whereas it clearly reflects total occlusion on inspiration. (From West P, Kryger MH. Sleep and respiration: terminology and methodology. *Clin Chest Med* 1985;6:706.)

change will occur. In such a case, inspiratory activity and a respiratory pause will not be differentiable.

Thermocouples also sense temperature change but use a different approach. Different metals expand at different rates when heated. This difference can be transduced to voltage alterations displayable on polygraph systems. Like thermistors, thermocouples are placed in the airflow path in front of the nares and mouth, where expired air heats the sensor and increases its resistance. The transduced signal reflects oscillation between exhaled warm air and cooled inhaled air, thus providing a trace roughly corresponding to respiratory airflow.

Nasal Airway Pressure

During inspiration, airway pressure is negative relative to atmosphere. By contrast, expiration produces a relatively positive pressure in the airway. The resulting alteration in nasal airway pressure can provide a surrogate estimate of airflow and correlates favorably with pneumotachographically recorded signals.[11] The nasal pressure signal also offers greater sensitivity than that of nasal-oral thermography for detecting subtle flow limitations (Figure 5-2) when patients breathe through their noses.[12] Airflow limitation shows as pressure trace plateauing during inspiration. A direct current (DC) amplifier provides optimal interface; however, long time-constant alternating current (i.e., a very slowly coupled signal) can suffice. By contrast, rapid coupling can create artifact (Figure 5-3).

Expired Carbon Dioxide Sensors

CO_2 concentration in air leaving the lungs far exceeds that in ambient air. Thus measuring CO_2 in front of the nose and mouth can detect expiration. Infrared analyzers can determine the concentration. Because exhaled CO_2 reflects physiologic chemical change, it offers several advantages compared with physical changes detected by thermistor, thermocouple, and nasal pressure recordings.

In some patients, the end-of-breath CO_2 concentration provides evidence of elevated end-tidal Pco_2. The catheters sampling CO_2 typically entrain some room air, making the measured CO_2 lower than actual end-tidal Pco_2. Therefore an elevated CO_2 indicates that true Pco_2 is even higher, thereby providing a noninvasive technique (merely sampling the air stream) for detecting hypoventilation. The shape of the expired CO_2 curve can also offer useful information. When the patient's baseline expired CO_2 curve shows a clear-cut plateau, the loss of this plateau (or the curve's becoming smaller or dome-shaped) indicates a change in breathing pattern, usually a reduction in expiratory volume.

During central apnea, a low-volume catheter system set at its most rapid response time can show cardiogenic oscillations in the CO_2 signal. These oscillations result from small volume displacements caused by the beating heart.[13] These heartbeat-synchronized oscillations signify upper airway patency (Figure 5-4).

Capnography can be used in the sleep labratory to titrate noninvasive ventilation in patients with hypoventilation syndromes.[14] In infants and children with upper airway obstruction, severe hypoventilation may occur during sleep without observable apnea or hypopnea. Measuring expired CO_2 provides evidence for hypoventilation not detectable using thermistors or thermocouples.[13]

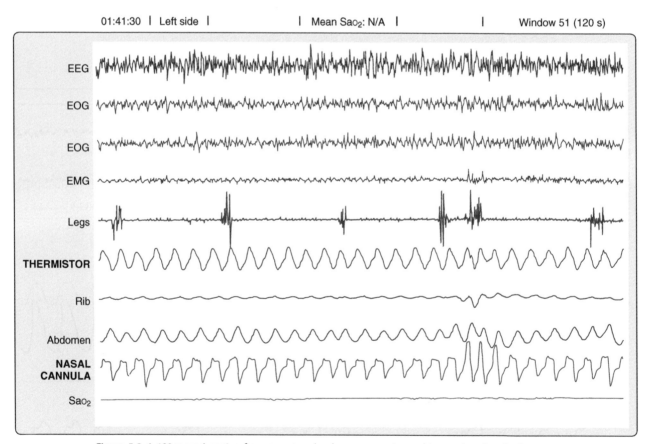

01:41:30 | Left side | | Mean Sao_2: N/A | | Window 51 (120 s)

EEG

EOG

EOG

EMG

Legs

THERMISTOR

Rib

Abdomen

NASAL CANNULA

Sao_2

Figure 5-2 A 120-second section from a nocturnal polysomnogram in a subject undergoing simultaneous recording with a conventional thermistor and with a nasal cannula used for recording pressure. Nothing in the thermistor tracing suggests a respiratory event, and subtle movement barely registers in the rib and abdominal inductance plethysmographic tracings. In the nasal cannula tracing, however, the end of one flow limitation episode and the beginning of another are easily detected. Note the plateaus (*chopped-off tops*) of the pressure traces during flow limitation. EEG, Electroencephalogram; EMG, electromyogram; EOG, electrooculogram; Sao_2, oxygen saturation in arterial blood. (Courtesy Dr. David Rappaport, New York University, New York.)

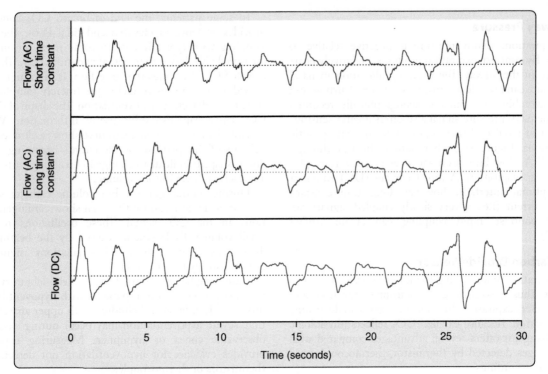

Figure 5-3 A flow limitation event recorded from the nasal cannula measuring pressure simultaneously amplified by three different amplifiers. The bottom signal is from a direct current (DC) amplifier with no filtering. The top two signals are from alternating current (AC) amplifiers with low-frequency filters, with time constants of 1.6 (*top*) and 5.3 (*middle*). The shorter time-constant filter (*top*) causes the flow signal to decay to baseline rapidly during a period of relatively constant flow (flow limitation plateau). The longer time-constant filter (*middle*) provides reasonably good reproduction of these constant flows.

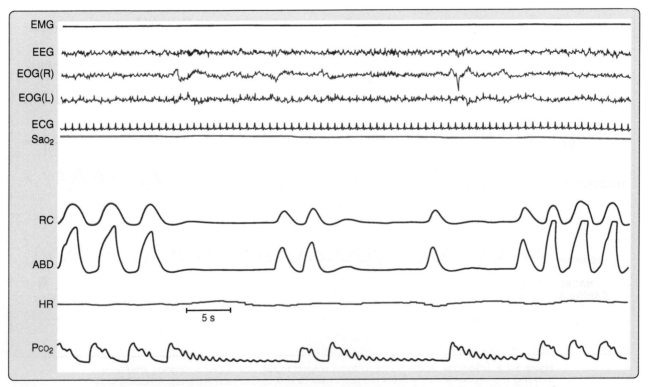

Figure 5-4 Cardiogenic oscillations in CO_2 are seen in the *bottom channel* of the recording in this example of central apnea. The presence of these oscillations, synchronous with the heartbeat, signifies that the upper airway is patent. ABD, Abdominal (movement); EEG, electroencephalogram; ECG, electrocardiogram; EMG, electromyogram; EOG, electrooculogram; HR, heart rate; RC, rib cage (movement); Pco_2, partial pressure of carbon dioxide; Sao_2, oxygen saturation in arterial blood.

Pneumotachography

Pneumotachography accurately and quantitatively measures airflow volume. The patient usually wears a face mask, and the procedure can be uncomfortable. In awake subjects, pneumotachography is known to alter breathing; it increases tidal volume and reduces respiratory rate. Some positive airway pressure machines contain an integrated pneumotachograph usable to monitor airflow during laboratory titration. Pneumotachography is seldom used for routine SRBD diagnostics.

Several types of pneumotachographs are available. These devices differ with respect to measurement technique: They use either (1) differential pressure airflow transducers, (2) ultrasonic flow meters, or (3) hot-wire anemometers. Discussion is limited here to differential pressure flow transducers because they are the most widely used. In this technique, airflow directed through a cylinder exits through a small resistive field, usually composed of small parallel tubes or a grill promoting laminar flow. The pressure drop across this resistive field is measured using a differential manometer. When flow is laminar, the relationship between the pressure differences and flow is linear. Changes in gas density, viscosity, and temperature alter the pressure-flow relationship. To prevent condensation on the resistive element requires heating, so calibration should be conducted when the pneumotachograph is heated. After correction for errors introduced by alterations in these physical factors, the flow signal is integrated to determine volume.

MEASURING RESPIRATORY EFFORT

Measuring respiratory effort provides information needed to distinguish between respiratory events of obstructive versus nonobstructive (central) etiology. Categorizing an apnea or hypopnea as obstructive, mixed, or central in origin derives from differential respiratory effort and airflow patterns. As reviewed next, several techniques are available to detect and/or measure respiratory effort, including rib cage and abdominal motion, electromyography, pleural pressure changes, movement detected by static charge sensors in or on the bed surface, movement detected by standing wave patterns in the bedroom, and digital video recording.

Rib Cage and Abdominal Motion

Currently, the most common polysomnographic technique for measuring respiratory effort involves detection and quantification of rib cage and abdominal movements. During normal breathing, the major inspiratory muscles produce rib cage expansion and a downward movement of the diaphragm. These movements cause the pressure around and in the lung to become negative (relative to atmospheric pressure). The pressure gradient between ambient air and the lung draws air through the airways into the alveoli. Thus a change in lung volume is the sum of the volume changes of the structures surrounding the lungs, the rib cage, and the abdomen.[15] Other respiratory muscles (e.g., intercostal, sternocleidomastoid) also play a role in stabilizing the thoracic cage. Some clinicians erroneously interpret the abdominal and rib cage motion changes as implying separate activities of abdominal and thoracic respiratory muscles, but this is not the case. Virtually all of the changes in abdominal and rib cage volumes (including paradoxical motion) can be explained by changes in the status of the respiratory muscles directly inserting onto the thoracic

---

> **Box 5-2 MECHANISMS UNDERLYING PARADOXICAL MOTION OF THE RIB CAGE AND ABDOMEN**
>
> **Loss of diaphragm tone.** When the diaphragm ceases to contract and becomes flaccid, it merely reacts to pressure changes around it instead of generating pressure changes. In this situation, when the other respiratory muscles contract, the rib cage is enlarged, and pleural pressure becomes negative, sucking the diaphragm into the chest. This condition results in an increase in rib cage volume and a reduction in abdominal volume.
>
> **Loss of accessory respiratory muscle tone.** When the accessory muscles lose tone, the rib cage, particularly the upper part of the rib cage, becomes unstable. When the diaphragm then contracts, the negative intrathoracic pressure causes the unstable part of the thorax to be sucked in during inspiration.
>
> **Partial upper airway obstruction.** With partial upper airway obstruction, the diaphragm must generate very strong negative pressures for inspiration to occur. As the diaphragm contracts, it both pushes out the abdomen and creates great negative intrathoracic pressure. This highly negative intrathoracic pressure can overcome the mechanisms maintaining chest wall stability (accessory muscle tone and rigidity of the cage), so that the least stable portions of the rib cage will tend to move inward with inspiration. This potential for inward movement of the rib cage is a problem mainly in the very young, in whom the rib cage is quite pliable.

---

cage. Paradoxical motion of the rib cage and abdomen can result from several changes, including loss of tone of the diaphragm, loss of tone of the other respiratory muscles, and upper airway obstruction (complete or partial). The mechanisms underlying this asynchronous motion of rib cage and abdomen are described in Box 5-2. Regardless of the pattern or its underlying mechanism, rib cage and abdominal movement reflect effort to breathe.

At a minimum, a single uncalibrated abdominal movement sensor can *detect* respiratory effort. Respiratory effort during airflow cessation usually signifies airway obstruction. Common approaches for *measuring* rib cage and abdominal movement use (1) strain gauges, (2) inductance plethysmography, and (3) piezoelectric transducers.

Strain gauges are sealed elastic tubes filled with conductive material through which an electric current is passed. When length is constant, current and resistance are constant. Stretching the strain gauge lengthens and narrows the cross-sectional area of the fixed-volume conductor. This deformation produces a proportional increase in electrical resistance. Current varies inversely in relation to the length of the gauge, thereby becoming an index of gauge length. A Whetstone bridge amplifier transduces this change to voltage for continuous display showing rib cage or abdominal expansion (depending on placement).

Inductance plethysmography electronically measures changes in the cross-sectional area of the rib cage and abdominal compartments by determining changes in inductance. Inductance is a property of electrical conductors characterized by the opposition to a change of current flow in the conductor.

Transducers are placed around the rib cage and abdomen—the physiologic equivalent of conductors. Each transducer consists of an insulated wire sewn into the shape of a horizontally oriented sinusoid and onto an elasticized band.

Piezoelectric transducers are used in yet another method of detecting movement. These sensors can be placed on the rib cage and abdomen and are sensitive to changes in length. When a piezoelectric crystal is squeezed, an electrical potential appears across its sides. The crystals can be arranged (usually as part of a belt) so that movement can be detected (see next).

Combined Sensors

Thermocouples, thermistors, and strain gauges are fairly old technologies. More recently, new materials such as polyvinylidene fluoride film have been introduced into the sleep laboratory. Such film has the interesting property of converting heat and mechanical energy into electrical energy that can be measured. Polyvinylidene fluoride films have both piezoelectric (responding to mechanical changes) and pyroelectric (responding to thermal changes) properties. The output from these films can be configured to measure airflow[16] (pressure and temperature), snoring[17] (pressure waveforms), and changes in length caused by abdomen and rib cage movement.[18-20]

Respiratory Muscle Electromyography

Recording intercostal muscle activity on the electromyogram (EMG) is one of the oldest polysomnographic techniques for detecting respiratory effort (Figure 5-5). These uncalibrated recordings are made using standard surface electrodes placed in pairs in the intercostal spaces on the right anterior chest. Obtaining an optimal signal requires practice, patience, and skill; recordings are prone to artifact, especially artifact from the electrocardiogram (ECG). Intercostal EMG activity, when recorded properly, can be extremely valuable for differentiating among central, obstructive, and mixed sleep-disordered breathing events. Furthermore, although signals are not calibrated, cascading increases in respiratory effort are readily apparent from recordings.

Pleural Pressure Changes

Some sleep centers use esophageal pressure to index inspiratory effort. In our experience, most patients undergoing all-night polysomnography find esophageal balloons unacceptable. However, the thin water-tip or catheter-tip piezoelectric transducers are better tolerated. Esophageal pressure measurements help verify central apnea or hypopnea episodes with a high degree of certainty. This technique also can detect very subtle respiratory events. However in subtle cases, a repeat

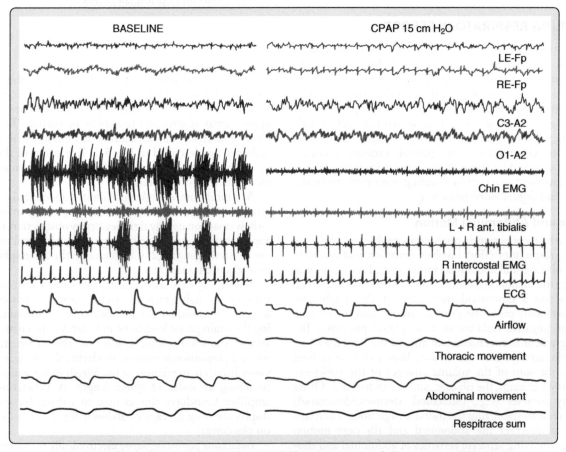

Figure 5-5 Surface respiratory (R intercostal) muscle EMG in sleep apnea. *Left,* The respiratory EMG signal is dramatically increased. *Right,* This signal is reduced on nasal continuous positive airway pressure (CPAP). A2, Right mastoid reference; C3, left central EEG; ECG, electrocardiogram; EEG, electroencephalogram; EMG, electromyogram; LE-fp, left eye referenced to frontal pole; L + R, linked left and right; O1, right occipital EEG; RE-fp, right eye referenced to frontal pole. (Courtesy Dr. J. Catesby Ware, Eastern Virginia Medical School, Norfolk, Virginia.)

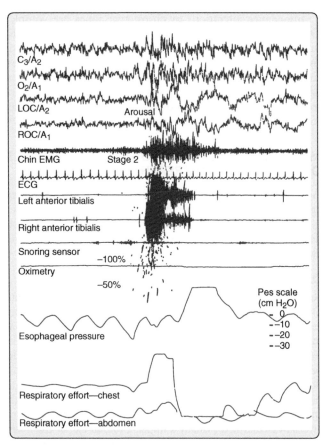

Figure 5-6 Esophageal pressure in the upper airway resistance syndrome. The esophageal pressure (Pes) swing was greatest just before the arousal. C3/A2, Left central EEG referenced to right mastoid; ECG, electrocardiogram; EMG, electromyogram; LOC, left outer canthus; O_2/A_1, right occipital lobe EEG referenced to left mastoid; ROC, right outer canthus. (From Butkov N. *Atlas of clinical polysomnography*. Ashland [Ore.]: Synapse Media; 1996, p. 224.)

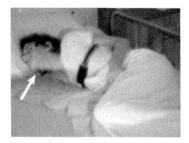

Figure 5-7 Synchronized digital video can be extremely helpful, as in this example in which a child with retrognathia slept with his neck arched and his mandible thrust forward (*arrow*). This sleep posture resulted in an unoccluded upper airway. The conventional polysomnography recording missed that a significant sleep breathing problem was present. (From Banno K, Kryger MH. Use of polysomnography with synchronized digital video recording to diagnose pediatric sleep breathing disorders. *CMAJ* 2005;173:28–30.)

polysomnogram may be preferable to using an esophageal catheter.[21]

In patients with *upper airway resistance syndrome*, the classic findings include progressively more negative pleural pressure until occurrence of a CNS arousal. The arousal is sometimes associated with an audible snort (Figure 5-6). After arousal, pleural pressure swings temporarily decrease until the next cycle begins, upon which pressure swings increase until another arousal occurs. Sometimes the CNS activation falls short of AASM duration criteria for arousal. However, the AASM's 3-second rule was established for determining reliability of spontaneous arousals using visual scoring.[22,23] On the electroencephalogram (EEG), signal changes of shorter duration are conceptually thought to represent CNS arousals, as are spectral analysis indices of alpha power loading, even when it is difficult to see on the raw data tracing.

Movement Detected by Static Charge and Pressure Sensors

The static charge–sensitive bed technology has been evaluated in sleep disorders.[24] The transducer is embedded within a thin mattress that responds to the slightest movement. Output from the bed is sensitive enough to detect heartbeat as a ballistocardiogram. Respiratory signal amplitude differs with body position changes; however, output is otherwise stable.

A similar but newer technology uses piezoelectric sensors embedded in a strip placed perpendicular to the sleeper's body. Changes in pressure resulting from breathing movement and heartbeat can be analyzed.[25]

Movement Detected by Wave Technologies

Several systems approach movement detection using microwaves, radar, and/or changes in standing wave patterns in the bedroom. One approach directs a beam at the bed surface and analyzes the returning signal to evaluate the sleeper's upper body movement. In one such system, laser radiation can be used. Microwave and other radar-like technologies also can be applied. Additionally, a series of sensors could be used to monitor movement. Application of some of these emerging technologies to sleep medicine for evaluating SRBD is an important aspect of ongoing developments in the field.

Polysomnography-Synchronized Digital Video

Digital video is now a common feature of computerized polysomnography. Although recordings are widely used to evaluate parasomnias and seizures, they can be helpful in assessing SRBD. When the recording is properly synchronized with polysomnography, ambiguous and difficult-to-interpret tracings often become obvious. For example, it is easy to recognize a small dip in arterial oxygen saturation (Sao_2) as a significant sleep-disordered breathing event when it is followed by oxygen resaturation after an audible snort, a repetitive moving forward of the jaw, an arching of the neck, or a closing of a gaping mouth. Video is especially helpful in children, whose polysomnographic recordings may be difficult to interpret (Figure 5-7). An Sao_2 dip, without the other visual information, is quite likely to be missed, ignored, or dismissed as artifact. Video recordings are particularly useful in thin persons, who might not experience oxygen desaturation with their abnormal respiratory events. Furthermore, showing the sleep study video to patients can be very effective for promoting understanding of the problem and an appreciation of its severity.

MEASURING CHANGES IN LUNG VOLUME

Several methods can estimate tidal volume. These measures provide semiquantitative data concerning presumed airflow while also documenting respiratory effort. Calibration is crucial in attempting to use these devices to gauge ventilation. Postcalibration movements, changes in body position, and shifting in placement of the recording device can introduce error. In sleep laboratories, strain gauges, inductance plethysmography, and impedance pneumography are sometimes used to measure volume changes. Other techniques include magnetometry, body plethysmography, canopy with neck seal, the barometric method, and pneumotachography; however, these are seldom used in a clinical setting.

Strain Gauges, Inductance Plethysmography, and Piezoelectric Transducers

In principle, length-sensitive devices can be used qualitatively to detect breathing abnormalities. If properly calibrated, these devices can be used quantitatively to measure dynamic volume changes.[26] Normally, the enlargement of the thorax and the outward movement of the abdominal wall occur together; that is, they are in phase. For a given change in lung volume, then, it is possible to quantify a change in rib cage volume and abdominal volume. For a given breath, the relative contributions of the rib cage and abdominal compartments also can be determined.

To quantify actual volume changes, the transducers must be calibrated against an independent volume-measuring system. In practice, two length-measuring devices are required for measuring changes in lung volume: one for the rib cage and one for the abdomen. The rib cage device is placed at the level of the axilla, and the abdominal device is placed just superior to the iliac crest. If it is assumed that the fractional contributions of the abdomen and the rib cage are constant, then changes in lung volume can be measured by calibrating transducers sensitive to rib cage and abdominal displacement. Once the transducers are calibrated, the sum of the rib cage and abdominal excursions will describe volume changes.

Unfortunately, the relative rib cage and abdominal contributions can change with posture and muscle tone occurring in sleep. Movement-related device migration from its original site and device deformability also must be considered. Such factors adversely affect calibration accuracy and stability. Nonetheless, calibrated inductance plethysmography appears to be sensitive enough to detect upper airway resistance syndrome events.[27]

Impedance Pneumography

Impedance defines the combined effects of two previously discussed properties of an electrical conductor: *resistance* and *inductance*. In physical terms, when impedance pneumography is used, the conductor is the thorax. Impedance is measured by applying a small current across the thorax using a pair of electrodes placed at the site of maximal thoracic excursion.

Transthoracic impedance changes reflect variations in the amount of conductive materials (liquids, including interstitial fluid, blood and lymph, and tissue) and nonconductive material (air) between the electrodes. The conductive and nonconductive materials affect the total impedance differently. Increased air in the lung increases impedance, and increased fluid in the thorax decreases impedance. A recording of the volume of air exchanged and the total of impedance changes can allow the differentiation between air-related and fluid-related changes in impedance. If total impedance is recorded in a single channel, changes related to air volume and fluid are measured.

Impedance alterations in obstructive apnea are complex. During apnea, lung volume decreases, whereas the negative intrathoracic pressure most likely temporarily pools blood in the pulmonary circulation. For these reasons, a precise measurement of respiratory volume and pattern may not be possible. Nonetheless, rate-adapting cardiac pacemakers using transthoracic impedance to drive ventilation have been used to screen for obstructive sleep apnea.[28]

MEASURING THE PHYSIOLOGIC CONSEQUENCES OF SLEEP-RELATED BREATHING DISORDERS

As previously mentioned, some SRBD events (e.g., hypopnea) are not intrinsically pathophysiologic; however, their consequences are. SRBD event consequences include oxyhemoglobin desaturations, carbon dioxide elevations, blood pressure changes, electrocardiographic abnormalities, and CNS arousals.

Oxygen and Carbon Dioxide Alterations

Routine clinical sleep evaluations require noninvasive, continuous, rapidly sampled measures to determine blood oxygen concentration. Thus directly measuring blood oxygen with an indwelling arterial catheter is ruled out on all counts. Pulse oximetry, however, serves the need well; consequently, it has become the standard technique for recording oxyhemoglobin desaturations during sleep. Pulse oximeters usually determine Sao_2 spectrophotoelectrically using a two-wavelength light transmitter and a receiver placed on either side of a pulsating arterial vascular bed (usually a finger, a toe, an ear, or the nose). Alternatively, in reflectance pulse oximetry, the light transmitter and the receiver are on the same surface. The light transmitted into the vascular bed is scattered, absorbed, and reflected. The amplitude of light detected in particular spectra by the receiver depends on the magnitude of the change in arterial pulse, the wavelengths transmitted through the arterial vascular bed, and the oxygen saturation of arterial hemoglobin (deoxygenated blood is bluer). These devices are sensitive only to pulsating tissues; consequently, venous blood, connective tissue, skin pigment, and bone theoretically do not hamper determination of Sao_2. Accurate measurement, however, requires a minimal pulse amplitude. Dyshemoglobinemias can cause problems.

Correct alignment of the light transmitter and receiver is critical to ensure measurement accuracy. If the sensor is applied to a digit, that digit must be immobilized. Significant bending of the digit can compromise detection of pulsatile flow and invalidate results. Although all pulse oximeters are based on similar technology, response characteristics differ both across manufacturers and even within a specific manufacturer's product line.[29] Sensor placement and device programming are crucial technical factors in obtaining optimal results. Reflectance oximeters also must contend with weaker pulse signals, because much less light is reflected back to the sensor. Differences in response characteristics and effect of sensor location cannot be overemphasized (Figure 5-8), because some oximeters appear to be completely insensitive to hypoxemia episodes clearly detected by other devices (Figure 5-9). Such devices can produce false-negative SRBD test outcomes.

A review of specific oximeters would be beyond the scope of this chapter; nonetheless, generalizations about (1) sensor location, (2) instrument filtering and sampling rates, and (3) potential pitfalls are worth noting here.

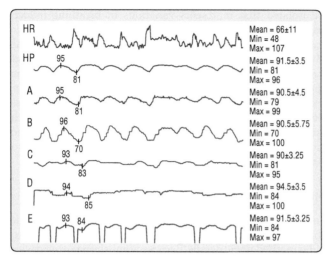

Figure 5-8 Heart rate (HR) and arterial oxygen saturation (SaO₂) during a 5-minute period in a patient with sleep apnea. The *top two traces* are for the HR monitor and a Hewlett Packard (HP) oximeter; A to E are traces for five different pulse oximeters. The scales for the six oximeters are identical. The *numbers* on the tracings represent the instantaneous SaO₂ measured during the peak and trough of an apneic episode. The data listed to the *right* of the figure are the mean, standard deviation, and minimum and maximum values for HR and SaO₂ for the six oximeters. Note that oximeters C and D do not track SaO₂, and that the recording for oximeter E has numerous artifacts.

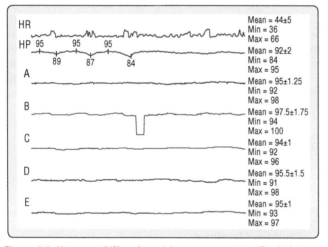

Figure 5-9 Heart rate (HR) and arterial oxygen saturation (SaO₂) during a 5-minute period in a patient with sleep apnea and bradycardia. Tracings are taken from six oximeters, as described in Figure 5-8. In this example, three apneic episodes are missed entirely by all of the pulse oximeters. This patient's problem would have gone completely undetected by pulse oximetry screening. HP, Hewlett Packard (oximeter).

Sensor Location

In our experience, the preferred sensor location in adults is the earlobe. Poor perfusion can be enhanced by applying a trace amount of vasodilator (e.g., nonylic acid vanillylamide plus nicotinic acid—Finalgon ointment [Boehringer Ingelheim, Ridgefield, Conn.]). Technicians must take care to avoid contact of the perfusion-enhancing agent with their own or the subject's eyes, because it is a powerful cutaneous vasodilator. When the ear site is not usable, reflectance pulse oximeter sensors placed on the forehead or another well-perfused surface will suffice. Recording from the ear also reduces circulator delay (compared with the finger). This advantage

becomes especially important for associating a respiratory event with its subsequent oxyhemoglobin desaturation in patients with congestive heart failure.

Instrument Filtering and Sampling Rate

Most pulse oximeters filter the signal, and some filter algorithms use the heart rate. The degree of filtering is inversely related to heart rate; brief, mild hypoxemic episodes may therefore be missed during periods of very low heart rate, because they are filtered more strongly. During polysomnographic recording, filtering should be minimized (i.e., by setting the oximeter to the fastest response or the highest sampling rate, or both) to reduce missing transient oxyhemoglobin desaturation events.

Potential Problems

Because pulse oximeters use two wavelengths of light to estimate SaO₂, they cannot distinguish three or more hemoglobin species. In the presence of carboxyhemoglobin (as in heavy smokers, in whom carboxyhemoglobin levels can reach 10% to 20%), SaO₂ is overestimated.[30] In the presence of a rising methemoglobin concentration, oximetry-determined SaO₂ will plateau at approximately 85%, regardless of whether true saturation is much higher or lower.[31] Because light is transmitted through tissue, pigment in the skin can degrade oximeter performance, producing incorrect "probe-off" or "perfusion-low" error reports.[32] Some finger-clip devices can produce pressure-related injuries when worn for an entire night.

Partial pressure of arterial oxygen (PaO₂) estimated from the skin's surface depends on oxygen flux through the skin, local oxygen consumption, and the skin's diffusion barrier.[33] This measurement technique is most commonly used in neonates, whose skin is thin. Accurate measurement of transcutaneous PO₂ (PO₂tc) requires maximal dilation of the local vasculature in the upper dermis. This is achieved by heating (to 43°C); however, heating shifts the oxyhemoglobin dissociation curve to the right, increases the resistance of the skin stratum corneum to oxygen permeation, increases the metabolic rate of the dermal tissue, and increases the rate of cutaneous blood flow. The shift in the oxyhemoglobin dissociation curve and the increase in metabolic rate effectively cancel each other out, leaving permeability and flow as the dependent factors in correlating PO₂tc and PaO₂. An important advantage of heating is that the amount of blood present is maximal, and PO₂tc is therefore unaffected by small changes in blood supply to the tissue.

The PO₂tc may be misinterpreted when the state of blood flow is unknown. When flow and PaO₂ are adequate, PO₂tc reflects PaO₂. Under conditions of compromised flow and adequate PaO₂, PO₂tc will change with flow. If SaO₂ and flow are compromised, PO₂tc tracks oxygen delivery. Transcutaneous measurement accuracy also depends on correct sensor application. To convert PO₂tc measurements to PaO₂ values precisely, a calibration curve for each subject is required, so this technique is too labor-intensive for use in routine clinical practice. In most laboratories, PO₂tc serves to track, in relative terms, arterial oxygenation status. Device responsiveness is too slow for tracking rapid blood gas changes associated with brief SRBD events (less than 30 seconds), because oxygen diffuses slowly across the skin. The conditions governing transcutaneous PCO₂ measurement are remarkably similar to those described for PaO₂. Although transcutaneous blood gas determinations are of greatest value in neonates and young children, Pco₂tc is useful for assessing hypoventilation in adults.

Central Nervous System Arousals and Awakenings

Awakenings and CNS arousals provide critical information concerning sleep disturbance and fragmentations. Standardized scoring derives from electroencephalographic activity, preferably recorded from occipital sites. CNS arousals often take the form of bursts of alpha (7 to 13 Hz) activity, and the term *EEG speeding* is sometimes used to describe the event. When scored visually, a 3- to 15-second burst of alpha activity in non–rapid eye movement (NREM) sleep is considered an arousal. During rapid eye movement (REM) sleep, when alpha bursts can be an ongoing part of background activity, the alpha intrusion must be accompanied by increased muscle tone. In any sleep stage, a burst exceeding 15 seconds in duration is scored as an awakening.

The CNS arousal represents a clinically significant sleep parameter because it is associated with (in cross-sectional studies) and provokes (in intervention studies) tiredness, fatigue, and sleepiness. As a pathophysiologic consequence of obstructive sleep apnea, the arousal is thought to result from increased respiratory effort (and accompanying increase in autonomic nervous system sympathetic activation) triggered by increased airway resistance. Presumably, the CNS arousal terminates the SRBD event, because the arousal returns ventilation to voluntary control. As a result, the airway can be dilated and breathing resumes. However, some controversy exists about resumption of breathing after an obstructive event without CNS arousal and about the presence of arousals at the termination of central events.

Blood Pressure Changes

Clinical laboratories do not routinely record sleep-related blood pressure. Nonetheless, many pulse oximeters also can track pulse pressure (a magnitude index of pulsation occurring at the oximetry sensor site). In addition, pulse transit times (PTTs) have been used to indirectly estimate blood pressure.[34] PPT represents the time interval from heartbeat (ECG R wave) to its pulse recorded in the periphery. Negative pleural pressure provokes a blood pressure drop and in so doing lengthens PTT. The progressive increase in pleural pressure during obstructive apnea correlates with rising oscillations in PTT amplitude. During central apnea, this does not occur. Thus it has been suggested that PTT might provide an opportunistic estimate of inspiratory effort and thereby provide a means to differentiate obstructive from central apnea.[35]

Automatic self-inflating arm-cuff sphygmomanometers have long been available but are problematic for routine clinical use because they disturb sleep. By contrast, miniature finger cuff systems disturb sleep much less. Devices obtaining data in alternating fashion from adjacent fingers reduce finger injury risk, and some systems automatically perform hydrostatic correction when arm movement occurs. Finger flexion artifacts, however, remain a problem.

Cardiopulmonary Coupling

Cardiopulmonary coupling uses a single-channel ECG recording to extract signal features modulated by breathing.[36] Respiration induces small alterations in heart rate and amplitude variations in R-wave amplitude. Using computerized frequency domain analysis, a high-frequency component can be isolated that represents variations in breathing-induced vagal sinus pressure heart rate. A low-frequency component can be extracted that provides data about interbreath intervals. By examining a weighted composite of these data (increased variability and the envelope of amplitude change), time-domain periods (usually 2 to 10 minutes) with breathing pauses can be discerned by examining coherence and cross-power spectrums. In general, normal breathing loads high-frequency bands, and SRBD events mass in low-frequency troughs. Few clinical sleep laboratories employ cardiopulmonary coupling analysis.

HOME SLEEP TESTING

In addition to standard attended polysomnography, guidelines for home sleep testing have been published.[37] Chapter 6 provides methodologic details. Because home sleep testing devices are less sensitive than laboratory polysomnography, the home test can rule in, but not rule out, SRBD.

To succeed diagnostically and economically, home sleep testing requires proper patient selection, appropriate portable recorder application, study interpretation by a qualified sleep specialist, readily available access to laboratory polysomnography when needed (as after a negative result on home sleep testing, or to investigate continuing problems despite treatment), and systematic follow-up assessments. Many health care coverage plans (including those administered by the Centers for Medicare and Medicaid Services) reimburse home sleep testing for diagnosing sleep apnea. Unattended studies are more prone to data loss as a consequence of uncorrected technical failures (e.g., electrode detachment) and patient tampering. Consequently, only patients with a high clinical suspicion for SRBD should be referred for HST.

CLINICAL PEARLS

- Detecting sleep-related breathing events and classifying each as obstructive, central, or mixed require measures of airflow, respiratory effort, and oxyhemoglobin saturation.
- Information about sleep-disturbing effects of SRBD events provides better sensitivity for the diagnosis of sleep-disordered breathing.
- Standardized guidelines developed by the AASM were developed to advance clinical practice and should not be construed as an impediment to advancing scientific inquiry.

SUMMARY

Evaluating patients with SRBDs is the most common application of laboratory and home sleep studies. Over the past four decades, some of the more frequently used procedures have evolved and become commonplace in clinical sleep laboratories. The American Academy of Sleep Medicine also published guidelines and a standards manual. Standard assessment for breathing disorders during sleep includes measures of airflow, respiratory effort, and oxyhemoglobin desaturation. Laboratory evaluation also includes sleep disturbance assessment. In this chapter we describe techniques to assess these and other, related physiologic activities. The underlying mechanism, advantages, and problems are also discussed.

Selected Readings

Berry RB, Brooks R, Gamaldo CE, et al; for the American Academy of Sleep Medicine. *The AASM Manual for the Scoring of Sleep and Associated Events: Rules, Terminology and Technical Specifications*, Version 2.3. Darien (Ill.): American Academy of Sleep Medicine; 2016 <www.aasmnet.org>.

Iber C, Ancoli-Israel S, Chesson A, Quan SF. *The AASM manual for the scoring of sleep and associated events: rules, terminology and technical specifications.* Westchester (Ill.): American Academy of Sleep Medicine; 2007.

Kushida CA, Littner MR, Morgenthaler T, et al. Practice parameters for the indications for polysomnography and related procedures: an update for 2005. *Sleep* 2005;**28**(4):499–521.

Mitterling T, Högl B, Schönwald SV, et al. Sleep and respiration in 100 healthy Caucasian sleepers—a polysomnographic study according to American Academy of Sleep Medicine standards. *Sleep* 2015;**38**(6): 867–75.

Zeidler MR, Santiago V, Dzierzewski JM, et al. Predictors of Obstructive Sleep Apnea on Polysomnography after a Technically Inadequate or Normal Home Sleep Test. *J Clin Sleep Med* 2015;**11**(11):1313–18.

A complete reference list can be found online at ExpertConsult.com.

Home Sleep Testing

Thomas Penzel

Chapter Highlights

- Home sleep testing for diagnosing sleep-disordered breathing outperforms attended cardiorespiratory polysomnography. Diagnostic sensitivity and specificity are high enough for effective clinical application.
- Home sleep testing protocols have been established in terms of required signals. Monitoring usually includes respiratory effort and airflow, oxygen saturation, and body position/activity. Visual scoring is a necessary component. Clinical symptom assessment and

home sleep testing should be combined to achieve high sensitivity and reliability.
- New developments are targeting use of fewer signals for diagnosing sleep-disordered breathing. Different systems achieve this with variable success. An economic benefit can be realized if sleep-disordered breathing can be diagnosed or managed using single-channel devices versus four- to six-channel devices, and such approaches currently are under investigation.

OVERVIEW AND BACKGROUND

Home sleep testing refers to portable monitoring for diagnosing sleep-disordered breathing. The term was introduced in the past decade. In 2014, a National Library of Medicine (NLM) PubMed database search for "home sleep testing" in all fields found 19 publications. The reference method for the diagnosis of sleep-disordered breathing is cardiorespiratory polysomnography. The recording technology and the scoring criteria used in home sleep testing are derived from this modality. Many studies on individual systems and a considerable number of evidence-based reviews indicate that home sleep testing for sleep-disordered breathing can be as specific and as reliable as sleep laboratory–based polysomnography recordings[1-3] in properly referred patients. Finally, adequate data are available to validate home sleep testing's use clinically, although it does have certain limitations.[4] A workshop consensus report presented the view of the participating medical societies (American Thoracic Society, American Academy of Sleep Medicine, American College of Chest Physicians, European Respiratory Society) on the use of this diagnostic procedure and provides directions for further research.[5] A clinical practice guideline from the American College of Physicians now recommends portable sleep monitors for diagnostic testing in patients suspected of having obstructive sleep apnea without serious comorbidity, and as an alternative to polysomnography when polysomnography is not available.[6] In Europe, home sleep testing has been widely used for several decades to diagnose sleep-disordered breathing.[7]

With respect to the guidelines and recommendations on home sleep testing, which are partially evidence-based, it is essential to consider the basis of the underlying studies used for evidence evaluation. The clinical studies evaluated for the guidelines usually are those performed by sleep centers on their patients, which correspond with clinical populations available in sleep centers.[8,9] Clinical populations differ from the general population in that the patients have been referred for evaluation for suspected sleep disorders. This selection leads to a high pretest probability for sleep disorders and for sleep apnea in particular.[1,10] Factors associated with this increased pretest probability include various physical examination measures and complaints reported by the patient or the bed partner, as follows:

- Loud and irregular snoring
- Observed or reported nocturnal cessation of breathing
- Excessive daytime sleepiness
- Nonspecific mental problems such as fatigue, low performance, or cognitive impairment
- Movements during sleep
- Morning dizziness, general headache, dry mouth
- Impaired sexual function
- Obesity
- Arterial hypertension and cardiac arrhythmias

A grading of the pretest probability factors could be useful to determine which patients may be more likely to suffer from sleep apnea or even from more severe sleep breathing disorder. This potential application has not been investigated in clinical practice.[11] Instead, clinicians commonly use a combination of validated questionnaires in conjunction with home sleep testing to confirm the suspected diagnosis.[12]

As revealed in a literature search, published reports are of several different types. Some papers describe new devices and comparative studies of such innovations with polysomnography. Reviews of data on existing devices are scarce. However, a good systematic review of data on existing systems that also provides categories for evaluation has been presented.[4] These categories are sleep, cardiovascular, oxygen saturation, position, effort of respiration, and respiratory flow—the SCOPER acronym. Sensors and systems are evaluated using these categories. A majority of published studies, however, focus on the role of home sleep testing in sleep apnea diagnosis. Some reports in the literature concentrate on general management of patients with sleep apnea, whereas other reports focus on home sleep testing. Presented next is a short technical overview of available systems, followed by a discussion of home sleep testing with respect to requirements and special considerations.

HOME SLEEP TESTING WITH FOUR- TO SIX-CHANNEL SYSTEMS FOR DIAGNOSING SLEEP-DISORDERED BREATHING

Systems for diagnosing sleep-disordered breathing generally fall into one of four classifications defined in an American Sleep Disorders Association (ASDA) standard of practice guideline.[13]

- level I: attended cardiorespiratory polysomnography with at least 7 signals
- level II: cardiorespiratory polysomnography at home with at least 7 signals, unattended
- level III: unattended portable sleep apnea testing with at least 4 signals including airflow, respiratory effort, oxygen saturation, ECG, or heart rate or pulse rate
- level IV: unattended one or two signal recording, such as actigraphy or oximetry

Most diagnostic systems for home sleep testing attain level III device status and record four to six physiologic signals but do not record the electroencephalogram (EEG). Evidence-based home sleep testing reviews commissioned by health technology assessment agencies[3] revealed limited reliability. Up to 17% false-negative and between 2% and 31% false-positive findings of sleep apnea have been reported. These high error rates compared with those for polysomnography are considered unacceptable, and Ross and colleagues[3] concluded that portable monitoring of sleep apnea is not recommended. A few years later, studies with revised recording systems showed substantial improvement.[9,14] If systems incorporate a thoughtful selection of physiologic measures, have good signal acquisition, and use good signal processing technique, the number of false-positive diagnoses declines considerably.[1] When studies sampling from the general population are compared with studies using clinical populations, the importance of a high pretest probability becomes clear. A high pretest probability reduces the number of false-positive diagnoses. Altogether, the specificity increases enough to permit a conclusion that home sleep testing for sleep apnea can be recommended under certain conditions[4,6]:

1. Systems should be used only by certified sleep physicians based in certified sleep centers. This recommendation attempts to improve quality control and quality assurance. An interview of the patient and assessment of complaints should be conducted before home sleep testing is performed. This screening increases the pretest probability as explained earlier.
2. Home sleep testing for obstructive sleep apnea is recommended when no other comorbid pulmonary, cardiovascular, mental, neurologic, and neuromuscular disorder, or heart failure or another sleep disorder, is present. Other sleep disorders to rule out include central sleep apnea, periodic limb movement disorder, insomnia, circadian sleep-wake disorders, and narcolepsy.
3. In the earlier published studies, home sleep testing systems could not distinguish between central and obstructive sleep apnea events.

4. Home sleep testing for diagnosing sleep apnea needs to record oronasal airflow (using a thermistor or nasal pressure sensor); respiratory effort (using inductive plethysmography); oxygen saturation (with a short averaging period over few [3 to 6] pulses; pulse or heart rate; and body position.
5. Evaluation of the recordings should incorporate visual scoring of respiratory events using the same rules specified for polysomnography.[15,16] Editing of recorded events is necessary to remove artifacts occurring during the recording period. Furthermore, the visual scoring should be performed by trained personnel.
6. The technical specifications and sampling rates for the digital recording should be the same as specified in the evidence-based recommendation for cardiorespiratory polysomnography.[16]

Today, many devices fulfill the requirements necessary to meet level III device criteria. The home sleep testing devices all include pulse oximetry technology to record oxygen saturation and pulse rate. Many systems record oronasal airflow, which reflects intranasal pressure. Few systems still use thermistors for flow recording. Most devices record respiratory effort using either piezo sensors or respiratory inductive plethysmography. Some devices use one belt for rib cage movements, whereas others use two belts (for recording abdominal movements as well). Most systems record body position to identify positional apnea. Very few systems record the raw electrocardiogram (ECG), but many report heart rate derived by other means. A number of systems offer specific options to record signals in sleep apnea patients under therapy. The options are the recording of CPAP mask pressure in addition or as an alternative to other airflow signals. The signal will be split into a CPAP pressure reading, corresponding to set pressure level and to a respiratory flow reading which may be observed superposed to the CPAP pressure set. This may vary depending on pressure mode selection (e.g., bilevel or flex modes). This option is an important feature for using home sleep testing for treatment follow-up studies. Some systems allow an option for recording additional electromyogram (EMG) tibialis activity to detect leg movements; thus far, however, no systematic studies on this option's utility have been conducted.

It remains an open question whether home sleep testing can reliably diagnose periodic limb movement disorder. Similarly, a few systems can add electroencephalography channels for recording the sleep EEG, but no systematic studies have evaluated this option for its potential added diagnostic value or validated its sleep-related parameters. Nonetheless, many systems have been validated for clinical use with their basic signal setup together with their scoring and analysis software. Ingeneral, most systems show good performance, with some minor differences. No overall preference for one or another system emerges from published studies.

HOME SLEEP TESTING WITH ONE- TO THREE-CHANNEL SYSTEMS FOR DIAGNOSING SLEEP-DISORDERED BREATHING

Systematic reviews of home sleep testing for diagnosing sleep-disordered breathing have revealed that systems with one to three channels (pulse oximetry, long-term ECG, actigraphy, and oronasal airflow) are not suitable for routine diagnostic use. Specifically, these devices yield too many false-negative (up to 17%) and too many false-positive (up to 31%) results.[3] This finding remained valid in the review by Collop and associates[1] and in a more recent systematic review using the new SCOPER criteria.[4] Therefore the application of these devices is not recommended for definitive diagnostic testing for obstructive sleep apnea, or to exclude the presence of obstructive sleep apnea.

Some of these devices, however, provide results in patients with severe sleep apnea that clearly suggest sleep-disordered breathing. Therefore high-quality recordings achieved with validated systems of this category can be used to increase the pretest probability before performance of cardiorespiratory polysomnography or even before four- to six-channel home sleep testing for sleep apnea.

Many technical innovations are currently emerging in this category of devices. A major challenge has been development of one- to three-channel devices that perform well and can diagnose sleep-disordered breathing. If reliable, such devices could facilitate diagnosis in new patient groups and provide tools for clinicians trained in other specialties with only basic knowledge of sleep medicine. Before initiation of therapy for sleep breathing disorders, however, a physician with a solid background in sleep-disordered breathing who is very familiar with the different treatment options should review the case.[17]

Described next are new technologies applicable with both one- to three-channel systems and four- to six-channel diagnostic devices.

NEW METHODS FOR HOME SLEEP TESTING

Different approaches are being explored for development of new technologies for diagnosing sleep-disordered breathing. Some approaches focus on developing new sensors to assess respiration for detecting breathing disturbances occurring during the night. Other technologies concentrate on assessing the patient's cardiovascular risk or sleep pathophysiology.

Assessment of Respiration

Several new sensors use surrogate signals to derive respiratory effort noninvasively. Some of these devices try to derive respiratory measures from direct respiration-related signals. These systems and concepts are discussed next.

A first-line approach entails recording respiratory airflow at the nose and the mouth. Usually these recordings are accompanied by pulse oximetry to determine oxyhemoglobin saturation. These simple screening devices provide a straightforward analysis for respiratory cessations. They even may distinguish obstructive from central respiratory events by analysis of flow limitation. Problems with obstructed nostrils, partial breathing through the mouth, blocked air tubes, and various artifacts pose logistical challenges to differentiating among the different types of apnea. Nevertheless, good validation studies are available,[18,19] with some limitations.

One approach tries to analyze respiratory sounds from the chest, with the goal of less obtrusive measures for detection of increased respiratory effort.[20] In other systems, respiratory sounds are recorded at the throat, and signal processing separates cardiac and movement signal first from breathing sounds and snoring. Together with oximetry, such recording quantifies respiratory measures, and snoring is tracked to detect respiratory cessations.[21,22]

Another approach involves recording midsagittal jaw movements based on magnetic distance determination.[23] A magnetic sensor is placed on the chin and another on the forehead to allow continuous determination of relative jaw movements. From this setup, it is possible to derive respiration and snoring. Analysis of this information is then used to detect respiratory events to diagnose sleep apnea.[24] By further analysis, a sleep wakefulness profile may potentially be estimated.[25,26] Combined with pulse oximetry and perhaps a cardiovascular parameter, this magnetic sensor–jaw movement detection feature is both simple and promising for clinical usefulness.

Pulse Wave Analysis

Many systems try to exploit the pulse wave on the finger or other peripheral sites. Such systems attempt to derive parameters from the pulse wave to assess cardiovascular event risk. The pressure wave may be detected with the photoplethysmograph already placed to measure oxygen saturation. In principle, this can be used to detect all forms of respiratory events[27] and cardiovascular event risk as associated with sleep apnea.[28,29]

Peripheral arterial tonometry[30] can be used to assess cardiovascular risk by measuring endothelial function during sleep-disordered breathing episodes. Arousals terminating sleep apnea events are accompanied by attenuated pulse amplitude. This decrease is due to peripheral vasoconstriction caused by sympathetic tone activation. If pulse rate also is analyzed, probability analysis can be used to distinguish between slow wave sleep and rapid eye movement (REM) sleep.[31] Several validation studies were published on use of the Watch-PAT, based on peripheral arterial tonometry, in patients with sleep apnea, with very good results.[29,32,33] A meta-analysis for this methodology is available and substantiates the diagnostic value of this device, even though it does not incorporate proximal sensors for effort and flow to record respiration, as recommended.[34]

Assessment of Electrocardiographic and Heart Rate Variability Parameters

ECG-derived respiratory parameters are very attractive for simple detection of sleep apnea owing to low costs and wide availability. To detect sleep apnea from the ECG alone does not require additional electrodes or additional hardware. The respiratory information is derived entirely from analytical software. This kind of analysis also could be performed retrospectively using previously recorded data. Sleep apnea is accompanied by a cyclic variation of heart rate, as already described many years ago.[35] Periodic changes in heart rate are related to the changes in sympathetic tone with apnea events.[36] Modern analysis of heart rate variability can satisfactorily derive cyclic variations of heart rate.[37,38] In addition, the morphology of the ECG wave itself is modulated by respiration. The derived respiratory curve—*ECG-derived respiration*[39]—correlates with respiratory effort and thus can be used to detect sleep-disordered breathing.[40,27] By combining ECG-derived respiration and sleep apnea–related heart rate variability, sleep apnea detection is possible.[41]

Electrocardiographic and Oximetry Assessments

A number of devices that use the ECG analysis techniques mentioned previously also try to link this approach to previous techniques. Early on, pulse oximetry was applied (with limited success) for portable diagnosis of sleep apnea. Pulse oximetry alone has large diagnostic limitations in patients with arrhythmias or with additional lung diseases such as chronic obstructive pulmonary disease. Combining ECG-based sleep apnea analysis and oximetry is therefore a very promising approach.[42] An early study using pulse rate in addition to oximetry[43] could show that this improves the detection of sleep apnea. One retrospective study showed the advantage over pulse oximetry alone when combined with ECG analysis.[44] In that study, the ECG from a parallel polysomnography recording was evaluated. Based on these results, a combined long-term ECG recording system with oximetry was tested prospectively and provided very convincing results in terms of sleep apnea detection.[42]

MANAGEMENT OF HOME SLEEP TESTING IN A SLEEP CENTER SETTING

Many new studies show high reliability of home sleep testing in detecting sleep apnea.[19] A number of open research questions needing clarification concerning the conditions and restrictions for using portable monitoring are now being addressed in recent studies.[1,5] The important parameters are no longer technical limitations but often study limitations such as the preselection of patients. The inherent screening process corresponds with the characteristic high pretest probability of sleep apnea. This aspect prohibits the use of portable monitoring as a screening tool to exclude sleep apneas, such as in professional drivers and people with supervision tasks (in which symptoms and complaints have not been assessed and may conflict with employability or other issues).

Diagnostic and therapeutic approaches to management of sleep-disordered breathing differ among countries worldwide.[45] The development of sleep medicine in some countries is very advanced. In others, economically affordable strategies constitute the primary consideration.[46,47] In certain settings, sleep medicine may be very basic, with only home sleep testing available for diagnosing sleep apnea.[45] One potential reason for this restriction to home sleep testing alone is the limited availability of sleep medicine centers owing to unmet needs for qualified experts and funding for polysomnography beds. This is the case in countries in which sleep medicine is a young discipline. A second reason is that even in countries with a long history of sleep medicine, and with enough sleep centers and polysomnography beds, an economic decision may be made to limit access to such studies to patients with comorbid illnesses, and those with regular sleep apnea are diagnosed with home sleep testing alone. With improvements in the knowledge base for sleep disorders and sleep-disordered breathing among general physicians, the individual clinician can decide whether a particular patient should be evaluated for suspected sleep apnea alone or exhibits some comorbidity or has other risk factors. Then the patient can be referred for either home sleep testing or cardiorespiratory polysomnography. This approach would allow economic and thoughtful management of patients with respect to diagnosis and subsequent treatment, as appropriate.[46] In Germany a debate was initiated on different levels of sleep medicine service that would include different levels of medical expertise and correspondingly different levels of equipment complexity. Family physicians may have some basic knowledge about

sleep-disordered breathing and already sometimes apply simple tests. A limited number of clinical centers would have clinical expertise, training, research, and other technical know-how as required in specialized sleep centers.[47] Many community-based centers may have basic sleep medicine knowledge and home sleep testing with four- to six-channel systems.

The other issue is health economy and patient care. A threshold regarding sleep apnea severity and assessing risk still remains to be established. How many apneas, how many hypopneas, what duration of apnea events, how much sleep fragmentation, or what degree of hypoxia represents substantial cardiovascular risk with increased mortality? How much increase in mortality justifies treatment with continous positive airway pressure (CPAP) or another lifelong therapy? In view of limited therapeutic adherence, how strict should researcher-clinicians be with respect to treatment follow-up studies? As the field of sleep medicine approaches the point at which diagnosis can be done easily with home sleep testing, a need is emerging for new clinical and economic decisions key for developing new strategies in managing sleep apnea.

Patients may be diagnosed and even treated at home. One home sleep testing study showed that the 4-week outcome in sleepiness and CPAP adherence was similar to that for sleep laboratory–based diagnosis and treatment.[48] An important limitation of the study was the short follow-up period.[49] Sleep-disordered breathing is a chronic condition, and long-term adherence with CPAP therapy may decline more at home. Thus more research is needed.

CONCLUSIONS

Attended cardiorespiratory polysomnography is the reference standard for diagnosing disordered breathing during sleep. Evidence-based literature, however, indicates that diagnosis of obstructive sleep apnea can be performed using home sleep testing under certain conditions in adults. The recording must include oxygen saturation, airflow, respiratory effort, heart or pulse rate, and body position. The SCOPER parameters summarize these requirements in a comprehensive and quantitative scheme.[4] Visual evaluation is needed to avoid misclassification of sleep apnea severity.[15] It is not possible to distinguish between central and obstructive respiratory events with certainty. Home sleep testing is reliable if it is performed under the supervision of personnel trained in sleep medicine and if screening has been adequate to achieve a high pretest probability among the study subjects of suffering from sleep-disordered breathing. In addition, the patients should not have other significant sleep or comorbid disorders (e.g., heart failure, stroke, diabetes mellitus, obstructive or restrictive lung diseases, or severe cardiac arrhythmias).

Home sleep testing systems with fewer channels can indicate the likelihood of sleep-disordered breathing but are not sufficiently validated for diagnostic purposes. Currently, these systems can point to the probable need for home sleep testing. Technological advances can be expected to improve these systems. Accordingly, it may well be that in the near future, systems with fewer channels may provide a sufficiently reliable diagnosis for disordered breathing during sleep. To prove the advanced usefulness of new technologies, good clinical studies, with sufficient sample size and testing of the new modality against a reference standard, are needed.

Technologic advances need to be accompanied by economy-driven strategies to diagnose and treat patients with sleep apnea. Recent approaches to diagnosing and even treating patients at home seem to provide effectiveness, in terms of outcome, similar to that for sleep laboratory–based studies. Economically proven home-based studies may be more feasible than sleep laboratory–based studies in light of the high prevalence of the disorders and the still-unmet clinical needs to recognize and treat patients with sleep-disordered breathing.

CLINICAL PEARLS

- Home sleep testing has been used for the portable diagnosis of sleep-disordered breathing for many years worldwide.
- Home sleep testing has been thoroughly compared against cardiorespiratory polysomnography.
- Sensitivity and specificity of home sleep testing are sufficient for a diagnosis if adult patients have a high pretest probability for sleep-disordered breathing.
- Home sleep testing requires monitoring of airflow, respiratory movement, oxygen saturation, pulse rate, and body position.
- Use of systems with fewer signals shows promising diagnostic results, but such streamlined systems require further validation.

SUMMARY

Home sleep testing is a well-validated technique to diagnose sleep-disordered breathing outside of the sleep laboratory and other clinical settings. Different devices are available. These devices usually record respiratory flow, respiratory effort, oxygen saturation, pulse or heart rate, and body position and/or activity. Some of these signals may be recorded indirectly and derived. The diagnostic sensitivity and specificity have been validated against those of polysomnography and generally show good agreement in patients with a high pretest probability for sleep-disordered breathing. Visual evaluation is needed to prevent misclassification of sleep apnea severity. Overall, the available evidence indicates that home sleep testing should be used in combination with a clinical assessment for factors and symptoms associated with sleep-disordered breathing. In view of the high prevalence of sleep-disordered breathing, methods to diagnose sleep apnea in a sufficiently accurate and economic way are urgently needed. Today, home sleep testing to assess sleep apnea is indispensable. In addition, home sleep testing offers a method for conducting therapy follow-up studies that may improve therapy compliance. Home sleep testing is developing an ever-more important role in the management of patients suffering from sleep-disordered breathing.

ACKNOWLEDGMENTS/DISCLOSURES

Several companies have furnished equipment for research or otherwise supported the work on which this chapter is based. Itamar Medical (Caesarea, Israel) provided sensors/consumables for research with the Watch-PAT device. Neuwirth Medical (Obernburg am Main, Germany) provided equipment to the Sleep Center for Research Studies. Cidelec (Sainte-Gemmes-sur-Loire, France) provided a grant for a validation study of its Pneavox system for laryngeal pressure and sound recording. Nomics (Liege, Belgium) provided a grant for a validation study of the Brizzy system. Somnomedics (Randersacker, Germany) provided Somnowatch equipment to the Sleep Center for Research Studies. Weinmann GmbH (Hamburg, Germany) provided Somnocheck equipment to the Sleep Center for Research Studies. Nox Medical (Reykjavik, Island) provided equipment and sensors for testing. Studies were done at the Interdisciplinary Sleep Medicine Center at Charite-Universitätsmedizin Berlin.

Selected Readings

Aurora RN, Putcha N, Swartz R, et al. Agreement between Results of Home Sleep Testing for Obstructive Sleep Apnea with and without a Sleep Specialist. *Am J Med* 2016;pii: S0002-9343(16)30203-0.

Aurora RN, Swartz R, Punjabi NM. Misclassification of OSA severity with automated scoring of home sleep recordings. *Chest* 2015;**147**:719–27.

Berry RB, Gamaldo CE, Harding SM, et al. *The AASM Scoring Manual*, Version 2.2. Updates: new chapters for scoring infant sleep staging and home sleep apnea testing. *J Clin Sleep Med* 2015;**11**(11):1253–4.

Collop N. Home sleep testing: appropriate screening is the key. *Sleep* 2012;**35**:1445–6.

El Shayeb M, Topfer LA, Stafinski T, et al. Diagnostic accuracy of level 3 portable sleep tests versus level 1 polysomnography for sleep-disordered breathing: a systematic review and meta-analysis. *CMAJ* 2014;**186**: E25–51.

Gozal D, Kheirandish-Gozal L, Kaditis AG. Home sleep testing for the diagnosis of pediatric obstructive sleep apnea: the times they are a-changing ...! *Curr Opin Pulm Med* 2015;**21**(6):563–8.

Kuna ST, Badr MS, Kimoff RJ, et al. An official ATS/AASM/ACCP/ERS Workshop report: research priorities in ambulatory management of adults with obstructive sleep apnea. *Proc Am Thorac Soc* 2011;**8**:1–16.

Pack AI. Sleep medicine: strategies for change. *J Clin Sleep Med* 2011; **7**:577–9.

Pereira EJ, Driver HS, Stewart SC, Fitzpatrick MF. Comparing a combination of validated questionnaires and level III portable monitor with polysomnography to diagnose and exclude sleep apnea. *J Clin Sleep Med* 2013;**9**:1259–66.

Qaseem A, Dallas P, Owens DK, et al. Diagnosis of obstructive sleep apnea in adults: a clinical practice guideline from the American College of Physicians. *Ann Intern Med* 2014;**161**:210–20.

A complete reference list can be found online at ExpertConsult.com.

Respiratory Physiology: Understanding the Control of Ventilation

Danny J. Eckert; Jane E. Butler

Chapter 7

Chapter Highlights

- In the absence of respiratory disease, the process of breathing typically is afforded little conscious thought. Yet it is clearly fundamental to survival.
- Multiple inputs are capable of regulating the rate and depth of breathing. These are regulated by feedforward and feedback mechanisms that control blood gas levels within relatively narrow limits to maintain homeostasis.
- The physiologic capacity to alter breathing is substantial. When metabolic demand decreases during sleep, even very low levels of ventilation can be tolerated. However, the major changes to the control of breathing that occur during sleep can cause breathing disruption.
- This chapter outlines the key neuroanatomic inputs to breathing, describes the changes that occur in the control of breathing during sleep, including differences between men and women, and highlights how abnormal control of ventilation can contribute to sleep-disordered breathing.

OVERVIEW OF THE CONTROL OF BREATHING

Breathing is controlled by means of highly effective feedforward and feedback mechanisms. Conceptually, the functional organization consists of three key elements: (1) brainstem neurons responsible for respiratory pattern generation (*central control*), (2) respiratory muscles that generate force to move airflow in and out of the lungs (*effectors*), and (3) multiple inputs that relay respiratory sensory information (*sensors*) to brainstem respiratory control centers to allow for adjustments according to the prevailing physiologic conditions (Figure 7-1). A breakdown in or damage to any one of these components can lead to breathing abnormalities. During wakefulness, however, additional inputs to breathing can compensate to maintain breathing and blood gas levels within acceptable levels despite damage to key elements that underlie the control of breathing. Accordingly, breathing problems often only emerge (or worsen) during sleep, when wakefulness compensatory mechanisms are either downregulated or absent. This chapter outlines the key components that underpin the control of breathing and highlights the major changes that occur during sleep. This chapter is a synthesis of many elements described in other chapters of this volume, with a perspective aimed at translating the information toward a more comprehensive understanding of respiration and sleep disturbances in humans.

CENTRAL CONTROL OF BREATHING

The precise neuroanatomic locations that contribute to respiratory pattern generation within the brainstem are incompletely understood. The central respiratory control network involves both inspiratory and expiratory neurons. Presented next is a brief summary of some of the key brainstem sites and their interconnections, based primarily on animal models.

Central respiratory control and rhythmicity occur within the pons and medulla. Within the medulla, the dorsal and ventral respiratory groups are particularly important (Figure 7-2). The *dorsal respiratory group* contains the nucleus tractus solitarius (nTS). The nTS is a key cardiorespiratory sensory integration site. Afferent information from phrenic, vagus, and peripheral chemoreceptors (by way of the glossopharyngeal nerve) arrive at the nTS. The nTS has numerous outputs contributing to important control of breathing centers, including the nearby retrotrapezoid nucleus[1,2] (see the following section on chemoreceptors). The ventrolateral region of the nTS is believed to be particularly important for inspiratory activity. Major projections also extend to other key respiratory control centers within the ventral respiratory group. Not yet known, however, is whether direct output to respiratory motoneurons occurs.

The pre-Bötzinger complex forms part of the *ventral respiratory group* (see Figure 7-2). The pre-Bötzinger complex is believed to be the major putative respiratory pacemaker. This stems from findings that show persistence of respiratory rhythmicity within these cells in minimal slice preparations.[3] In support of the importance of this region to respiratory control, the pre-Bötzinger complex has multiple projections to other known respiratory control sites within the brainstem.[4] Adjacent to the pre-Bötzinger is the Bötzinger complex. This area plays an active role during expiration by inhibiting respiratory motor neurons to modulate the overall motor output. The rostral ventral respiratory group also includes inspiratory pre-motoneurons such as those located in the nucleus ambiguus. The nucleus ambiguus provides respiratory motor output to the larynx and pharynx by way of the vagi. The nucleus

63

retroambiguus also may contribute to respiratory rhythm generation.[5]

Although respiratory rhythm generation neurons are located predominantly within the medulla, the *pontine respiratory group* (previously referred to as the pneumotaxic center) also is importantly involved in central respiratory control[6] (see Figure 7-2). The pontine respiratory group includes the nucleus parabrachialis medialis, containing expiratory active neurons. The parabrachialis lateralis and the Kölliker-Fuse

nucleus in the upper pons contain inspiratory neurons. Pontine respiratory group activation can decrease inspiratory activity within the dorsal respiratory group, leading to a decrease in inspiratory time. This "inspiratory-expiratory phase transition" can increase breathing frequency.

CHEMICAL CONTROL OF BREATHING

Chemical control is the most important regulator of breathing in healthy persons during quiet breathing. This is true during both wakefulness and sleep. All cells are capable of modifying their activity in response to extreme changes in the chemical environment. Certain cells, however, are highly sensitive to quite minor changes. These chemically sensitive areas can regulate the control of breathing directly or have projections to central control of breathing sites. Accordingly, these groups of cells, known as *chemoreceptors*, are fundamentally important to the control of breathing.

Peripheral versus Central

Chemoreceptors are located peripherally and centrally (Figure 7-3). The main peripheral chemoreceptors lie at the bifurcation of the common carotid arteries. The carotid bodies have long been known to respond to changes in oxygen, carbon dioxide, and hydrogen ion concentration.[7] Detection of these stimuli can lead to rapid alterations in breathing (within 1 or 2 breaths). In addition, recent findings show that the carotid bodies respond to a wide range of other stimuli including potassium, norepinephrine, temperature, glucose, insulin, and immune-related cytokines.[7,8] Repeated exposure to hypoxia can cause plasticity within the carotid bodies.[8] The changes that occur can contribute to pathologic states including an increased propensity for breathing instability during sleep.[7,8] In addition to the carotid bodies, the nearby aortic bodies are also capable of responding to changes in oxygen and other

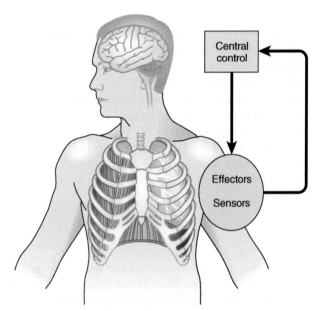

Figure 7-1 Control of Breathing Overview. Breathing is controlled by means of feedforward and feedback mechanisms involving central control, effectors, and sensors. Refer to text for further details.

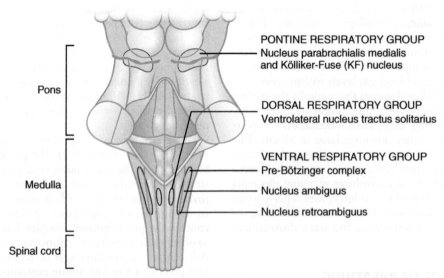

Figure 7-2 Central Control of Breathing. Major regions involved in the central control of breathing lie within the pontine respiratory group, comprising the nucleus parabrachialis medialis and the Kölliker-Fuse nucleus; the ventral respiratory group, consisting of the pre-Bötzinger complex, nucleus ambiguus, and nucleus retroambiguus; and the dorsal respiratory group, comprising the ventrolateral nucleus tractus solitarius. Refer to text for further details. (From Eckert DJ, Roca D, Yim-Yeh S, Malhotra A. Control of breathing. In: Kryger M, editor. *Atlas of clinical sleep medicine*, vol. 2. 2nd ed. Philadelphia: Saunders; 2014, p. 45–52.)

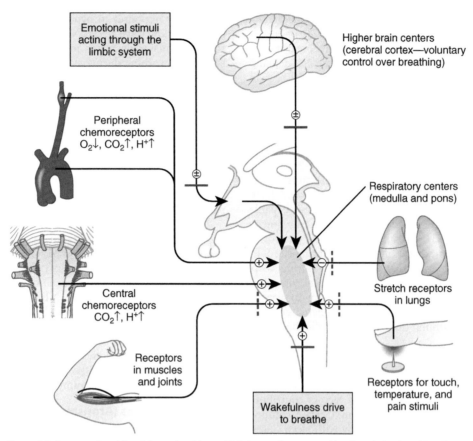

Figure 7-3 Inputs to Breathing. Schematic of the multiple inputs that are capable of regulating breathing. During sleep, many of these inputs are either substantially diminished (*dashed red lines*) or absent (*solid red lines*). Thus the predominant inputs to breathing during sleep are the chemoreceptors, which themselves also are downregulated and affected by state. *Note:* For simplicity, voluntary control of breathing is shown to act by way of the respiratory centers. Whether this is in fact the case or whether voluntary control acts directly on the respiratory motoneurons, however, has not been established. Refer to text for further details. (Modified from Kehlmann GB, Eckert DJ. Central sleep apnea due to a medical condition not Cheyne Stokes. In: Kushida CA, editor. *Encyclopedia of sleep*, vol. 1. 1st ed. San Diego: Elsevier; 2013, p 244–52; and Eckert DJ, Roca D, Yim-Yeh S, Malhotra A. Control of breathing. In: Kryger M, editor. *Atlas of clinical sleep medicine*, vol. 2. 2nd ed. Philadelphia: Saunders; 2014, p. 45–52).

chemical stimuli. Although the peripheral chemoreceptors are important for moment-to-moment modulation of breathing, the most powerful input to breathing during quiet wakefulness is from the central chemoreceptors.

Located on the ventral surface of the medulla, adjacent to the ventral respiratory group, lies the retrotrapezoid nucleus. This region is particularly important for central chemoreception.[9,10] The retrotrapezoid nucleus has major projections to key respiratory control centers including to the nTS within the dorsal respiratory group.[1,2] The central chemoreceptors respond to Pco_2 through changes in the pH of the extracellular fluid. CO_2 diffuses across the blood–brain barrier to increase hydrogen ion concentration in the cerebrospinal fluid. Thus, compared with the relatively fast-responding peripheral chemoreceptors, central chemoreceptors can take up to a minute to respond to changes in chemical stimuli. As discussed later, chemoreceptor response delays are critically important in mediating cyclicbreathing instability during sleep.[11-13]

Although the peripheral and central chemoreceptors are anatomically distinct and have different response characteris-

tics, recent findings indicate complex interconnectivity.[7,8,14] Specifically, the activity of the central chemoreceptors is critically dependent on the activity of the peripheral chemoreceptors, and vice versa.[7,8,14]

OTHER INPUTS TO BREATHING

In addition to input from the chemoreceptors, other important inputs and sensors can contribute to the rate and depth at which we breathe (see Figure 7-3). Receptors in the limb muscles and joints can respond to movement to increase minute ventilation. Similarly, when receptors responsible for touch, temperature, and pain are stimulated, breathing increases. An independent stimulus to breathing known as the *wakefulness drive to breathe* also may be recruited.[15] Conversely, overinflation or excess lung stretch can inhibit minute ventilation by means of the Hering-Breuer reflex.[16] Other inputs can either stimulate or inhibit breathing. These inputs include limbic system input in response to emotional stimuli or voluntary cortical control. It remains uncertain, however, if voluntary override of breathing acts indirectly through changes in central respiratory pattern generation or directly by way of phrenic motoneurons, or by a combination of both.[17] Nonetheless, the physiologic capacity to alter breathing is substantial. As highlighted later, when metabolic demand decreases during sleep, very low levels of ventilation (less than 5 L/minute) can be tolerated. Conversely, during intense exercise, ventilation can increase to greater than 200 L/minute.

STATE-RELATED CHANGES IN THE CONTROL OF BREATHING

Major changes in the control of breathing occur from wakefulness to sleep. The most significant change that occurs from wakefulness to sleep is that a majority of the inputs capable of modifying breathing are either absent or markedly downregulated (see Figure 7-3). Accordingly, chemical control of breathing is the dominant driver of breathing during sleep. In particular, CO_2 is critical in mediating breathing during sleep. Certain disease states adversely affect the chemical control of breathing and can cause sleep-disordered breathing in susceptible persons. This section outlines key state-related changes in the control of breathing that underlie cyclic breathing instability during sleep.

Sleep Onset

Respiratory control is inherently unstable during the transition from wakefulness to sleep.[18] Several factors contribute to respiratory instability at sleep transition. Certain components of respiratory control change rapidly with sleep onset, whereas others require more time. Mismatch in timing combined with downregulation in important respiratory control mechanisms underlies breathing disturbances during the sleep-onset period. Indeed, brief breathing stoppages at sleep onset are very common, even in otherwise healthy persons.

With respect to mechanical factors, the wakefulness drive to breathe and behavioral influences cease with sleep onset.[19] Movement and excitatory input to breathe from other external sensors become minimal or completely absent. Chemosensitivity also decreases[20] (see Figure 7-3). Accordingly, respiratory pump muscle tone is reduced, leading to a reduction in minute ventilation.[21] An abrupt reduction in upper airway muscle tone and protective reflexes also occurs with sleep onset.[21-25] These changes contribute to increased upper airway resistance.[23] The timing and magnitude of these changes vary among individual subjects. Rapid withdrawal of excitatory drive to breathing, in and of itself, can cause respiratory events as a consequence of the delay required to elicit a compensatory response from the chemoreceptors.[26] Patients who experience sleep apnea appear to be more prone than healthy control subjects to major reductions in the wakefulness drive to breathing.[27] As indicated by these findings, sleep onset affects all components of respiratory control and can cause major "state instability."

Stable Sleep

The removal of most excitatory inputs to breathing that occurs with sleep onset is a feature of stable sleep as well. Respiratory load compensation also is reduced during stable sleep compared with wakefulness.[28] Thus minute ventilation decreases during stable sleep, and the control of breathing becomes dominated by chemical input. However, downregulation in chemosensitivity is not isolated to the sleep-onset period.

Ventilatory responses to hypoxia are reduced during stage 2 (N2) and slow wave sleep (N3), compared with wakefulness, such that major decreases in oxygen levels are required to stimulate breathing during sleep.[29-31] Accordingly, CO_2 is the main regulator of breathing during sleep. However, ventilatory responses to hypercapnia also are reduced during sleep compared with wakefulness, albeit to a lesser extent than for hypoxia.[32] Consequently, people can tolerate lower levels of minute ventilation and higher levels of CO_2 during sleep than in wakefulness. Typically, depending on the prevailing metabolic conditions, minute ventilation is reduced by 1 to 2 L/minute, and the partial pressure of carbon dioxide in the blood ($Paco_2$) increases by 3 to 8 mm Hg during stable sleep, compared with wakefulness[33] (Figure 7-4, *A*).

In the absence of respiratory disease, breathing is quite regular during stable non–rapid eye movement (NREM) sleep. Rapid eye movement (REM) sleep, by contrast, is characterized by breathing irregularity. Many medullary central control-of-breathing regions exhibit increased activation during REM compared with NREM sleep.[34] In humans, breathing frequency increases, and major variations are seen in breath-to-breath tidal volume. Active eye movements during REM sleep are associated with inhibition of upper airway dilator muscle activity and decreased tidal volume.[28,35] Protective upper airway reflexes also are inhibited.[36] Accordingly, obstructive apnea is common during REM sleep.

Brief Awakenings (Arousal from Sleep)

Brief cortical arousals from sleep lasting less than 15 seconds occur between 10 to 20 times per hour in healthy subjects. Arousal frequency increases with age.[37] Arousals can occur spontaneously or in conjunction with a sleep disorder such as sleep apnea or periodic limb movement disorder. Historically, arousals were believed to be essential for reopening the upper airway during obstructive breathing events.[38] Indeed, arousal can be beneficial in certain circumstances to rapidly resolve blood gas disturbances and to alleviate the increased work of breathing during flow-limited breathing.[39] However, although the initial physiologic changes associated with arousals may be beneficial for respiratory homeostasis, the rapid switch from sleep to wakefulness and the subsequent resumption of sleep can be highly destabilizing for respiratory control.[39] The extent to which arousals destabilize breathing and contribute to central or obstructive breathing events is dependent on two key features: (1) the subject's threshold for arousal—the *arousal threshold*—and (2) the ventilatory response to arousal.

Arousal Threshold

Whether an arousal occurs spontaneously, with a periodic limb movement, or in association with a respiratory disturbance, a person who wakes up easily (i.e., has a *low arousal threshold*) may be susceptible to sleep-state breathing instability. Specifically, a predisposition to sleep-onset breathing instability coupled with a low arousal threshold may lead to repetitive breathing disturbances as the affected person oscillates between wakefulness and sleep.[11] Approximately one third of patients with obstructive sleep apnea arouse to modest levels of respiratory stimuli (negative airway pressure less than 15 cm H_2O).[39,40] This relatively low threshold is likely to contribute to their sleep-disordered breathing.[39] Increasing the arousal threshold in these at-risk patients can stabilize

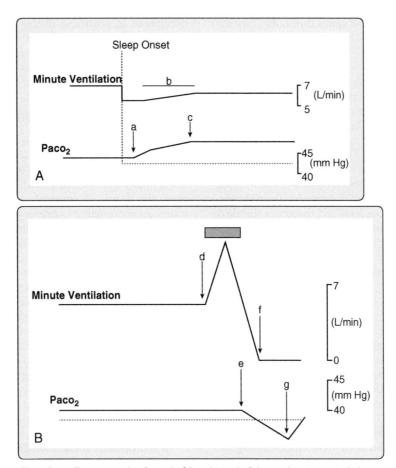

Figure 7-4 Sleep State Changes to the Control of Breathing. **A,** Schema showing typical changes in minute ventilation and $PaCO_2$ from wakefulness to sleep. At sleep onset (*dashed vertical line*), a rapid reduction in minute ventilation (from 7 to 5 L/min) occurs. A delay between the reduction in ventilation and changes in $PaCO_2$ (sleep onset to point a) also is seen. As CO_2 rises, upper airway muscles may be recruited, and minute ventilation may increase somewhat (period b), until a new eucapnic sleeping minute ventilation (5.5 L/min) and $PaCO_2$ (45 mm Hg) are reached (point c). The *horizontal red line* represents the theoretical apnea threshold (in this case, 39 mm Hg). **B,** Schematic representation of a central apnea after an arousal from sleep. At point d, a brief arousal from sleep occurs (arousal duration represented by the *gray box*). Hyperventilation occurs in association with reintroduction of wakefulness stimuli (ventilatory response to arousal). The hyperventilation lowers $PaCO_2$. However, a delay between the change in ventilation and the change in $PaCO_2$ can be seen (point d to point e). As the patient returns to sleep, the reduction in $PaCO_2$, caused by the ventilatory response to arousal, falls below the apnea threshold (which in this example is very close to the eucapnic sleeping $PaCO_2$ level), and apnea occurs (point f). The apnea leads to an increase in $PaCO_2$ until either an arousal occurs, and the cycle is repeated, or the apnea threshold is crossed and breathing resumes. Refer to text for further details. (From Kehlmann GB, Eckert DJ. Central sleep apnea due to a medical condition not Cheyne Stokes. In: Kushida CA, editor. *Encyclopedia of sleep*, vol. 1. 1st ed. San Diego: Elsevier; 2013, p. 244–52).

breathing.[41] Indeed, although the precise mechanisms remain uncertain, the arousal threshold and upper airway muscle activity increase in deeper stages of sleep, and sleep-disordered breathing severity decreases.[42-44] Not known, however, is whether deeper stages of sleep are intrinsically more stable in terms of respiratory control or if breathing stability allows sleep to deepen.

Ventilatory Response to Arousal

In much the same way in which rapid changes in respiratory control occur during sleep onset, arousal from sleep causes a rapid change in the homeostatic control of breathing. As highlighted, during stable sleep, lower levels of minute ventilation and higher levels of CO_2, compared with wakefulness

(~3 to 8 mm Hg higher), can be tolerated. With arousal, the wakefulness chemical control of breathing is reinstated, and the increased levels of CO_2 that were tolerated during sleep suddenly become excessive. Upper airway motoneurons are activated, and sleep-related upper airway resistance is rapidly resolved.[45] The wakefulness drive to breath also is reintroduced. Accordingly, arousal from sleep is associated with a rapid increase in breathing. The magnitude of the ventilatory response to arousal is dependent on the integrative effects of the various aforementioned factors and may be further augmented by an independent wakefulness reflex.[46] Indeed, this ventilatory arousal response varies substantially among subjects.[47] As outlined next, on the resumption of sleep, the previous ventilatory response to arousal can drive $PaCO_2$ levels below a critical level known as the apnea threshold[48] (see also Figure 7-4, *B*).

APNEA THRESHOLD

Multiple compensatory mechanisms act to oppose breathing cessation even with quite major reductions in $Paco_2$ during wakefulness (see Figure 7-3). During sleep, however, this is not the case. Specifically, if $Paco_2$ falls below a critical level during sleep, breathing ceases. The apnea threshold ranges between 2 and 6 mm Hg below the stable sleep $Paco_2$ level. Evidently, then, the apnea threshold is similar to the wakefulness $Paco_2$ level[49,50] (see Dempsey[51] for details). The difference between the wakefulness $Paco_2$ level and the apnea threshold often is termed the CO_2 reserve. The reduction in $Paco_2$ required to cause apnea is importantly dependent on the peripheral chemoreceptors.[52] Schematic examples outlining important state-related changes in the control of breathing are displayed in Figure 7-4.

Loop Gain

As outlined in this chapter, many inputs contribute to the control of breathing. Loop gain is one approach to conceptualize and quantify the overall sensitivity of the ventilatory control system. Specifically, the gain of the ventilatory control feedback loop can be quantified as the ratio of a ventilatory response to a ventilatory disturbance.[11,26,53] Loop gain has three major components: (1) *plant gain* (the efficiency of breathing to remove CO_2, which is determined by the properties of the lungs, blood, and body tissues), (2) *mixing and circulation delays* (the time required for a change in alveolar CO_2 to mix with the blood in the heart and the arteries before reaching the chemoreceptors), and (3) *controller gain* (the sensitivity of the chemoreceptors). Because CO_2 is the predominant modifier of ventilatory control during sleep, determining the loop gain during sleep provides important insight into the overall sensitivity of the ventilatory control system and allows for comparisons to be made between individual subjects and patient groups. Accordingly, techniques have been developed to quantify the steady state loop gain during sleep.[54,55] If certain elements that contribute to loop gain are abnormal (e.g., plant or controller gain), breathing instability can occur. Circulation delay is an integral component of breathing instability; without it, cyclic breathing would not occur. Of note, however, is that although increasing circulation delay increases the length and duration of breathing instability, increased circulation delay alone does not cause breathing instability.

Sex Differences

Sleep-disordered breathing in adults is more common in men than in women. Respiratory control differences between the sexes may contribute to this difference, at least in part. Progesterone is a respiratory stimulant, and sleep-disordered breathing is more common in women after menopause. Although ventilatory responses to CO_2 and hypoxia vary throughout the menstrual cycle, ventilatory responses during sleep to chemical stimuli do not appear to be systematically different between the sexes.[56,57] Consistent with these earlier observations, overall steady state loop gain is not different between men and women.[58,59] In accordance with increased vulnerability to breathing instability, however, important differences in breathing during sleep onset, the ventilatory response to arousal, and the apnea threshold have been observed between men and women.[18,60-62] Whether or not men have systematically lower arousal thresholds remains unclear.

CLINICAL MANIFESTATIONS

Altered respiratory control can contribute to various forms of sleep-disordered breathing and clinical syndromes. Many causes of abnormal respiratory control have been recognized. These topics are covered elsewhere in this volume and have been the focus of comprehensive reviews.[11-13,63,64] Briefly stated, an abnormality in one or more of the components that importantly contribute to respiratory control as outlined in this chapter can cause breathing instability during sleep. Damage to central respiratory control centers or drugs that impair its function (e.g., certain brain tumors, Chiari type I malformation, and drugs that can depress breathing such as morphine) can directly affect central respiratory control.[11-13] Congenital central hypoventilation syndrome is associated with major loss of chemosensitive neurons within the retrotrapezoid nucleus.[12] Heart failure is associated with heightened peripheral chemosensitivity and increased vulnerability to onset of apnea (i.e., crossing the apnea threshold). Conversely, patients with obesity-hypoventilation syndrome have blunted ventilatory responses to chemical stimuli and experience sustained hypoventilation and major blood gas disturbances during sleep.

As indicated by these findings, high and low loop gain can be problematic and can contribute to both obstructive and central breathing instability during sleep.[63] Indeed, approximately one third of patients who experience obstructive sleep apnea demonstrate abnormally high loop gain, which is likely to be an important contributor to the pathogenesis of their obstructive apnea.[40]

CLINICAL PEARL

Sleep is a particularly vulnerable time for respiratory control instability. Many of the potential compensatory inputs to breathing are markedly diminished or absent during sleep. Accordingly, regardless of the underlying cause, abnormality in one or more of the important contributors to respiratory control can cause sleep-disordered breathing. The sleep-related breathing instability that ensues is dependent on the extent to which the respiratory control system is altered and on which of the components of the respiratory control system are involved.

SUMMARY

An understanding of the control of ventilation provides important insight into the causes of various forms of sleep-disordered breathing. Ventilatory control is regulated by means of highly effective feedforward and feedback mechanisms that control blood gas levels within relatively narrow limits to maintain homeostasis. Many inputs have been recognized to regulate ventilatory control. Although these processes are predominantly under autonomic control, voluntary modulation of breathing also is possible in various circumstances.

The dorsal, ventral, and pontine respiratory groups are key regions within the medulla and pons responsible for central respiratory control. Central (e.g., retrotrapezoid nucleus) and peripheral (e.g., carotid bodies) chemoreceptors provide essential sensory information to modify breathing. Other sensory systems also can provide input to alter the rate and depth of breathing. Most such systems, however, are either downregulated or absent during sleep. Accordingly, the chemical control of breathing—in particular, by CO_2—is the dominant input to ventilatory control during sleep. Sleep onset is particularly destabilizing to ventilatory control. Arousal from sleep and high loop gain can lead to marked fluctuations in CO_2 and to breathing cession during sleep if the apnea threshold is crossed. Abnormalities in one or more of the components that contribute to ventilatory control can contribute to both central and obstructive breathing events during sleep.

ACKNOWLEDGMENT

DJE and JEB are supported by the National Health and Medical Research Council of Australia.

Selected Readings

Burke PG, Kanbar R, Basting TM, et al. State-dependent control of breathing by the retrotrapezoid nucleus. *J Physiol* 2015;**593**(13):2909–26.

Carberry JC, Hensen H, Fisher LP, et al. Mechanisms contributing to the response of upper-airway muscles to changes in airway pressure. *J Appl Physiol* 2015;**118**:1221–8.

Deacon NL, Jen R, Li Y, Malhotra A. Treatment of Obstructive Sleep Apnea. Prospects for Personalized Combined Modality Therapy. *Ann Am Thorac Soc* 2016;**13**(1):101–8.

Dempsey JA, Smith CA. Pathophysiology of human ventilatory control. *Eur Respir J* 2014;**44**:495–512.

Dempsey JA, Smith CA, Blain GM, et al. Role of central/peripheral chemoreceptors and their interdependence in the pathophysiology of sleep apnea. *Adv Exp Med Biol* 2012;**758**:343–9.

Eckert DJ, Roca D, Yim-Yeh S, Malhotra A. Control of breathing. In: Kryger M, editor. *Atlas of clinical sleep medicine*, 2nd ed. Philadelphia: Elsevier; 2014. p. 45–52.

Guyenet PG, Stornetta RL, Bayliss DA. Central respiratory chemoreception. *J Comp Neurol* 2010;**518**:3883–906.

Javaheri S, Dempsey JA. Central sleep apnea. *Compr Physiol* 2013;**3**:141–63.

Kehlmann GB, Eckert DJ. Central sleep apnea due to a medical condition not Cheyne Stokes. In: Kushida CA, editor. *Encyclopedia of sleep*, vol. 1. 1st ed. San Diego: Elsevier; 2013. p. 244–52.

Khoo MC, Kronauer RE, Strohl KP, Slutsky AS. Factors inducing periodic breathing in humans: a general model. *J Appl Physiol* 1982;**53**:644–59.

Kumar P, Prabhakar NR. Peripheral chemoreceptors: function and plasticity of the carotid body. *Compr Physiol* 2012;**2**:141–219.

A complete reference list can be found online at ExpertConsult.com.

Physiology of Upper and Lower Airways

Raphael Heinzer; Frédéric Sériès

Chapter Highlights

- Sleep has an impact on ventilation and gas exchanges mediated through an increase in airway resistance and a decrease in lung volume and thoracopulmonary compliance.
- Upper airway stability can be altered during sleep because of its effects

- on upper airway muscle control and chest mechanics.
- When upper airway anatomy is compromised, these sleep-related effects can trigger obstructive disordered breathing.

This chapter focuses on the physiologic determinants of respiration used to estimate breathing function in normal persons. The ultimate goal is to allow readers who are not familiar with the field of respiratory medicine to benefit from the more subtle concepts that will help them to better understand sleep-disordered breathing. Chapter 7 describes the basis of the physiology and applied concepts of respiratory function during wake and sleep.

The dual aim of breathing is to provide oxygen to the different body parts and to eliminate carbon dioxide resulting from cell metabolism. This is achieved through continuous gas exchange between inspired and exhaled air and the blood in the pulmonary circulation. After blood coming from the right side of the heart has been loaded with oxygen, it passes to the left side of the heart, which sends it to every part of the body through the arterial system. The different organs then take up oxygen from the arterial blood and remove carbon dioxide. Blood loaded with carbon dioxide travels through the venous system to reach the pulmonary circulation, where carbon dioxide passively diffuses through the alveolocapillary membrane into the airway, whence it is exhaled. Survival depends on the integrity of this physiologic process, and death can occur if respiratory function stops for more than a few minutes. Maintenance of normal arterial blood gases involves several physiologic systems—control of breathing, thoracopulmonary mechanics, circulatory components, and blood transport—that are intimately linked to one another. This chapter considers only the mechanical properties of the chest and the upper and lower airways, which influence ventilation during sleep (Box 8-1).

ANATOMY AND PHYSIOLOGY

The upper airway, which includes the nasal cavities, pharynx, and larynx, serves to moisten and warm the air and conduct it to the trachea and lungs. Upper airway muscles also are involved in phonation and swallowing. A very subtle regulation of vocal cord tension also allows humans to speak and sing during exhalation. It is hypothesized that the evolution

of speech, which requires substantial mobility of the pharynx, led to a loss of the rigid support of the upper airway, which makes it more collapsible in humans than in most mammals.

Breathing is possible through either the nose or the mouth, but nasal breathing is the physiologic breathing route. The lower airway includes the trachea and the lungs (bronchi and alveoli). Thin blood vessels, the capillaries lining the alveoli, allow gas exchange between inspired air and blood. The rib cage provides protection for the lungs and also allows them to change volume from a minimum of approximately 1.5 L to a maximum of 6 to 8 L, depending on the height and sex of the person.[1]

The ribs articulate with the transverse processes of the thoracic vertebrae and have flexible anterior cartilaginous connections with the sternum. The lungs are covered by thin visceral pleura. The inner aspects of each hemithorax are lined with parietal pleura. The virtual space between the visceral and the parietal pleura contains a few milliliters of lubricating fluid, which allows these layers to slide against each other easily during ventilation. Owing to its proximity to the pleural tissue, the esophageal pressure varies in parallel with the changes in pleural pressure and often is used to quantify respiratory efforts.

Respiratory Muscles

The diaphragm is the main muscle of respiration. It is a dome-shaped muscle that separates the thoracic and abdominal cavities. The diaphragm is innervated by the phrenic nerves. During inspiration, the neural outflow coming from the central respiratory centers leads to diaphragm contraction; the shortening of those muscle fibers flattens the diaphragm, with consequent loss of its dome shape, thereby increasing intrathoracic volume. Intercostal muscles also can increase the intrathoracic volume by elevating ribs and increasing the anteroposterior diameter of the thorax (Figure 8-1). Accessory breathing muscles such as the scalene or sternocleidomastoid are not active during normal breathing, but they can be recruited during an effort or in the presence of thoracopulmonary disorders.

Box 8-1   SOME DEFINITIONS USED IN RESPIRATORY MECHANICS

Chest or Lung Compliance
Change in volume per change in pressure: $\Delta V/\Delta P$

Minute Ventilation
Tidal volume times respiratory rate: $Vt \times RR$

Laminar Flow
Change in pressure per resistance: $\Delta P/R$

Turbulent Flow
Pressure drop along the airway is proportional to flow and its square values: $\Delta P \propto aV + bV^2$ (V is air flow, and a and b are constants)

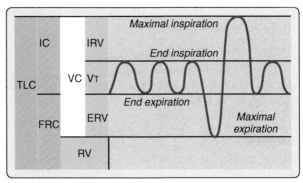

Figure 8-2 Schematic illustration of the static lung volumes determined by a spirometer in which airflow velocity does not play a role. Lung capacity is estimated by the sum of two or more lung volume subdivisions. ERV, Expiratory reserve volume; FRC, functional residual capacity; IC, inspiratory capacity; IRV, inspiratory reserve volume; RV, residual volume; TLC, total lung capacity; VC, vital capacity; VT, tidal volume. (Reproduced with permission from American Association for Respiratory Care. AARC clinical practice guideline: static lung volumes: 2001 revision & update. *Respir Care* 2001;46:531–9.)

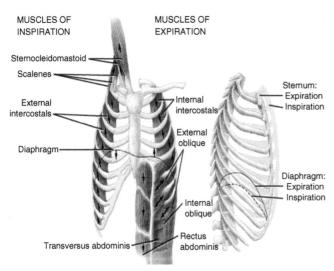

Figure 8-1 Drawing of inspiratory and expiratory muscles from abdomen to neck. The main inspiratory muscles include the diaphragm and external intercostal muscles. Accessory inspiratory muscles include the scalene and sternocleidomastoid muscles. Expiration usually is a passive process. However, internal intercostals and abdominal muscles are recruited during forced expiration. (Reproduced from Netter FH. *Atlas of human anatomy.* Philadelphia: Saunders; 2006.)

Elastic Forces and Lung Volumes

An isolated lung (not surrounded by the thoracic cage) will tend to contract until it eventually collapses owing to the large amount of elastic fibers inside the lung tissue. The lung is thus submitted to a constant recoil force. By contrast, the isolated thoracic cage tends to expand to a volume approximately 1 L more than its natural, in vivo resting position. In a relaxed subject with an open airway and no airflow, the inward elastic recoil of the lungs will be balanced by the outward resting force coming from the thoracic cage. *Lung compliance* or *distensibility* is defined as the change in lung volume per unit change in transmural pressure gradient:

$$compliance = \Delta V/\Delta P$$

where V is volume and P is pressure.

The lung volume, in the natural resting end-expiratory position, is its *functional residual capacity* (FRC). *Total lung*

capacity (TLC) is reached when the thoracic cage and lungs are fully expanded (maximal inspiratory effort). *Residual volume* (RV) represents the volume remaining in the lungs at the end of a forced expiration. *Vital capacity* (VC) is the maximum amount of air that can be expelled after the lungs have been fully inflated. *Tidal volume* (VT) is the volume of air inspired or expired during each quiet breathing cycle (Figure 8-2). The typical VT value is 500 mL, but it can dramatically increase during exercise. Only approximately two thirds of inspired air participates in oxygen and carbon dioxide exchange, because the volume corresponding to upper airway, trachea, and bronchi does not contribute to gas exchange; this area is the *dead space* (VDS) of the respiratory tract.[1]

Breathing Cycle and Minute Ventilation

Air always flows from an area of higher pressure to one of lower pressure, to achieve equilibrium. The pressure inside the pleural space is generated by the forces developed during inspiration and expiration and is proportional to the amount of respiratory effort. The pleural pressure represents the driving pressure. During inspiration, the diaphragm and intercostal muscles contract and the pressure inside the thorax decreases below the atmospheric pressure (negative transpulmonary pressure gradient). This gradient is responsible for air movement from the nose (atmosphere) to the tracheobronchial tree down to the alveoli. During expiration, the inspiratory muscles relax, making resting expiration a passive phenomenon. However, during active expiration (volitional or during exercise), the contraction of abdominal and external intercostal muscles enhances the changes in intrathoracic pressure. This causes an abrupt increase in pleural pressure to a less-negative value, with a corresponding rise in alveolar pressure by the same amount. These changes generate a positive pressure gradient from the alveoli to the mouth, which is responsible for exhalation. Lung and chest volume decrease as air flows out, causing lung recoil pressure to fall until a new equilibrium is reached at FRC.

Respiratory rate, or breathing frequency, represents the number of breaths per minute. Average respiratory rate in a healthy adult subject at rest is approximatelyt 12 (range, 10 to

18) breaths/minute. Minute ventilation ($\dot{V}$) can be calculated using the following equation:

$$\dot{V} = V_T \times RR$$

where RR is the respiratory rate. During quiet breathing, a typical value is 6 L/minute, but the volume can rise to 180 L/minute during exercise.

Resistance

Different profiles of airflow may be observed inside the airways, depending on airway anatomy (in accordance with the specific division of the tracheobronchial tree) and mechanical properties (caliber, shape, collapsibility) of the airway structures and on the amount of driving pressure. With a constant laminar flow regimen, the resistance is directly proportional to the pressure gradient along the tube:

$$flow = \Delta P / R$$

where ΔP is the pressure difference and R is the resistance. Airflow is described as *turbulent* when the pressure drop along the airway is proportional to flow and its square values:

$$\Delta P \propto aV + bV^2$$

where ΔP is the pressure difference and V is the airflow. Airflow along airways is complex and usually consists of a mixture of laminar and turbulent flow. In normal lungs, respiratory resistance depends mainly on airway diameter. The velocity of airflow and airway diameter decrease in successive airway generations, from a maximum in the trachea to almost zero in the smallest bronchioles.

A third flow regimen is represented by flow limitation, whereby flow plateaus once the driving pressure has reached a given level. In this regimen, the flow value depends on the difference between intraluminal and extraluminal pressures, as well as on the compliance of the specific airway. Flow limitation can occur during expiration when the pressure generated by expiratory forces increases intraluminal pressure and induces an external compression of the airway walls at the same time. This pattern of flow is, however, more prone to be seen during inspiration at the level of the upper airway. Upper airway resistance depends on nasal and pharyngeal anatomy, position of the vocal cords, and lung volume (see later).

EFFECTS OF OBESITY AND BODY POSTURE ON LUNG VOLUMES

In an awake normal and healthy subject, a reduction in FRC and TLC is observed in the supine position in comparison with the upright position, both in adults[2] and in children.[3] This reduction is thought to be due to an increase in intrathoracic blood volume or to the gravitational effect of abdominal contents pushing the relaxed diaphragm into a more rostral position.[4] The change in diaphragm position reduces its ability to contract, as suggested by a decreased maximal inspiratory pressure in the supine posture relative to that in the upright and sitting positions.[5] Moreover, this restrictive defect in lung volume increases the work of breathing and deteriorates gas exchange by decreasing the ventilation-perfusion ratio in the dependent parts of the lungs. Decreased lung volume also can increase upper airway resistance by reducing the caudal traction of the mediastinum and trachea on the pharyngeal walls, making them more collapsible during inspiration (as discussed further later on).[6-9]

In obese subjects, a restrictive defect in lung volume also is observed in the sitting position. A further small decrease of 70 to 80 mL from approximately 2.4 L (for an average-sized man) in FRC and TLC occurs when obese subjects lie supine.[2] In view of the effects of abdominal volume on lung function in sitting obese subjects, a greater reduction in lung volume with adoption of the supine position compared with that in lean persons might be expected. However, a lesser decline in FRC and TLC in obese subjects in the supine position has been documented.[2,4,10] One possible explanation is that in sitting obese subjects, the diaphragm is already shifted in a more rostral position and cannot move much farther in the supine position. Two experimental studies also suggest a possible protective or adaptive mechanism against large changes in end-expiratory lung volume during wakefulness[11] and sleep.[12]

Maximal minute ventilation, expiratory reserve volume, FVC, and, to a lesser extent, forced expiratory volume in 1 second (FEV_1) also are affected by obesity.[13] The estimated reduction of FVC is 17.4 mL/kg weight gain for men and 10.6 mL/kg weight gain for women.[14] Men show more impairment of FVC with weight gain than women, possibly because of differential patterns of fat deposition: Waist circumference is negatively associated with FVC and FEV_1. On average, a 1-cm increase in waist circumference was associated with a 13-mL reduction in FVC.[15] All of these effects observed with change from the upright to the supine position and in obese persons may contribute to the exacerbation of respiratory disturbances in the presence of sleep-disordered breathing, as described in later chapters of this volume.

EFFECTS OF SLEEP ON LUNG VOLUME

A modest but significant decrease in FRC occurs during sleep in most healthy subjects. FRC decreases by approximately 200 mL in stage 2 non–rapid eye movement (NREM) sleep and by 300 mL during slow wave sleep and rapid eye movement (REM) sleep when measured with a helium dilution technique, in comparison with normal FRC obtained with the subject awake (approximately 2.4 L for an average-sized man).[16] When plethysmography is used to measure differences in lung volume, a 440- to 500-mL decrease in lung volume has been reported in NREM sleep (stages 2 to 4), with a similar decrease in REM sleep.[17] Possible mechanisms of the decrease in FRC during sleep are rostral displacement of the diaphragm secondary to diaphragmatic hypotonia, alteration of the respiratory timing from the central generator of breathing, decrease in lung compliance, decrease in thoracic compliance, and central pooling of blood.

A reduction in tidal volume by approximately 6% to 15% has been reported during NREM sleep (stages N2 and N3), with a further decrease during REM sleep (approximately 25% lower than during wakefulness).[18,19] Minute ventilation is significantly lower during all NREM sleep stages compared with wakefulness and decreases further during REM sleep, especially during phasic REM (approximately 84% of the level during wakefulness)[18-21] (Figure 8-3). The decrease presumably is due to a faster and shallower breathing pattern in all sleep stages with a lower tidal volume, especially during REM sleep. This explanation is, however, controversial, because another study showed no significant change in V_T between wakefulness and any sleep stage and suggested that the decrease in minute ventilation (8% in NREM and 4% in REM sleep) is due to a decrease in respiratory rate.[22] Nevertheless, most studies agree that during NREM sleep, the rib cage's contribution to V_T increases, in association with an approximately 34% increase in the activity of intercostal muscles.[21-23] There is thus an apparent contradiction between the increase in electromyogram (EMG) activity of thoracic muscles and a decrease in minute ventilation. A possible explanation is that even though muscle activity increases, the actual negative thoracic pressure decreases because of a decrease in the efficiency of muscle contraction during NREM sleep.[24] During REM sleep, the relative contribution of the rib cage and abdomen is not significantly different from that during wakefulness.[21] Age and sex do not seem to significantly alter sleep-related changes in lung volume.

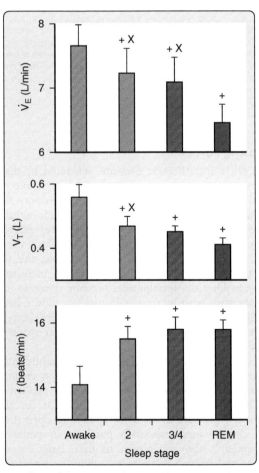

Figure 8-3 Effects of sleep on ventilation and lung volumes. Minute ventilation ($\dot{V}E$), tidal volume (V_T), and breathing frequency (f) during wakefulness and different sleep stages are illustrated. $\dot{V}E$ is reduced during NREM sleep, with a further reduction in REM sleep. +, $P < .05$ versus awake; X: $P < .05$ versus REM sleep. (Reproduced with permission from Douglas NJ, White DP, Pickett CK, et al. Respiration during sleep in normal man. *Thorax* 1982;37:840–4.)

EFFECTS OF SLEEP ON BREATHING PATTERN AND BLOOD GASES

During NREM sleep, the decrease in minute ventilation induces a drop in Pao_2 of 3 to 9 mm Hg and an increase in $Paco_2$ and $PAco_2$ levels ranging from 2 to 4 mm Hg.[25,26] During stable NREM sleep, the breathing pattern usually is regular. However, periodic breathing with waxing and waning ventilation commonly is observed at sleep onset (unstable NREM sleep).[27,28] Complete cessation of breathing for more than 10 seconds with respiratory effort (obstructive sleep apnea) or without respiratory effort (central sleep apnea) can even occur at this time in healthy persons. In these circumstances, the transient periodic breathing seems to be due to an unstable ventilatory feedback loop (loop gain). A low arousal threshold during this stage also can induce instability in the sleep-wake cycle and contribute to unstable breathing. Because of the higher CO_2 set point during sleep, arousals are associated with a sudden increase in ventilation, which will then decrease CO_2 level. If the CO_2 level is below the apnea threshold (below which the central respiratory drive is abolished) when sleep resumes, an apneic interval can occur and breathing will resume only when the CO_2 level again reaches the sleep set point. The magnitude and the breathing fluctuation depend on several factors such as chemoreceptor sensitivity (controller gain), lung-to-chemoreceptor circulation delay, and the efficiency of the respiratory system in inducing changes in CO_2 level (plant gain) (see also Chapter 7).[29] The relative effects of each loop gain component can be evaluated using a validated model.[30]

During REM sleep, ventilation is notably variable in both amplitude and frequency. This heterogeneity seems to be directly related to the intensity of phasic activity, as indicated by bursts of eye movements. Specifically, phasic REM activity, characterized by a high density of rapid eye movements and muscle twitches, seems to have an inhibitory influence on ventilation.[19] Overall alveolar ventilation tends to fall by approximately 20% compared with wakefulness, mainly because of a fall in tidal volume.[21]

Upper Airway

Among the mechanical determinants of ventilation just summarized, the upper airway plays a unique role because its mechanical properties are dramatically affected by sleep.

The airway can be divided into intrathoracic and extrathoracic components. These include the upper part of the trachea, the larynx, and the different pharyngeal (nasopharynx, velopharynx, orophrarynx, hypopharynx) segments. The upper airway corresponds to the pharyngeal and laryngeal structures. The airway should remain open throughout the respiratory cycle. The intrathoracic, tracheal, and laryngeal airway structures are supported by cartilaginous structures that prevent them from collapsing during tidal breathing in normal persons. Pharyngeal airways do not have such rigid support and are prone to close in conditions of imbalance between the forces that tend to dilate or close them.

From a mechanical standpoint, the upper airway behaves as a Starling resistor, in which the pharyngeal airway represents the collapsible segment and is situated between two noncollapsible structures (larynx and nasopharynx). The flow

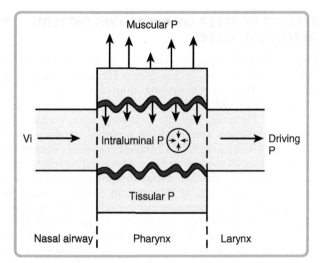

Figure 8-4 Schematic representation of the upper airway (UA) and of the forces applied to the pharyngeal airway. The muscular pressure represents the dilating force coming from the tonic and phasic activity of UA dilator muscles. The intraluminal pressure and the tissue pressure both tend to occlude the UA. P, Pressure; Vi, inspiratory flow volume.

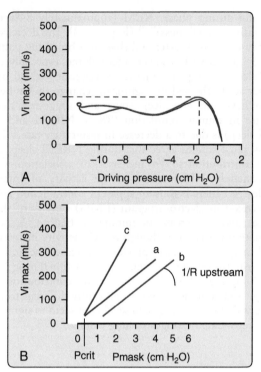

Figure 8-5 A, The *upper panel* is a representative example of the relationship between the respiratory flow over the driving pressure during a flow-limited breath. The instantaneous flow value reaches a maximum value and then plateaus despite the continuous decrease in driving pressure. **B,** Typical relationship between flow and upstream pressure during a series of flow-limited breaths. An increase in the instability of the upper airway will be accompanied by a right shift of the flow-pressure curve (slope b). A decrease in upstream resistance will increase the slope of the flow-pressure curve (slope c). Pcrit, Critical pressure; Pmask, mask pressure; 1/R upstream, reciprocal of upstream resistance; VImax, maximal inspiratory flow.

pattern depends on the forces applied inside and outside the collapsible segment. The transmural pressure gradient is the net pressure difference between all of these opposite forces. The collapsing forces are represented by the negative inspiratory transmural pressure gradient and the pressure applied by upper airway tissue (Figure 8-4). The contraction of upper airway stabilizing muscles (upper airway dilators) is the main dilating force, the other being represented by tracheal traction (Figure 8-4). Therefore the amount and timing of the neuromuscular activation process of upper airway stabilizing muscles and the mechanical properties of upper airway tissues play a pivotal role in determining upper airway stability.

According to the Starling resistance model,[31] inspiratory flow increases with rising inspiratory efforts (driving pressure) up to a maximal value and then plateaus independently of respiratory efforts (Figure 8-5, *A*). These features of the flow-pressure relationship characterize a flow limitation regimen. The steepness of the initial rise in flow depends on the resistance upstream and downstream of the collapsing site. The pressure at which flow begins to plateau depends on upper airway mechanical properties. The critical pressure (Pcrit) represents the pressure at which the dilating forces cannot overcome the collapsing ones, leading to upper airway closure. The changes in maximal inspiratory flow with modifying upstream pressure can be used to determine Pcrit and resistance upstream to the collapsing site. A linear positive relationship between these variables can be shown (Figure 8-5, *B*). The slope of the relationship corresponds to the reciprocal of upstream resistance, and the pressure at which flow is zero represents Pcrit. In a given subject, an increase in the propensity for the upper airway to occlude translates the flow-pressure relationship to the right, without changes in slope (i.e., slope a to slope b), making the Pcrit value more positive. In the situation of a decrease in upstream resistance, the steepness of the slope will rise (greater changes in flow occur with changing upstream pressure), but the Pcrit value will remain unchanged (i.e., slope a to slope c on Figure 8-5, *B*).

Collapsing Forces

The negative intrathoracic pressure generated by diaphragmatic contraction is transmitted to the whole airway, from the alveoli to the nose, to create inspiratory flow. At the pharyngeal level, the difference between intraluminal and peritissue pressures (transmural pressure) represents a suction force that tends to dynamically close the upper airway. According to the Bernoulli principle, the pressure along the walls of a tube drops with the increase in its velocity, making the intraluminal pressure decrease (become more negative) with increasing inspiratory flow. Changes in flow from a laminar to a turbulent pattern increase air velocity near airway walls, which will further reduce intraluminal pressure.

The weight of upper airway tissue significantly influences upper airway stability. In animals, upper airway critical pressure increases proportionally to the weight applied to the hyoid arch.[32] This correlation could account for the fact that positive pressure needs to be applied to open the upper airway during anesthesia with paralysis in patients with sleep apnea,[33] who are known to have large amounts of muscular and adipose tissue surrounding the upper airway.[34] See Chapter 20 for more information on anaesthesia effects in sleep apnea patients. On the other hand, negative pressure applied around the neck significantly unloads the upper airway,[35] and resection of upper airway tissue improves Pcrit in patients with sleep apnea.[36]

MUSCLES OF PHARYNX: LATERAL VIEW

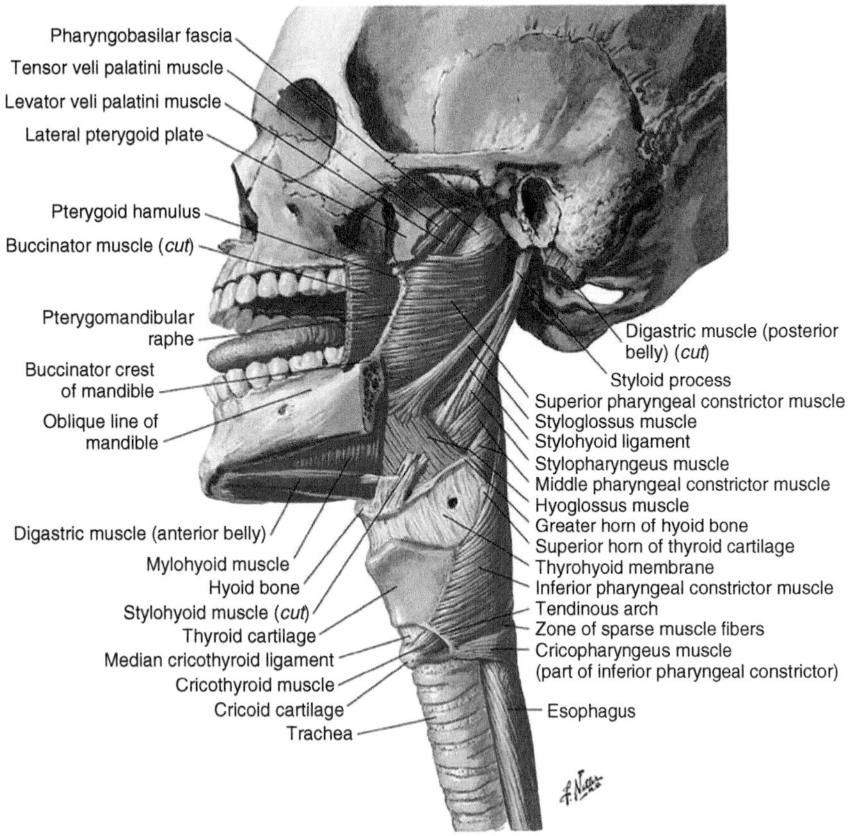

Figure 8-6 Drawing of upper airway muscles. (Reproduced from Netter FH. *Atlas of human anatomy.* Philadelphia: Saunders; 2006.)

Dilating Forces

Contraction of inspiratory muscles—diaphragm, intercostals, and accessory muscles—leads to lung inflation. The downward movement of the diaphragm produces a longitudinal traction of the bronchi and of the trachea. This traction is transmitted to the upper airway, where it contributes to unloading of that region.[37] From a dynamic perspective, tracheal traction improves upper airway stability by unfolding upper airway soft tissue and by decreasing extraluminal airway pressure.[38,39]

Numerous upper airway stabilizing muscles (such as the genioglossus, levator palatini, tensor palatini, geniohyoid, musculus uvulae, and palatopharyngeus) contribute to the maintenance of upper airway patency (Figure 8-6). Activation of masseter and pterygoid muscles also may contribute to stabilizing the upper airway by their influence on the position of the mouth and the mandible.[40] The activation profile of the upper airway muscles is characterized by their tonic activity and the respiratory-related and afferent reflex–mediated phasic activities.[41] This last factor is an important determinant of activity of the upper airway muscles, the negative pressure developed inside the upper airway having a positive feedback on muscle activity through activation of tensoreceptor and mechanoreceptor pathways.[42]

Tonic activity contributes to the maintenance of the upper airway aperture, its obligatory fall during sleep leading to a reduction in upper airway volume.[43,44] Inspiratory phasic activity has an automatic component that is linked with the central respiratory activity through projections of premotor inspiratory neurons to the hypoglossal motor nucleus.[45] Neuromodulators—serotonin, norepinephrine, glutamate, thyrotropin-releasing hormone, and substance P—play a key and complex role in the activity of upper airway muscles.[46-49] In lean animals, resting tonic and phasic activities of the genioglossus muscles mainly depend on endogenous norepinephrine, rather than serotonin drive on hypoglossal motor nucleus,[50,51] but these neuromodulators have similar stimulating effects.[50]

However, the influence of the serotonin drive on upper airway stabilizing muscle activity may be enhanced if upper airway patency is compromised, as demonstrated by the detrimental effects of serotonin antagonists (ritanserine) on upper airway caliber and stability, and on the occurrence on breathing abnormalities in animal models of obstructive sleep apnea.[52,53] Such changes in the balance of the norepinephrine-serotonin drive could result from facilitating hypoglossal nerve activities induced by intermittent hypoxia,[54] or from the relative vulnerability of norepinephrine and serotonin neurons to intermittent severe hypoxia.[55,56] Stimulation of peripheral chemoreceptors by intermittent hypoxia can lead to a prolonged rise in minute ventilation (long-term facilitation)[57,58] and a decrease in upper airway resistance (see also Chapter 7).[59,60] These ventilatory and upper airway facilitation effects are thought to be mediated by the serotonin-driven changes in activity of the phrenic and hypoglossal nerves[54,61] through plasticity. In humans, posthypoxia upper airway facilitation is observed during sleep in conditions of flow-limited breathing (as in snorers and persons with sleep apnea)[60,62] but is not observed during wakefulness[63-65] unless periodic desaturation is associated with hypercapnia.[66]

Apart from the influence of the extent of phasic activation of upper airway muscles, the dynamic profile of this phasic activity plays a key role in the maintenance of upper airway patency. Phasic activation of upper airway muscles precedes and reaches its peak value earlier than that of respiratory muscles.[67,68] Phasic activity and the preactivation delay increase with increasing central respiratory activity[67,69] and with decreasing upper airway pressure.[70] This activation pattern decreases upper airway resistance and prevents upper airway inspiratory collapse. The occurrence of upper airway obstruction in normal awake subjects when this preactivation of upper airway stabilizing muscles is lost (as with diaphragmatic pacing, phrenic nerve stimulation, or iron lung ventilation)[71] further supports the importance of the upper airway muscle preactivation pattern in maintaining upper airway patency. The link that exists between ventilatory and upper airway stability (see later on) could result from the common activation process of respiratory and upper airway stabilizing muscles originating from the central pattern generator that would be responsible for the fine tuning in the amplitude and activation pattern of these different muscle groups.

Another phasic component comes from the reflex activation of upper airway muscles linked with the decrease in upper airway pressure during inspiration.[70] Upper airway mechanoreceptor afferents contribute to modulation of the different components of upper airway muscle activity, as suggested by the effects of local anesthesia on tonic and phasic activities[72] and on genioglossus reflex–mediated negative pressure response.[73,74] Accordingly, modulating any of these components of the upper airway muscle activation profile can have an influence on upper airway patency[75,76] and stability.[77-80]

EFFECTS OF SLEEP ON UPPER AIRWAY MUSCLE ACTIVITY

The loss of wakefulness stimulus contributes to the sleep-induced decrease in upper airway muscle activity.[81] Tonic and phasic upper airway activities are significantly altered during sleep.[82-84] The impact of sleep on the activation profile of upper airway muscles differs among the various muscles. The tensor palatini has a tonic activity, but the genioglossus, palatoglossus, and levator palatini demonstrate phasic activities. These activity levels are higher during wakefulness, but only tensor palatini activity consistently falls at sleep onset.[85] The decrease in tensor palatini activity correlates with the sleep-induced rise in upper airway resistance, and a compensatory rise occurs in genioglossus activity.[85]

The tensor palatini and genioglossus muscles strongly differ in their response to negative airway pressure during both wakefulness and sleep,[86] with no correlation being found between tensor palatini activity and driving pressure. Even if tensor palatini and genioglossus activities are governed by different efferent motor fibers (trigeminal motor nucleus versus hypoglossal motor nucleus), both activities depend on central neuromodulator drive.[87,88] The preferential decrease in upper airway muscle tonic activity observed during sleep[89]

may relate to decrease in central excitatory drive to upper airway motor nuclei stemming from the loss of the awake corticomotor-stimulating drive and from a decrease in the stimulating effects of neuromodulators.[50,51,90,91] Sleep also may compromise upper airway stability by altering the pattern of preactivation of upper airway muscles.[92] The loss of such preactivation is associated with the rise in upper airway resistance and upper airway closure. The reappearance of alpha activity on the electroencephalogram (EEG) restores the normal preactivation pattern with a parallel drop in upper airway resistance and ventilatory resumption.

The neuromuscular activation processes of upper airway and respiratory muscles are closely linked. Tidal inspiration has a facilitating effect—increase in amplitude and reduction in latency of motor response—on diaphragm bulbospinal activity that is enhanced during sleep. This can be attributed to the loss of a wakefulness-related tonic depolarization of phrenic motor neurons, with secondary unmasking of the role of the bulbospinal command on the corticomotor excitability of the diaphragm. It is not known how sleep interacts with the facilitating effect of inspiration on upper airway muscle excitability.[93] On the other hand, some evidence indicates that breathing instability during sleep may promote upper airway closure.

Obstructive breathing disorders are mainly observed during stages N1 and N2 of NREM and REM sleep, when ventilation is physiologically unstable, and rarely during slow wave sleep, when breathing amplitude and frequency are particularly regular.[94] Breathing remains unstable (periodic) after resumption of upper airway obstruction with tracheostomy in patients with obstructive sleep apnea.[95] In normal sleeping subjects, the induction of periodic breathing can lead to partial upper airway obstruction.[96] Ventilatory stimulation with CO_2 decreases the occurrence of obstructed breaths in patients afflicted with sleep apnea.[97] In patients with a moderate increase in upper airway collapsibility, the frequency of obstructive sleep-disordered breathing correlates with the degree of breathing instability.[98]

FACTORS INFLUENCING STABILIZING AND COLLAPSING FORCES

For a given amount of upper airway neuromuscular outflow, the net mechanical effect of the neuromuscular activation process depends on the mechanical effectiveness of the contraction of upper airway stabilizing muscles.[99] Such function depends on factors such as the shape and dimensions of the upper airway. In fact, the amount of phasic activity required to maintain a given upper airway cross-sectional area increases when the upper airway axis converts from a transverse to an anteroposterior orientation.[100,101] Lung volumes influence upper airway dimension, as demonstrated by the decrease in pharyngeal cross-sectional area and the increase in upper airway resistance and collapsibility when lung volume decreases from TLC to residual volume.[102-104] Upper airway dimension also varies throughout the respiratory cycle, being maximal at the beginning of expiration and minimal at end expiration.[105] Vascular tone also interacts with upper airway collapsibility through its effect on upper airway dimension; the decrease in vascular tone or increase in vascular content decreases upper airway caliber but not upper airway collapsibility.[106] In these physiologic situations, various factors as described can interact with upper airway patency to favor obstruction of the upper airway if upper airway stability is already compromised (i.e., with a highly compliant upper airway).

The mechanical conditions that prevail during muscle contraction also determine the force the involved muscles can develop. The suctioning effect of negative intraluminal pressure can result in a lengthening of upper airway muscles during inspiration (eccentric contraction)[107] that interferes with their ability to dilate the upper airway and leads to upper airway muscle fatigue and structural damage.[108-110] The characteristics of the soft tissues surrounding the upper airway muscles also influence the ability of these muscles to improve upper airway patency, the increase in tissue stiffness impeding the transmission of the dilating force to the upper airway structure.[111]

CONCLUSIONS

Numerous factors are involved in the regulation of normal breathing, including a predominant role of different muscles such as respiratory and upper airway muscles as well as the mechanical conditions that determine the effectiveness of their contraction. Sleep can interfere with several determinants of normal ventilation such as ventilatory control, skeletal muscle activity, and lung volumes. Therefore, because of the influence of thoracopulmonary mechanics on upper airway patency and the close link between respiratory and upper airway muscles, sleep also has a strong impact on upper airway aperture and mechanical properties. Careful delineation of sleep-related changes in respiratory physiology is key to improving our knowledge of sleep-disordered breathing, because these principles are involved in all nocturnal breathing disturbances: hypoventilation, periodic breathing, central apnea, and upper airway closure.

CLINICAL PEARL

Numerous factors contribute to ventilation and mechanical properties of the thoracopulmonary system. Because sleep interacts with several of these factors, it has an impact on ventilation and gas exchanges through its effect on airway resistance, thoracopulmonary compliance, and lung volumes. As a consequence of its effect on upper airway muscle control and chest mechanics, sleep has a strong influence on upper airway stability. Accordingly, persons with compromised upper airway anatomy are at increased risk for development of obstructive sleep-induced disordered breathing, especially during the transition between wakefulness and sleep.

SUMMARY

The respiratory system can be divided into two compartments, the upper and lower airways. The mechanics of both compartments are strongly influenced by sleep. Lung volume, rib cage muscle activity, and minute ventilation tend to decrease during sleep, as does the activity of upper airway stabilizing muscles. The upper airway also plays a critical role in determining ventilation and breathing pattern during sleep. Its patency is influenced not only by pharyngeal and orofacial muscle activity but also by thoracopulmonary mechanics. Sleep therefore has a strong impact on upper airway aperture and mechanical properties. Even though obesity and susceptible pharyngeal anatomy are important contributors to the development of sleep-induced disordered breathing, sleep plays a key role in generating upper airway instability and therefore in determining the underlying pathophysiology.

Selected Readings

Bokov P, Essalhi M, Delclaux C. Loop gain in severely obese women with obstructive sleep apnoea. *Respir Physiol Neurobiol* 2016;**221**:49–53.

Deacon NL, Catcheside PG. The role of high loop gain induced by intermittent hypoxia in the pathophysiology of obstructive sleep apnoea. *Sleep Med Rev* 2015;**22**:3–14.

Deacon NL, Jen R, Li Y, Malhotra A. Treatment of Obstructive Sleep Apnea. Prospects for Personalized Combined Modality Therapy. *Ann Am Thorac Soc* 2016;**13**(1):101–8.

Dempsey JA, Veasey SC, Morgan BJ, O'Donnell CP. Pathophysiology of sleep apnea. *Physiol Rev* 2010;**90**:47–112.

Gederi E, Nemati S, Edwards B, et al. Model-based estimation of loop gain using spontaneous breathing: a validation study. *Respir Physiol Neurobiol* 2014;**201**:84–92.

Heinzer RC, Stanchina ML, Malhotra A, et al. Lung volume and continuous positive airway pressure requirements in obstructive sleep apnea. *Am J Respir Crit Care Med* 2005;**172**(1):114–17.

Horner RL, Hughes SW, Malhotra A. State-dependent and reflex drives to the upper airway: basic physiology with clinical implications. *J Appl Physiol* 2014;**116**:325–36.

Kim KT, Cho YW, Kim DE, et al. Two subtypes of positional obstructive sleep apnea: Supine-predominant and supine-isolated. *Clin Neurophysiol* 2016;**127**(1):565–70.

Series F, Cormier Y, Desmeules M. Influence of passive changes of lung volume on upper airways. *J Appl Physiol* 1990;**68**(5):2159–64.

Stanchina M, Robinson K, Corrao W, et al. Clinical use of loop gain measures to determine continuous positive airway pressure efficacy in patients with complex sleep apnea. A pilot study. *Ann Am Thorac Soc* 2015;**12**(9):1351–7.

Trinder J, Whitworth F, Kay A, Wilkin P. Respiratory instability during sleep onset. *J Appl Physiol* 1992;**73**(6):2462–9.

White DP, Younes MK. Obstructive sleep apnea. *Compr Physiol* 2012;**2**:2541–94.

A complete reference list can be found online at ExpertConsult.com.

Chapter

9

Sleep-Related Breathing Disorders: Classification

Richard B. Berry

Chapter Highlights

- This chapter presents a classification and clinical overview of sleep breathing disorders based on the recently published *International Classification of Sleep Disorders*, third edition (ICSD3).

- Diagnostic criteria for sleep-related breathing disorders in adults, including the obstructive sleep apnea disorder, central sleep apnea disorders, and sleep-related hypoventilation disorders, are provided based on the ICSD3.

- New additions to the ICSD3 classification of sleep-related breathing disorders include diagnostic criteria for the obesity

hypoventilation syndrome and treatment-emergent central sleep apnea.

- Out-of-center sleep testing (home sleep apnea testing) is now included in the diagnostic criteria for obstructive sleep apnea disorder in adults.

- Central sleep apnea with Cheyne-Stokes breathing is uniquely defined in the ICSD3 based on symptoms and comorbid conditions as well as polysomnographic findings.

- Areas of controversy and unresolved issues relating to the ICSD3 diagnostic classification of sleep-related breathing disorders are discussed.

This chapter presents a classification and clinical overview of sleep breathing disorders based on the recently published *International Classification of Sleep Disorders*, third edition (ICSD3).[1] The term *Sleep Related Breathing Disorders* is used throughout the text and tables of this chapter to conform to the ICSD3 terminology. The goal is to provide a summary of diagnostic criteria for the major disorders, with brief illustrative clinical cases for selected disorders. Box 9-1 lists the ICSD3 sleep related breathing disorder classification in adults; the *International Classification of Diseases*, 9th (ICD-9) and 10th (ICD-10) revisions' codes for each diagnosis are also listed. The ICSD3 provides a timely update of diagnostic criteria for sleep-related breathing disorders because the ICSD2 (second edition) was published in 2005. Where

appropriate, areas of controversy and unresolved issues are discussed.

Of note, the ICSD3 does not itself define sleep-related respiratory events, but instead refers to the most recent version of the *American Academy of Sleep Medicine (AASM) Manual for the Scoring of Sleep and Associated Events* (hereafter referred to as the AASM scoring manual).[2] Where relevant for understanding diagnostic criteria, the definition of selected respiratory events is reviewed. The fact that patients may fit into more than one diagnostic category of sleep-related breathing disorders is emphasized in the ICSD3.

The ICSD3 often uses the term *disorder* rather than *syndrome*. A disorder usually refers to a disease process for which a cause is known. In contrast, a syndrome is a

Obstructive Sleep Apnea Disorders
Obstructive Sleep Apnea, Adult (327.23) [G47.33]

Central Sleep Apnea Disorders*
Central Sleep Apnea with Cheyne-Stokes Breathing (786.04)
  [R06.3]
Central Sleep Apnea Due to a Medical Disorder without
  Cheyne-Stokes Breathing (327.27) [G47.37]
Central Sleep Apnea Due to High Altitude Periodic Breathing
  (327.22) [G47.32]
Central Sleep Apnea Due to a Medication or Substance
  (327.29) [G47.39]
Primary Central Sleep Apnea (327.21) [G47.31]
Treatment-Emergent Central Sleep Apnea (327.29) [G47.39]

Sleep-Related Hypoventilation Disorders
Obesity-Hypoventilation Syndrome (278.03) [E66.2]
Idiopathic Central Alveolar Hypoventilation (327.24) [G47.34]
Sleep Related Hypoventilation Due to Medication or Substance
  (327.26) [G47.36]
Sleep Related Hypoventilation Due to a Medical Disorder
  (327.26) [G47.36]

Sleep Related Hypoxemia Disorders
Sleep-Related Hypoxemia (327.26) [G47.36]

*In ICSD3, Central Sleep Apnea Syndromes (here, "disorders" is used for consistency).
ICD-9, *International Classification of Diseases*, 9th revision; ICD-10, *International Classification of Diseases*, 10th revision; ICSD3, *International Classification of Sleep Disorders*, 3rd edition.

constellation of symptoms. In general, use of disorder versus syndrome is somewhat arbitrary and often variable in the medical literature. For example, the term *congenital central hypoventilation syndrome* continues to be used in the literature although the genetic cause has been identified (mutation in *PHOX2B* gene).

OBSTRUCTIVE SLEEP APNEA DISORDERS

In the ICSD3, obstructive sleep apnea (OSA) disorders are classified separately as adult and pediatric. However, this chapter refers solely to adult disorders. OSA is classified as a disorder in the ICSD3. One could argue that OSA is better described as a syndrome because the pathophysiology may be structural in one patient and due to unstable respiratory control in another patient.[3] It is to be noted that the term *obstructive sleep apnea syndrome* is frequently used in the literature.

The adult OSA diagnostic criteria currently include a provision for use of both in-center polysomnography (PSG) and out-of-center sleep testing (OCST), in which sleep is usually not recorded. OCST has also been termed *portable monitoring*, *home sleep testing*, and *home sleep apnea testing*. Obstructive respiratory events in sleep that account for the diagnosis of adult OSA include obstructive and mixed apneas, hypopneas, and respiratory effort–related arousals (RERAs). The ICSD3 does not provide a definition for these events. A summary of such respiratory event definitions as defined by the AASM scoring manual is provided in Box 9-2. There are currently two hypopnea definitions in the manual ("recommended" and "acceptable"). Of note, if sleep is not recorded, hypopneas must be scored based on airflow attenuation and arterial

Apnea
1. Score a respiratory event as an apnea when *both* of the following criteria are met:
   a. There is a drop in the peak signal excursion by ≥90% of pre-event baseline using an oronasal thermal sensor (diagnostic study), positive airway pressure (PAP) device flow (titration study), or alternative apnea sensor (diagnostic study).
   b. The duration of the ≥90% drop in sensor signal is ≥10 seconds.
2. Score an apnea as obstructive if it meets apnea criteria and is associated with continued or increased inspiratory effort throughout the entire period of absent airflow.
3. Score an apnea as central if it meets apnea criteria and is associated with absent inspiratory effort throughout the entire period of absent airflow.
4. Score an apnea as mixed if it meets apnea criteria and is associated with absent inspiratory effort in the initial portion of the event, followed by resumption of inspiratory effort in the second portion of the event.

Hypopnea
1A. Score a respiratory event as a hypopnea if *all* of the following criteria are met (**RECOMMENDED**):
   a. The peak signal excursions drop by ≥30% of pre-event baseline using nasal pressure (diagnostic study), PAP

device flow (titration study), or an alternative hypopnea sensor (diagnostic study).
   b. The duration of the ≥30% drop in signal excursion is ≥10 seconds.
   c. There is ≥3% oxygen desaturation from pre-event baseline, or the event is associated with an arousal.
1B. Score a respiratory event as a hypopnea if *all* of the following criteria are met (**ACCEPTABLE**):
   a. The peak signal excursions drop by ≥30% of pre-event baseline using nasal pressure (diagnostic study), PAP device flow (titration study), or an alternative hypopnea sensor (diagnostic study).
   b. The duration of the ≥30% drop in signal excursion is ≥10 seconds.
   c. There is a ≥4% oxygen desaturation from pre-event baseline.

Respiratory Effort–Related Arousal
Score a respiratory event as a respiratory effort-related arousal (RERA) if there is a sequence of breaths lasting ≥10 seconds characterized by increasing respiratory effort or by flattening of the inspiratory portion of the nasal pressure (diagnostic study) or PAP device flow (titration study) waveform leading to arousal from sleep when the sequence of breaths *does not meet criteria for an apnea or hypopnea.*

Adapted from Berry RB, Brooks R, Gamaldo CE, et al, for the American Academy of Sleep Medicine. *The AASM manual for the scoring of sleep and associated events: rules, terminology and technical specifications.* Version 2.2. www.aasmnet.org. Darien, Illinois: American Academy of Sleep Medicine, 2015.

oxygen desaturation criteria alone because there is an inability to score arousals from sleep without documentation of sleep.

The most recent version of the AASM scoring manual defines the apnea-hypopnea index (AHI) as the number of apneas and hypopneas per hour of sleep; the respiratory disturbance index is defined as the AHI plus the number of RERAs per hour of sleep. If OCST is performed, sleep is usually not recorded, and the diagnostic metric is the number of apneas and hypopneas per hour of monitoring time (sometimes called the *respiratory event index*). The ICSD3 does not define the terms *AHI*, *RDI*, or *respiratory event index*.

Diagnostic criteria for OSA (Box 9-3) require either 15 or more obstructive respiratory events per hour of sleep using PSG (or per hour of monitoring using OCST) *or* a combination of symptoms, manifestations, and comorbidities (see later) and at least 5 but less than 15 obstructive respiratory events per hour of sleep (PSG) or per hour of monitoring if OCST is used. The rationale is that patients with 15 or more obstructive respiratory events per hour are thought to have a clinically significant disorder even if symptoms are absent. The best evidence for increased risk for cardiovascular morbidity is in patients with more than 30 obstructive respiratory events per hours of sleep.[4] In the case of at least 5 but less than 15 obstructive respiratory events per hour, the clinician may be concerned about overdiagnosis in an asymptomatic patient without a significant clinical disorder. The requirement of symptoms in the milder range of an increased AHI (or RDI) will exclude asymptomatic patients. The clinical significance of an AHI (or respiratory disturbance index

[RDI]) in the mild range must be evaluated by the clinician, taking into account symptoms as well as comorbid cardiovascular conditions. Certainly, symptomatic patients with an AHI (RDI) in the mild range may experience benefit from treatment of OSA.[4]

Identification of RERAs is adjudicated based on associated arousal rather than oxygen desaturation and therefore requires the recording of sleep (i.e., PSG). Hypopneas are included as OSA respiratory events without specific determination as to whether they are obstructive or nonobstructive (i.e., central). It is emphasized that symptoms and comorbid conditions thought to be associated with or adversely affected by the presence of OSA are required for the diagnosis if the index of obstructive events is equal to or greater than 5 per hour but less than 15 per hour (see Box 9-3). Such comorbid conditions qualifying a patient for a diagnosis of OSA include systemic hypertension, a mood disorder, cognitive dysfunction, coronary artery disease, stroke, congestive heart failure, atrial fibrillation, type 2 diabetes mellitus, nocturia, and erectile dysfunction.

Although a major study published in 1993 found OSA prevalence (defined as symptoms *and* AHI ≥5 per hour) to be 2% in women and 4% in adult men,[5] the current prevalence of OSA is believed to be much higher, likely because of increased prevalence of obesity.[6] The prevalence of OSA, in fact, varies with the characteristics of the population studied and respiratory event definitions.[4] Note that although patients with obesity-hypoventilation syndrome are currently classified under the sleep-related hypoventilation disorders (see later), 80% to 90% of patients so classified also meet diagnostic criteria for OSA.

There is continuing controversy concerning the most appropriate definition of hypopnea.[4] The current AASM scoring manual *acceptable* definition of hypopnea, a 30% or greater drop in airflow plus 4% or greater arterial oxygen desaturation (see Box 9-2), is consistent with that accepted by the Centers for Medicare and Medicaid Services. The recommended definition of hypopnea is based on a lesser degree of oxygen desaturation (≥3%) or the presence of an associated arousal, or both. The AHI-acceptable and AHI-recommended terminology will be used here to denote the AHI determined using either the acceptable hypopnea (H-acceptable) or recommended hypopnea (H-recommended) definition. Note that, because RERAs by definition do not meet diagnostic criteria for hypopnea,[2] classification of a given event as RERA versus hypopnea often depends on the definition of hypopnea that is used to score events. For example, an event characterized by flattening of the airflow profile with a 30% reduction in flow for 15 seconds followed by a 2% arterial oxygen desaturation and an arousal would meet diagnostic criteria for H-recommended but not H-acceptable. If hypopneas are scored based on criteria for H-acceptable, the event would meet criteria for RERA. If one uses the ICSD3 criteria, which include the RERA index as part of the diagnostic metric (e.g., AHI-acceptable + RERA index), a wider spectrum of patients will be diagnosed as having OSA than using AHI-acceptable. The addition of the RERA index will diagnose patients often labeled as having the upper airway resistance syndrome as having OSA. These patients report symptoms due to respiratory arousals but do not have significant arterial oxygen desaturation.[4] Of note, upper airway resistance syndrome is not included in the ICSD3 diagnostic criteria; such patients are

---

Box 9-3 ICSD3 DIAGNOSTIC CRITERIA: OBSTRUCTIVE SLEEP APNEA, ADULT

(A and B) or C satisfy the criteria.
A. The presence of one or more of the following:
   1. The patient complains of sleepiness, nonrestorative sleep, fatigue, or insomnia symptoms.
   2. The patient wakes with breath holding, gasping, or choking.
   3. The bed partner or other observer reports habitual snoring, breathing interruptions, or both during the patient's sleep.
   4. The patient has been diagnosed with hypertension, a mood disorder, cognitive dysfunction, coronary heart disease, stroke, congestive heart failure, atrial fibrillation, or type 2 diabetes mellitus.
B. Polysomnography (PSG) or out-of-center sleep testing (OCST*) demonstrates:
   1. Five or more obstructive respiratory events[†] (i.e., obstructive or mixed apneas, hypopneas, or respiratory effort–related arousals [RERAs])[‡] per hour of sleep during PSG or per hour of monitoring (OCST*)
   or
C. PSG or OCST* demonstrates:
   1. Fifteen or more obstructive respiratory events[†] (i.e., obstructive or mixed apneas, hypopneas, or RERAs)[‡] per hour of sleep during PSG or per hour of monitoring (OCST*)

*OCST may underestimate the true number of obstructive respiratory events per hour because actual sleep is not usually recorded.
[†]Respiratory events defined according the latest version of the *AASM Manual for the Scoring of Sleep and Associated Events*.
[‡]RERAs cannot be scored using OCST because arousals cannot be identified.

thought to have a variant of OSA (see Chapter 14, Snoring and Pathologic Upper Airway Resistance Syndromes). If the H-recommended definition is used, most events scored as RERAs when using H-acceptable would meet criteria for H-recommended such that AHI-acceptable + RERA index ≈ AHI-recommended.[4] Data indicate that using a diagnostic metric including RERAs or an AHI-recommended will identify an increased percentage of individuals studied as having OSA.

The following clinical case illustrates the hypopnea definition issue. A thin 30-year-old man reported loud snoring and daytime sleepiness. A diagnostic PSG recorded 420 minutes of sleep, during which there were 10 obstructive apneas, 10 hypopneas (H-acceptable definition) and 40 RERAs. The AHI was therefore 2.8/hour, and the RDI was 8.6 per hour. Many of the events scored as RERAs were associated with a 1% or 2% drop in the oxygen saturation. Using the AHI-acceptable as a diagnostic metric, the patient does not have the OSA disorder. If the same sleep study were scored using the recommended rather than the acceptable hypopnea definition, 10 obstructive apneas, 45 hypopneas, and 5 RERAs would be scored, and the AHI would be 7.8 per hour (the RDI would have continued to be 8.6 per hour). A diagnosis of OSA would then be possible (if associated with symptoms/comorbidity). This assumes that 35 of the 40 RERA events were associated with a 30% or greater drop in flow as well as inspiratory flattening for at least 10 seconds.

CENTRAL SLEEP APNEA DISORDERS

Patients with the central sleep apnea (CSA) disorders are a diverse group with a wide spectrum of etiologies.[7,8] Many of the diagnostic entities associated with CSA are associated with either unknown or multiple etiologies. The common finding is absence of airflow and respiratory effort (central apnea) or reduced airflow and respiratory effort without clear evidence of partially obstructed breathing (e.g., inspiratory airflow signal flattening or paradoxic thoracoabdominal respiratory effort [central hypopnea], or both). In the AASM scoring manual,[2] scoring hypopneas as central or obstructive is noted as an option, with the following specifications: hypopnea is scored as obstructive if any of the following are present: there is snoring during the event; there is increased inspiratory flattening of the nasal pressure or positive airway pressure (PAP) device flow signal compared with baseline breathing; or there is an associated thoracoabdominal paradox that occurs during the event but not during pre-event breathing. A hypopnea is scored as central if none of these are present. The option for scoring hypopneas as central was added because some patients with CSA have a significant proportion of events that are central hypopneas.[4,9,10] Further, a number of large clinical trials of patients with CSA have included central hypopneas in the inclusion criteria.[9,10]

Some clinicians have proposed that the CSA disorders can be categorized on the basis of the disorder being associated with awake- or sleep-associated hypocapnia (i.e., high ventilatory drive) and normocapnia or hypercapnia (i.e., normal or low ventilatory drive).[7] Primary CSA, CSA with Cheyne-Stokes breathing (CSB), CSA due to high-altitude periodic breathing, and treatment emergent CSA are thought to occur because the sleeping arterial partial pressure of carbon dioxide ($Paco_2$) is below the apneic threshold (AT)—the $Paco_2$ value below which there is no ventilatory effort.[7] High hypercapnic ventilatory drive (both awake and during sleep) characterizes such patients and is associated with a small difference between the sleeping $Paco_2$ and the AT (delta $Paco_2$). While awake, such patients have a normal or low $Paco_2$. The low awake or sleeping $Paco_2$ does not cause the small delta $Paco_2$ but rather is a marker of high ventilatory drive. CSA due to a medical disorder without CSB and CSA due to a medication or substance are thought to be associated with normal or low ventilatory drive.

Central Sleep Apnea with Cheyne-Stokes Breathing

In the ICSD2,[11] this entity was listed as CSB pattern without a requirement for symptoms or associated conditions. One could argue that diagnostic criteria for a breathing *pattern* would be more appropriately defined in the scoring manual rather than in the classification of sleep disorders. As defined in the ICSD3, central sleep apnea with Cheyne-Stokes breathing (CSA-CSB) is a clinical disorder rather than simply a PSG finding (Box 9-4),[1] with the main rationale being that the identification of patients with CSA-CSB, which is a very common disorder, has clinical implications, including etiology (most have congestive heart failure) and prognosis.[12] Thus symptoms (sleepiness, insomnia, awakening short of breath, snoring, witnessed apneas) or the presence of comorbid conditions (atrial fibrillation, congestive heart failure, or a neurologic disorder), or both, are required in the ICSD3 for a diagnosis of CSA-CSB. CSA-CSB is common in patients with both stable and decompensated congestive heart failure[13] and can occur following a cerebrovascular accident.[14-16] Renal failure has also been associated with CSA-CSB, although such documentation in the literature is very limited.[17] Patients with idiopathic CSA-CSB have also been reported.[18]

Box 9-4   ICSD3 DIAGNOSTIC CRITERIA: CENTRAL SLEEP APNEA WITH CHEYNE-STOKES BREATHING

(A or B) + C + D satisfy the criteria.
A. The presence of one or more of the following:
   1. Sleepiness
   2. Difficulty initiating or maintaining sleep, frequent awakenings, or nonrestorative sleep
   3. Awakening short of breath
   4. Snoring
   5. Witnessed apneas
B. The presence of atrial fibrillation/flutter, congestive heart failure, or a neurologic disorder
C. Polysomnography (PSG) (during diagnostic or positive airway pressure titration) shows all of the following:
   1. Five or more central apneas or central hypopneas per hour of sleep
   2. The total number of central apneas and/or central hypopneas is >50% of the total number of apneas and hypopneas
   3. The pattern of ventilation meets criteria for Cheyne-Stokes breathing
D. The disorder is not better explained by another current sleep disorder, medication use (e.g., narcotics), or substance use disorder

In the current AASM scoring manual,[2] CSA-CSB (the respiratory event, not the clinical disorder) is scored when both of the following criteria are met:

1. Three or more consecutive central apneas or central hypopneas, or both, separated by a crescendo and decrescendo change in breathing amplitude with a cycle length of at least 40 seconds
2. Five or more central apneas or central hypopneas, or both, per hour of sleep associated with the crescendo and decrescendo breathing pattern recorded over at least 2 hours of monitoring.

The ICSD3 criteria for CSA-CSB are listed in Box 9-4. If central apneas of CSB morphology as defined previously are *not* frequent enough to be more than 50% of the total respiratory events, CSB is simply listed as a PSG finding. Note that CSA-CSB and OSA diagnoses may coexist in a patient who meets PSG and clinical criteria for both. Further, as per the ICSD3, diagnostic criteria for CSA-CSB may be met during *either a diagnostic PSG or PAP titration.* Many patients with CSA-CSB associated with heart failure have a significant number of both obstructive and central apneas,[13] and the predominance of obstructive versus central events may vary over time or during the night[19] in a given patient. If a patient with a mixture of obstructive and central events is placed on continuous positive airway pressure (CPAP), with titration specifically for the OSA, central events, including outright CSA-CSB, may persist after obstructive events have resolved.

A typical clinical example is the following. A 50-year-old man with a history of witnessed apnea, snoring, atrial fibrillation, and congestive heart failure underwent diagnostic and therapeutic PSG. During the diagnostic portion of the study, 120 minutes of sleep were recorded. The AHI was 30/hour with 40 obstructive apneas, 10 mixed apneas, and 10 central apneas. Typical obstructive and mixed events in this patient are shown in Figure 9-1, *A.* During the CPAP titration portion of the PSG, 300 minutes of sleep were recorded, with an AHI of 15/hour, 15 obstructive apneas, 50 central apneas, and 10 hypopneas (adjudicated as obstructive). The central AHI was 10/hour, and central events composed more than 50% of the respiratory events on CPAP. A typical period of

central apnea, in fact central apnea with CSB, in this patient is shown in Figure 9-1, *B.* This patient meets diagnostic criteria for OSA (diagnostic portion) and CSA-CSB (the CPAP titration portion). The clinical implications of such results remain to be defined; presumably, the patient continues to carry the cardiovascular morbidity and mortality associations of CSA-CSB in this setting.

Central Sleep Apnea Due to a Medical Disorder without Cheyne-Stokes Breathing

CSA that is attributed to a medical disorder, but does not have the characteristic periodic breathing pattern of CSB, is classified as CSA due to a medical disorder without Cheyne-Stokes breathing (Box 9-5). Here the term *medical disorder* is used as an all-inclusive nomenclature that includes cardiovascular, respiratory, and neurologic conditions; however, most of these patients have brainstem lesions of developmental, vascular, neoplastic, degenerative, demyelinating, or traumatic origin. Examples of such neurologic conditions that are typically associated with CSA without CSB include prior cerebrovascular accident (CVA),[14-16] Chiari malformation,[20] brainstem neoplasms, and multiple system atrophy.[21] A predominance of OSA versus CSA is more common after a CVA.[15] However, many post-CVA patients have a mixture of OSA and CSA; CSA following CVA can be present with and without a pattern of CSB.

Patients classified in the diagnostic category of CSA without CSB may have awake or sleep-related hypoventilation, or both. Further, in such patients, if diagnostic criteria for CSA and sleep-related hypoventilation are met (see later), both diagnoses are made (i.e., CSA *and* sleep–related hypoventilation).

Central Sleep Apnea Due to High-Altitude Periodic Breathing

Periodic breathing during sleep is a common response to altitude. Typically, an altitude of at least 2500 meters (8202 feet) is required for such periodic breathing to be present. However, some individuals may exhibit the disorder at

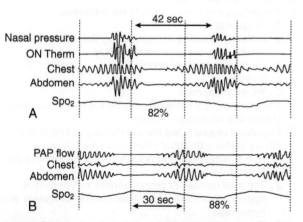

Figure 9-1 Respiratory events during a diagnostic **(A)** and positive airway pressure sleep study **(B).** The middle event in the top tracing is a "mixed" apnea; the flanking events are "obstructive" apneas. Central apneas with Cheyne-Stokes breathing are shown in the lower tracing. The patient was on continuous positive airway pressure of 12 cm H_2O. ON Therm, Oronasal thermal flow sensor; PAP, positive airway pressure.

Box 9-5   ICSD3 DIAGNOSTIC CRITERIA: CENTRAL APNEA DUE TO MEDICAL DISORDER WITHOUT CHEYNE-STOKES BREATHING

Criteria A to C must be met:
A. The presence of one or more of the following:
   1. Sleepiness
   2. Difficulty initiating or maintaining sleep, frequent awakenings, or nonrestorative sleep
   3. Awakening short of breath
   4. Snoring
   5. Witnessed apneas
B. Polysomnography (PSG) shows all of the following:
   1. Five or more central apneas and/or or central hypopneas per hour of sleep
   2. The number of central apneas and/or central hypopneas is >50% of the total number of apneas and hypopneas
   3. Absence of Cheyne-Stokes breathing
C. The disorder occurs as a consequence of a medical or neurologic disorder but is not due to medication use or substance use.

> **Box 9-6 ICSD3 DIAGNOSTIC CRITERIA: CENTRAL SLEEP APNEA DUE TO HIGH-ALTITUDE PERIODIC BREATHING**
>
> Criteria A to D must be met:
> A. Recent ascent to high altitude*
> B. The presence of one or more of the following:
>   1. Sleepiness
>   2. Difficulty initiating or maintaining sleep, frequent awakenings, or nonrestorative sleep
>   3. Awakening with shortness of breath or morning headache
>   4. Witnessed apnea
> C. The symptoms are clinically attributable to high-altitude periodic breathing, or polysomnography, if performed, demonstrates recurrent central apneas or hypopneas primarily during non–rapid eye movement sleep at a frequency of ≥5/hour.
> D. The disorder is not better explained by another current sleep disorder, medical or neurologic disorder, medication use (e.g., narcotics), or substance use disorders.
>
> *Typically at least 2500 meters (8202 feet), although some individuals may exhibit the disorder at altitudes as low as 1500 meters.

> **Box 9-7 ICSD3 DIAGNOSTIC CRITERIA: CENTRAL SLEEP APNEA DUE TO A MEDICATION OR SUBSTANCE**
>
> Criteria A to E must be met:
> A. The patient is taking an opioid or other respiratory depressant.
> B. The presence of one or more of the following:
>   1. Sleepiness
>   2. Difficulty initiating or maintaining sleep, frequent awakenings, or nonrestorative sleep
>   3. Awakening short of breath
>   4. Snoring
>   5. Witnessed apneas
> C. Polysomnography (PSG; diagnostic or on positive airway pressure) shows all of the following:
>   1. Five or more central apneas and/or central hypopneas per hour of sleep (PSG)
>   2. The number of central apneas and/or central hypopneas is >50% of the total number of apneas and hypopneas
>   3. Absence of Cheyne-Stokes breathing
> D. The disorder occurs as a consequence of an opioid or other respiratory depressant.
> E. The disorder is not better explained by another current sleep disorder.

altitudes as low as 1500 meters. There are no specified levels of central AHI (central apneas or central hypopneas per hour) nor frequency of episodes of periodicity of breathing that clinically separate a normal from an abnormal response to altitude. The ICSD3 diagnostic criteria require 5 or more central events per hour of sleep *and* associated symptoms to make the diagnosis of CSA due to high-altitude periodic breathing (Box 9-6). The cycle length of this periodic breathing is commonly less than 40 seconds and often as short as 12 to 20 seconds.[22,23] The periodic breathing present at altitude does *not* specifically meet the criteria for CSB as defined earlier. A diagnosis of CSA due to high-altitude period breathing may be made concomitantly with a diagnosis of OSA if criteria for each of these are clearly present. A study by Pagel and colleagues[24] of sleep study results at three sleep centers at progressively higher altitudes found that central apnea becomes significantly more common at increasing altitude in both the diagnostic and treatment portions of PSG in patients with OSA, with an apparent exponential increase in the percentage of OSA patients with a central apnea index greater than 5 occurring with increasing altitude.

Central Sleep Apnea Due to a Medication or Substance

Patients with this diagnosis have CSA adjudicated as secondary to an opioid medication or other respiratory depressant (Box 9-7). The condition has been described in patients taking methadone and long-acting forms of morphine or oxycodone as well as individuals being treated with fentanyl patches or continuous narcotic infusions.[25] Suboxone (a combination of buprenorphine and naloxone) is often used for treatment of patients with narcotic dependence and pain and can also be associated with central apnea. Patients taking these medications can also manifest OSA and ataxic breathing. In addition, some patients may exhibit mostly obstructive respiratory events during a diagnostic study but mainly central events on positive airway pressure, and the required frequency of central events to meet diagnostic criteria for this entity may be present

on either a diagnostic or PAP PSG. Although most patients with this disorder have normal or only mildly elevated awake values of $Paco_2$, some manifest sleep-related hypoventilation (see later) as well as central apneas. If sleep-related hypoventilation is present, a diagnosis of sleep-related hypoventilation due to a medication or substance is made *in addition to* a diagnosis of CSA due to a medication or substance.

Primary Central Sleep Apnea

Primary CSA, which has also been referred to as *idiopathic CSA*, is a disorder of unknown etiology and is characterized by recurrent central apneas that do not have CSB morphology (Box 9-8) or a specific known etiology. Primary CSA is believed to occur because the sleeping arterial $Paco_2$ is below the AT,[26,27] as discussed previously. High hypercapnic ventilatory drive (both awake and during sleep) characterizes such patients; while awake, they therefore have a normal or low $Paco_2$. The reason for the high ventilatory drive in patients with primary CSA is unknown.

Clinical manifestations of primary CSA typically include daytime sleepiness, insomnia, awakening short of breath, and witnessed apneas. PSG diagnostic criteria include the requirement that there must be 5 or more central apneas or central hypopneas per hour of sleep and that central, rather than obstructive, events make up greater than 50% of the total number of scored respiratory events. Further, the central apneas or hypopneas cannot, by definition, occur with the periodic breathing morphology of CSB. If the central apnea is believed to be due to a medical or neurologic condition or to a medication, then a diagnosis of primary CSA is not made. Primary CSA is a diagnosis based on *exclusion of identifiable causes of this pattern of breathing*. Clinical implications regarding etiology and sequelae of this disorder are not clear.

A typical clinical example is the following. A 30-year-old man underwent a PSG to evaluate complaints of snoring, witnessed breathing pauses, and mild daytime sleepiness. The PSG showed a total sleep time of 420 minutes and an AHI of 15/hour. There were 20 obstructive apneas and 85 central apneas. The central apneas did not have a Cheyne-Stokes morphology, although runs of central apneas did occur, most commonly associated with stages 1 and 2 non–rapid eye movement sleep (Figure 9-2). The patient was taking no medications and was otherwise healthy. Magnetic resonance imaging revealed no structural lesion of the brainstem (note that such a lesion would define the disorder as CSA due to a medical disorder without CSB).

Treatment-Emergent Central Sleep Apnea

Treatment-emergent CSA as defined in the ICSD3 is similar to a phenomenon described in the medical literature as complex sleep apnea. In this situation, a patient with predominantly obstructive respiratory events (obstructive and mixed apneas or hypopneas) during a diagnostic PSG manifests predominantly central respiratory events (persistent or emergent) on PAP treatment (CPAP, or bilevel PAP without a backup rate) after the obstructive events have resolved.[28]

This remains an area of controversy[29] because some clinicians consider all patients manifesting the pattern described previously as having complex sleep apnea (or TE-CSA), whereas others reserve the diagnosis of TE-CSA for patients in whom a clear diathesis for CSA is not present. A diagnosis of treatment emergent CSA as defined in ICSD3 (Box 9-9) is more specific than the typically applied terminology of complex sleep apnea because it requires that the CSA present during a PAP sleep study *not be* better explained by another CSA disorder or diathesis (e.g., CSA-CSB or CSA due to a medication or substance). Perhaps a more accurate term would be *idiopathic treatment emergent CSA*, when a reason or even risk for the phenomenon is unclear; in any event, the current term has clinical importance and specificity in that CSA has been reported to be present in 2% to 20% of patients in whom PAP is initiated,[28-29] whereas the TE-CSA as defined by the ICSD3 is believed to resolve with chronic PAP treatment in most patients.

In contrast, patients with complex sleep apnea associated with opioids and patients with CSB-CSA and heart failure each are less likely to experience resolution of CSA with chronic CPAP.[30,31,32] Although about 50% of patients with CSA-CSB due to heart failure will respond to the first night of exposure to CPAP, after 3 months about 43% still have an AHI greater than 15/hour.[30] However, the long-term

---

Box 9-8   ICSD3 DIAGNOSTIC CRITERIA: PRIMARY CENTRAL SLEEP APNEA

Criteria A to D must be met:
A. The presence of at least one of the following:
   1. Sleepiness
   2. Difficulty initiating or maintaining sleep, frequent awakenings, or nonrestorative sleep
   3. Awakening short of breath
   4. Snoring
   5. Witnessed apneas
B. Polysomnography demonstrates all of the following:
   1. Five or more central apneas or central hypopneas per hour of sleep
   2. The total number of central apneas and/or central hypopneas is >50% of the total number of apneas and hypopneas
   3. Absence of Cheyne-Stokes breathing
C. There is no evidence of daytime or nocturnal hypoventilation.
D. The disorder is not better explained by another current sleep disorder, medical or neurologic disorder, medication use, or substance use disorder.

Box 9-9   ICSD3 DIAGNOSTIC CRITERIA: TREATMENT EMERGENT CENTRAL SLEEP APNEA

Criteria A to C must be met:
A. Diagnostic polysomnography (PSG) shows five or more predominantly obstructive respiratory events (obstructive or mixed apneas, hypopneas, or respiration effort–related arousals [RERAs]) per hour of sleep.
B. PSG during use of positive airway pressure without a backup rate shows significant resolution of obstructive events and emergence or persistence of central apnea or central hypopnea with all of the following:
   i. Central apnea–central hypopnea index [CAHI] ≥5/hour
   ii. Number of central apneas and central hypopneas is ≥50% of total number of apneas and hypopneas
C. The central sleep apnea (CSA) is not better explained by another CSA disorder (e.g., CSA with Cheyne-Stokes breathing or CSA due to a medication or substance).

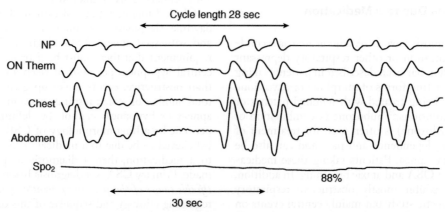

Figure 9-2 Central apneas in a patient without an apparent cause of central apnea. Note that the cycle length of the central events is less than 30 seconds. NP, Nasal pressure; ON Therm, oronasal thermal flow sensor.

morbidity associated with the diagnosis of treatment emergent CSA (ICSD3 criteria) and the pathophysiology have not been defined. Patients with persistent CSA on chronic CPAP treatment may not experience benefit from PAP treatment and may fail to be adherent to CPAP.

An illustrative clinical example of treatment emergent CSA is follows. A 50-year-old man underwent a PSG to evaluate complaints of snoring, daytime sleepiness, and witnessed apnea. He was being treated for systemic hypertension, had no history of heart failure, and was not taking opioid medications. During the diagnostic portion of the PSG, 120 minutes of sleep were recorded, with an AHI of 40/hour, including 55 obstructive apneas, 5 central apneas, and 20 hypopneas. During the CPAP titration, 300 minutes of sleep were recorded, with a final overall AHI of 20/hour. Respiratory events consisted of 10 obstructive apneas, 10 hypopneas (uncharacterized as central or obstructive), and 80 central apneas. The central apneas did not have Cheyne-Stokes morphology. A diagnosis of OSA and treatment emergent CSA was made.

SLEEP-RELATED HYPOVENTILATON DISORDERS

The sleep-related hypoventilation disorders are listed in Box 9-1. The current criteria for scoring hypoventilation during sleep for adults are addressed by the most recent version of the *AASM Manual for the Scoring of Sleep and Associated Events*,[2] as follows:

1. Score hypoventilation during sleep if *either* of the following occur:
   a. Increase in the arterial Pco_2 (or surrogate) to a value >55 mm Hg for ≥10 minutes
   b. Increase of ≥10 mm Hg in arterial Pco_2 (or surrogate) during sleep (in comparison to an awake supine value) to a value exceeding 50 mm Hg for ≥10 minutes

Because monitoring of arterial Pco_2 during sleep is not practical and is not widely done during PSG, acceptable surrogates include end-tidal Pco_2 and transcutaneous Pco_2. Arterial oxygen desaturation is often present but is not required for the diagnosis.

The rationale for the previous definition of sleep-related hypoventilation is discussed in a review paper[4] and is based on limited "consensus" evidence. A normal increase in $Paco_2$ during sleep compared with awake has been described, with a range of about 2 to 8 mm Hg. The criteria attempt to define both an abnormal increase in $Paco_2$ and an absolute $Paco_2$ level considered to represent hypoventilation. Note that criterion 1a, although stated as an increase, in fact represents an absolute value during sleep rather than a comparison to awake and therefore not necessarily an effect of sleep in a person with awake hypoventilation. On the other hand the arterial Pco_2 invariably increases during sleep, irrespective of the presence or absence of daytime hypoventilation. The ICSD3 diagnostic criteria for sleep-related hypoventilation are simply those as defined in the AASM scoring manual.

Obesity-Hypoventilation Syndrome

The obesity-hypoventilation syndrome (OHS) is the only sleep-related hypoventilation disorder that requires documentation of awake hypoventilation ($Paco_2$ >45 mm Hg) (Box 9-10). In the other ICSD3 defined sleep-related hypoventilation disorders, awake hypoventilation may or may not be present.

> **Box 9-10 ICSD3 DIAGNOSTIC CRITERIA: OBESITY-HYPOVENTILATION SYNDROME**
>
> Criteria A to C must be met:
> A. Presence of hypoventilation during wakefulness ($Paco_2$ >45 mm Hg) as measured by arterial Pco_2, end-tidal Pco_2, or transcutaneous Pco_2.
> B. Presence of obesity (body mass index >30 kg/m²; >95th percentile for age and sex for children).
> C. Hypoventilation is not primarily due to lung parenchymal or airway disease, pulmonary vascular pathology, chest wall disorder (other than mass loading from obesity), medication use, neurologic disorder, muscle weakness, or a known congenital or idiopathic central alveolar hypoventilation syndrome.

During PSG, if a noninvasive estimate of the $Paco_2$ is measured in OHS patients, sleep-related hypoventilation is invariably present (i.e., criterion 1a for scoring hypoventilation during sleep), with increases in the $Paco_2$ from awake to sleep typical (i.e., criterion 1b for scoring hypoventilation during sleep). Arterial oxygen desaturation in usually present during sleep and may be present during wakefulness, but neither is required for a diagnosis of OHS. In 80% to 90% of OHS patients, a diagnosis of OSA can also be made.[33] The other 10% to 20% manifest awake hypoventilation that worsens during sleep in association with reduced tidal volume. In OHS, by definition, the etiology of the hypoventilation is not primarily due to lung parenchymal or airway disease, pulmonary vascular pathology, chest wall disorder (other than mass loading from obesity), medication use, neurologic disorder, muscle weakness, or a documented congenital or idiopathic central alveolar hypoventilation syndrome.

The etiology of OHS also likely varies among individuals. In clinical practice there is often uncertainty concerning the most appropriate diagnosis in an obese individual with OSA, obstructive lung disease, and awake hypoventilation; for example, does the patient have OHS or the "overlap syndrome" (OSA + chronic obstructive pulmonary disease [COPD])? Such clinical considerations affect the optimal treatment of the awake- and sleep-related hypoventilation disorder. If a patient diagnosed with OHS undergoes CPAP treatment for the OSA component, normalization of the awake $Paco_2$ can occur; similarly, treatment of the OSA in the overlap syndrome can favorably affect both OSA and COPD outcomes. An unresolved issue concerning the nosology is the recommended exclusion of a diagnosis of OHS in the presence of "a known idiopathic central hypoventilation syndrome" (see later); such a diagnosis in an obese patient would require that the clinician affirm that the hypoventilation developed before obesity or persisted after resolution of obesity, an unlikely clinical possibility.

Idiopathic Central Alveolar Hypoventilation

In this disorder, the cause of sleep-related alveolar hypoventilation is unknown (Box 9-11). It is a diagnosis of exclusion, and the disorder appears to be rare. By definition, the hypoventilation is *not* primarily due to an identifiable cause of hypoventilation such as lung parenchymal or airway disease, pulmonary vascular pathology, chest wall disorder, medication use, neurologic disorder, muscle weakness, obesity, or

---

> **Box 9-11   ICSD3 DIAGNOSTIC CRITERIA: IDIOPATHIC CENTRAL ALVEOLAR HYPOVENTILATION**
>
> Criteria A and B must be met:
> A. Sleep-related hypoventilation is present.
> B. Hypoventilation is not primarily due to lung parenchymal or airway disease, pulmonary vascular pathology, chest wall disorder, medication use, neurologic disorder, muscle weakness, or obesity or congenital hypoventilation syndromes.

congenital hypoventilation syndromes. The congenital central hypoventilation syndrome usually manifests at birth, but late-onset cases have been described. The definitive diagnosis of congenital central hypoventilation syndrome requires demonstration of a mutation in the *PHOX2B* gene.[34]

Sleep-Related Hypoventilation Due to a Medication or Substance

In this disorder, the sleep-related hypoventilation is due to a medication or substance that inhibits ventilatory drive (Box 9-12). Hypoventilation may be present during wakefulness but is not required for the diagnosis. The medications associated with the closely related diagnosis of CSA due to medication or substance (see earlier) may also be associated with sleep-related hypoventilation. Hypoventilation is not primarily due to another identifiable cause of hypoventilation, such as lung parenchymal or airway disease, pulmonary vascular pathology, chest wall disorder, neurologic disorder, muscle weakness, OHS, or a known congenital central alveolar hypoventilation syndrome. Although obstructive and central apneas may be present, the predominant respiratory pattern is usually one of reduced tidal volume or ataxic breathing and associated arterial oxygen desaturation. However, some patients may manifest frequent central apneas and also meet the criteria for sleep-related hypoventilation. When relevant criteria are met, as defined previously, a diagnosis of OSA or CSA, or both, due to a medication or substance, as well as sleep-related hypoventilation due to a medication or substance, may be made.

Sleep-Related Hypoventilation Due to a Medical Disorder

In this disorder of breathing during sleep, sleep-related hypoventilation is believed to be due to a defined medical disorder (Box 9-13). Here the term "medical disorder" is inclusive and includes disorders of the lung parenchyma, airways, or pulmonary vasculature; chest wall disorders (other than mass loading for obesity); neurologic disorders such as neuromuscular disorders (disorders of the brain, spinal cord, or phrenic nerve); and myopathies.[35,36] By definition, hypoventilation is *not* associated with OHS or a central alveolar hypoventilation syndrome. Although awake hypoventilation may be present, this is not required for this diagnosis. The predominant respiratory pattern is one of reduced tidal volume or ataxic breathing and associated arterial oxygen desaturation, rather than a predominant pattern of central or obstructive apnea. However, if appropriate criteria are met, as defined previously, a diagnosis of OSA or CSA, or both, due to a medical or neurologic condition, as well as sleep-related hypoventilation due to a medical disorder, may be made.

> **Box 9-12   ICSD3 DIAGNOSTIC CRITERIA: SLEEP-RELATED HYPOVENTILATION DUE TO A MEDICATION OR SUBSTANCE**
>
> Criteria A to C must be met:
> A. Sleep-related hypoventilation is present.
> B. A medication or substance known to inhibit respiration and/or ventilatory drive is believed to be the primary cause of sleep-related hypoventilation.
> C. Hypoventilation is not primarily due to lung parenchymal or airway disease, pulmonary vascular pathology, chest wall disorder, neurologic disorder, muscle weakness, obesity-hypoventilation syndrome, or a known congenital central alveolar hypoventilation syndrome.

> **Box 9-13   ICSD3 DIAGNOSTIC CRITERIA: SLEEP-RELATED HYPOVENTILATION DUE TO A MEDICAL DISORDER**
>
> Criteria A to C must be met:
> A. Sleep-related hypoventilation is present.
> B. A lung parenchymal or airway disease, pulmonary vascular pathology, chest wall disorder, neurologic disorder, or muscle weakness is believed to be the primary cause of hypoventilation.
> C. Hypoventilation is not primarily due to obesity-hypoventilation syndrome, medication use, or a known congenital central alveolar hypoventilation syndrome.

> **Box 9-14   ICSD3 DIAGNOSTIC CRITERIA: SLEEP-RELATED HYPOXEMIA**
>
> Criteria A and B must be met:
> A. Polysomnography, out-of-center sleep testing, or nocturnal oximetry shows the arterial oxygen saturation (SpO_2) during sleep of ≤88% in adults or ≤90% in children for ≥5 minutes.
> B. Sleep-related hypoventilation is not documented.

SLEEP-RELATED HYPOXEMIA DISORDER

This disorder has also been referred to as *nocturnal oxygen desaturation* and is based on either PSG, OCST, or oximetry findings (Box 9-14). Note that a diagnosis of sleep-related hypoventilation with such hypoxemia cannot be made if Pco_2 is not measured during sleep or, if measured, remains within normal limits. Conversely, if sleep-related hypoventilation is documented (as measured by arterial blood gas, transcutaneous Pco_2, or end-tidal CO_2 sensors), the disorder is classified as sleep-related hypoventilation rather than sleep-related hypoxemia disorder. OSA or CSA may be present, but such events are not directly associated with the majority of the sleep time spent with hypoxemia. Physiologic causes, if known, should be indicated (e.g., shunt, ventilation-perfusion [V/Q] mismatch, low mixed venous oxygen, and low partial pressure of inspired O_2, as with high altitude). In the ICSD3, sleep-related hypoxemic disorder is listed separately from the sleep-related hypoventilation disorders. Note, however, that most disorders associated with a diagnosis of sleep-related hypoventilation due to a medical disorder will be classified as sleep-related hypoxemia disorder if the sleeping $Paco_2$ or a surrogate has not been measured, or if such a measure does not meet criteria for sleep-related hypoventilation. For example, a patient with COPD (whether or not awake $Paco_2$ is elevated) undergoing nocturnal oximetry without a CO_2 measure may show significant nocturnal arterial oxygen desaturation; such a patient would fit criteria for sleep-related hypoxemia disorder. One could argue that this diagnostic category should be combined with the sleep-related hypoventilation disorders. In fact, the ICD-9 (International Classification of Diseases) diagnostic code 327.26 denotes sleep-related hypoxemia or hypercapnia associated with a condition classified elsewhere. Further, such hypoxemia during sleep may also be associated with sleep-related hypoventilation not clearly documented by a CO_2 sensor because of limitations in the technology of CO_2 sensors, which typically substitute for direct arterial blood gas measurement.

OTHER SLEEP-RELATED BREATHING DISORDERS

As may be expected, a number of sleep-related breathing disorders do not fit easily into the previous diagnostic categories. Many types of lung disease, including COPD, cystic fibrosis, asthma, interstitial lung disease, and pulmonary vascular disease (often with pulmonary arterial hypertension), may result in hypoxemia during sleep with or without documented awake or sleep-related hypoventilation. If sleep-related hypoventilation is not documented but nocturnal hypoxemia is present, a diagnosis of sleep-related hypoxemic disorder is made. Further, many of these clinical entities may "overlap" with either CSA or OSA. The most classically described overlap syndrome,[37] consisting of the combination of OSA and COPD, is a common condition that clearly does not fit easily into a diagnostic category. These patients may have episodes of obstructive events (apnea, hypopnea, or both) superimposed on a low baseline sleeping arterial oxygen saturation. Patients with the overlap syndrome would by definition meet diagnostic criteria for OSA, but the recognition of the role of COPD is important because patients benefit from treatment of both components. It has also been increasingly shown that treatment of the OSA component when present in combination with the previously noted pulmonary and pulmonary vascular disorders may also be necessary for optimal treatment of each entity.

CLINICAL PEARL

Sleep-related breathing disorders encompass a wide and clinically important spectrum of disordered breathing and related medical morbidities, which often overlap. The ICSD3 has published new diagnostic criteria for sleep-related breathing disorders. Separate diagnostic criteria are now available for CSA with CSB, OHS, and treatment emergent CSA. Definitions of specific respiratory events are not provided in the ICSD3, and the clinician must use the *AASM Manual for the Scoring of Sleep and Associated Events: Rules, Terminology and Technical Specifications* for such definitions. A diagnosis of treatment emergent CSA requires that the CSA during positive-pressure initiation is *not* better explained by another CSA disorder. In this sense, *treatment emergent CSA* is more specific than the widely used term *complex sleep apnea*. A diagnosis of sleep-related hypoventilation disorders requires measurement of $Paco_2$ or a surrogate of $Paco_2$ during sleep.

SUMMARY

A diagnosis of OSA in adults requires either 15 or more obstructive events (obstructive or mixed apneas, hypopneas, and RERAs) per hour or the combination of symptoms or comorbid conditions and 5 or more obstructive events per hour. The diagnoses of CSA with CSB, CSA due to a medical disorder without CSB, CSA due to a medication or substance, and primary CSA all require 5 or more central apneas or central hypopneas per hour of sleep, with at least 50% of the total number of respiratory events present during sleep being central apneas or central hypopneas. A diagnosis of sleep-related hypoventilation disorders requires demonstration of hypoventilation during sleep (in practice, usually assessed by a surrogate measure of arterial Pco_2 such as end-tidal Pco_2 or transcutaneous Pco_2 monitoring). OHS requires demonstration of awake hypoventilation; most of these patients also have OSA. In the other sleep-related hypoventilation disorders, daytime hypoventilation may or may not be present. A diagnosis of sleep-related hypoventilation due to a medical disorder requires that hypoventilation is primarily due to a disorder of the lung parenchyma, airways, or pulmonary vasculature; chest wall disorders (other than mass loading for obesity); neurologic disorders (disorders of the brain, spinal cord, or phrenic nerve); or myopathy.

Selected Readings

Aboussouan LS. Sleep-disordered breathing in neuromuscular disease. *Am J Respir Crit Care Med* 2015;**191**(9):979–89.

American Academy of Sleep Medicine. *International classification of sleep disorders*. 3rd ed. Darien, IL: American Academy of Sleep Medicine; 2014.

Berry RB, Brooks R, Gamaldo CE, et al, for the American Academy of Sleep Medicine. *The AASM Manual for the Scoring of Sleep and Associated Events: Rules, Terminology and Technical Specifications*, Version 2.3. Darien, Illinois: American Academy of Sleep Medicine; 2016 <www.aasmnet.org>.

Eckert DJ, Jordan AS, Merchia P, Malhotra A. Central sleep apnea: pathophysiology and treatment. *Chest* 2007;**131**:595–607.

Escourrou P, Grote L, Penzel T, et al; ESADA Study Group. The diagnostic method has a strong influence on classification of obstructive sleep apnea. *J Sleep Res* 2015;**24**(6):730–8.

Javaheri S, Dempsey JA. Central sleep apnea. *Compr Physiol* 2013;**3**:141–63.

Jordan AS, McSharry DG, Malhotra A. Adult obstructive sleep apnoea. *Lancet* 2014;**383**(9918):736–47.

A complete reference list can be found online at ExpertConsult.com.

Sleep Breathing Disorders: Clinical Overview

Reena Mehra; Douglas E. Moul; Kingman P. Strohl

Chapter Highlights

- Sleep breathing disorders (SBDs) is an umbrella term used to describe a range of breathing disorders of sleep that include obstructive sleep apnea, central sleep apnea, periodic breathing, and sleep-related hypoventilation.

- Overall, SBDs are highly prevalent in adults, with each type of disturbance having distinct pathophysiologic and clinical features. The widespread prevalence and scope of SBDs, afflicting more than 50 million Americans alone, along with the compounding adverse effects on medical, mental health, quality-of-life, and productivity outcomes, provides compelling motivation to design and engage in strategies to optimize their diagnosis and management.

- SBDs uniquely intersect with a host of medical, surgical, and neurologic comorbid conditions and directly affect health outcomes. Optimal

management strategies for SBDs therefore must involve not only multidisciplinary expertise but also a team-based approach incorporating efforts from primary care physicians, medical and surgical subspecialists, and sleep specialists.

- Novel therapeutics will likely be forthcoming based on addressing the specific pathophysiologic attributes of SBDs, including critical closing pressure of the upper airway, upper airway muscle recruitment, arousal threshold, and loop gain.

- From a holistic standpoint, it is imperative to take into account the health status and life course of the patient when tailoring treatment strategies for an SBD such that these are effectively incorporated in the patient's personal life narrative.

The broad impact of disorders of respiration in sleep on human health and disease has spurred the development of major new conceptual frameworks and treatments over the past 50 years.[1] We now know in much greater detail how sleep is a critical biologic function for brain development and maintenance, behavioral vigilance, memory, and general well-being. Respiratory disturbances during sleep dramatically interfere with not only brain but also other organ functions, resulting in accompanying cardiovascular, endocrine, neurologic, and psychiatric disorders. The functional benefits of sleep reside in the amount and continuity of sleep and its various stages, effects that are inevitably disrupted in those with sleep breathing disorders (SBDs).

The purpose of this overview to the section on SBDs is to orient and represent a broad view of pulmonary-related sleep medicine and to provide a framework for consideration of the SBDs in a clinical preventative paradigm. More detailed and annotated work on each aspect of what we will cover will be found in the subsequent chapters of this section.

HISTORICAL PERSPECTIVE

SBD is an umbrella term used to describe a range of sleep-related breathing disorders that includes obstructive sleep apnea (OSA), central sleep apnea (CSA), periodic breathing (including Cheyne-Stokes breathing), and sleep-related

hypoventilation (see Chapter 9). Historically, recurrent central or nonobstructive events (airflow and effort absent) were clinically identified as part of the pathobiology of congestive heart failure and central nervous system disorders, including stroke. Now OSA (airflow absent but efforts persist) is considered more prevalent, with each apnea type exhibiting somewhat different clinical presentations

OSA as a clinical entity began to be recognized in the 1960s when several groups in Europe reported observations on sleep in patients with excessive daytime sleepiness.[2] Suspecting upper airway obstruction as the cause for disturbed sleep, several groups took a radical step by performing tracheostomy as treatment. This regularized breathing during sleep, with the signs and symptoms of awake-time sleepiness[3] and cardiopulmonary disease resolving.[4] Other centers soon used the same diagnostic and therapeutic approach, confirming the disease ("upper airway apnea") in adults and children. In the 1970s, case series of OSA were reported, and the term *polysomnography* became widely used to describe the process of monitoring sleep and its associated movements and cardiopulmonary functions. Motta and colleagues in 1978 reported success with tracheostomy for OSA in a large case series.[5] In the 1980s there was an emphasis on the neurophysiology of respiratory control and the anatomic features of a vulnerable upper airway, the interactions of which created recurrent nonobstructive and obstructive apneas and hypopneas, respectively.[6] OSA was still considered a rare and curious disease, to be considered when other causes for polycythemia, pulmonary hypertension, or extreme inability to stay awake were excluded. OSA treatments first described in 1981 included positive airway pressure (PAP)[7] and uvulopalatopharyngoplasty surgery[8] directed at abnormalities of the size and compliance of the nasopharynx and oropharynx.

In 1993, the first organized epidemiologic investigation published the figure of a 2% to 4% prevalence of OSA syndrome (elevated apnea-hypopnea index [AHI] with symptoms) in adults, placing OSA in the United States among common chronic medical conditions such as asthma and diabetes.[9] Since then, established clinical pathways for management have been developed in addition to improved methods of positive-pressure therapy delivery and to the alternative of oral appliance therapy. Outcomes of both the untreated and the treated state of OSA have been described in enough detail to articulate general thresholds for OSA severity: mild (AHI, 5 to 15), moderate (AHI, 15 to 30), and severe (AHI, >30).

Central sleep apnea and Hunter-Cheyne-Stokes breathing are among the SBDs that received initial attention in the early nineteenth century. Although these disorders are less prevalent than OSA, the symptom-based characteristics and physiologic perturbations are perhaps more readily apparent. In 1818, John Cheyne, a physician in Dublin, was one of the first to describe the disorder in a 60-year-old patient with breathing oscillations that he observed during sleep in the latter phases of the patient's illness. On postmortem examination, Cheyne discovered that the patient's heart was enlarged with fatty tissue invasion of the cardiac muscle.[10] In 1854 another physician from Dublin, William Stokes, went further and attributed the abnormal breathing pattern to a "weakened state of the heart."[11] For the purposes of historical accuracy, it should be noted that 37 years before Cheyne's report, John Hunter, an English surgeon, was the first to describe the classic crescendo-decrescendo breathing pattern: "The patient's respiration was extraordinary. He ceased to breathe for twenty or thirty seconds and then started breathing again. First faintly, and then with increasing force until the climax, after which his breathing again weakened until it disappeared completely."[12] Treatment options for CSA associated with Hunter-Cheyne-Stokes breathing initially included stabilization of the underlying contributing condition (e.g., optimizing heart failure management) and some drugs. More advanced technologies are currently available, including novel PAP approaches.

OVERVIEW OF THE PATHOPHYSIOLOGIC BASIS OF SLEEP BREATHING DISORDERS INFORMING THE TREATMENT APPROACH

Our review in 1987 described the clinical understanding of sleep apnea and the intent of different therapies to address suspected anatomic and neural factors in SBDs and the elements of clinical risk gleaned in the examination of the patient.[6,13] Although long-term prognostic generalizability has leapt forward in the past 25 years regarding SBDs more generally, the fine-grained understanding about findings on sleep studies still has areas of substantial ambiguity, particularly when patient-specific findings and preferences need to be incorporated into treatment planning. For example, two clinically salient domains of ambiguity concern treatment emergent CSA and residual sleepiness in the OSA patient

who is fully compliant with continuous positive airway pressure (CPAP). Accordingly, the field has moved to more fundamental issues,[14-16] including the development of a process of separating and measuring features during sleep that correlate with the expression of recurrent apneas in an individual patient.[17,18] These features include (1) the pharyngeal critical closing pressure (Pcrit), (2) the recruitment (or "gain") function of muscles that keep the airway patent, (3) the threshold for arousal from sleep, and (4) the tendency for a disturbance to "set up" the person for a subsequent apnea ("loop gain") (see Chapters 7 and 12).

The pressure at which the compliant upper airway closes can be measured during sleep and calculated as the Pcrit. A positive pressure needed to keep the airway open is called a positive Pcrit and is the principle for using CPAP; if closing requires a negative pressure (as in a healthy person or in those with nonobstructive apneas or hypopneas), it is a negative Pcrit. Moving Pcrit to a more negative level is therefore beneficial in terms of treating OSA. Upper airway muscles can keep an airway open through brainstem activation using reflex mechanisms and direct actions on size or stiffness of the airway wall. Sleep reduces both activation and reflex recruitment, and in severe OSA there are additional reductions in reflex activations.[19-21] Another factor is the inherent gain of recruitment with the increasing chemoreceptor stimulation.[22] Furthermore, muscle efferent output must be translated into mechanical changes in the airway, which may be more difficult in the presence of edema.[23]

Arousal thresholds operate in SBDs in two ways.[24,25] Arousals are a mechanism that not only shorten events but also rapidly increase ventilation for any given carbon dioxide level. However, a longer time to arousal is thought to increase the chance for a person to increase drive to upper airway muscles, improve ventilation, maintain oxygenation, and reduce arousals during sleep,[24,26] permitting muscle activation to rise up to open the airway.

The fourth mechanism to discuss is loop gain, which is the propensity of the respiratory feedback control system to oscillate in response to a perturbation like a nonobstructive or obstructive apnea. A high loop gain indicates a relative inability for a person's control system to return to steady breathing after a disturbance such as an apnea, and a number of studies indicate that high loop gain is a factor in OSA and in the recurrent nonobstructive apneas of Cheyne-Stokes breathing. One major aspect of this control system relates to the effectors for ventilation (nerves, muscles, chest wall); another is related to the response organized by the brainstem to the disturbance. Oxygen administration can decrease loop gain and reduce OSA in some patients who have a high loop gain,[27] and indomethacin can increase loop gain and increase the tendency for apneas to reoccur.[28] CPAP itself will lower loop gain,[29] as the ventilatory response to CO_2 decreases (i.e., ventilation becomes less oscillatory) following treatment with CPAP.[22,30] Thus an individuality of and change in loop gain could be a mechanism of the appearance of emergent nonobstructive apnea, the variability among individuals in drug trials, the success of oxygen therapy, and obstructive and nonobstructive tendencies in disease presentation.

In summary, the anatomy of an apnea in sleep is determined in the following manner. There is a reduction in global respiratory muscle drive to create opportunity for an apnea. The nonobstructive apnea occurs when the upper airway has a negative Pcrit, whereas the obstructive apnea occurs when there is a mechanical collapse with a reduction in drive to upper airway dilator muscles. In the middle of the apnea, drive increases to one degree or another, with both negative pressure and chemoreflex stimulus, until there occurs either an arousal or sufficient muscle activation to reopen the airway. The degree of overshoot in ventilation sets up the opportunity for a reduction in drive to set up the next apneas. Less well known are the factors that lead to the length of an apnea, the interapneic interval, and the cycle length between the onset of one apnea and the onset of the next.

All of these four factors contribute alone and in combination to the development and level of severity of both nonobstructive and obstructive apneas and will affect the response to therapy. There is some prospect that these elements will be ultimately measurable using a CPAP interface to clamp the airway pressure and initiate interventions to collect values related to muscle recruitment, arousals, and loop gain.[26] Currently, longitudinal studies of these factors and how they influence the development of sleep apneas over time are absent, and the collected traits at presentation are more epidemiologically oriented (e.g., obesity, hypertension) than based on data on causes (e.g., Pcrit, loop gain). In addition to the functional factors just discussed, some supportive evidence for risks associated with molecular markers associated with sympathetic activity, oxidative stress, and inflammation are present in some but not all cross-sectional studies in the presence of hypoxiareoxygenation with recurrent obstructive and nonobstructive apneas.[31] Genetic and epigenetic factors will undoubtedly emerge, but currently the genetic studies are underpowered for common alleles and inconclusive for rare alleles sought in family studies.[32] Although some causal generalizability has arisen epidemiologically about the effects of SBDs, and etiologic frameworks have undergone robust clarifications, the current level of knowledge leaves the sleep clinician with limited guidance, relying mainly on modification of an abnormal Pcrit, and clinical management is based on algorithms rather than measures of the four pathophysiologic causes.

CLINICAL ASSESSMENTS AND DECISION MAKING

Detection of SBDs is at a historical inflection point. Rather than "rare, curious, or untreatable," SBDs are inevitably present in any clinical cohort. Treating SBDs improves quality of life and reduces cardiovascular risks. SBDs are common, treatable, and likely to some extent preventable. Because OSA is itself as common as asthma or diabetes, the sleep medicine specialist cannot take care of all SBD patients. The role of the specialist, like that of the diabetes or asthma specialist, is to assist in diagnosis and treatment of more complex cases and, in the future, to institute care paths to serve as a guide for the primary care physician or subspecialist for informed management of SBDs.

The prevalence and scope of SBDs, afflicting more 50 million Americans alone, along with its compounding effects on adverse medical, mental health, behavioral, and quality-of-life outcomes, as well as loss of productivity,[33] provides compelling motivation to engage in strategies to optimize the diagnosis and management of these conditions. SBDs have been notably underrecognized, with 85% to 90% of cases estimated to be undiagnosed.[34] This is partly attributable to limited awareness and understanding of the relevance of SBDs and to suboptimal guides and tools available for practitioners to efficiently diagnose and treat SBDs. A challenge facing many primary care physicians, our first-line "gatekeepers," is to choose which health problem to address for each patient, given clinical time constraints and patients' own health care preferences. In contrast, subspecialists face the challenges of addressing focused domains of care in a targeted and comprehensive manner, but not necessarily the composite of a patient's comorbidities. In the middle zone, treatment of SBDs encompasses somewhat specialized aspects of respiratory care but, owing to the prevalence and protean effects of untreated SBDs, necessitates the involvement of a wide range of medical specialties.

Hence there exist multiple opportunities to identify SBDs not only in everyday settings of health maintenance and disease prevention but also along the patient's trajectory through acute inpatient settings and subsequent outpatient follow-up. For example, while addressing a variety of common medical issues such as blood pressure and diabetes control, the patient and clinician may not prioritize or view SBD symptoms (e.g., snoring, daytime sleepiness) as clinically relevant or important. Nonetheless, a systematic approach for identifying and managing respiratory and nonrespiratory sleep disorders can have strategic importance for the effective longitudinal control of cardiovascular and cardiometabolic health consequences. Treatment of SBDs is part of a holistic approach of medical management and optimization of health care.

The clinical evaluation of a person suspected of having an SBD or being assessed after initiation of treatment requires a multisystem assessment. Because sleep patterns and preferences are determined by embodiments of personal, occupational, and social goals, effective care of SBDs can take on a complexity and richness not often needed for other organspecific specialty assessments. Certain instruments, such as the Berlin Questionnaire and the STOP-BANG questionnaire, are designed to provide risk factor analysis as well as a psychometrically valid, generalizable suspicion of OSA. The Berlin Questionnaire is geared toward recognition of OSA in the primary care office, and it best considered for its negative predictive value, rather than as a predictor of severity of disease.[35] The STOP-BANG was developed for preoperative screening for general anesthesia in a population particularly at risk for OSA because of many chronic illnesses,[36] and it is gaining increasing use primarily because of ease of implementation; note, however, that the original STOP-BANG includes neck size measurement, which is often overlooked. These instruments highlight that the clinical skill set for the sleep specialist has come to include understanding of self-report scales and their utility, appropriate context, and limitations, especially in regard to determining the need for clinical management. Similarly, assessments of diagnostic tests such as polysomnography require a skill set in evaluating the plausibility of the test compared with pretest probability, the risk and difficulty of testing, the ability to initiate a treatment decision based on its result, and patient collaboration. Interpreting information, scales, and tests related to SBDs requires topic-related skills in identifying a study question, interpreting study design, and data analysis. Insurance providers and patients are asking tough questions about process and value. Sleep medicine specialists have to acquire these skills in communication, but translating some of these issues to other specialties remains a challenge for sleep clinicians.

Growing attention has been paid to research in health services and quality improvement in the treatment of SBDs. This trend has engaged funding agencies, health care delivery systems, and the government, and each has increasingly emphasized this as an area of focus as population-level health impacts become better known. Such research will increasingly shape the financing and administration of SBD-associated health care. As the volume of systematic research studies increases, assessing the nature and quality of the studies, particularly when they suggest contrasting findings, is essential for the development of wise clinical practices. Meta-analyses and systematic reviews can be helpful to integrate findings from several studies and appraise biases. Cost-effectiveness and comparative effectiveness analyses attempt to scale the real-world benefit of new interventions to current standards of care while simultaneously evaluating associated costs.

Incorporating proven state-of-the-art innovations at the bedside will continue to be an ethical priority in evaluating and treating SBDs in a clinical system that embraces continuous quality improvement. Important outcomes commonly evaluated include reduction of cost, reduction of morbidity and mortality, and improvement in patient satisfaction. A vital part of quality improvement is sustainability—creating systems to ensure the desired outcomes are regularly achieved. Accordingly, SBD specialists will need to oversee quality improvement projects to better understand how the process works, how to improve individual practice, and how to sustain successful practice in the changing health care environment.

SLEEP BREATHING DISORDERS IN DISEASE-SPECIFIC POPULATIONS

SBDs are uniquely comorbid with a whole host of major, common clinical conditions and medical settings, spanning, but not limited to, cardiac disease, obstructive and restrictive pulmonary disease, neurologic conditions, kidney disease, and the perioperative and anesthesia setting. The common clinical scenarios discussed in this section and highlighted in Table 10-1 provide a sense of the need for high-level awareness of SBDs and a low threshold for testing for, and managing, associated SBDs in such conditions and settings because an SBD often represents a modifiable risk factor for adverse health outcomes related to these.

Cardiovascular Disease

SBDs and cardiac disease have clear bidirectional relationships. As an example, a family medicine practitioner evaluates a patient with recalcitrant hypertension who meets the criteria for resistant hypertension. The practitioner notes that the patient snores and has a history of witnessed apneas. In this clinical scenario, it must be considered that concomitant and sustained increases in blood pressure are observed in OSA, likely through pathways involving hypoxia as a potent stimulus for sympathetic activation, hypercapnia, reductions in baroreflex sensitivity, and direct increases in sympathetic nervous system activation.[37,38] OSA-induced increases in activation of the renin-angiotensin-aldosterone system may in particular play a role in resistant hypertension. Results pooled across many randomized controlled trials designed to examine the effect of OSA reversal with CPAP on blood pressure outcomes consistently demonstrate statistically significant and clinically meaningful reductions in office systolic and diastolic

blood pressure levels.[39] In fact, the Joint National Committee has recognized OSA as a secondary contributor to hypertension.[40] OSA has also been associated with nocturnal nondipping patterns[41,42] (i.e., does not undergo a standard dipping pattern of blood pressure reduction of at least 10% of the wake value), which is predictive of future cardiovascular risk.[43-45] Furthermore, resistant hypertension (approximately 15% of the hypertensive population[46]), which involves blood pressure above goal despite at least three antihypertensive medications,[47] is an entity in which OSA represents an important promulgating contributor. In fact, a large randomized clinical trial has demonstrated 3-month improvement in mean and diastolic blood pressure in those with resistant hypertension and OSA treated with CPAP versus no therapy.[48]

As another example, an internist admits a patient for management of acute non-ST elevation myocardial infarction; the patient undergoes coronary catheterization. Phenotypic characterization in this case most likely involves a background risk for dyslipidemia, hypertension, and diabetes mellitus. In terms of how undiagnosed SBD fits into this clinical paradigm, it should be recognized that SBD prevalence is greater than 70% in acute coronary syndrome and appears to be characterized by mainly obstructive respiratory physiology.[49] Furthermore, compared with patients without OSA, those with OSA and coronary artery disease have a higher degree of late lumen loss,[50] a marker for coronary restenosis after percutaneous coronary intervention, and there is evidence that OSA inflicts direct cardiac injury.[51] The prevalence of OSA exceeds that of other known risk factors for coronary artery disease on those who are revascularized and therefore represents a key modifiable therapeutic target to consider after coronary intervention.[52] Untreated severe OSA also predicts increased mortality and subsequent myocardial infarction in patients who have experienced an ST elevation myocardial infarction.[53] Similarly, CPAP treatment in those with cardiovascular risk appears to reduce cardiac event risk[54] and minimizes need for revascularization.[55] The treating physician also needs to consider the benefits of SBD treatment on cardiovascular risk factors (e.g., hypertension) to mitigate future adverse cardiovascular events.

Down the hall from the catheterization laboratory, in the heart failure unit, a cardiologist is managing a patient with acutely decompensated reduced ejection fraction heart failure (left ventricular ejection fraction of 30%) with diuresis and afterload reduction pharmacologic therapy. A high index of suspicion for SBD in systolic heart failure should be in place given the known high prevalence in this setting (ranging from 50% to 75%[56,57]), and a combination of OSA and CSA with Cheyne-Stokes breathing is typically represented. Symptom-based screening for SBDs in heart failure patients poses a challenge because standard symptoms of SBD such as excessive daytime sleepiness are often not present. This is likely because of the overall enhanced sympathetic nervous system state inherent in heart failure. Moreover, symptoms of nocturnal awakenings due to shortness of breath and nocturia may be attributed to heart failure rather than an SBD, potentially leading to underdiagnosis of an SBD. Hypoxia-induced impairments in myocardial oxygen delivery and increased cardiac strain from sympathetic activation are likely factors in the initiation and progression of SBD-related heart failure. The dire importance of the detection and treatment of an SBD in those admitted with acute decompensated heart

Table 10-1 Key Considerations in Specific Clinical Conditions and Settings

Clinical Condition	Key Considerations
Hypertension	• Sleep breathing disorder prevalence of 50% to 60% is driven predominantly by obstructive sleep apnea.[40] • Elevation in blood pressure in obstructive sleep apnea occurs both awake and in the sleep period. • Nondipping blood pressure patterns are observed in obstructive sleep apnea, which is predictive of adverse cardiovascular sequelae.[43-45] • More than 15 randomized controlled trials have demonstrated improvement in blood pressure profiles with continuous positive airway pressure.[39] • The Joint National Committee recognizes obstructive sleep apnea as a secondary contributor to systemic hypertension.[40]
Resistant hypertension	• Obstructive sleep apnea is associated with resistant hypertension (prevalence of 60% to 90%)[86] and biologic plausibility for modulation by a hyperaldosteronism state. • Interventional trial data support blood pressure improvement with treatment of obstructive sleep apnea with continuous positive airway pressure in resistant hypertension.[48]
Coronary artery disease	• The prevalence of sleep breathing disorders is approximately 70%, and they primarily involve obstructive physiology.[49] • Obstructive sleep apnea is associated with late lumen loss (marker for restenosis) after coronary intervention[50] and appears to inflict direct myocardial injury (i.e., increased troponin-I levels).[51] • The prevalence of obstructive sleep apnea as a risk factor in coronary artery disease exceeds that of other traditional risk factors such as hypertension and diabetes mellitus.[52] • Untreated severe obstructive sleep apnea is associated with increased cardiovascular-specific mortality in several large scale epidemiologic studies.[87,88]
Heart failure	• Sleep breathing disorder prevalence of 50% to 75% is characteristic; a combination of obstructive sleep apnea, central sleep apnea, and Cheyne-Stokes breathing is represented.[56,57] • Clinical presentation is a challenge because typical symptoms of excessive daytime sleepiness are not present (presumably owing to sympathetic nervous system activation) and symptoms of sleep-related nocturnal dyspnea overlap with symptoms characteristic of fluid overload and paroxysmal nocturnal dyspnea characteristic of heart failure. • Sleep breathing disorders in acute decompensated heart failure are associated with a 50% to 60% increase in mortality after discharge and increased hospital readmissions.[58] • The effect of improvement of sleep breathing disorders with adaptive servoventilation in heart failure on mortality and other outcomes is biologically tenable and is currently the focus of study in large multicenter interventional trials.
Atrial fibrillation	• The prevalence of sleep breathing disorders in atrial fibrillation is estimated to be approximately 50%, with a stronger magnitude of association with central than with obstructive sleep apnea.[63] • Autonomic nervous system fluctuations are strongly implicated in atrial arrhythmogenesis based on experimental data, as are the mechanisms of intermittent hypoxia, the resolution phase of hypercarbia, and intrathoracic pressure alterations resulting in direct mechanical effects on the thin-walled atria. • Several retrospective studies have demonstrated a significant decrease in atrial fibrillation recurrence after ablation or cardioversion with the treatment of sleep breathing disorders compared with no treatment.[60,61]
Chronic obstructive pulmonary disease	• The presence of concomitant chronic obstructive pulmonary disease and obstructive sleep apnea has been termed overlap syndrome. • Patients with overlap syndrome experience more profound hypoxia and pulmonary vasoconstriction compared with either disorder in isolation. • REM sleep likely represents a particular state of vulnerability for obstructive lung disease given enhanced cholinergic mediated bronchoconstriction and further blunting of the hypoxic and hypercapnic ventilatory drives. • Continuous positive airway pressure and bronchodilators should be used along with supplemental oxygen in overlap syndrome because this strategy appears to confer a survival advantage.[67]
Obesity-hypoventilation syndrome	• This is defined by obesity (body mass index >30 kg/m^2), resting hypercapnia, and is characteristically associated with sleep-related hypoventilation in the presence or absence of obstructive sleep apnea. • Obesity-hypoventilation syndrome is important to recognize because it is associated with right-sided heart failure and increased mortality compared with obstructive sleep apnea alone.[68]

Table 10-1	Key Considerations in Specific Clinical Conditions and Settings—cont'd
Clinical Condition	**Key Considerations**
Stroke	• The prevalence of sleep breathing disorders is approximately 50% to 70% in the setting of acute ischemic stroke, with representation by both obstructive and central sleep apnea.[69,70] • Sleep breathing disorders tend to improve over time after stroke; however, half of these individuals continue to have sleep breathing disorders 3 months after stroke.[69,70] • Moderate to severe sleep breathing disorders in stroke that remain untreated may hinder the poststroke recovery process and also impair cognitive function and have an association with depression, with apparent improvement with continuous positive airway pressure use.[76]
Renal insufficiency	• Sleep breathing disorder–related intermittent hypoxia contributes to activation of the systemic and renal-specific renin-angiotensin-aldosterone system. • Recognition of sleep breathing disorders in renal insufficiency remains a diagnostic challenge because of the often atypical presentation of symptoms. • The prevalence of sleep breathing disorders is approximately 50%, with obstructive and central disordered breathing contributions.[78] • In end-stage renal disease, there is evidence that nocturnal hemodialysis is more effective than traditional hemodialysis in the improvement of sleep breathing disorder parameters.[80]
Perioperative anesthesia	• Anesthetics may result in a particular disadvantage to a vulnerable upper airway in patients with obstructive sleep apnea owing to effects of anesthesia in terms of blunting the hypoxic and hypercapnic ventilatory drives and also reducing upper airway muscle tone.[81] • Data are accruing that suggest the importance of identifying sleep breathing disorders preoperatively in an effort to improve outcomes, including perioperative and postoperative morbidity and mortality, and of enhancing anesthesiology preparedness for handling a compromised upper airway and blunted ventilatory drive during intubation and anesthesia administration.

failure is underscored by a large study noting a 50% to 60% increase in postdischarge mortality in those with an SBD compared with those without.[58] Although treatment of SBDs in patients with heart failure has not unequivocally demonstrated mortality benefit,[59] existing data are limited given suboptimal reversibility of Cheyne-Stokes breathing pathophysiology in response to CPAP. On the other hand, improvement in secondary outcomes, including left ventricular function and exertional capacity, has been observed with CPAP, with potential advantages in terms of mitigating heart failure progression. Larger ongoing clinical trials using more sophisticated treatment modalities such as adaptive servoventilation (using variable pressure support delivery to stabilize oscillatory breathing patterns) in patients with CSA and Cheyne-Stokes breathing are underway to address this question more definitively.

Meanwhile, in the electrophysiology laboratory, an electrophysiologist prepares to perform pulmonary vein isolation ablation in a patient with atrial fibrillation. In addressing the important issue of sustainability of normal sinus rhythm after such ablation in a patient with a predisposed substrate, the possibility of an SBD should be strongly considered given numerous data that have accrued supporting reduced recurrence of atrial fibrillation with SBD treatment.[60,61] Albeit, to date, these data are based on retrospectively designed studies, the consistency and reproducibility of these findings are sufficiently compelling to lead the clinician here to assess and investigate the possibility of an SBD. Epidemiologic data indicate a stronger association of CSA compared with OSA as the SBD related to atrial fibrillation, independent of underlying self-reported heart failure,[62] with an overall prevalence of about 50%.[63] Autonomic nervous system fluctuations have a strong biologic basis in terms of arrhythmogenic propensity[64] and have been implicated in experimental models of obstructive apneas and also appear to exert effects in central

apnea physiology given the accompanying sympathetic excitation observed.

Pulmonary Disease

A pulmonologist treating a patient with chronic obstructive pulmonary disease (COPD) also needs to be cognizant of the potential for a concomitant SBD, that is, the "overlap syndrome" (see Chapter 29), so coined given the prevalent merging of these two common pulmonary disorders and the distinctness of the pathophysiology occurring as a result of this overlap above and beyond each disorder alone.[65] Patients with overlap syndrome have more profound hypoxia and resultant nocturnal oxygen desaturation than those with either disorder alone and thereby theoretically have higher risk for pulmonary vasoconstriction and pulmonary hypertension. A modest degree of pulmonary hypertension in general has been observed in OSA, with immediate temporal influences of apneic events resulting in acute rises in pulmonary artery pressure from initiation to termination of the apneic event.[66] Rapid eye movement (REM) sleep, characterized by predominance during the latter part of the sleep cycle, in particular represents a state of vulnerability given the physiology of REM-related reduction in hypoxic and hypercapnic ventilatory drive, reduced muscle tone, and enhanced likelihood for bronchoconstriction due to REM-related parasympathetic tone. Consideration of nocturnal bronchodilators for the COPD and CPAP therapy for the OSA is warranted in light of data demonstrating that these modalities when used together confer a survival advantage compared with supplemental oxygen (long-term oxygen therapy) alone.[67]

Obesity-hypoventilation syndrome (OHS; see Chapter 30) is characterized by morbid obesity and awake resting hypercapnia accompanied by sleep-related hypoventilation with or without the presence of OSA. Importance of recognition of an SBD in OHS lies in its association with right-sided heart failure and, if left untreated, increased mortality risk.[68] The degree of hypoxia is more profound and extensive in OHS with OSA than in OSA alone.

Other Comorbid States

A neurologist evaluates a middle-aged woman in the office subsequent to the patient suffering right-sided lacunar stroke with failure of improvement in functional outcome and depressed mood. An SBD (primarily OSA and/or CSA) in this setting is not only an independent predictor of ischemic stroke but also highly prevalent after stroke and accompanied by worse post-stroke outcomes. An SBD is common after ischemic stroke, affecting 50% to 70% of patients, and although over time the degree of SBD may improve, at least half of patients will have an SBD 3 months after the stroke.[69,70] Although both OSA and CSA may occur after a stroke, improvement over time is more pronounced for CSA than for OSA.[71] CSA represents a negative prognostic indicator after stroke[71] and is related to stroke severity as well as topography.[72,73] Although some epidemiologic data support a stronger association of SBDs and incident ischemic stroke in men,[74] other data in an Asian population suggest that younger women may be at higher stroke risk.[75] When of moderate or severe degree, SBDs can hinder the recovery and rehabilitation process. Identification and treatment of an SBD are important given associations of SBDs with depressed mood, cognitive dysfunction, and impairment of the ability to perform activities of daily living. Data suggest that treatment of SBDs may thwart compromise of neurologic and cognitive function in the stable poststroke phase.[76] Interestingly, stroke etiology subtypes, including cardioembolic, large artery, and small artery strokes, are not variable in terms of association with SBDs or their severity.[77]

Similarly, an elderly man with daytime sleepiness and snoring in the setting of chronic renal insufficiency is being seen by a nephrologist in clinic. Although sleep symptoms are common among patients with chronic renal insufficiency, there are challenges in terms of specificity of these symptoms in the detection of SBDs in this setting. It also appears that there are a fair number of patients with an SBD and chronic renal insufficiency who do not have standard symptoms but do have an SBD. Insults to the kidney occur because of SBD-related intermittent hypoxia, which activates not only the systemic but also the renal-specific renin-angiotensin system, resulting in progression of renal disease and thereby underscoring the importance of the detection and treatment of SBDs. In end-stage renal disease, an estimated 50% of patients are afflicted with an SBD.[78] In end-stage renal disease, both OSA and CSA are observed, with a prevalence apparently concordant to that observed in the setting of heart failure[79] and with a potential overlap in pathophysiology in terms of contribution of rostral neck edema. Nocturnal versus conventional hemodialysis has been demonstrated to improve both OSA and CSA physiology.[80]

A middle-aged obese man with hypertension and a neck circumference of 18 inches is being prepared to undergo an appendectomy under general anesthesia. He undergoes standard preoperative anesthesia testing. Per the STOP-BANG screening questionnaire, he meets high pretest probability for OSA (more than three items positive). Patients with OSA may exhibit anesthesia medication–related reduction in hypoxic and hypercapnic ventilatory, with increased sensitivity

to sedatives and opioids. A detailed airway assessment should be performed in these cases, with preparedness tactics in place, including airway adjuncts such as oral, nasal, and laryngeal mask airways as well as use of the ramped-up position, which enhances visualization of the glottic aperture during intubation. Attention to postoperative management is also of critical importance; descriptive data indicate elevated residual neuromuscular blockade effect, postoperative hypoxia, and increased length of stay in patients at high risk for OSA compared with those without high pretest probability for OSA.[81]

ECOLOGIC FEATURES

Holistically speaking, SBDs will have a bearing on one's health status and life course. In relation to the project of understanding patients' personal narratives and reactions concerning SBDs and their treatment, it is evident that generalizing about the life course narratives of persons with SBDs is epidemiologically not feasible. Treating SBDs will always remain a practical art.

Patients individually fit suspected or diagnosed SBDs into personal narratives. On the population-level of understanding the effects of SBDs, one may certainly appreciate how compliance with treatment may be partially determined by social or cultural contexts, to yield different rates for morbidities and mortality across groups.

In considering the course of OSA and its treatment, for example, it is essential to appreciate that although the cardiovascular and cerebrovascular outcomes are typically "hard" (i.e., not subject to reappraisal),[82] the decision to accept an identity (here the issue is having an SBD) or a treatment (such as CPAP) is "soft" (i.e., continually subject to reevaluation).

There are many patients who have sleep studies, and who even go on to use CPAP (or other non-PAP therapies) for a period of time, but then stop using treatment, only to come back to consider treatment years later. The implication is that the goal for the clinician need not exclusively be immediate treatment compliance (although this is certainly a main issue for insurers and a worthy goal for a practitioner), but instead to place some credence on identifying with the patient's personal narrative as the patient confronts the diagnosis of an SBD. For many days' clinical work, doing the medical art well is measure enough, irrespective of the patient's decision or indecision. This is the approach taken with motivational interviewing,[83] which, curiously, turns out to be highly effective in interacting with patients across a broad range of clinical presentations, severity, and response to treatment suggestions.

It should also be appreciated that the chronic sleep deprivation and neurocognitive sequelae associated with chronic OSA have an effect on patients' comprehension and treatment compliance. The frontal lobes are the most affected by sleep deprivation. In clinical practice, lowering of frontal functioning from chronic sleep deprivation has been observed to degrade a patient's capacity for maintaining personal morale, regulating affect in response to daily events, thinking more reflectively, remembering well, and relating to others. Anecdotally, some SBD patients can thus present as having psychiatric or personality disorders in clinical encounters, leading to a delayed or missed diagnosis of an SBD. Many presenting patients have impaired comprehension of health care information and physician recommendations. Additionally, it has been long known that for some patients, sleep deprivation may increase anxiety. This anxiety might be generalized or conditioned to nighttime and sleep stimuli; for example, for OSA patients, each breath could be a choking experience. The sleepy patient may not have sufficient judgment and free will when making health care decisions about OSA treatments. Yet, for some who are diagnosed and treated, the mental health symptoms will be substantially improved and occasionally cured, owing to the benefits of getting uninterrupted wholesome sleep and reduced oxidative stress.

The clinician should also consider that comorbid disorders may disturb sleep to such an extent that compliance with treatment for an SBD becomes difficult if not impossible. This may arise, for example, if the patient has comorbid insomnia. However, other comorbidities can likewise provide the context for impairing good sleep. These include psychiatric conditions, cardiorespiratory conditions, pain, aging, and the use of particular medications such as alerting agents (e.g., stimulants, with some such as pseudoephedrine even available over the counter), anticholinergics, corticosteroids, and adrenergic inhalers.

The aging process presents interesting clinical issues regarding the SBDs. As middle age advances into older age, populations become increasingly biologically and clinically diverse throughout this span of time in relation to the burden of comorbidities, including those that an SBD might affect. Additionally, there is the consideration that the major measure of the sleep apneas, the AHI, may have normative ranges that increase with aging in adults. Reynolds and colleagues noted that in a cohort of patients advancing though the age span from 50 to 80 years, the AHI according to 1980s scoring rules increased per decade to a plateau at about 70 years of age.[84] These studies of recruited samples of healthy aging would give the impression that aging populations have AHIs that are biologically normal for their age although elevated for younger age groups. Indeed, there is debate about the optimal approach to treatment of SBDs, particularly OSA, in aging populations, including whether there might be an acceptable AHI level, perhaps 15 events per hour, which could be medically insignificant in older patients. However, although in practice it seems likely that some increase in AHI might be overall benign in some patients; aging patients should be considered to require the same attention to clinical symptoms and the comorbid milieu as younger populations in considering the diagnosis and treatment of the various SBDs. The recent literature on reduced sleep, SBDs, and hypoxemia playing an initiating or amplifying role in the development of Alzheimer disease and other dementias (including ischemia-related stroke)[85] reinforces such a clinical strategy.

CLINICAL PEARLS

- SBDs are a modifiable risk to be considered in numerous cardiologic settings, including treatment of resistant hypertension, minimization of risk for restenosis after percutaneous coronary intervention, mitigation of progression of heart failure and its adverse outcomes, and reduction in atrial fibrillation recurrence after intervention.
- SBDs also contribute to morbidity accompanying pulmonary disorders, including COPD, pulmonary hypertension, and OHS.
- SBDs are increasingly recognized as not only an independent predictor of acute stroke but also an obstacle in the poststroke recovery and rehabilitation process.

- Assessment of an SBD in the preoperative anesthesia setting is imperative to ensure implementation of optimal preparedness strategies for the perioperative and postoperative settings, including providing availability of adjunct airways and postoperative respiratory monitoring.
- Upper airway and central physiologic characteristics that predispose to the propagation of apneas and hypopneas in OSA include the critical closing pressure of the upper airway, upper airway muscle recruitment, arousal thresholds, and loop gain.

SUMMARY

In the past 30 years, treating the SBDs has developed from a medical curiosity to an epidemiologic mandate. Such a mandate for sleep medicine encompasses not only OSA but also other numerous forms of sleep-related respiratory disturbances (see Chapter 9). Despite the evidence base, however, patients and many medical professionals still have a dim appreciation of current knowledge about SBDs, their recognition, and their response to therapy. Even as physiologic knowledge of SBDs advances, there remains a continuing need for the expansion of public and medical education about SBDs and a continuing need for developing decision supports about SBDs for nonsleep clinicians as well as sleep specialists. That said, there is every reason to be confident that the physiologies of SBDs will continue to be explored in ever-increasing depth and sophistication. The four-factor functional model for OSA as discussed earlier will motivate attempts to apply a causal, systematic analysis of SBDs, based on measurable physiologic variables. Biochemical, genetic, and epigenetic variables related to the SBDs will also need to be explored more broadly, particularly those that have tie-ins to other highly prevalent cardiovascular, respiratory, and metabolic health conditions.

Selected Readings

Dempsey JA, et al. Pathophysiology of sleep apnea. *Physiol Rev* 2010; **90**(1):47–112.

Dewan NA, Nieto FJ, Somers VK. Intermittent hypoxemia and OSA: implications for comorbidities. *Chest* 2015;**147**(1):266–74.

Institute of Medicine Committee on Sleep Medicine and Research, Colten HR, Altevolgt BM, editors. *Sleep disorders and sleep deprivation: an unmet public health problem.* Washington DC: National Academies Press; 2006. p. 3, Extent and Health Consequences of Chronic Sleep Loss and Sleep Disorders. Available from: <http://www.ncbi.nlm.nih.gov/books/NBK19961/>.

Kapur V, et al. Underdiagnosis of sleep apnea syndrome in U.S. communities. *Sleep Breath* 2002;**6**(2):49–54.

Malhotra A, Orr JE, Owens RL. On the cutting edge of obstructive sleep apnoea: where next? *Lancet Respir Med* 2015;**3**(5):397–403.

Mansukhani MP, Wang S, Somers VK. Chemoreflex physiology and implications for sleep apnoea: insights from studies in humans. *Exp Physiol* 2015;**100**(2):130–5.

Somers VK, et al. Sympathetic neural mechanisms in obstructive sleep apnea. *J Clin Invest* 1995;**96**(4):1897–904.

Strohl KP. Sleep medicine training across the spectrum. *Chest* 2011;**139**(5):1221–31.

Strohl KP, Cherniack NS, Gothe B. Physiologic basis of therapy for sleep apnea. *Am Rev Respir Dis* 1986;**134**(4):791–802.

Wolf J, Drozdowski J, Czechowicz K, et al. Effect of beta-blocker therapy on heart rate response in patients with hypertension and newly diagnosed untreated obstructive sleep apnea syndrome. *Int J Cardiol* 2016; **202**:67–72.

A complete reference list can be found online at ExpertConsult.com.

Obstructive Sleep Apnea: Phenotypes and Genetics

Susan S. Redline

Chapter Highlights

- There is clear evidence that a positive family history of obstructive sleep apnea (OSA) is an important risk factor for an elevated apnea-hypopnea index (AHI) and associated symptoms such as snoring, daytime sleepiness, and apneas. Patients with OSA often have relatives—parents, siblings, and children—who have similar symptoms, a diagnosis of OSA, or both. The familial aggregation of OSA has been quantified through use of twin and cohort studies, which conservatively estimate that risk for OSA is increased by 50% in individuals with an affected first-degree relative.

- Overall heritability estimates (the proportion of the variance in a trait attributable to genetic factors) for the AHI are 0.30 to 0.40. Although there is a strong correlation between OSA and obesity, only 35% of the genetic variance in the AHI may be accounted for by genes that influence obesity (with 65% of the genetic

variance likely due to genetic variants in other etiologic pathways). Other potentially inherited risk factors for OSA include craniofacial structural traits that influence upper airway patency; body fat distribution, including propensity for airway fat deposition; chemoreflex ventilatory control; and arousability to ventilator stimuli.

- Pedigree studies analyzed using linkage analysis have identified several areas where biologically plausible candidate genes are located, including candidates for ventilatory control and obesity. A number of association studies and emerging meta-analyses of candidate and genome-wide association studies also provide evidence for increased susceptibility to OSA in persons who inherit variants for genes in pathways implicated in ventilatory control, inflammation, body fat distribution, and craniofacial structure.

DEFINITION OF THE OBSTRUCTIVE SLEEP APNEA PHENOTYPE

As is the case with many other complex disorders, variable definitions have been used to characterize obstructive sleep apnea (OSA) in genetic analyses. Clinically, OSA is recognized by the occurrence of repetitive episodes of complete or partial upper airway obstruction during sleep that result in oxygen desaturation or arousal and that are usually accompanied by symptoms of loud snoring and daytime sleepiness. However, there can be substantial variability in identification and characterization of OSA because of variations in how specific respiratory events are identified and defined, the threshold level for frequency of events during sleep considered pathologic, and to what extent other clinical and polysomnographic data are thought necessary for characterizing disease status.

Most family and genetic studies of OSA have used the apnea-hypopnea index (AHI) to define phenotype. The advantages of using the AHI include its ability to be readily calculated from data obtained from overnight sleep apnea tests with moderate to high night-to-night reproducibility[1] and from widespread clinical use. In addition, it is often followed as a key outcome in OSA treatment research studies.

Because the AHI has been shown to be moderately correlated with other indexes of OSA severity, such as nighttime oxygen desaturation and sleep fragmentation, it may provide information about several correlated traits that are important in disease expression. All genetic studies of OSA that use the AHI as the outcome measure have demonstrated significant familial aggregation, suggesting that this measure captures useful information for quantifying genetic associations. All candidate gene studies conducted to date also have defined "case" and "controls" on the basis of threshold levels of AHI (either >5 or >15/hour of sleep).

Additional metrics of OSA that provide more specific information on patterns of respiratory disturbances during sleep have been reported to be heritable and thus have potential for use in genetic studies. These include measures of AHI specific to rapid eye movement (REM) and non–rapid eye movement (NREM) sleep, average levels of nocturnal oxygen desaturation, and average duration of sleep-related respiratory disturbances. The latter metric, which is related to respiratory arousability, has been reported to have a heritability of almost 0.60[2] (indicating as much as 60% of the variance in this trait is explained by familial factors acting additively) and thus may be useful for identifying genes influencing ventilatory control.

A multidimensional OSA phenotype can be derived by combining polysomnographic data with information related to symptoms, signs, and outcome data. In the Cleveland Family Study, a stronger relationship between familial risk and OSA was observed when OSA was defined by an AHI greater than 15/hour plus reported daytime sleepiness than when disease was defined by AHI alone.[3] Additional power may be gained in future genetic studies of OSA that use multidimensional phenotypes. For example, alternatives to the AHI, such as indexes of flow limitation during sleep and critical airway closing pressure, may prove to be superior markers for genetic studies. However, a phenotype must be feasible for use in the large numbers of subjects who are needed for genetic epidemiologic studies of complex traits. The choice of phenotype for use in genetic and other research studies will be influenced by the cost, degree of invasiveness, and individual burden required for identifying and quantifying the phenotype and by applicability across the spectrum of age and body mass index (BMI), as well as by its accuracy and reliability.

INTERMEDIATE DISEASE PATHWAYS AND PHENOTYPES

OSA is a complex disorder that is defined using a combination of clinical and physiologic measures, such as symptoms and data from overnight sleep apnea testing. However useful such an approach may be for clinical diagnosis, such definitions may be insufficiently specific for use in genetic analyses. An alternative approach for studying the genetic basis of OSA is to study intermediate traits that confer increased risk for the disorder. Such intermediate traits may be more closely associated with specific gene products and may be less influenced by environmental modification than more complex (and downstream) phenotypes (Figure 11-1).

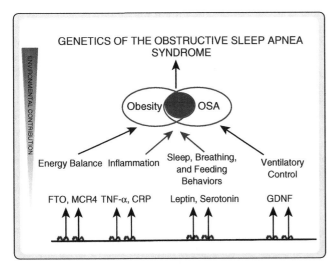

Figure 11-1 Schema showing the influence of genes on obstructive sleep apnea (OSA) from four intermediate pathways (energy balance, inflammation, sleep-feeding overlap, and ventilatory control) may be influenced by specific genes, and individually or together may influence obesity and/or OSAH. CRP, C-reactive protein gene; FTO, fat mass and obesity–associated gene; GDNF, glia-derived growth factor; Leptin: leptin or leptin receptor genes; MCR4, melanocortin-4 receptor gene; Serotonin: genes in the serotonin pathways (e.g., *HTR2A*); TNF-α, tumor necrosis factor-α gene. As one moves from the gene to the complex phenotype, the relative influence of specific genes decreases while the influence of environmental factors increases.

A number of risk factors likely interact to increase propensity for the repetitive upper airway collapse that occurs during sleep in patients with OSA. In a given person, the relevant attributes may be determined by anatomic and neuromuscular factors that influence upper airway size and function. Strong OSA risk factors are obesity and male gender. Although it has been argued that the genetics of obesity cannot be separated from the genetics of OSA, careful statistical modeling of AHI and BMI indicates that only about 35% of the genetic variance in AHI is shared with BMI, suggesting that a substantial portion of the genetic basis for OSA is in fact independent of obesity.[4] Other pathogenic pathways include those that influence upper airway size, ventilatory control mechanisms, and possibly elements of sleep and circadian rhythm control.

Thus it is useful to consider at least four primary intermediate pathogenic pathways through which genes might act to increase susceptibility to OSA: obesity and body fat distribution and related metabolic syndrome and inflammatory phenotypes, craniofacial and upper airway morphology, control of ventilation, and control of sleep and circadian rhythm[5]; these are discussed in more detail in the following sections. The limitation of this approach is that the genes so identified might not be sufficient to describe the clinically important phenotype, which might only occur in the context of other genetic and environmental factors. Specifically, susceptibility genes for intermediate traits associated with OSA might not be equivalent to the susceptibility genes for OSA.

Obesity and Body Fat Distribution

Obesity increases risk for OSA by 2- to 10-fold, with the strongest associations observed in middle age.[6] There are several pathways through which obesity predisposes to OSA. Fat deposition in the parapharyngeal fat pads may directly narrow the upper airway and predispose it to collapse when neuromuscular activation of upper airway muscles declines with sleep (see Chapters 7 and 13). Fat deposition in the thorax and abdomen (i.e., visceral fat) can increase the mechanical work of breathing, which can produce hypoventilation and reduce lung volumes, which in turn reduces parenchymal traction on the trachea, making the airway more collapsible. Reduced lung volumes also can increase propensity for oxygen desaturation to occur, increasing the likelihood that any given reduction in airflow may be classified as a "hypopnea," thus operationally increasing the severity of the adjudicated AHI, as well as physiologically increasing the severity of a hypopnea-associated disturbance. In addition, low lung volumes can reduce oxygen stores and alter "loop gain," which in turn can promote ventilatory instability. Finally, adipose tissue secretes hormones such as leptin that can influence ventilatory drive (see later).

Heritability estimates for obesity-associated phenotypes such as BMI, skinfold thickness, regional body fat distribution, fat mass, and leptin levels range between 40% and 70%, consistent with moderate to strong influences of genetic factors on these traits.[6-8] Approximately 7% of cases of early-onset obesity have been estimated to be attributable to the effects of mutations in a small number of genes involved in the leptin-melanocortin signaling pathway (i.e., melanocortin-4 receptor, leptin, leptin receptor, and pro-opiomelanocortin [POMC]), which are believed to influence weight largely through alterations in appetite regulation.[7] Mutations in melanocortin-4 receptor, the most common mutation, increase risk for severe childhood obesity by approximately 30% and also have been implicated in 0.5% to 1% of adult cases of obesity.[8]

The genetic etiology of obesity in the general population has been studied intensively in large populations that have undergone genotyping. Meta-analyses of genome-wide association studies, which examine the variation of frequency of thousands of alleles with disease status, have led to the discovery and replication of 36 genetic loci that associate with BMI.[9] However, all risk alleles together explain only 6% to 11% of the phenotypic variation.[10] The locus with the largest effect size is in the *FTO* (fat mass and obesity–associated gene),[11] which explains 0.34% of the variation in BMI among adult populations. An association between *FTO* and BMI has been replicated across populations and indicates that homozygotes for the risk allele weigh on average 3 to 4 kg more than persons without the risk allele and have an associated 1.67-fold increased risk for obesity compared with persons without the allele. Although the functioning of this gene is not well understood, *FTO* is expressed in the hypothalamus, and there is some evidence that it confers a risk for increased obesity through regulation of food intake and possibly through mechanisms that influence stress responses. Distinct genetic variants have been associated with waist-to-hip ratio,[12] which may be particularly relevant to OSA given the strong association between central obesity and OSA.

Craniofacial Morphology

Craniofacial morphology, which encompasses both bony and soft tissues, predisposes to OSA by reducing upper airway dimensions. Soft tissue structures that vary with OSA include elongation of the soft palate, macroglossia, and hypertrophy of adenoids and tonsils. Magnetic resonance imaging (MRI) has specifically shown that the lateral pharyngeal wall and tongue are larger in OSA patients compared with matched controls.[13] Cephalometry also has shown that patients with OSA compared with those without OSA have reduction of the anterior-posterior dimension of the cranial base, increased lower facial height, mandibular retrognathia or micrognathia, and inferior displacement of the hyoid[14-16] (see Chapters 3 and 13). A brachycephalic head form, measured by anthropometry, is often found in association with reduced upper airway dimensions. This head form is associated with a small but significant increased risk for OSA in those of European ancestry, and it also identifies families at risk for both OSA and sudden infant death.[17] In African Americans, this head form is uncommon and does not appear to increase risk for OSA. It is possible that a brachycephalic head form may contribute to increase risk for OSA among individuals of Asian ancestry.

In the Cleveland Family Study, both hard tissue (e.g., head form, intermaxillary length) and soft tissue (e.g., soft palate length, tongue volume) factors predicted the AHI level in European Americans. In African Americans, soft tissue factors also predicted AHI levels, but hard tissue anatomic features appeared to be only weakly associated with OSA.[18] These data support the importance of structural features in increasing susceptibility to OSA, but they also suggest that the anatomic underpinnings and the genes for upper airway anatomy might differ among ethnic groups.

Facial morphogenesis and patterning are complex processes that involve multiple signaling pathways. In humans, the genetic basis for craniofacial features is supported by both twin and family studies.[19,20] Heritability estimates (the proportion of the variance in the trait explained by additive genetic factors) for facial features such as facial height and mandibular position have been reported to be high as 0.80. A genome-wide association study has identified loci in five genes associated with facial morphology,[21] the most robust of which was in the paired box 3 gene (*PAX3*), which encodes a developmentally important transcription factor expressed in neural crest cells. There are also at least 50 syndromes in which congenital malformations of mandibular and maxillary structure occur, many of which also are associated with respiratory impairment and upper airway obstruction. These include Pierre-Robin syndrome and Treacher Collins syndrome.[22,23] Studies of various syndromes and genetic defects suggest potential roles of genes belonging to the fibroblast growth factor (e.g., *FGFR1*, *FGFR2*, *FGFR3*), transforming growth factor-β (e.g., *TGFBR1*, *TGFBR2*), homeobox (e.g., *MSX1*, *MSX2*), and sonic hedgehog (e.g., *PTCH*, *SHH*) pathways. Other potentially relevant candidate genes are those that have been implicated in craniofacial development, including genes on the endothelin pathway (e.g., *ECE1*, *EDN1*, *EDNRA*),[24-26] and *TCOF1*, the cause of Treacher Collins syndrome.[27] Further understanding of homeobox genes and genes controlling growth factors might contribute to our clarifying the origins of craniofacial dysmorphisms found in OSA.

Inherited abnormalities of craniofacial structure appear to explain at least some of the familial aggregation of OSA. Relatives of patients with OSA have been shown to have a more retropositioned mandible and smaller posterior-superior airway space compared with normative data.[28] Relatives of OSA probands also have been shown to have decreased total pharyngeal volume and glottic cross-sectional area, retropositioned maxilla and mandible, and a longer soft palate compared with relatives of controls.[29] In subjects both with and without OSA, acoustic reflectometry has demonstrated that more than 30% of the variance in the minimal cross-sectional area of the pharynx is heritable.[30] MRI has further demonstrated significant heritability for both the volume of soft tissue airway structures (including the tongue and lateral pharyngeal walls)[20] and hard tissue craniofacial dimensions (e.g., mandibular length and width).[31]

Although MRI precisely describes anatomic characteristics, its cost limits its utility for large-scale genetic epidemiology studies. Future research needs to assess the ability of reproducible and noninvasive techniques to identify subgroups of persons who inherit polymorphisms associated with genes relevant to craniofacial compared with other etiologic OSA pathways. There is also a need to further investigate how anatomic measurements performed awake and in the sitting position predict collapsibility during sleep and how anatomy interacts with physiology to influence susceptibility to OSA. Anatomic compromise may also be inferred from measurement of the pharyngeal critical closing pressure (Pcrit),[32] an index that can be derived during attended polysomnography with measurement of airway responses to progressive decreases in the delivery of therapeutic continuous positive airway pressure.

Ventilatory Control

Potentially inherited abnormalities of ventilatory control may predispose to OSA or central sleep apnea by affecting ventilation, ventilatory drive, and upper airway patency. These inherited ventilatory control abnormalities may include neuromuscular responses to the influences of state (sleep-wake), chemical drive (e.g., ventilatory response to hypoxia and hypercapnia), sensitivity of ventilatory load compensation (the degree to which an individual defends the tidal volume or minute ventilation in the presence of an imposed mechanical load to breathing such as an increased resistance or elastance), and arousal threshold. They can result in different ventilatory responses to sleep-related stresses and shape both the magnitude of ventilation and ventilatory pattern and the propensity for respiratory oscillations in sleep. The relative contribution of these ventilatory control factors varies among individuals, and such variability likely contributes to genetic heterogeneity in OSA. According to a multiple-risk factor model, OSA is likely to manifest as severe anatomic compromise, regardless of nonanatomic risk factors. In the presence of a lesser degree of anatomic compromise, OSA occurs when there are coexistent abnormalities in arousal threshold, loop gain (sensitivity of the ventilatory control system to feedback loops, such as due to changes in CO_2), or muscle responses.

Experimental data indicate that there is substantial interindividual variation in the contributions of these physiologic factors to OSA.[33] Further, the magnitude of ventilatory chemoresponsiveness appears to be subject to major genetic control; for example, heritability estimates for chemoresponsiveness to oxygen saturation levels range from approximately 30% to 75%.[34] Ventilatory responses are more strongly correlated between monozygotic than dizygotic twins.[35-37,38] Population differences in ventilatory patterns and hypoxic sensitivity have been identified for populations that have adapted to living at high altitude.[39,40] Abnormalities in hypoxic or hypercapnic ventilatory responsiveness have been described in the first-degree relatives of probands with unexplained respiratory failure,[41] chronic obstructive pulmonary disease,[42,43] and asthma.[44] There is a growing understanding of the molecular bases for ventilatory responses, with identification of a number of respiratory chemoreceptors in the carotid body and lower brainstem, including the nucleus solitaries, retrotrapezoid nucleus, locus coeruleus, and raphe.[45]

Although the contributions of the previously noted population and genetic data to OSA-related phenotypes are not clear, there is some evidence that absence of the retrotrapezoid nucleus causes severe central apneas in congenital central hypoventilation syndrome.[46] Additionally, a potential role for inherited impairments of ventilatory control in influencing susceptibility to OSA has been suggested by several studies of carefully characterized families of OSA patients, which have demonstrated blunted hypoxic responses and impairment in load compensation compared with controls.[47-51]

As referred to earlier, the potential impact of deficits in ventilatory control on OSA susceptibility is likely magnified in persons with anatomically compromised upper airways. With sleep onset, the central inspiratory drive to upper airway motor neurons, a major determinant of airway patency, is reduced or fluctuates.[52,53] Any given reduction in central inspiratory drive results in greater increases in upper airway resistance in persons with anatomically compromised airways than in others.[54] Conversely, persons with greater degrees of upper airway resistance (due to craniofacial or obesity risk factors) can require a high level of compensatory drive to overcome sleep-associated airway collapse, and thus they may be especially vulnerable to the influence of genetically determined ventilatory control deficits.

These observations underscore the potential importance of considering the interaction of genetic risk factors that influence more than one etiologic pathway. Similarly, systematic characterization of ventilatory control pathophysiology and clinical phenotypes could accelerate discovery of genes that influence specific mechanistic pathways in humans, similar to mouse models which have allowed genes to be identified that determine respiratory timing, frequency, awake ventilation, chemosensitivity, and load responses. Clear strain differences have been observed for many of these phenotypes, with evidence of quantitative trait loci near plausible candidate genes. Knockout and transgenic mice also have helped identify the role of specific proteins and receptors in ventilatory chemoreception, neuromuscular transmission, and neural integration. Candidate genes identified from such studies include genes that sense O_2[55-57] and CO_2[58,59]; genes that modulate serotonin signaling[60]; genes on the endothelin pathway,[61,62] which also are important in craniofacial development; and genes that regulate neural crest migration, including *PHOX2B*, mutations of which are associated with congenital central hypoventilation.[63,64]

Control of Sleep and Circadian Rhythm

Given the effect of sleep-wake state on respiratory motor neuron activation, insights into the susceptibility of upper airway muscles to collapse during sleep may require delineation of the genetics of sleep-wake control. Orexins, neuropeptides that play a fundamental role in the regulation of appetite and sleep-wake states,[65,66] also influence arousal and muscle tone.[65] Orexin A levels are reported to be reduced in OSA.[67] Thus abnormalities in orexin genes may be relevant to OSA because of their influence on arousal, muscle tone, ventilatory control, and weight.

It may similarly be useful to consider how respiratory motor neuron control is influenced by genetic processes that determine circadian clocks, which are known to drive important metabolic and behavioral rhythms. Genes influencing circadian rhythm have been identified in animal models and in humans[68] and have been shown to influence metabolism, inflammation, and aging.[69] The relevance of these findings to OSA is unclear. However, genetic variation in circadian rhythm determination may influence apnea number and duration by affecting the distribution of REM and NREM sleep and the associated neuromuscular responses across the sleep period. Genes that influence regulation of sleep-wake rhythm may also influence the phenotypic expression of OSA (e.g., ability to compensate for sleepiness in response to recurrent apneas and sleep disruption).

FAMILIAL AGGREGATION OF OBSTRUCTIVE SLEEP APNEA

In addition to the specific heritability and genetic associations of OSA discussed to this point, significant familial aggregation of AHI or of symptoms of OSA have been observed in studies from the United States, Finland, Denmark, the United Kingdom, Israel, and Iceland.[28,29,70-72] Such studies have used a variety of designs, including cohorts, small and large pedigrees, twins, and case-control studies; they have included adults and children; and they have employed varying

	Partially Adjusted* Familial Correlation		BMI-Adjusted† Familial Correlation	
Relationship	Coefficient	Relationship P Value	Coefficient	P Value
Parent-offspring	0.21	.002	0.17	.017
Sibling-sibling	0.21	.003	0.18	.008

Table 11-1 — **Familial Correlations for Apnea-Hypopnea Index**

*Adjusted for age, age squared (age²), ethnic group, and gender.
†Adjusted for body mass index (BMI), age, age², ethnic group, and gender.
From Redline S, Tishler PV, Tosteson TD, et al. The familial aggregation of obstructive sleep apnea. *Am J Respir Crit Care Med* 1995;151:682–7.

approaches for assessing phenotype. Despite study design and population differences, these studies have consistently shown familial aggregation of the AHI level and symptoms of OSA in children and adults and in obese and nonobese subjects. These studies have provided clear evidence that a positive family history of OSA is an important risk factor for an elevated AHI and for associated symptoms such as snoring and daytime sleepiness, although the estimated magnitude of effects has varied greatly.

Several large twin studies have shown that concordance rates for snoring, a cardinal symptom of OSA, were significantly higher in monozygotic twins than in dizygotic twins.[71,73,74] A study of adult male twins has shown significant genetic correlations for daytime sleepiness as well as snoring, with models consistent with common genes underlying both symptoms.[71] A subsequent report from this cohort showed significant heritability for objectively measured AHI levels in this twin population.[75] A large Danish cohort study showed that the age, BMI, and comorbidity-adjusted risk for snoring were increased threefold when one first-degree relative was a snorer and were increased fourfold when both parents were snorers.[76]

The prevalence of objectively measured OSA among first-degree relatives of OSA probands has been reported to vary from 22% to 84%.[28,29,70-72] Among the studies that included controls, the odds ratio, which relates the odds of a person with OSA in a family with affected relatives to that for someone without an affected relative, has varied from 2 to 46.[3,28,29,70] Pedigree studies from the United States and Iceland have shown consistent associations; the overall risk for OSA in a family member of an affected proband compared with an individual without affected relatives is approximately 2. This is lower than that reported from case-control studies, which may be subject to biases depending on the appropriateness of the selection of cases and controls. Heritability estimates for the AHI from both pedigree[77,78] and twin studies[75] are approximately 35% to 40%. Similar parent-offspring (correlations of approximately 0.20) have been observed, and they are greater than spouse-spouse correlations.[3]

OSA has been described as occurring more commonly as a multiplex (affecting at least two members) than as a simplex (occurring in a single family member) disorder. Further evidence for a genetic basis for OSA is derived from the observation that the odds of OSA syndrome, defined as AHI greater than 15/hour and self-reported daytime sleepiness, increases with increasing numbers of affected relatives.[3] Table 11-1 show the odds for OSA syndrome given one, two, or three affected relatives with these findings, adjusted for age, gender, ethnicity, and BMI, compared with OSA patients who have

no affected relatives, These results support the utility of ascertaining family history as part of the evaluation of the patient for OSA. Information on snoring, apneas, and sleepiness among first-degree relatives can be used to refine the likelihood of OSA in a given patient. Such information can also be used to help identify the need for other family members to seek sleep evaluations.

Several studies have reported a coaggregation of OSA with sudden infant death syndrome (SIDS) and acute life-threatening events.[70,79,80] Members of families with both OSA and SIDS cases have been reported to have a relatively increased prevalence of brachycephaly, an anatomic feature that is associated with upper airway narrowing, as well as reduced hypoxic ventilatory responsiveness.[80] These observations suggest that the two sleep-related breathing disorders have a shared genetic predisposition acting through ventilatory control or craniofacial structure pathways. The demonstration of widespread serotoninergic brainstem abnormalities in SIDS victims and the putative role of this pathway in respiratory drive[81] suggest a biologic basis for the potential genetic link between these disorders.

In children, both OSA and adenotonsillar hypertrophy (the chief risk factor for pediatric OSA) have been elevated in the siblings of children with OSA.[82] Pedigree studies show that the disease is transmitted across generations,[83] suggesting that common risk factors might influence OSA susceptibility in children and adults. Although hypertrophy of the tonsils is a major risk factor for childhood OSA, children of OSA probands more often have residual OSA after tonsillectomy compared with the offspring of adults without OSA,[84] suggesting the importance of underlying genetic susceptibility as a determinant of treatment response as well.

GENETIC ANALYSES

Candidate Gene Studies

The molecular genetics of OSA have been investigated using candidate gene approaches. In these association studies, the frequency of genetic variants thought to relate to disease susceptibility are compared in groups with and without OSA or are assessed in relationship to the severity of a quantitative phenotype (e.g., AHI). A number of plausible candidate genes are also found in pathways that influence the intermediate traits of obesity, craniofacial structure, and ventilatory control (Box 11-1). Candidate genes that have been examined in relationship to OSA in humans include those for apolipoprotein E (*APOE*), angiotensin-converting enzyme (*ACE*), serotoninergic pathways, leptin pathways, obesity, and inflammation. The largest single multiple-candidate gene

---

Box 11-1   CANDIDATE GENES* FOR INTERMEDIATE PHENOTYPES FOR OBSTRUCTIVE SLEEP APNEA

Obesity

FTO (fat mass and obesity–associated gene)
Melanocortin-4 receptor
Leptin
Pro-opiomelanocortin
Melanocyte-stimulating hormone
Neuropeptidase Y
Prohormone convertase
Neutrophic receptor TrkB
Insulin-like growth factor
Glucokinase
Adenosine deaminase
Tumor necrosis factor-α
Glucose regulatory protein
Agouti signaling protein
β-Adrenergic receptor
Carboxypeptidase E
Insulin-signaling protein
Resistin
Ghrelin
Adiponectin
Gamma-aminobutyric acid transporter
Orexin

Ventilatory Control

RET protooncogene
PHOX2B
HOX IIL2
KROX-20
Receptor tyrosine kinase
Neurotrophic growth factors
• Brain-derived neurotrophic factor
• Glia-derived neurotrophic factor
• Neurotrophic factor-4
• Platelet-derived growth factor
Neuronal synthase
Acetylcholine receptor
Dopaminergic receptor
Substance P
Glutamyl transpeptidase
Endothelin-1
Endothelin-3
Leptin
EN-1
GSH-2
Orexin

Craniofacial Structure

Class I homeobox genes
Growth hormone receptors
Growth factor receptors
Retinoic acid
Endothelin-1
Collagen types I and II
Tumor necrosis factor-α

*Includes related proteins and receptors.

study analyzed more than 1000 single nucleotide polymorphisms (SNPs) from 53 candidate genes representing key intermediate pathways in approximately 1500 individuals of European or African ancestry.[85] In European Americans, variants within the C-reactive protein (*CRP*) and glia-derived

neurotrophic factor (*GDNF*) were significantly associated with OSA, with suggestive associations observed for several SNPs in the 5-hydrotrypamine receptor 2A (*5-HTR2A*) gene and endothelin-1 (*EDN1*) gene. In African Americans, a variant in the serotonin receptor 2a (*5-HTR2A*) gene was associated with approximately twofold increased odds of OSA, with suggestive associations observed for variants in the leptin receptor and hypocretin receptor 2. Genetic associations frequently reflect false-positive findings and require replication in independent samples. However, smaller candidate gene studies, summarized later, provide additional support implicating serotoninergic, leptin signaling, and inflammatory pathways.

Serotoninergic Pathways

Serotonin (5-hydroxytryptanmine [5-HT]) receptors are found in the carotid body and in the brainstem near ventilatory control centers important for chemoreception, as well as in hypoglossal neurons. Research in animals suggests that serotoninergic neurotransmission, through peripheral actions at the level of the carotid body or hypoglossal nerve, or centrally, at medullary respiratory control centers, influences a wide range of functions relevant to OSA, including upper airway reflexes, ventilation, and arousal, as well as sleep-wake cycling.[60] Although the pharmacology is complex, with at least 14 receptor subtypes, this pathway has been implicated in the pathogenesis of SIDS, which, as discussed earlier, might share common genetically determined risk factors with OSA.

Polymorphisms in three genes—*5-HTT* (5-hydroxytryptamine transporter; encoding a serotonin transporter protein that clears serotonin from the synaptic space), *HTR2A* (encoding the 5-HT$_{2A}$ receptor), and *HTR2C* (encoding the 5-HT$_{2C}$ receptor)—each have been studied in relationship to OSA.[86-88] Several meta-analyses have been conducted that have pooled data on variants in these genes for approximately 500 to 700 cases and controls, each from three to six studies conducted in Japan, China, Turkey, and Brazil.[89-91] These analyses indicate than an approximately twofold increased OSA risk is associated with a variant in *5-HT2A* (an allele of 5-HT2A 148G/A) and 20% and 200% increased risks are associated with variants in the *5-HTT* gene (intron-2 variable numbers of tandem repeats and *5-HTT* gene–linked polymorphic region, respectively). Although requiring further replication, these findings are noteworthy given that the HTR2A receptor appears to be the predominant excitatory receptor subtype at the hypoglossal motor neuron and thus is a strong biologic candidate for an association with OSA.

Leptin Signaling

Animal and human studies suggest that leptin, an adipose-derived circulating hormone that influences appetite regulation and energy expenditure, not only influences body weight but also has important effects on central ventilatory drive mediated by brainstem receptors in the nucleus tractus solitarius and hypoglossal motor nucleus.[92,93] Mice homozygous for a knockout mutation in leptin hypoventilate and have a blunted ventilatory response to hypercapnia. Leptin replacement improves the ventilatory responses to hypercapnia in both wakefulness and sleep in leptin-deficient mice.[94] In obese women, increases in circulating levels of leptin have been shown to correlate with the magnitude of compensatory upper airway neuromuscular responses to experimental airway occlusion.[59] The stimulatory effects of leptin on hypercapnic ventilatory response appear to be mediated through melanocortin, which is produced from a precursor polyprotein, POMC. As described earlier, the Cleveland Family Study reported suggestive evidence for linkage to an area on chromosome 2p that houses the POMC locus,[77] an area also reported by others to be strongly linked to serum leptin levels.[95] An association of OSA with the leptin receptor LEPR also has been reported in candidate gene studies.[85,91] Thus hypothalamic and pituitary pathways involved in leptin signaling may influence OSA susceptibility.

Inflammatory Pathways

Genes in inflammatory pathways may contribute to OSA by influencing upper airway patency through effects on pharyngeal edema, tonsillar hypertrophy, and pharyngeal neuropathic changes[96] or through effects of adipokines such as leptin that influence central respiratory drive. Given the reported associations between tumor necrosis factor-α (TNF-α) levels and OSA severity and sleepiness, a functional polymorphism in the TNF-α gene has been examined in several case-control studies of OSA[97,98] (including one study that compared genetic variants in affected and unaffected sibling pairs[98]) that have reported an elevated risk for OSA in association with a variant associated with higher TNF-α levels. A more recent population-control study by some of the same investigators did not report a significant difference between controls and subjects with OSA in the frequency of that single nucleotide polymorphism of TNF-α or other alleles of TNF-α.[98a] Other studies have reported associations with variants in genes for interleukin-6 and CRP.[85,99] Variants in the nitric oxide synthase (NOS) and endothelin (EDN) pathways have been reported to be elevated in children with OSA compared with snoring controls.[100] These genes have been implicated in cardiovascular disease, which is common in OSA. These findings suggest that either there are common genetic mechanisms which predispose to both OSA and cardiovascular disease or that individuals with OSA who harbor these variants may be at increased risk for cardiovascular disease.

Apolipoprotein E. An allele of the apolipoprotein E ε4 gene (APOE) gene associated with increased risk for both cardiovascular disease and Alzheimer disease was reported to be associated with OSA in two cohort studies of predominantly white subjects.[101,102] Two other studies, however, did not replicate this finding.[103,104] The Cleveland Family Study reported evidence for linkage to AHI near the APOE locus on chromosome 19.[86] However, the APOE genotype did not explain the linkage findings and was not associated with OSA status. These findings suggested that the susceptibility locus for OSA is not to APOE but another locus close to it. A candidate gene in this area is hypoxia-inducible factor 3, which plays a role in oxygen sensing.

APOE e4 has also been examined as a disease-modifying risk factor. Several studies have shown that individuals with moderate to severe OSA who carry one or more APOE e4 variants have greater cognitive impairment than individuals with OSA without such a risk allele.[87,88] It has been hypothesized that the APOE e4 allele increases the likelihood of brain injury to oxidative or other stresses.

Angiotensin II Converting Enzyme. Angiotensin II, an important vasoconstrictor, also appears to modulate afferent activity from the carotid body chemoreceptor and thus might influence ventilatory drive.[105] Angiotensin II levels are regulated by the actions of ACE, which is encoded by the ACE gene. Several studies of Chinese cohorts have reported an association between polymorphisms in the ACE gene and OSA, particularly in persons with hypertension.[106-110] Data from the Wisconsin Sleep Cohort and the Cleveland Family Study did not show an association between ACE genotype and OSA but did show an association between hypertension and OSA severity, which varied in strength by ACE genotype.[111,112]

Linkage Analysis

Linkage analysis quantifies the cosegregation of a disease locus and a marker locus among family members. Typically, the strength of genetic associations is expressed as an LOD score (the log-odds quantifying the probability of receiving alleles at two loci). A LOD score of 3 or more is considered strong evidence for linkage. By identifying alleles that cosegregate in related individuals, areas of the genome are identified that have an increased probability of harboring risk alleles for a given trait. Although linkage analysis has limited resolution to identify specific genetic variants, linkage signals can help prioritize areas of the genome likely to harbor risk variants, and this information can then be integrated into tests of genetic association to increase the statistical power for discovering genetic variants. Linkage analysis can also be used to identify families likely to carry risk alleles, particularly rare mutations that may have large effects. A whole-genome screen for OSA-related traits has been performed in the Cleveland Family Study.[77,78] In one set of analyses including 1275 members of 237 families, linkage analysis was used to identify genetic regions that were uniquely associated with OSA (modeling the AHI) and other regions that associated with AHI through genetic associations with BMI.[113] Several areas of significant linkage to AHI were identified that were not associated with coincident linkage for BMI. Notably, significant linkage was observed on chromosome 6 for the BMI-adjusted AHI level (LOD score of 3.5). A linkage peak on chromosome 13 near the serotonin 2a receptor was observed in African Americans for both AHI and BMI, providing supportive evidence that variants in HTR2A may influence both OSA and obesity.

Genome-Wide Association Analyses

Marked advances in technology permit dense mapping of genetic markers across the genome, with some assays providing coverage of more than 1 million genetic variants (SNPs), providing the opportunity to discover genetic variants for a trait without prior knowledge of candidate genes. Such whole-genome scans can be applied to family members and analyzed with linkage analysis. The first study to report a broad analysis of genetic variants for OSA used an assay ("chip") that contained 45,237 SNPs from more than 2000 genes selected to be relevant to heart, lung, blood, and sleep phenotypes.[114] In 3551 participants from three cohort studies, significant associations were identified for several novel loci with OSA. Evidence of replication in independent cohorts was found for a variant in the lysophosphatidic acid receptor (LPAR1), a gene expressed in the embryonic cortex with proinflammatory effects. Craniofacial abnormalities have been observed in an *LPAR1* knockout mouse. Another replicated association was in the prostaglandin E_2 receptor (*PTGER2*), which also is expressed in neuronal tissues and previously was associated with hypertension. Preliminary findings from more recent genome-wide studies of more than 20,000 individuals studied with assays of more than 500,000 SNPs have been reported. It is expected that, as such findings are replicated, genetic loci and their corresponding pathophysiologic pathways, relevant in the pathogenesis of OSA, will be identified.

CLINICAL PEARL

A positive family history of OSA (or of related symptoms) is useful in identifying patients at increased risk for the disorder. Craniofacial abnormalities and obesity can each have a genetic basis and are risk factors for OSA. Clinicians should ask about OSA symptoms in family members, including offspring. Individuals from families with more than one affected member may harbor genetic variants for OSA and may benefit from close follow-up after interventions to ensure their OSA is adequately treated.

SUMMARY

Despite the challenges in studying an inherently complex trait, there is strong evidence from clinical and epidemiologic studies supporting the importance of familial, and specifically genetic, factors in influencing OSA susceptibility. The largest pedigree and twin studies consistently estimate heritability for the AHI to be between 35% and 40%, with recurrent risk factors of approximately 2. Although obesity is the strongest risk factor for OSA and has a clear genetic basis, causal modeling suggests that only 35% of the genetic variance in the AHI of persons with OSA is shared with pathways that determine body weight. Thus most of the genetic variance for the AHI is likely due to the influence of genes that influence other pathways, including those that influence craniofacial structure, ventilatory control, and possibly sleep-wake patterns. Molecular studies of OSA still lag behind those of

other chronic diseases. However, data from candidate gene studies, linkage analyses, and emerging genome-wide association analyses implicate variants in genes in the serotonin and leptin pathways, as well as genes in novel inflammatory and development pathways, relevant to the pathogenesis and possible treatment of OSA. Further investigations of the genetic etiology of OSA should provide a means of better understanding its pathogenesis, with the goal of improving preventive strategies, diagnostic tools, and therapies.

Selected Readings

Bielicki P, MacLeod AK, Douglas NJ, Riha RL. Cytokine gene polymorphisms in obstructive sleep apnoea/hypopnoea syndrome. *Sleep Med* 2015;**16**(6):792–5.

Carmelli D, Bliwise DL, Swan GE, Reed T. Genetic factors in self-reported snoring and excessive daytime sleepiness: a twin study. *Am J Respir Crit Care Med* 2001;**164**:949–52.

Eckert DJ, White DP, Jordan AS, et al. Defining phenotypic causes of obstructive sleep apnea: identification of novel therapeutic targets. *Am J Respir Crit Care Med* 2013;**188**:996–1004.

Gislason T, Johannsson JH, Haraldsson A, et al. Familial predisposition and cosegregation analysis of adult obstructive sleep apnea and the sudden infant death syndrome. *Am J Respir Crit Care Med* 2002;**166**:833–8.

Larkin EK, Patel SR, Elston RC, et al. Using linkage analysis to identify quantitative trait loci for sleep apnea in relationship to body mass index. *Ann Hum Genet* 2008;**72**:762–73.

Larkin EK, Patel SR, Goodloe RJ, et al. A Candidate gene study of obstructive sleep apnea in European Americans and African Americans. *Am J Respir Crit Care Med* 2010;**182**:947–53.

Patel SR, Goodloe R, De G, et al. Association of genetic loci with sleep apnea in European Americans and African-Americans: the Candidate Gene Association Resource (Care). *PLoS ONE* 2012;**7**:e48836.

Patel SR, Larkin EK, Redline S. Shared genetic basis for obstructive sleep apnea and adiposity measures. *Int J Obes (Lond)* 2008;**32**(5):795–800.

Qin B, Sun Z, Liang Y, et al. The Association of 5-Ht2a, 5-Htt, and Lepr polymorphisms with obstructive sleep apnea syndrome: a systematic review and meta-analysis. *PLoS ONE* 2014;**9**:e95856.

Redline S, Tishler PV, Tosteson TD, et al. The familial aggregation of obstructive sleep apnea. *Am J Respir Crit Care Med* 1995;**151**:682–7.

Schwab RJ, Pasirstein M, Kaplan L, et al. Family aggregation of upper airway soft tissue structures in normal subjects and patients with sleep apnea. *Am J Respir Crit Care Med* 2006;**173**:453–63.

Yalcmkaya M, Erbek SS, Babakurban ST, et al. Lack of association of matrix metalloproteinase-9 promoter gene polymorphism in obstructive sleep apnea syndrome. *J Cranio-Maxillo-Facial Surgery* 2015;**43**:1099–103.

A complete reference list can be found online at ExpertConsult.com.

Chapter 12

Central Sleep Apnea: Definitions, Pathophysiology, Genetics, and Epidemiology

Madalina Macrea; Eliot S. Katz; Atul Malhotra

Chapter Highlights

- The various clinical entities comprising sleep breathing disorders are the result of pathophysiologic mechanisms that frequently overlap. Defining the types of central sleep apnea (CSA) within the sleep breathing disorder spectrum is essential for a common language among clinicians, educators, and researchers.

- CSA includes several heterogeneous syndromes, many heavily represented in day-to-day medical practice. Recent scientific evidence allows a more comprehensive understanding of CSA

epidemiology, genetics, pathophysiology, and associated morbidity and mortality.

- Several mechanisms participate in the control of breathing. Chemical, mechanical, and neural pathophysiology involved in CSA, and their clinical implications, are detailed.

- Considerable progress has been made in our understanding of control of breathing related to CSA, with major implications of these new findings for patient care. Only by further mechanistic research are new therapeutic strategies likely to emerge.

Sleep breathing disorders (SBDs) is characterized by repetitive periods of cessation in breathing (i.e., apneas) or reductions in breathing (i.e., hypopneas) that occur during sleep. The various clinical entities belonging to SBDs are the result of pathophysiologic mechanisms that frequently overlap; centrally driven events are primarily due to a temporary loss of output from the pontomedullary pacemaker that generates breathing rhythm, resulting in loss of the respiratory pump muscles (diaphragm, thorax, abdomen). Alternatively, obstructive events are primarily due to inward collapse of the oropharynx when the pharyngeal dilator muscles are relaxed, resulting in loss of airflow because of upper airway narrowing.[1] Both obstructive and central respiratory events converge in their symptoms of frequent nocturnal awakenings and excessive daytime sleepiness.

Defining the end points of SBDs polysomnographically (i.e., central sleep apnea [CSA] and obstructive sleep apnea [OSA]), is often a straightforward process. In CSA, both oronasal flow and thoracoabdominal excursions are absent; that is, there is an absence of respiratory effort during the cessation of airflow, whereas in OSA, there are ongoing respiratory efforts during the absence of oronasal flow. In contrast, differentiating rigorously between events within the SBD spectrum (i.e., "central" and "obstructive" hypopnea) is difficult without quantification of respiratory effort as recorded by esophageal pressure monitoring. Because esophageal manometry is mildly invasive and rarely employed clinically, thoracic and abdominal excursions assessed by respiratory inductance plethysmography are widely used to detect asynchrony of

these excursions during hypopnea (consistent with obstruction) or in-phase breathing (consistent with decreased central drive). Thus, central hypopnea is characterized by a proportional and synchronous decrease in thoracic and abdominal excursions, whereas obstructive hypopnea is characterized by paradoxical inward rib cage movement or asynchronous decrease in the thoracic and abdominal excursions (Figure 12-1). Nasal pressure recordings are sometimes used as a surrogate for upper airway narrowing because inspiratory flattening has been shown to correspond with inspiratory flow limitation. Additionally, obstructive and central apneas may overlap within the same event: such "mixed" apneas have features of both conditions, when an apnea begins with loss of central drive to breathe ("central" apnea) but then proceeds with increasing effort against an occluded upper airway ("obstructive" apnea).

DEFINITIONS

As defined by the *International Classification of Sleep Disorders*, third edition (ICSD3), CSA includes six heterogeneous adult syndromes (Box 12-1).[2,3] Several of these have in common a waxing and waning ventilatory pattern.

1. *Cheyne-Stokes breathing* (CSB) is an abnormal pattern of breathing characterized by oscillations of tidal volume between apnea or hypopnea at the nadir of ventilation and hyperpnea at the height of ventilation, with a spindle-like crescendo-decrescendo pattern in the depth of breathing.[4] According to the American Academy of Sleep Medicine

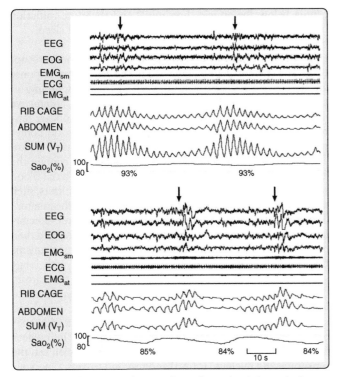

Figure 12-1 Polysomnographic recordings of central and obstructive hypopneas from patients with heart failure with use of respiratory inductance plethysmography. The *upper panel* shows a central hypopnea during stage 2 NREM sleep in a patient who has central sleep apnea with Cheyne-Stokes breathing. Note in-phase gradual waxing and waning of tidal volume during hyperpnea and only minimal O_2 desaturation during hypopnea. Arousal occurs several breaths after termination of the hypopnea. The *lower panel* shows an obstructive hypopnea in a patient with obstructive sleep apnea. Note that in contrast to central hypopnea, rib cage and abdominal motion are out-of-phase and O_2 desaturation is greater during hypopnea, and the rise in ventilation following its termination is more abrupt and hyperpneas are shorter. In addition, arousals occur earlier at hypopnea termination. ECG, Electrocardiogram; EEG, electroencephalogram; EMG_{sm}, submental electromyogram; EMG_{at}, anterior tibial EMG; EOG, electrooculogram. Arrows (↓) indicate arousals. (From Central Sleep Apnea and Cheyne-Stokes Respiration, Volume 5, Issue 2, The Proceedings of the American Thoracic Society.)

Box 12-1   HETEROGENEOUS ADULT SYNDROMES OF CENTRAL SLEEP APNEA

Central sleep apnea with Cheyne-Stokes breathing
Central sleep apnea due to a medical disorder without Cheyne-Stokes breathing
Central sleep apnea due to high-altitude periodic breathing
Central sleep apnea due to a medication or substance
Primary central sleep apnea
Treatment emergent central sleep apnea

(AASM),[5] CSB in adults is scored when both of the following are met: (1) there are episodes of three or more consecutive central apneas or central hypopneas, or both, separated by a crescendo and decrescendo change in breathing amplitude with a cycle length of at least 40 seconds (typically 45 to 90 seconds), and (2) there are five or more central apneas or central hypopneas, or both, per

hour associated with the crescendo and decrescendo breathing pattern recorded over a minimum of 2 hours of monitoring. In terms of nocturnal oxygen desaturation, there is generally less desaturation during central apnea and hypopnea than during obstructive events in patients with heart failure.[6]

2. *Primary CSA* resembles CSA-CSB except that the cycle duration is shorter, arousals occur earlier (at the termination of apnea versus during or near the peak ventilatory effort), and resumption of breathing is more abrupt and not crescendo, typically with a large-volume breath. The patient must not be hypercapnic while awake ($Paco_2$ greater than 45 mm Hg). The diagnostic polysomnography (PSG) shows five or more apneic episodes per hour of sleep, the number of central apneas or central hypopneas more than 50% of the total number of apneas and hypopneas, and absence of CSB.

3. *High-altitude periodic breathing* is seen in normal persons at elevations greater than 7600 meters and in some at lower altitudes. This ventilatory pattern is characterized by periods of alternating hyperpnea and apnea,[7] the cycle length typically being between 12 and 34 seconds. PSG, if performed, demonstrates recurrent central apneas or hypopneas primarily during NREM sleep at a frequency of five or more per hour.

4. *CSA due to a medical condition, without CSB* is encountered in individuals with cardiac, renal, and neuromuscular disease who have CSA without the CSB.

5. *Central sleep apnea due to a medication or substance* is commonly seen in patients with long-term opioid use that causes respiratory depression by acting on the μ receptors of the ventral medulla. PSG demonstrates lack of CSB and five or more central apneas or central hypopneas, or both,[1] per hour of sleep, with the number of central apneas or central hypopneas, or both, greater than the total number of apneas and hypopneas.

6. *Treatment emergent central apnea* (or "complex" sleep apnea) is included in the ICSD3 and refers to CSA not explained by another CSA disorder (e.g., CSA with CSB or CSA due to a medication or substance). The diagnostic PSG shows five or more predominantly obstructive respiratory events per hour of sleep. The titration PSG without a backup rate shows resolution of obstructive events and emergence or persistence of central apnea or central hypopnea with both a central apnea-central hypopnea index (CAHI) of five or more per hour and number of central apneas and central hypopneas 50% or greater than total number of apneas and hypopneas.

PATHOPHYSIOLOGY

As Cherniack[8] noted in the early 1980s, breathing in an awake healthy person involves a smooth and regularly recurring sequence of inspiration and expiration without pauses. The rate and depth of breathing are regulated by a negative-feedback control system aimed at maintaining arterial partial pressures of carbon dioxide ($Paco_2$) and oxygen (Pao_2) at relatively constant levels. When diseases of the lung or chest wall produce hypoxemia and hypocapnia or hypercapnia, they usually do so without affecting the regularity of breathing. Several mechanisms and their corresponding controls influence the rhythmicity of breathing. A synopsis of the following roadmap we used in the discussion of CSA pathophysiology and its clinical translation is detailed in Tables 12-1 and 12-2.

Mechanisms

Several types of receptors and their associated afferent and efferent pathways are involved in maintaining the regular normal breathing.

Chemical Aspects of Ventilation

Ventilatory responses vary widely between the awake and asleep state, as well as between rapid eye movement (REM) and non–rapid eye movement (NREM) sleep. Ventilation during sleep is largely regulated by the same mechanisms that drive breathing while awake,[9] except that behavioral influences[10] become suppressed in transition to, and during, sleep. Therefore central apneic events are rarely present during the awake state[11,12] or REM sleep.[13] During NREM sleep, however, changes in the respiratory pattern are primarily controlled chemically, being the result of a fine balance among a critical $Paco_2$ level, below which there is a central cessation of breathing (i.e., apneic threshold); its triggering factors (mainly hypocapnia); and respondent receptors (i.e., central and peripheral chemoreceptors). Additionally, the level of ventilation in respiratory dysrhythmias is augmented by arousals from sleep, resulting in transient hyperventilation with hypo-

Table 12-1 Common Non-cardiac Conditions Associated with Central Sleep Apnea Events

Medical Condition	Prevalence (%)	Authors
Multiple sclerosis	18	Braley et al.[147]
Central nervous system tumor survivors	12.9	Mandrell et al.[148]
Cerebrovascular accident	7	Johnson et al.[149]
Congenital muscular dystrophies	55	Pinard et al.[150]
End-stage renal disease on hemodialysis	17	Tada et al.[151]
Diabetes	3.8	Resnick et al.[152]

Table 12-2 Roadmap Used in Discussion of the CSA Pathophysiology

Mechanism	Control	Clinicopathophysiologic Translation
Chemical	Metabolic	Cheyne-Stokes breathing OHS Sleep transition Apnea CCHS
Mechanical	Metabolic Neural	Muscular degenerative Postarousal/postsigh central apnea
Neural	Neural	Stroke CCHS

capnia below the apneic threshold[14] and therefore initiation of central apneic events, primarily during NREM sleep.

Hypoxic Stimulus and Peripheral and Central Chemoreceptors. The chemoreceptors involved in the ventilatory response are both peripheral and central, each of them responding to changes in arterial Po_2 *and* Pco_2 in a complex, interactive manner. In mammals, the peripheral chemoreceptors are represented by the aortic and carotid bodies. The carotid bodies represent the main drive of the ventilatory stimulation due to acute, chronic,[15,16] and intermittent[17] hypoxia and contain the glomus cells that respond to the changes in the arterial blood oxygen concentration through several neurotransmitters, such as acetylcholine, substance P, and adenosine triphosphate.[18] The aortic bodies, on the other hand, likely become upregulated only if the carotid bodies are chronically absent, and then respond to changes in the arterial Po_2[19] through mechanisms that are less known. Notably, studies in patients with longstanding OSA demonstrated the possibility of the carotid bodies becoming desensitized with extended exposure to intermittent hypoxia.[20-22] In comparison with the peripheral chemoreceptors, the central chemoreceptors have a wide anatomic distribution in the brainstem (especially in nucleus tractus solitarius [NTS], locus coeruleus, raphe nuclei, and the retrotrapezoid nucleus [RTN]) and respond to central nervous system–specific hypoxia by augmentation of alveolar ventilation during both wakefulness[23] and sleep.[24]

Hypercapnic Stimulus and Peripheral and Central Chemoreceptors. In addition to responding to hypoxia, the carotid bodies also act as a sensitive detector of the adequacy of alveolar ventilation,[25] as seen in the prompt ventilatory response to small increases in arterial Pco_2 and insensitive feedback to decreasing arterial Po_2 until it reaches the critical value of 50 to 60 mm Hg.[26] Quantitatively, assuming a purely additive model, Forster estimated that 40% of the steady-state ventilatory CO_2 response belongs to the carotid body and 60% to the central chemoreceptors, the carotid body providing its response prompter.[27,28] In the absence of an exact biologic definition for the central chemoreceptors, most consideration is given to the possibility that these cells are glial or vascular cells that regulate the activity of surrounding neurons through paracrine mechanisms and respond promptly to the changes of the local neuronal pH.[29,30] Anatomically, the RTN is considered to be the predominant location of integration of the central chemoreceptor drive.[31]

Apneic Threshold and Implications for Central Sleep Apnea. During NREM sleep, motor output to respiratory muscles is dramatically reduced compared with wakefulness, causing mild to moderate sustained hypoventilation in all healthy subjects (+2 to +8 mm Hg $Paco_2$). If relative hyperpnea occurs and $Paco_2$ falls below a characteristic value for each individual (the apneic threshold), a central apnea occurs (see Fig. 12-2).[32] The hypocapnia-induced apneic threshold is not a constant value but usually occurs at a level very close to the eupneic $Paco_2$ present during wakefulness following a very small reduction in $Paco_2$, from 2 to 5 mm.

Mechanistically, to reach the apneic threshold, transient ventilatory overshoots are necessary, commonly provided by transient arousals with consequent brief hyperpnea with hypocapnia. Alternatively, to overcome the apneic threshold

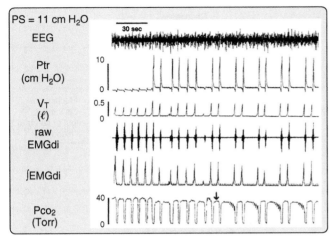

Figure 12-2 Polygraph record of one pressure support (PS) trial (11 cm H_2O) in which ventilatory instability was achieved in dogs. A reduced diaphragmatic EMG (EMGdi) and inspiratory effort on the seventh ventilator cycle was insufficient to trigger a ventilator breath. Clear periodicity developed after the ninth ventilator cycle. The *arrow* marks the petCO2 considered to be the apneic threshold. Ptr, Tracheal pressure. (Modified from Nakayama H, Smith CA, Rodman JR, et al. Effect of ventilatory drive on carbon dioxide sensitivity below eupnea during sleep. *Am J Respir Crit Care Med* 2002;165:1251–61.)

and therefore reinitiate the breathing rhythm, a $Paco_2$ higher by 1 to 4 mm Hg than the apneic threshold is needed; this difference reflects a postapneic control system termed *inertia*, aimed at enhancing the chemoreceptor stimulus after the ventilatory overshoot.

Interactions between the Central and Peripheral Chemoreceptors.

Several anatomic and functional connections (e.g., the RTN receives direct input from the NTS and, thus, the carotid body)[33] serve a dual chemotactic role (peripheral and central), raising the question of interdependence between the two types of chemoreceptors. Failing to demonstrate unequivocally the existence of only one model because of variations in the experimental protocol, the literature describes three possible interactions: additive (the two responses simply sum), hyperadditive (the two responses multiply), or hypoadditive (the sum of each response is less than their mathematical sum). Regardless of the specifics of the final augmentative response, it is postulated that carotid chemoreceptors act as the immediate hypocapnic sensors,[34] given the lack of short-term response of the central chemoreceptors to systemic hypocapnia when normocapnia and normoxia are maintained at the level of the carotid bodies.[35] However, peripheral receptors do not primarily induce hypocapnic apnea by themselves, as demonstrated by experimental models involving isolated carotid body hypocapnia that fails to result in apnea.[36] Therefore it appears that both central and peripheral chemoreceptors must interact and respond to hypocapnia for the ventilatory overshoot to induce central apnea during sleep.

Mechanical Aspects of Ventilation

Dysfunction of upper airway mechanics represents the basis of OSA pathophysiology. Such dysfunction, however, is also observed in CSA because of upper airway collapsibility resulting in ventilatory instability.

The two primary collapsing forces of the upper airway are intraluminal negative pressure (generated by the diaphragm during inspiration) and extraluminal soft tissues (e.g., generated by fat deposition within bony structures surrounding the airway). These forces are opposed primarily by the pharyngeal dilator muscles, whose activity either varies from breath to breath (phasic respiratory muscles such as genioglossus) or stays similar throughout the respiratory cycle (tonic muscle, such as the tensor palatini). Additionally, activity of these muscles is dependent on mechanoreceptor and chemoreceptive influences. Studies in animals have shown that chemoreceptor activation resulted in an augmented depolarization of the inspiratory and expiratory hypoglossal motoneurons, thus providing evidence for the arterial chemoreceptors' contribution to maintaining upper airway patency throughout the respiratory cycle.[37] Additionally, the activity of the most important pharyngeal dilator muscle, the genioglossus, is accentuated by hypoxia and abolished by hyperoxia.[38] Alternatively, hypercapnia at the level of peripheral and central chemoreceptors leads to increased afferents to hypoglossal motoneurons and decreased threshold of the genioglossus activation. Comparing the quantitative participation of mechanoreceptors with chemoreceptors as modulators of upper airway activation, it has been suggested that chemoreceptors are stronger, although the two stimuli in combination may interactively augment upper airway muscle activity more than either stimulus alone.[39] Besides the upper airway muscles, the fluctuations in chemical stimuli also affect the diaphragm. Animal studies demonstrate a linear chemoreceptor-driven recruitment of the diaphragm electromyogram.[40] Endoscopy performed during both induced and naturally occurring central apnea demonstrated that upper airway obstruction occurs without evidence of an inspiratory effort in the first 10 seconds of a CSA episode.[41] Consequently, neuromuscular respiratory pathology overlaps in these different types of SBDs, making a clear adjudication between obstructive and central events difficult in many cases.

Neural Aspects of Ventilation

The respiratory neurons are divided into two groups, inspiratory and expiratory. The former belong to the dorsal respiratory group localized in the area of the NTS; the latter belong to the ventral respiratory group localized adjacent to the nucleus ambiguous.[42] Although the hypoxic and hypercapnic afferent responses of the peripheral and central chemoreceptors activate certain populations of respiratory neurons, the details of such intricate processes are still missing; likewise, the relative contribution of each neuronal population to central apnea pathogenesis is also unknown.[43] Studies of several congenital disorders have provided information on the central apnea neuronal ventilatory impairment and helped in understanding better the sudden infant death syndrome. Such rare congenital diseases include Leigh syndrome, a mitochondrial encephalopathy whose manifestations include frequent post-sigh apneic episodes due to lung stretch receptors ending their vagal afferents into abnormal NTS[44]; and Fukuyama-type congenital muscular dystrophy, in which sudden death is commonly encountered as a result of migration defects of the brainstem structures involving pathology of the arcuate nucleus that acts as a central chemoreceptor sensitive to hypercapnia.[45]

As Harper and colleagues[46] reviewed recently, however, CSB with or without CSA affects the brain structure and function beyond the rhythmicity of breathing and includes hormonal, autonomic, and behavioral (affect, memory, and cognition) functions. Neural injuries of the ventrolateral and dorsal medullary areas are common in heart failure patients who demonstrate CSB patterns with or without CSA, affecting the final pathway of sympathetic outflow and sympathetic tone regulation.[47] Congenital central alveolar hypoventilation syndrome (CCAHS) neuropathology also involves the ventrolateral medulla, with subsequent dysfunction of the respiratory phase switch.[48] Neurotransmitter system injuries have been also recognized in CCAHS, in the raphe system, locus coeruleus (noradrenergic neurons), ventral midbrain, hypothalamus, and basal ganglia (dopaminergic fibers).[49] The cerebral cortex is not spared in either of these conditions; ischemic damage to the right insula is significantly accentuated in heart failure patients who have a high prevalence of OSA and CSB.[50] Essentially, because of hippocampal injury, short-term memory and cognitive impairments are also common in CCAHS.

Ventilatory Control in Central Sleep Apnea

Metabolic Control of Ventilation

Normal respiratory rhythmicity during sleep is maintained by a complex feedback mechanism best described by the concept of "loop gain," with CO_2 responsiveness between the eupnea and apneic threshold contributing.[51] *Loop gain* is an engineering term that describes the dynamic feedback of several stabilizing ventilatory mechanisms composed of three elements: (1) the controller gain (chemoresponsiveness, including ventilatory response to Pao_2 and $Paco_2$ above and below eupnea); (2) the plant gain (effectiveness of CO_2 excretion from such ventilatory response); and (3) mixing gain (e.g., from circulation delay between the lungs and the peripheral and central chemoreceptors). Simplistically, the loop gain could be defined as the ratio of the amplitude of the ventilatory response to a ventilatory disturbance. A loop gain of less than 1 accompanies a stable ventilatory system with low respiratory variability because disturbances lead to smaller responses, assuring a rapid return to a stable pattern. On the contrary, a loop gain of greater than 1 accompanies an unstable ventilatory system with high respiratory variability, in which disturbances lead to disproportionately large responses, resulting in a perpetual waxing and waning pattern. The ventilatory control system is dynamic, with both chemical and nonchemical inputs contributing to the breath-by-breath variability, as detailed by Khoo[52] (Figure 12-3).

Ventilatory variability is due to the feedback instability of the hypoxic and hypercapnic chemosensitivities. For example, a transient episode of hyperpnea leads to an eventual decrease in ventilation, but given the lag in the chemical response due to the circulation time, the initial correcting ventilatory response occurs well into the hyperpneic episode. This brief episode of hypopnea or apnea elicits a similarly delayed response, resulting in an ongoing oscillatory pattern of hyperpnea-hypopnea, whose magnitude and duration depends heavily on the *net effects* of the ventilatory control system. Several factors influence each of the gains: (1) the controller gain is affected by the sensitivity of the peripheral chemoreceptors to changes in gas partial pressure, sensitivity of central centers to peripheral chemoreceptors, and the excitability and integrity of the lower motor neurons supplying the respiratory muscle; (2) the plant gain is determined by the respiratory cycle frequency, $Paco_2$, Pao_2, ventilation-perfusion matching,

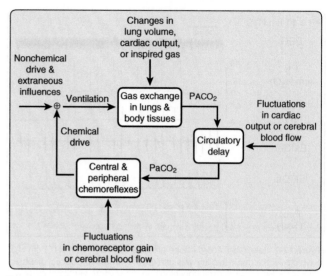

Figure 12-3 Chemical and nonchemical inputs contributing to the breath-by-breath variability.

and dead-space ventilation[53]; (3) the mixing gain is dependent on the circulatory delay time, thoracic blood volume, and brain extracellular fluid volume. In addition to the loop gain, another factor affecting ventilatory stability is the $Paco_2$ reserve, that is, the difference between the eupneic $Paco_2$ and the $Paco_2$ at the apneic threshold. The lower the $Paco_2$ reserve, the smaller the increase in the ventilation required for reaching the apneic threshold and developing central apnea. Conversely, when the apneic threshold for $Paco_2$ is far away from the eucapnic $Paco_2$, large ventilatory changes are necessary to lower the $Paco_2$ below the apneic threshold, decreasing the likelihood of developing central apnea.

The theoretical applications of the concepts of ventilatory instability and loop gain have been translated clinically by several clinical experiments. Common to all of them is the pathophysiologic relationship between alveolar ventilation (V_A) and alveolar Pco_2 described best by several authors[54-56]; a compiled explanation is given by Dempsey and colleagues[51] and depicted in Figure 12-4.

In hypoxic and normoxic acetazolamide-induced metabolic acidosis, the accompanying hyperventilation results in an increase in the V_A required to reduce the $Paco_2$ to the apneic threshold, protecting against apnea and respiratory instability. Despite a similar conceptual pathway of *reduced plant gain* for both hypoxic and normoxic hyperventilation, in hypoxia the slope of the ventilatory response increases and therefore the CO_2 reserve below eupnea is decreased, predisposing to ventilatory instability compared with nonhypoxic hyperventilation (Figure 12-5).[54]

Ventilatory instability is also promoted by *increasing plant gain*, such as is seen with $NaHCO_3$-induced metabolic alkalosis that narrows the CO_2 reserve without a change in the slope of the CO_2 response below eupnea.[58] For the controller gain, both increased and decreased controller gain have been demonstrated using pharmacologic manipulations of the peripheral chemoreceptor sensitivity; intravenous administration of dopamine resulted in a fall in ventilation and reduced O_2 sensitivity[59] (i.e., *reduced controller gain*), whereas administration of the dopamine D_2-receptor antagonist domperidone

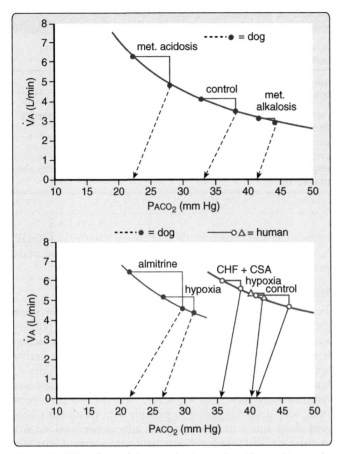

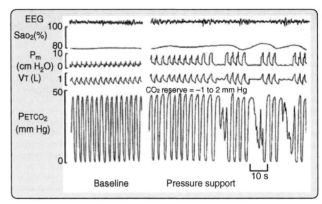

Figure 12-5 Hypoxia reduces the CO_2 reserve. A healthy human is exposed to moderate hypoxia (PaO_2 80%) for 15 to 20 minutes during NREM sleep, causing mild hyperventilation. When pressure support ventilation is subsequently applied, note that a transient reduction of only 1 or 2 mm Hg in $PaCO_2$ is required to cause apnea and periodic breathing. This effect contrasts with the 3- to 5-mm Hg $\Delta PaCO_2$ required in the normoxic control condition. The CO_2 reserve is markedly reduced in hypoxia despite the reduced $PaCO_2$ and plant gain because the slope of the $\Delta \dot{V}_A$–$\Delta PaCO_2$ relationship below eupnoea is significantly increased. EEG, Electroencephalogram; P_m, Mean airway pressure. (From Braley TJ, Segal BM, Chervin RD. Sleep-disordered breathing in multiple sclerosis. *Neurology* 2012;28:929–36.)

Figure 12-4 The effects of changing background ventilatory drive on the gain of the ventilatory responsiveness to CO_2 below eupnoea, on "plant gain," and on the CO_2 reserve ($\Delta PETCO_2$ eupnoea – apnea) in sleeping dogs and humans. Data are plotted on separate isometabolic lines for dogs [CO_2 flow ($\dot{V}CO_2$) = 150 mL/min^{-1}] and for humans ($\dot{V}CO_2$ = 250 mL/min^{-1}). The *diagonal dashed* or *continuous lines* join eupneic and apneic points, and their slopes indicate the gain below eupnoea of the ventilatory response to hypocapnia in each condition. The height of the *vertical bar* above the isometabolic line indicates the increase in $\dot{V}_A$ required to reduce the $PaCO_2$ to the apneic threshold (i.e., the inverse of plant gain). The CO_2 reserve is the difference in $PaCO_2$ between eupnoea and the apneic threshold. CHF, Congestive heart failure; CSA, central sleep apnea.

resulted in increased carotid body sensitivity to O_2 (i.e., *increased controller gain*).[60] As detailed in Figure 12-5, the steeper the slope of the $\dot{V}ACO_2$–$PaCO_2$ relationship, the smaller the change in $PaCO_2$ required to reach the apneic threshold, and therefore the higher the controller gain. Numerous clinical entities are associated with one or more abnormalities of loop gain, as summarized in Table 12-3.

Neural Control of Ventilation

Neural mechanisms of ventilatory control in central apnea are likely as important as the metabolic pathways, dictating behavior during wakefulness, affecting airway patency, and controlling respiratory plasticity. The wakefulness stimuli to breathe include tonic excitatory inputs from the so-called reticular formation, brainstem aminergic systems, and hypothalamic orexin neurons.[61] Younes,[62] using correlational analysis, demonstrated that an effective neural control of the upper airway and chest wall respiratory muscles was more important than the inherent passive collapsibility of the airway.

Respiratory plasticity translates into *long-term facilitation* (LTF), a term used to describe the increase in the respiratory activity that persists after the conclusion of an acute episode of intermittent hypoxia.[63] Mediated through several receptors, including serotonergic and *N*-methyl-D-aspartate, this response in sleeping humans is aimed at stabilizing ventilation through increased minute ventilation (i.e., ventilatory LTF),[64] decreased inspiratory upper airway resistance,[65] and increased genioglossus electromyographic activity (i.e., upper airway LTF).[66] However, concentrating on central apnea pathophysiology, Chowdhuri and colleagues[67] demonstrated that, in healthy participants undergoing nasal noninvasive ventilation for promoting hypocapnic central apnea, the increase in hypocapnic ventilatory response resulted in a significant decrease in the CO_2 reserve, thus offsetting the protective effect of LTF.

Examples of Pathophysiologic to Clinical Applications

Cheyne-Stokes Breathing with or without Central Sleep Apnea

CSB is characterized by a destabilizing interplay of several gains: specifically, controller and plant, with CSA presenting when this destabilization is most accentuated. A *high controller gain* is due to a hypersensitive ventilatory chemoreflex response to CO_2. Although the exact mechanism for this increase in chemosensitivity is not yet known, both congestive (i.e., pulmonary edema[68] and left atrial stretch[69]) and noncongestive factors (reduced carotid arterial blood flow[70]) result in vagal afferents that stimulate central respiratory control centers and fail to allow the $PaCO_2$ to increase at sleep onset.[71] Ventilatory control is also affected in congestive heart failure (CHF) patients because of an attenuated cerebrovascular reactivity to the changes in $PaCO_2$ levels.[72] The *mixing gain* is a concept sometimes used to define how a delay in the circulation can be destabilizing for ventilation. The fact that the chemoreceptors are in the carotid bodies and brainstem rather than in the lung is one factor that can

Table 12-3   Loop Gain Abnormalities in Clinical Disorders

Increased Plant Gain	Decreased Plant Gain	Increased Controller Gain	Decreased Controller Gain	Increased Mixing Gain
Obesity-hypoventilation syndrome (OHS)	Congenital central hypoventilation syndrome	Cheyne-Stokes breathing (CSB)	OHS	CSB
Neuromuscular weakness	Hypercapnic chronic obstructive pulmonary disease	High-altitude periodic breathing Treatment emergent central apnea		Idiopathic pulmonary hypertension

contribute to instability because periodic breathing would be unlikely if chemoreceptors were in the lung. Circulatory delay was induced in classic experiments by Guyton and colleagues,[73] who showed that delays of several minutes (beyond what could occur clinically) were sometimes required to induce periodic breathing in animals. Subsequent studies suggested that circulatory delay was similar in patients with CSB with CHF compared with patients without CSB matched for the severity of heart failure. However, some studies have shown that improvements in circulatory delay are associated with improvement in loop gain (and hence improved AHI). Thus, in aggregate, the data suggest that circulatory delay is necessary but not sufficient to destabilize ventilation in most cases. Therefore the overall response in CSB is that of an increased loop gain manifesting as increased ventilatory instability.

CSB with CSA had been also noted in individuals with cerebrovascular accident (CVA) and chronic renal failure. Among patients with CVA and CSA, the presence of CSB with long hyperpnea and cycle durations, and a gradual rise to peak tidal volume during hyperpnea, was associated with left ventricular systolic dysfunction, but was not related to the location or type of stroke. The authors indicated that the presence of CSA with CSB was more closely associated with left ventricular systolic dysfunction than it was with the stroke itself.[74] Similarly, Yamamoto and Mohri,[75] studying the influence of chronic renal insufficiency on SBDs in patients with symptomatic chronic heart failure, found that most of these patients had unspecified central events, with estimated glomerular filtration rate comparable between non-SBD and SBD groups. The authors suggested that renal dysfunction played a relatively minor role in determining breathing abnormalities in chronic heart failure.[75]

High-Altitude Periodic Breathing

High-altitude periodic breathing is another example of ventilatory instability that occurs during sleep in individuals during ascent to moderate and high altitude. Individual susceptibility to high-altitude periodic breathing is driven by multiple genetic factors; polymorphisms in numerous genes, including the hypoxia-responsive transcription factor subunit EPAS1/HIF2α and additional genes in the HIF pathway linked to hemoglobin level, have been associated with differences in susceptibility to or severity of acute mountain sickness associated conditions.[76,77] In this case, high-altitude periodic breathing is the result of ambient hypoxia inducing hyperventilation (*increased controller gain*), which further leads to

hypocapnia and consequently to *decreased plant gain*. Overall, however, the controller gain dominates the decreased plant gain, resulting in periodic breathing.[78]

Treatment Emergent Central Sleep Apnea

Treatment emergent central sleep apnea develops in some patients both during titration and after continuous positive airway pressure (CPAP) therapy initiation. This phenomenon is associated with *increased controller gain* due to lowering upper airway resistance with perhaps a contribution of the air leak washing out the anatomic dead space.[79] It usually resolves spontaneously with ongoing CPAP therapy. As in a pilot study, loop gain was higher in patients with treatment emergent sleep apnea in whom central apneas persisted after 1 month of CPAP therapy; loop gain measurement in these patients may enable an a priori determination of those who need alternative modes of PAP.[79a]

Obesity-Hypoventilation Syndrome

Obesity-hypoventilation syndrome (OHS) is characterized by a combination of obesity (body mass index >30 kg/m^2) and arterial hypercapnia during wakefulness (Paco$_2$ >45 mm Hg) (see Chapter 30). OHS is the result of an interplay between respiratory mechanics and ventilatory drive, with leptin, a circulating protein produced mainly by adipose tissue, playing a role. A deficiency of this adipokine, as seen in the leptin-deficient *ob/ob* mouse mode, results in impaired respiratory mechanics, depressed ventilatory responsiveness, and awake hypercapnia.[80] Because leptin replacement in these mice reverses their OHS, recent work has focused on the potential role of leptin in individuals with OHS. It is presumed that the development of central leptin resistance or relative leptin deficiency in OHS could contribute to the development of awake hypoventilation by altering respiratory drive output as well, affecting the mechanical properties of the lungs and chest wall and attenuating the normal compensatory mechanisms used by individuals to cope with obesity-related respiratory loads.[81] These patients have decreased ventilatory responsiveness to hypoxia and hypercapnia compared with similarly obese non-OHS patients and also respond with large increases in Paco$_2$ to small decreases in ventilation (*increased plant gain*), increasing overall the probability of developing central apneic events.[82]

Congenital Central Alveolar Hypoventilation Syndrome

CCAHS is a rare congenital disease caused by mutation in *PHOX2B* gene leading to lack of central drive and decreased ventilatory response to $Paco_2$ (decreased controller gain) despite normal lungs and respiratory muscle function.

Hypercapnic Chronic Obstructive Pulmonary Disease

Although not characterized by frank central sleep apneas or as a CSA disorder, advanced chronic obstructive pulmonary disease (COPD) is associated with progressive hypercapnia due to impaired lung mechanics, with renal compensation toward a physiologic pH (by increasing serum bicarbonate). Prognosis in individuals with advanced COPD has been reported to be negatively affected by hypercapnia,[83,84] and degree of hypercapnia is not correlated with survival after hypercapnia has developed.[85] The long-term optimal management of the hypercapnia in these patients remains unclear. Recent data by Köhnlein and colleagues demonstrated that the addition of long-term noninvasive positive pressure ventilation to standard treatment improved 1 year survival of patients with hypercapnic, stable COPD when noninvasive positive pressure ventilation was targeted to reduce hypercapnia.[86] Patients with COPD and concomitant OSA may be referred to as having "overlap syndrome" (see Chapter 29), and large series have shown that patients with overlap syndrome who did not receive treatment with nocturnal CPAP had a lower survival rate than patients who suffered from either COPD[87] or OSA[88] alone. However, data regarding optimal management of overlap syndrome are lacking.

Opioid-Induced Central Sleep Apnea

The exact pathophysiologic mechanism of opioid-induced apnea remains poorly understood but is likely related to opioid-induced suppression of inspiration generated by the pre-Bötzinger complex in the brainstem.[89] Both a periodic, non-waxing waning breathing pattern, and a cluster-type breathing pattern, each with central apneas, have been reported during NREM sleep in individuals receiving chronic opiates.[90] Chronic opioid use is a risk factor for the development of central sleep apnea and ataxic breathing,[91] but it is only rarely associated with daytime hypercapnia.[92]

GENETICS

Congenital Central Alveolar Hypoventilation Syndrome

Most CSA disorders in adults have not been linked to specific genotypes. The one clear exception is CCAHS, which is a monogenetic disorder of central respiratory control associated with diffuse autonomic dysregulation[93] and, at times, Hirschsprung disease and tumors of neural crest origin.[94] CCAHS is characterized by a specific facial phenotype, such as boxy facies and an inferior inflection of the lateral segment of vermillion border on the upper lip.[95] CCAHS has a familial presentation, and the *PHOX2B* mutation located on chromosome 4p12 has been identified and confirmed as the disease-defining gene.[96-99] CCAHS, a lifelong disease, is diagnosed in the absence of other systemic pathology and a positive *PHOX2B* screening test or whole-gene *PHOX2B* sequencing test.[100] Clinically, CCAHS is defined by an inability to adapt appropriately to needed ventilatory changes; these patients have altered or absent perception of shortness of breath when awake and profound and life-threatening hypoventilation during sleep.[101] Patients with CCAHS develop apnea or severe bradypnea during NREM sleep.

However, expression of the disease is highly variable, with some patients presenting as neonates and others presenting in adulthood, largely depending on the genotype. Approximately 90% of mutations involve excessive polyalanine repeats of the *PHOX2B* gene beyond the normal 20/20 pattern observed in the normal population. Polyalanine repeat patterns of 20/25 to 20/33 typically present at birth with hypoventilation. By contrast, people with a 20/24 pattern may present after the neonatal period, including as adults. Approximately 10% of CCHAS patients have nonpolyalanine repeat mutations (frameshift, missense, or nonsense), and they are typically affected at birth with hypoventilation during wakefulness and sleep. Therapeutically, CCAHS patients require intratracheal or noninvasive positive pressure ventilation during sleep, and about one third also require additional ventilator support during wakefulness, including positive pressure ventilation or diaphragmatic pacing.[102] Generally, adults present with the 20/24 CCAHS genotype, which typically involves only mild hypoventilation that can be managed with noninvasive ventilation during sleep only.

EPIDEMIOLOGY

Risk Factors

Several independent risk factors have been established for CSA-CSB. In patients with CHF and reduced left ventricular ejection fraction, risk factors for CSA-CSB include age older than 60 years, male gender, presence of atrial fibrillation, and hypocapnia.[103-105] For patients with treatment emergent CSA, a high baseline AHI or arousal index, hypertension, opioid use, coronary artery disease, stroke, and CHF all appear to be risk factors.[106]

Prevalence

CSA is estimated to account for 5% to 10% of patients with SBDs that, according to ICSD3, includes OSA, sleep-related hypoventilation disorders, and sleep-related hypoxemia disorder.[107] Additionally, variations in the hemodynamic profile of CHF patients predispose them to alterations day to day and sometimes within the same night of the predominant type of apnea—from OSA to CSA, and vice versa.[108,109]

Cheyne-Stokes Breathing

CSA-CSB is highly prevalent in patients with left ventricular dysfunction regardless of the etiology (ischemic vs. idiopathic), type (preserved or low ejection fraction), New York Heart Association (NYHA) class, and acuity of event (acute or chronic heart failure).[110] CSA-CSB can present during both sleep and wakefulness. Nocturnal CSA-CSB has been studied mostly in stable compensated heart failure and is present in up to 44% of patients who have heart failure with a reduced ejection fraction (HFREF)[111,112] and in up to 27% of patients who have heart failure with a preserved ejection fraction (HFPEF).[113] CSA-CSB during wakefulness is less common, occurring in 16%[114] of patients with HFREF NYHA class II or III; however, because it emerges in the early afternoon and evening and evidence of nocturnal CSA-CSB correlates only weakly with its presence, its reported prevalence could be underestimated. CSA-CSB has been demonstrated after myocardial infarction and unstable angina; in both situations, it is a common occurrence, being present in more than 60%[115] of these patients.

Primary Central Sleep Apnea

Primary CSA, formerly categorized as "idiopathic" CSA, is uncommon. The general population prevalence of primary CSA is not known. However, within the sleep center population, the prevalence has been reported to be 4% to 7%. A higher prevalence of idiopathic CSA has been reported in older patient populations.[116] These individuals usually complain of excessive daytime sleepiness, insomnia, or difficulty breathing during sleep.[117]

High-Altitude Periodic Breathing

Despite considerable heterogeneity in the susceptibility to altitude illness, periodic breathing in the form of cyclic central apneas and hypopneas occurs in almost all individuals at a sufficiently high altitude.[118]

Treatment Emergent Central Sleep Apnea

When treatment emergent CSA (or "complex" CSA) is simply defined as the emergence of central apneas and hypopnea both during and after the application of PAP therapy in patients with OSA, its estimated prevalence in the general sleep center patient population is between 10% and 15%.[119] Treatment emergent CSA is a dynamic process, and its prevalence decreases with ongoing PAP therapy within 2 to 3 months in most patients.[120]

Central Sleep Apnea Due to a Medical Disorder

A synopsis of several common noncardiac medical conditions associated with CSA events is described in Table 12-1. In cardiac conditions not related to left heart disease, CSA events were identified by PSG in 10.6%[121] of a cohort of such patients who developed NYHA class II or III disease due to variety of conditions such as idiopathic pulmonary hypertension, chronic thromboembolic disease with pulmonary hypertension, COPD, and interstitial lung disease. PSG and ambulatory cardiorespiratory sleep studies documented concomitant CSA in up to 39% of patients with idiopathic pulmonary hypertension and NYHA class II to IV chronic thromboembolic disease with pulmonary hypertension[122] and in up to 20% of patients with hypertrophic cardiomyopathy.[123]

Central Sleep Apnea Due to a Medication or Substance

Opioid-induced CSA has only been recognized since about 2000,[124] with a reported prevalence, for example, of 30% of patients in a methadone pain program.[125] Given the progressive increase in opioid use for symptom management in both neoplastic and chronic diseases, it is expected that such CSA will be increasingly identified in clinical sleep practice.

Age

In both general and heart failure populations, CSA-CSB seems to be more commonly encountered in patients of advanced age. In children with CHF, CSA-CSB is quite rare,[126] whereas in a random sample of men aged 20 to 100 years, using sleep laboratory evaluation subsequent to a telephonic survey, Bixler and colleagues[127] noted CSA in 0.4% of those 45 to 64 years old and in 1.1% for those 65 to 100 years old. Others[128] have reported an even higher occurrence of 17% in a population aged 71 years and older.

Gender

Among healthy middle-aged adults, CSA syndromes are overall much more common in men (7.8%) than in women (0.3%).[129] For example, a study including a large proportion of women with stable HF reported unspecified CSA in only 0.05% of those with HF and in none of those with preserved ejection fraction heart failure.[130] Although OSA is increasingly recognized in postmenopausal women, similar consistent data for CSA are lacking.

Race

No data are available on the racial distribution of CSA syndromes to our knowledge.

Morbidity

Central Sleep Apnea and Cardiac Hemodynamics

In CSA-CSB, intermittent surges in blood pressure and heart rate occur in association with oscillations in ventilation. Such surges can be precipitated by cyclic increases in sympathetic nervous system activity targeting the heart and peripheral vasculature.[131,132] Studies concentrating on these hemodynamic responses have confirmed that the frequency and peaks of heart rate and blood pressure oscillations are dependent primarily on periodic oscillations in ventilation.[133] The clinical significance of this finding is not certain, but surges in blood pressure during hyperpnea may be one factor related to the poorer prognosis in patients with heart failure with CSB compared with those without it.[134] More recently, Yumino and colleagues[135] assessed the beat-to-beat stroke volume from before until the end of central respiratory events during sleep in patients with HFREF and demonstrated an increase in stroke volume by a mean of 2.6% (P <.001 for the difference).

Central Sleep Apnea and Cardiac-Related Hospital Readmission

The only study to date[136] that prospectively evaluated cardiac readmission associated with SBD in a cohort of hospitalized patients with acutely decompensated HFREF demonstrated CSA-CSB to be a predictor of both 1-month and 6-month readmission (univariable rate ratios of 1.5 and 1.63, respectively). Ongoing studies are evaluating whether treating CSA-CSB prevents such readmission.

Central Sleep Apnea and Cerebrovascular Accident

Using near-infrared spectroscopy in individuals with acute and subacute CVA, Pizza and colleagues documented asymmetrical patterns of cerebral hypoxia during unspecified CSA events, with significantly larger changes on the unaffected compared with the affected hemisphere.[137]

Mortality

As the oxyhemoglobin desaturations, arousals, increased sympathetic output, and negative intrathoracic pressure (during hyperpnea that follows central apnea in CSA-CSB) contribute to myocardial ischemia, CSA-CSB could contribute to excess mortality in patients with heart failure. Relatively large studies looking specifically at the mortality associated with unspecified CSA and CSA-CSB have provided divergent results, some likely deriving from the lack of a strict definition for CSA or for CSA-CSB. Javaheri and associates[138] evaluated survival in HFREF (ejection fraction <45%) over a period of 51 months and demonstrated that patients with unspecified CSA had half the survival time of those without such CSA, 45 and 90 months, respectively ($P = .01$), independent of systolic function, NYHA functional class, heart rate, serum digoxin and sodium concentrations, hemoglobin, and age. In contrast, Andreas and colleagues[139] noted that, in patients with HFREF, nocturnal CSA-CSB had no prognostic impact. Both Andreas and colleagues[139] and Lange and Hecht[140] reported that awake CSA-CSB was associated with a high likelihood of death within 1 to 24 months. Roebuck and associates[141] noted that systolic heart failure patients with unspecified CSA had decreased survival at 500 days but similar long-term survival compared with those without such CSA. Luo and colleagues[142] demonstrated that unspecified CSA had no effect on the prognosis of middle-aged patients with CHF, whereas Bakker and associates[143] provided contrasting evidence by demonstrating a significantly lower survival rate in patients with heart failure and unspecified CSA compared with both heart failure and OSA (mean survival time difference, 3.8 years; $P = .005$) and those with heart failure only (mean survival time difference, 4 years; $P = .01$). Additionally, within the group of patients with HFREF and unspecified CSA, mortality is reported to be significantly higher in the "severe" (AHI >22.5/hour) unspecified CSA group compared with the "mild" unspecified CSA group (AHI <22.5/hour; 38% vs. 16%; unadjusted $P = .002$ and adjusted for the confounders age and NYHA class $P = .035$).[144] Notably, all of these studies have focused on understanding mortality in untreated patients with heart failure and CSA with or without CSB, and definitive outcome data on the impact of PAP therapy on the natural progression of unspecified CSA and CSA-CSB in patients with heart failure are still lacking. To date, the largest randomized controlled multicenter trial, the Canadian Continuous Positive Airway Pressure for Patients with Central Sleep Apnea and Heart Failure Trial (CANPAP)[145] and its post hoc analysis,[146] showed that death and heart transplantation events did not differ between the control group and the CPAP group. The post hoc analysis showed improved survival without heart transplantation in the CANPAP group when CPAP therapy was associated with a reduced frequency of CSA-CSB events to fewer than 15 events per hour.

CLINICAL PEARLS

- Centrally driven respiratory events are primarily due to a temporary loss of output from the pontomedullary pacemaker that generates breathing rhythm, resulting in loss of diaphragmatic activity.
- CSA with CSB is a form of periodic breathing, commonly observed in patients with heart failure, in which central apneas alternate with hyperpneas that have a waxing-waning pattern of tidal volume.

- Nocturnal CSB has been studied mostly in stable compensated heart failure and is present in up to 44% of patients with low ejection fraction and in up to 27% of patients with preserved ejection fraction. However, variations in the hemodynamic profile of heart failure patients predispose them to day-to-day and sometimes within-night alterations of the predominant type of apnea—OSA to CSA, and vice versa.
- Ventilatory control in CSA is largely chemically driven, especially during NREM, and is the result of a fine balance between a critical $PaCO_2$ level, below which there is a central cessation of breathing (i.e., apneic threshold); its ventilatory triggering factors (mainly hypocapnia); and respondent receptors (i.e., central and peripheral chemoreceptors). This complex feedback mechanism is best described by the concept of loop gain.
- CSA-CSB is likely an independent risk for increased mortality or cardiac transplantation in patients with heart failure.
- Definitive outcome data on the effect of PAP therapy on the natural progression of CSA and CSA-CSB in patients with heart failure are still lacking.

SUMMARY

In CSA, both oronasal flow and thoracoabdominal excursions are absent; that is, there is an absence of respiratory effort during the cessation of airflow. CSB and treatment emergent (or "complex") CSA are the most common clinical CSA patterns. CSA with CSB is characterized by oscillations of ventilation between apnea and tachypnea, with a waxing and waning crescendo-decrescendo pattern in the depth of respirations, and is highly prevalent in patients with heart failure. Treatment emergent CSA most commonly refers to the development of CSA with the application of CPAP in patients with OSA; in most cases, this breathing pattern resolves spontaneously with ongoing therapy. CSA-CSB is likely associated with increased mortality in treated patients with systolic heart failure. It remains unclear whether improving the frequency of CSA-CSB in sleep improves clinical outcomes in this setting or, conversely, resolution of the CSA-CSB is simply a marker of a good prognosis.

Selected Readings

Costanzo MR, Khayat R, Ponikowski P, et al. Mechanisms and clinical consequences of untreated central sleep apnea in heart failure. *J Am Coll Cardiol* 2015;**65**(1):72–84.

Dempsey JA. Crossing the apneic threshold: causes and consequences. *Exp Physiol* 2004;**90**:13–24.

Eckert DJ, Jordan AS, Merchia P, et al. Central sleep apnea: pathophysiology and treatment. *Chest* 2007;**131**:595–607.

Javaheri S, Dempsey JA. Central sleep apnea. *Compr Physiol* 2013;**3**:141–63.

Jordan AS, McSharry D, Malhotra A. Adult obstructive sleep apnea. *Lancet* 2014;**383**:736–47.

Nishino T, Lahiri S. Effects of dopamine on chemoreflexes in breathing. *J Appl Physiol* 1981;**50**:892–7.

A complete reference list can be found online at ExpertConsult.com.

Chapter 13

Anatomy and Physiology of Upper Airway Obstruction

James A. Rowley; M. Safwan Badr

Chapter Highlights

- Upper airway patency is determined by craniofacial structure, surrounding tissues, intrinsic properties of the upper airway, and the neuromuscular function of the upper airway.
- With sleep, the loss of the wakefulness drive to breathe is associated with decreased neuromuscular activity of the upper airway, and in particular decreased afferent reflexes, and is further modified by such factors as lung volume, hypercapnia, and age. Upper airway caliber decreases, with a resultant increase in upper airway resistance and compliance and upper airway collapsibility.

- In patients with obstructive sleep apnea (OSA), there is evidence of histologic changes to upper airway tissues, which may explain abnormalities in sensorimotor and reflex activity in the upper airway in patients with OSA.
- This chapter describes and discusses the factors that influence the determinants of upper airway obstruction in humans. However, further research is needed to understand how these determinants interact to maintain upper airway patency.

Although investigations into the pathogenesis of obstructive sleep apnea (OSA) have been underway since the disorder was first described, the mechanisms underlying an increased propensity to sleep-related upper airway obstruction in some individuals are not well understood. This chapter reviews the anatomy and physiology of the upper airway as they relate to upper airway patency and propensity to obstruct during sleep. The occurrence of collapse during sleep and not wakefulness implicates the removal of the wakefulness drive to breathe as a key factor underlying sleep-related upper airway obstruction. The determinants of upper airway patency—upper airway neuromuscular activity and nonneuromuscular factors including craniofacial structure, surrounding tissues, and intrinsic properties of the upper airway itself—are discussed.

This chapter additionally reviews the effect of sleep on upper airway properties such as patency, resistance, compliance, and collapsibility. Within each area, the factors that influence these properties, including host factors (e.g., gender and body mass index [BMI]), disease (e.g., tonsillar hypertrophy, fluid overload), and OSA, are examined.

BASELINE DETERMINANTS OF UPPER AIRWAY PATENCY

Upper Airway Function and Structure

The human upper airway is unique in that it serves as a multipurpose passage. It both transmits air to the lungs (through the nose and mouth) and liquids and solids to the esophagus (through the mouth). The upper airway, particularly the nose, also serves as a heat exchanger. In humans, the upper airway, particularly the larynx and lips, is important for vocalization. However, because it serves multiple purposes, portions of

the upper airway lack rigid support, and hence are prone to collapse.

The upper airway is classically divided into five regions based on anatomic structures (see Figure 13-1, *A*). Each of these regions is either rigid and resistant to collapse or semirigid and susceptible to collapse. Whether rigid or semirigid, however, each region can become occluded because of other anatomic variants or abnormalities. Although the nose is a rigid section of the upper airway because of its bony components, it can become obstructed owing to nasal congestion and polyps, altering upper airway mechanics. The nasopharynx is defined as the area from the posterior aspect of the nasal turbinates to the horizontal plane of the soft palate. Thus the proximal portion of the nasopharynx tends to be rigid, but the distal region is semirigid. Nasopharyngeal patency can be compromised by local mass lesions and palatal and uvular hypertrophy or edema. The oropharynx is defined as the area from the soft palate to the base of the tongue and is semirigid. It can be further divided into an area posterior to the soft palate (retropalatal) and tongue (retroglossal). Oropharyngeal patency is generally compromised from tonsil hypertrophy, palatal or uvular enlargement, or macroglossia. Because the nasopharynx and oropharynx are semirigid, these two areas are the site of collapse in most patients with OSA. The hypopharynx extends from the base of the tongue to the larynx and is relatively rigid and resistant to collapse. Finally, the larynx, the most distal portion of the upper airway, is rigid, composed of both cartilage and muscle.

Upper airway caliber can be measured by a variety of methods, including computed tomography (CT) scanning, magnetic resonance imaging (MRI), nasopharyngoscopy, and acoustic imaging. These methods allow researchers to measure

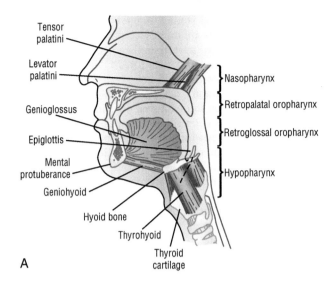

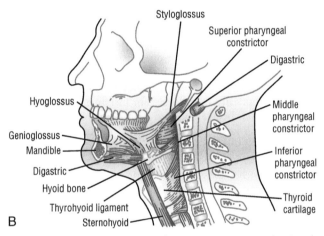

Figure 13-1 **A,** Schematic diagram of upper airway anatomy showing the classic divisions of the pharynx and key upper airway muscles. **B,** Schematic diagram of upper airway muscles and other key landmarks such as the hyoid.

upper airway caliber either at one point in the respiratory cycle (a static measurement) or dynamically throughout the respiratory cycle.

Neuromuscular Function of the Upper Airway

The upper airway musculature consists of 24 pairs of striated skeletal muscles extending from the nares to the larynx (see Figure 13-1, *B* for major anatomic landmarks and muscles).[1,2] These pharyngeal muscles have complex anatomic relationships but can generally be classified into groups that regulate the position of the soft palate, tongue, hyoid bone, and pharyngeal walls. The muscles are generally activated in groups to control the major functions of the upper airway such as phonation and swallowing.

There are two general patterns of electrical discharge from upper airway muscles when these are studied with multiunit electromyograms (EMGs): tonic (constant) activity, independent of phase of respiration; and phasic activity, occurring during one part of the respiratory cycle. There are at least 10 upper airway muscles that may be classified as pharyngeal "dilators," innervated by multiple cranial nerves. Some, such as the genioglossus, are classified as dilators by virtue of their phasic inspiratory activity. Others, such as the tensor palatini,

do not clearly have a dilating effect but demonstrate activity throughout the respiratory cycle (tonic activity) and are presumed to "stiffen" the upper airway wall and decrease pharyngeal collapsibility. It is widely accepted that upper airway dilators play a critical role in preserving pharyngeal patency.[3] There is evidence from EMG studies that activity of upper airway dilators begins about 200 milliseconds before onset of thoracic pump activity in normal subjects.[4,5]

Upper airway narrowing or obstruction during sleep is associated with a sleep-related decrease in upper airway muscle activity. The effect of non–rapid eye movement (NREM) sleep on upper airway muscle function is complex and difficult to study because of the challenges in isolating the many other influences on upper airway muscle activity, such as changes in air flow, magnitude of negative pressure in the pharyngeal airway, and lung volume. Available evidence indicates that NREM sleep is associated with a reduction in tonic or phasic EMG activity in numerous upper airway muscles,[2] including the levator palatini,[6] tensor palatini,[7] palatoglossus,[6] and geniohyoid.[8] Studies measuring single motor unit activity of the genioglossus muscle also noted decreased activity of the phasic inspiratory motor units at sleep onset[9] and NREM stage 2 sleep with increased discharge frequencies and duration in NREM stage 3 sleep.[10] The EMG changes are accompanied by upper airway narrowing and increased upper airway resistance.

The effect of rapid eye movement (REM) sleep on upper airway muscle activity is more clearly documented. Activity of antigravity muscles is reduced during REM sleep, and there is strong evidence that activity of phasic upper airway dilating muscles, such as the genioglossus, is greatly attenuated during REM sleep,[11,12] particularly during periods of phasic rapid eye movements.[13,14] Reduced activity has also been shown for the alae nasi[13] and geniohyoid muscles.[8] Similar findings have been reported for single motor unit activity of the genioglossus.[15] In summary, the sleep state is associated with decreased upper airway muscle activity.

The response of upper airway muscles to chemical and mechanical perturbations during sleep may be relevant physiologically and clinically to such reduced activity. Negative pressure applied to the upper airway results in a brisk reflex response in upper airway muscle activity. This reflex is attenuated with application of topical lidocaine, indicating mediation through local mechanoreceptors.[16] Studies of reflex activity in the genioglossus, palatoglossus, and tensor palatini muscles show that this negative pressure reflex response is attenuated during NREM[17-19] and REM sleep[20] compared with wakefulness. Similarly, responsiveness of the genioglossus muscle to hypercapnia is attenuated during sleep.[21] This reflex response has also been shown to be attenuated with aging during both wakefulness and sleep.[22] These data suggest that upper airway dilator muscles are less able to maintain upper airway patency in the face of chemical or mechanical perturbations. Furthermore, there is evidence that lung volumes alter genioglossus muscle activity during NREM sleep, with decreases in endexpiratory lung volume being associated with increased genioglossus activity above baseline.[23]

The large number of upper airway muscles and their complex interactions mandate caution in extrapolating findings from studies focusing on the genioglossus or hypoglossal nerve activity alone, particularly because measurement of electrical activity of the muscle is not necessarily an appropriate surrogate for muscle fiber shortening or indeed for upper airway dilation. In fact, there is evidence that upper airway muscle activation is not necessarily sufficient to dilate the upper airway under either physiologic or loading conditions, including resistive loading due to airway resistance[24] or elastic loading due to either increased soft or fat tissue[25-27] or small mandibular enclosure.[28] Nor may such activation be necessary; for example, in sleeping humans, increased end-expiratory lung volume has been found to result in decreased upper airway resistance and increased retropalatal cross-sectional area in association with *reduced* EMG activity of the genioglossus.[29] In patients with OSA, increased lung volume causes a substantial decrease in sleep-disordered breathing during NREM sleep,[30] and an inverse correlation between continuous positive airway pressure (CPAP) requirements and lung volume in patients with OSA has been found.[31]

It is also unclear whether complete atonia of the pharyngeal muscles increases upper airway collapsibility. For example, the pharyngeal airway becomes more collapsible in dead infants,[32,33] but not in paralyzed animal preparations.[34,35] In addition, REM sleep, associated with decreased neuromuscular stimulation, is not associated with changes in upper airway compliance or collapsibility in human studies of upper airway physiology.[36,37] Likewise, increased pharyngeal compliance in patients with sleep apnea cannot be attributed to decreased upper airway dilating muscle activity per se because patients with OSA show increased activity of the genioglossus muscle during wakefulness[38] and sleep,[39] perhaps as a compensation for anatomically reduced caliber. Similarly, when the pharyngeal airway is narrowed during hypocapnic central apnea,[40] more pronounced narrowing (or even closure) occurs in patients with OSA relative to normal control subjects despite complete inhibition of upper airway dilating muscle activity in both groups.

A related question is the role of upper airway dilating muscles in stabilizing the upper airway and therefore preventing upper airway obstruction, apart from activity that is directly associated with increased or decreased upper airway patency. There is evidence, for example, that stimulation of the hypoglossal nerve results in decreased collapsibility (i.e., a stiffer airway) and decrease surrounding pressure in animal models.[41,42] Existing studies indicate that supraphysiologic electrical stimulation of the hypoglossal nerve using a surgically implanted upper airway stimulation device in patients with OSA lead to significant improvements in the severity of the sleep-disordered breathing in a select group of patients.[43,44]

Nonneuromuscular Factors Contributing to Upper Airway Patency and Obstruction

Upper Airway Muscle Histology

There is a large body of research examining upper airway muscle histology in patients with OSA, based on the hypothesis that pathologic changes in upper airway muscle histology may promote upper airway obstruction by increasing propensity to upper airway muscle fatigue or delay reopening through impairment of sensorimotor function. Studies have shown a variety of histologic changes, including edema and mucosal gland hypertrophy,[45] neurogenic injury,[46] changes in muscle enzyme activity,[47,48] and leukocytic inflammation.[49,50] A consistent finding across studies is an increase in type 2 fast-twitch fibers in the genioglossus muscle of patients with OSA.[46,51-53] Because type 2 fibers are more likely to fatigue

than type 1 fibers, these studies suggest that upper airway muscles in OSA patients are more susceptible to fatigue than in normal subjects. In contrast, there is no consistent finding for differences in tongue protrusive force[54,55] in patients with OSA compared with normal subjects.

Changes in sensorimotor activity of the upper airway in OSA patients have been studied based on evidence that upper airway sensory receptors contribute to apnea-terminal arousal and that topical anesthesia impairs these responses. In patients with OSA, changes in two-point discrimination, vibratory sensation, upper airway muscle reflex response to short air pulses, and sensory perception to varying air flow rates have been observed.[56-58] These changes may explain the observation that inspiratory load sensation is decreased in patients with OSA.[59,60] Such impairment of upper airway sensorimotor function may contribute to decreased upper airway muscle activity in response to upper airway obstruction, loading, or collapse.

Although the previous studies indicate changes in upper airway neuromuscular histology and sensorimotor function in patients with OSA, there is only minimal evidence linking specific histologic changes or sensorimotor changes to changes in upper airway mechanics or propensity of the upper airway to collapse. In fact, the noted histologic changes, if secondary to recurrent airway collapse, may not be contributing to an increased propensity to collapse. For instance, treatment with nasal CPAP has been associated with improvement in genioglossus muscle force production[52] and vibratory thresholds.[56] Thus further investigation is necessary to determine to what extent changes in upper airway histology and function seen in patients with OSA are primary or secondary and whether and how such changes, primary or secondary, contribute to the noted increased propensity to collapse in sleep in patients with OSA.

Craniofacial Structure

Craniofacial structure is an important determinant of upper airway patency. This is most evident in children with craniofacial abnormalities such as Pierre Robin sequence and Treacher Collins syndrome, each of which are associated with an increased prevalence of OSA.[61] In adults, several anatomic abnormalities have been associated with OSA, including retrognathia, micrognathia, overjet, and a high arched palate.[62-64]

Several investigations have used lateral cephalometry to analyze the contribution of craniofacial structure to the development of OSA (Figure 13-2).[65-73] These studies vary widely in methodology, sample size, gender ratios, and the presence and degree of obesity. In these studies, common craniofacial abnormalities that have been associated with increased severity of sleep apnea include (1) smaller airway dimensions, particularly those involving the maxilla and mandible; (2) mandibular retrognathia; (3) decreased posterior airspace; (4) an inferiorly placed hyoid bone; and (5) increased soft palate dimensions and length. These abnormalities decrease the dimensions of the nasopharynx and oropharynx, likely increasing the risk for upper airway obstruction. In one study in 57 male patients with OSA, airway collapsibility[74] was correlated with soft palate length, hyoid bone distance, and an inferiorly placed hyoid bone.

MRI has also been used to compare upper airway craniofacial structure and soft tissue between subjects with and

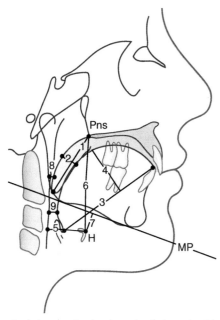

Figure 13-2 Cephalometric landmarks and soft tissue, hyoid position, and airway size variables frequently used in cephalometric studies. Landmarks: Pns, posterior nasal spine; H, hyoid bone; MP, mandibular plane (tangent line from the symphysis to the inferior border of the mandibular angle). Variables: (1) SPl, the length of the soft palate; (2) Spw, the width of the soft palate; (3) Tl, the length of the base of the tongue; (4) Tw, the width of the tongue; (5) H-Ph, the distance from the hyoid bone to the posterior wall of the pharynx; (6) H-Pns, the distance from the hyoid bone to Pns; (7) H-MP, the distance from the hyoid bone to the mandibular plane; (8) SPAS, the upper posterior pharyngeal space; (9) IPAS, the lower posterior pharyngeal space. In one study, critical closing pressure was predicted by the length of the soft palate (1), distance from hyoid bone to posterior wall of the pharynx (5), and the distance from the hyoid bone for the posterior nasal spine (6). (From Sforza E, Bacon W, Weiss T, et al. Upper airway collapsibility and cephalometric variables in patients with obstructive sleep apnea. *Am J Respir Crit Care Med* 2000;161[2 Pt. 1]:347–352.)

without OSA (Figure 13-3). Important differences have been found in men and include a wider mandibular divergence, smaller mandibular length, and smaller area at the mandibular plane being associated with OSA.[75,76] Although the hyoid bone was inferiorly placed in these studies in subjects with OSA, it was not a primary determinant of upper airway obstruction.

Craniofacial indexes derived from both cephalometric and MRI data have been used to compare OSA susceptibility between races. Redline and colleagues found that bony and soft tissue factors and brachycephaly were associated with OSA in whites, whereas only soft tissue factors were similarly associated in African Americans.[66,77] In contrast, Polynesian men with OSA were shown to have more mandibular retrognathia and larger nasal aperture width than white men, whereas neck circumference, tongue, and soft palate dimensions were associated with the respiratory disturbance index in the white subjects.[78] Finally, Japanese subjects with OSA have upper airway bony dimensions, whereas obesity and upper airway soft tissue and volume are less important.[76,78a] Taken together, these data indicate that race-specific craniofacial and neck structural factors contribute to the likelihood of having OSA.

Only one study has specifically compared gender differences in craniofacial and structural factors that could contribute to a propensity for OSA. Using MRI, Malhotra and colleagues[79] found that men had increases in airway length, soft palate cross-sectional area, and airway volume, presumably contributing to a diathesis for upper airway obstruction.

It should be noted that in many of these craniofacial studies, obesity remained the predominant etiologic factor for OSA, with abnormal craniofacial structure most important in nonobese patients with OSA. However, in a recent study in a large sample of men, obesity alone explained only 26% of the variance in the apnea-hypopnea index (AHI), and obese patients with unfavorable airway dimensions were susceptible to larger increases in OSA severity.[67]

Surrounding Tissues and Pressures

A collapsing upper airway transmural pressure can be generated either by a negative intraluminal pressure or a collapsing surrounding pressure. The role of negative intraluminal pressure in the pathogenesis of upper airway obstruction is widely hypothesized,[3] whereby a subatmospheric intraluminal pressure generated by the thoracic pump muscles causes upper airway collapse by "sucking" the hypotonic upper airway. However, there are no data showing that such subatmospheric intraluminal pressure causes upper airway obstruction in sleeping humans. In addition, upper airway narrowing and obstruction do not appear to require negative pressure. For example, studies using fiberoptic nasopharyngoscopy have shown that the upper airway narrows during hypocapnia mediated central inhibition.[40,80] Isono and colleagues[81] compared the mechanics of the pharynx in anesthetized and paralyzed normal subjects and in patients with OSA. The pharynx was patent at atmospheric intraluminal pressure in normal subjects and required negative intraluminal pressure for closure. In contrast, patients with OSA had a positive closing pressure; that is, the pharynx was occluded at atmospheric intraluminal pressure. Similarly, the critical closing pressure in patients with OSA has been generally found to be positive, as opposed to the negative critical closing pressure in normal subjects.[82, 83]

The disconnect between the occurrence of upper airway obstruction and of negative intraluminal pressure supports the possibility that upper airway patency is, in part, determined by the extrinsic or surrounding pressure contributed to by properties of soft tissue structures of the upper airway. Using MRI technology, three factors have been found to be most significantly associated with an increased risk for OSA: increased tongue size, increased size of lateral pharyngeal walls, and increased total soft tissue volume (Figure 13-4).[84] The association of increased tongue and lateral pharyngeal wall size with OSA has also been noted in CT and cephalometric studies of the upper airway[65,85] as well as in clinical studies.[62] Subsequent work has shown that these same factors show familial aggregation, even after correction for confounding factors such as gender and age.[86] Thus the known familial predisposition to OSA[87] may be in part explained by heritable soft tissue factors.

Enlarged tonsils have also been shown to be associated with an increased risk of OSA even after correction for BMI and neck circumference.[62] Enlarged tonsils are particularly noted as a causative factor in children and thin adults, who may have resolution of OSA after tonsillectomy.[88]

CT and MRI of the upper airway have also demonstrated evidence of increased soft tissue volume and pharyngeal fat at

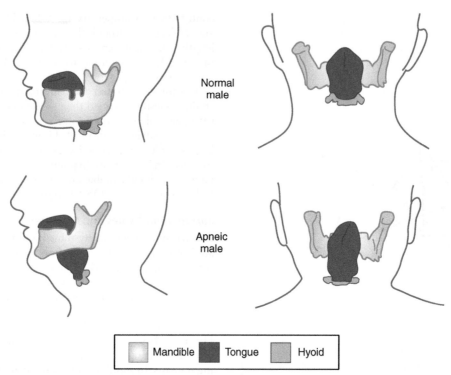

Figure 13-3 Three-dimensional reconstruction of hyoid, tongue, and mandible in a patient with obstructive sleep apnea (*bottom:* male, apnea-hypopnea index [AHI] 86 events/hr; body mass index [BMI] 31 kg/m²; 49 years of age) and a normal subject (*top:* male, AHI 5 events/hr; BMI 25 kg/m²; 44 years of age) illustrating the inferior-posterior positioning of hyoid and enlarged tongue volume. Note that the hyoid is more inferior-posteriorly positioned in the apneic subject than in the normal subject; tongue volume is greater in the apneic subject than in the normal subject. (From Chi L, Comyn FL, Mitra N, et al. Identification of craniofacial risk factors for obstructive sleep apnoea using three-dimensional MRI. *Eur Respir J* 2011;38[2]:348–58.)

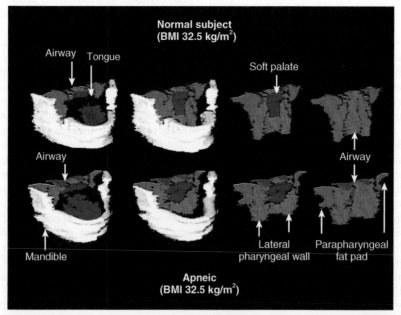

Figure 13-4 Volumetric reconstruction of axial magnetic resonance images in a normal subject and a patient with sleep apnea, both with an elevated body mass index of 32.5 kg/m². The mandible is depicted as *gray*, tongue as *orange/rust*, soft palate as *purple*, lateral parapharyngeal fat pads as *yellow*, and lateral/posterior pharyngeal walls as *green*. Note that the airway is larger in the normal subject than in the apneic subject. The tongue, soft palate, and lateral pharyngeal walls are larger in the patient with sleep apnea. (From Schwab RJ, Pasirstein M, Pierson R, et al. Identification of upper airway anatomic risk factors for obstructive sleep apnea with volumetric magnetic resonance imaging. *Am J Respir Crit Care Med* 2003;168[5]:522–30.)

the level of the nasopharynx in males,[89] which could explain, in part, their higher prevalence of OSA. Pharyngeal fat volume was found to correlate with the AHI in one study,[27] but not in other studies.[84,85] Further investigations are needed to better determine the role of pharyngeal fat volume in particular, and extrinsic tissue volume and pressures overall, in the generation of a collapsing transmural pressure and the pathogenesis of upper airway obstruction in sleeping humans.

Intrinsic Properties of the Upper Airway

The collapsing effect of transmural pressure on upper airway patency is subject to modification by the intrinsic compliance of the pharyngeal wall. In addition to the Isono and colleagues[81] data noted previously, it has been shown that, in the isolated upper airway model of collapsibility, critical closing pressure is negative during complete paralysis, indicating that at normal atmospheric pressure, the normal upper airway remains open.[90,91] These studies suggest that the pharyngeal wall has an intrinsic "stiffness" or resistance to collapse. The determinants of such intrinsic stiffness have not been fully elucidated but likely involve complex interactions among many of the pharyngeal components already discussed, including muscles (which may have different properties in a passive state compared with a stimulated state), bony structures (particularly in the nasopharynx), soft tissues, and vascular properties, with such interactions affecting pressure and cross-sectional area relationships.

In the passive or paralyzed nasopharynx, the relationship between pharyngeal transmural pressure and cross-sectional area is curvilinear, implying that the airway becomes more compliant as the cross-sectional area decreases, that is, the "tube law" (Figure 13-5). Therefore baseline decreased airway cross-sectional area is likely a determinant of diathesis for upper airway obstruction, supported by evidence that the pharyngeal airway is smaller during wakefulness in patients with OSA relative to that of normal subjects.[92-94] However, it has been shown that under the dynamic conditions of inspiratory flow limitation, airway compliance decreases at more negative driving pressures (associated with a smaller cross-sectional area), indicating that static airway properties may

not be as physiologically or clinically relevant during dynamic conditions.[94a]

In association with such intrinsic properties of the upper airway, increased inspiratory lung volume is associated with increased upper airway caliber and decreased collapsibility. Potential mechanisms through which the increased caudal traction works include increased longitudinal tension, increased subatmospheric pressure through the trachea, and decreased transmural pressure.[42,95-97] Therefore caudal traction appears to influence upper airway collapsibility by both dilating and stiffening the pharyngeal airway as well as decreasing extramural tissue pressure. It is likely that patients with OSA are more dependent on such increased lung volume–associated dilatation or stiffening because of their relatively compliant upper airway.[81,98,99]

Vascular perfusion of the upper airway is also a potential determinant of intrinsic pharyngeal wall stiffness. Vasoconstriction and vasodilation have been shown to cause a decrease and increase in upper airway resistance, respectively.[100-102] More recently, a series of experiments have investigated the relationship between rostral fluid shifts and upper airway properties, demonstrating an association between reduction in leg fluid volume and increased neck circumference. In awake subjects, such rostral body fluid shift is associated with increased pharyngeal resistance,[103] decreased upper airway cross-sectional area,[104] and increased upper airway collapsibility.[105,106] Similar results have been found in patients with drug-resistant hypertension[107] and end-stage renal dialysis,[108,109] two groups in which there is evidence of an increased prevalence of OSA.[110] Interestingly, despite similar changes in leg total fluid volume and neck circumference with lower body positive pressure, men have a larger increase in collapsibility than women,[106] suggesting that a differential response to fluid shifts between men and women could contribute to the difference in gender prevalence in OSA.

When upper airway closure occurs, surface mucosal forces may impede subsequent upper airway opening.[35] In awake humans, surfactant and other topical lubricants have been shown to decrease the opening and closing pressures of the upper airway and to decrease upper airway resistance in sleeping normal subjects.[111,112] Mucosal lining forces may be particularly important in patients with OSA with mucosal inflammation from repeated trauma,[111] in whom the AHI in sleep decreases with the use of such soft tissue lubrication.[112,113]

In summary, upper airway patency is determined by multiple factors that are present during wakefulness and sleep, all typically further compromised during sleep compared with awake, leading to changes in upper airway function that contribute to sleep-related upper airway obstruction. The four primary factors include neuromuscular activity of the upper airway, craniofacial structure, tissues surrounding the upper airway, and the intrinsic properties of the airway (Figure 13-6). The following section reviews the sleep-specific effects on these factors and associated upper airway resistance and patency.

SLEEP EFFECTS ON UPPER AIRWAY PATENCY AND COLLAPSIBLITY

The sleep state is a challenge, rather than a period of rest, for the ventilatory system. In addition to the reduced activity

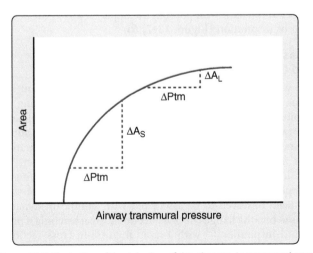

Figure 13-5 Illustration of the tube law of the pharynx. As transmural pressure (P_{tm}) increases, so does cross-sectional area (A). The slope of the tube law represents compliance of the pharynx. Note that compliance decreases as the area of the pharynx increases.

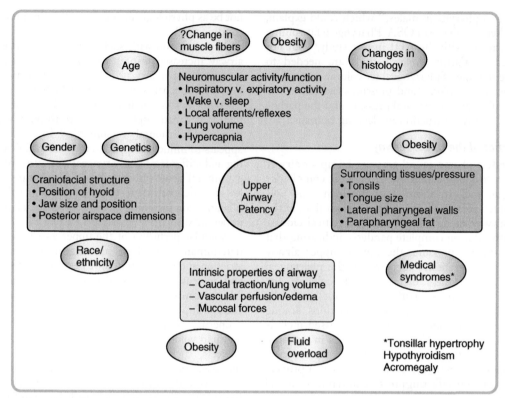

Figure 13-6 Summary showing the major determinants of upper airway patency and other factors that modify these main determinants.

of upper airway dilators discussed previously, consequences of the loss of wakefulness on the upper airway include reduced upper airway caliber, increased upper airway resistance, increased pharyngeal compliance, and collapsibility. Ultimately, these changes lead to reduced tidal volume and hypoventilation.

Upper Airway Caliber and Resistance

The sleep state is associated with upper airway narrowing and a corresponding increase in upper airway resistance. Using nasopharyngoscopy during sleep in normal subjects, Rowley and colleagues[46,126] have shown that, during NREM sleep, both retropalatal and retroglossal cross-sectional area decreases to approximately 70% of awake cross-sectional area, with further narrowing of the retroglossal airway during REM sleep. Decreased cross-sectional area corresponds with the pattern of decreased upper airway dilator muscle activity during NREM sleep and further reduction of the genioglossus during REM sleep. In REM sleep, retroglossal but not retropalatal cross-sectional area decreases further compared with NREM sleep.[36,114]

The evidence for increased upper airway resistance during sleep is compelling, even in normal subjects.[36,114-116] In fact, increased upper airway resistance occurs as early as sleep onset and continues to increase, reaching highest values in slow wave sleep. Most evidence indicates that there are no further increases in upper airway resistance during REM sleep compared with NREM sleep in normal humans.[36,114,117] In summary, the sleep state is associated with upper airway narrowing, which manifests as increased upper airway resistance and decreased pharyngeal caliber.

It is important to note that upper airway resistance is not an independent measure of the dynamic behavior of the pharyngeal airway during sleep. Many subjects exhibit inspiratory flow limitation, in which the pressure-flow graph demonstrates a changing relationship between driving pressure and inspiratory flow, culminating in complete dissociation between pressure and flow; that is, pressure continues to decrease with no further increase in flow (Figure 13-7, *A*). Thus the optimal physiologically meaningful measurement of upper airway resistance is the slope of the linear portion of the pressure-flow loop, which likely reflects upper airway caliber at the narrowest point in the upper airway at the beginning of inspiration (Figure 13-7, *B*).

Measurements and Meanings of Compliance and Collapsibility

The walls of the pharyngeal airway consist of compliant soft tissue structures, amenable to changes in pressure during the respiratory cycle. During wakefulness, upper airway caliber is constant during inspiration, with a decreased caliber during expiration, returning to inspiratory values at end-expiration. This finding has been observed in both normal subjects[92,118] and in patients with OSA[118] using either CT scanning or nasopharyngoscopy. Using nasopharyngoscopy, NREM sleep has been observed to be associated with significant dynamic within-breath changes in cross-sectional area, reaching a nadir at mid-inspiration,[118] with a rapid increase in cross-sectional area during expiration (Figure 13-8).[40] In addition, in subjects with OSA, there is progressive upper airway narrowing before the onset of apnea, which is primarily seen during expiration.[119] BMI appears to be a determinant of the degree of

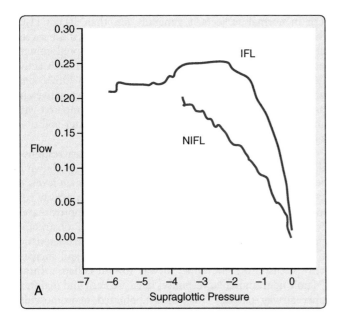

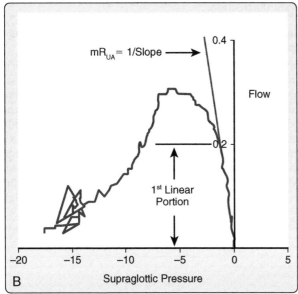

Figure 13-7 A, Pressure-flow loops illustrating a non–flow-limited (NIFL) and a flow-limited (IFL) breath. **B,** Illustration of a flow-limited breath and measurement of resistance along the first linear portion of the pressure-flow loop.

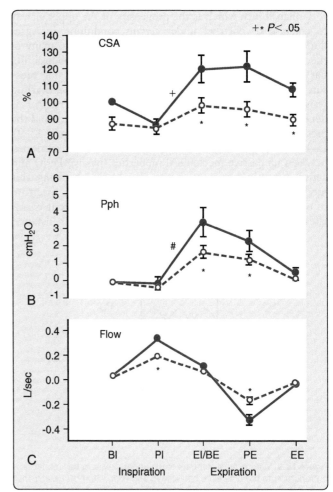

Figure 13-8 Retropalatal cross-sectional area (CSA) **(A)**, pharyngeal pressure (Pph) **(B)**, and flow **(C)** during control (*closed circles*) and hypocapnic hypopnea (*open circles*). Note the significant CSA change throughout the respiratory cycle within the control breaths compared with the hypopnea breaths. BE, Beginning expiration; BI, beginning inspiration; EE, end expiration; EI, end inspiration; PE, peak expiration; PI, peak inspiration. (Modified from Sankri-Tarbichi AG, Rowley JA, Badr MS. Expiratory pharyngeal narrowing during central hypocapnic hypopnea. *Am J Respir Crit Care Med* 2009;179:313–9.)

airway narrowing seen in these studies.[40,118] The sleep reversal in the pattern of change in upper airway cross-sectional area is thought to be due to sleep-related increase in upper airway compliance, a decrease in pharyngeal caliber, and subsequently, decreased (more negative) inspiratory intraluminal pressure.

The changes in upper airway patency during sleep can be investigated using compliance as a measurement. Compliance of the pharyngeal wall is an important modulator of the effect of pressure changes on upper airway patency. The occurrence of pharyngeal narrowing and flow limitation suggests, although does not prove, increased pharyngeal compliance during sleep. Using a methodology that measures changes in cross-sectional area at different levels of applied pressure, it has been demonstrated that compliance is increased as the pharyngeal caliber decreases[81,120,121] and that the upper airway of patients with

OSA is more compliant than that of normal subjects,[81,98,121,122] consistent with an increased propensity to collapse. Using a methodology that combines measurement of cross-sectional area using fiberoptic nasopharyngoscopy and measurement of intraluminal pressure at the same level in normal subjects has confirmed that retropalatal compliance is increased during NREM sleep compared with wakefulness, with no difference between REM sleep and wakefulness.[36] At the retroglossal level, however, compliance is not increased during either NREM or REM sleep compared with wakefulness.[114] The dissociation between compliance and reported muscle activity in these studies is consistent with studies in patients with OSA demonstrating that increased pharyngeal compliance occurs despite an increased activity of the genioglossus muscle during wakefulness[38] and sleep,[39] perhaps as a compensation for anatomically reduced caliber. This finding again suggests a major role for nonneuromuscular factors, as referred to previously, as determinants of pharyngeal compliance.

Collapsibility, which is the propensity of the upper airway to collapse or obstruct under certain conditions, increases during sleep compared with awake, likely owing to many of the factors discussed previously. Upper airway collapsibility has been primarily measured using the critical closing pressure, Pcrit, which is based on the concept of the Starling resistor,[123] whereby maximal flow through the resistor is dependent on the resistance of the upstream segment and the pressure surrounding the collapsible segment (Figure 13-9). In humans, the critical closing pressure can be partitioned between its passive mechanical properties (passive Pcrit) and active dynamic responses (active Pcrit).[124,125] Applying this model to humans, it has been shown that across the spectrum of obstructive sleep-disordered breathing, active Pcrit correlates with propensity for airway collapse.[82,83,126] For instance,

Pcrit in normal subjects is generally less than 10 cm H_2O, whereas in patients with predominant hypopneas, it is between zero and –5 cm H_2O, and in patients with predominant apneas, it is more than zero cm H_2O. Although both active and passive Pcrit are increased in patients with OSA compared with control subjects, the difference between active and passive Pcrit is greater in non-OSA controls compared with those with OSA, likely associated with the greater ability of normal subjects to maintain airway patency.

The roles of mechanical loads and compensatory responses related to Pcrit are summarized in Figure 13-10. As shown in the left-hand bar with graded shading, approximate levels of Pcrit measurements define a continuum of upper airway collapsibility from health to disease. A Pcrit of approximately –5 cm H_2O represents the level above which obstructive hypopneas and apneas will occur. Structural characteristics of the upper airway impose mechanical loads and increase Pcrit, predisposing the upper airway toward collapse. Intact dynamic neuromuscular responses decrease Pcrit and maintain upper airway patency. In contrast, blunted neuromuscular responses increase Pcrit and predispose the upper airway toward obstruction.

Phase of the Respiratory Cycle: Inspiratory Versus Expiratory Narrowing

Upper airway obstruction during sleep is characteristically attributed to inspiratory narrowing owing to a collapsing subatmospheric pressure against a hypotonic pharyngeal airway. However, several lines of evidence implicate expiratory narrowing as a possible mechanism of the initial narrowing. First, ventilatory motor output is an important determinant of upper airway patency. Oscillation of ventilatory motor output, during the characteristic periodic breathing of OSA, is associated with pharyngeal narrowing or obstruction at the nadir of the motor output, especially in individuals with a highly

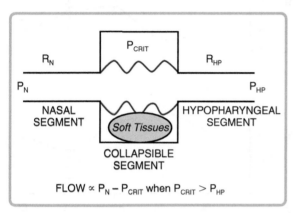

Figure 13-9 Starling resistor model of the upper airway. In this model, flow is proportion to the difference between P_N and Pcrit, with Pcrit greater than P_{HP}. P_N, Nasal (upstream) pressure; P_{HP}, hypopharyngeal (downstream) pressure; R_N, resistance in the nasal segment; R_{HP}, resistance in the hypopharyngeal segment.

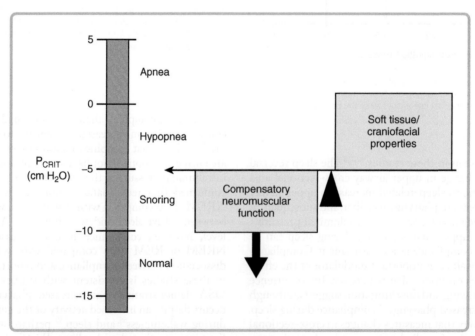

Figure 13-10 Role of mechanical loads and compensatory neuromuscular responses in the context of critical pressure measurements. See text for explanation. (From Patil SP, Schneider H, Marx JJ, et al. Neuromechanical control of upper airway patency during sleep. *J Appl Physiol* 2006;102:547–56, with permission.)

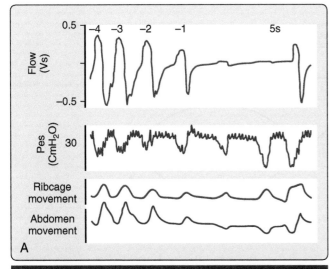

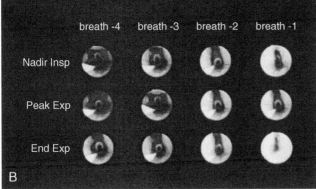

Figure 13-11 A, A recording of air flow (flow; inspiration positive), esophageal pressure (Pes), and rib cage and abdominal movements. Tracings show four breaths leading to an obstructive apnea (breaths -4, -3, -2, and -1). During the apnea, respiratory effort is indicated by the negative swings in the esophageal pressure and paradoxical rib cage and abdominal movements. **B,** Fiber-optic images of the retropalatal airway during the four breaths shown in **A** where breath-1 is the breath immediately preceding the apnea and breath-4 is the breath farthest away from the apnea. Within each breath the images selected correspond to the smallest cross-sectional area (CSA) that occurred during inspiration (Nadir Insp), the largest CSA during expiration (Peak Exp), and the CSA at end-expiration (End Exp). Note that progressive narrowing is occurring in both inspiration and expiration. Within each image the *dark area* is the airway lumen, the *lighter horseshoe shape* is the epiglottis, and the *white triangular shape* in the *bottom left corner* is the esophageal pressure catheter. (From Morrell MJ, Arabi Y, Zahn B, Badr MS. Progressive retropalatal narrowing preceding obstructive apnea. *Am J Respir Crit Care Med* 1998;158[6]:1974–81.)

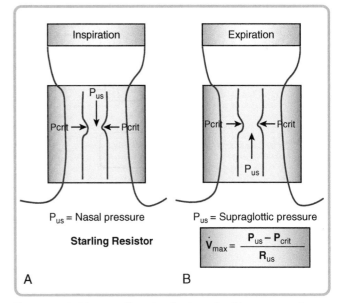

Figure 13-12 Schematic illustration for the collapsible segment of upper airway during hypocapnic hypopnea as a Starling resistor. In this model, flow is determined by the gradient between the upstream segment and critical closing pressure (Pcrit). During inspiration **(A),** when upstream pressure (P_{us}) (i.e., nasal pressure) is below the Pcrit, the collapsible segment is closed, and no flow occurs. During expiration **(B),** when P_{us} in the supraglottic area is below the Pcrit, the collapsible segment is closed, and no flow occurs. During hypocapnic hypopnea, expiratory flow is limited, correlating with the gradient between the supraglottic pressure and Pcrit. Hence this pressure gradient is an important determinant of pharyngeal narrowing. R_{us}, Upstream resistance; $\dot{V}_{max}$, maximal flow. (From Sankri-Tarbichi AG, Rowley JA, Badr MS. Expiratory pharyngeal narrowing during central hypocapnic hypopnea. *Am J Respir Crit Care Med* 2009;179[4]:313–9.)

collapsible airway.[127] Second, an obstructive apnea is often preceded by expiratory narrowing of the upper airway as evidenced by increased expiratory resistance[128] or progressive expiratory narrowing, detected by fiberoptic imaging (Figure 13-11).[119] Finally, although upper airway narrowing or occlusion occurs during a spontaneous or induced hypocapnic central apnea[80] or induced hypocapnic hypopnea,[40] pharyngeal narrowing during central hypopnea occurs during the expiratory phase only and is associated with increased expiratory upper airway compliance. Therefore upper airway obstruction may occur in either inspiration or expiration (Figure 13-12). Individuals with a high surrounding tissue pressure may be particularly susceptible to expiratory pharyngeal narrowing during such low ventilatory motor output and driving pressure.

Gender, Body Mass Index, and Weight Effects on Upper Airway Structure and Function

Potential determinants of upper airway mechanics during sleep include many variables known to be associated with an increased prevalence of OSA, such as gender, BMI, and age.

Most studies indicate no consistent difference in upper airway caliber, or compliance, between men and women without OSA. Upper airway resistance during NREM sleep is also similar in both genders,[117,129] although one study[130] demonstrated higher upper airway resistance in men during slow wave NREM sleep. REM sleep has not been similarly studied. Likewise, studies during wakefulness demonstrate no significant difference in upper airway cross-sectional area or smaller airway in women.[92,131-133] In addition, sleep-related narrowing is similar in men and in women (approximately a 40% decrease in cross-sectional area for both genders) from wakefulness to NREM sleep.[134] However, it appears that men have increased retropalatal compliance compared with women[134] because of gender difference in neck circumference, again indicating that factors other than gender are important in explaining such gender differences in upper airway function. Finally, there is no demonstrated gender difference in Pcrit under active conditions.[129] Thus the available studies taken together do not suggest a gender difference alone in upper airway mechanics during wakefulness or sleep, except for higher retropalatal compliance in men compared with women, in subjects without OSA. However, gender has been found to modulate the effect of BMI on Pcrit, and thus upper airway collapsibility, with men, with or without OSA,

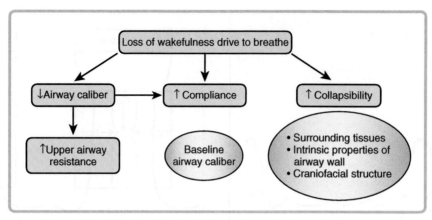

Figure 13-13 Effect of the loss of wakefulness drive to breathe on the upper airway.

increasing passive Pcrit in relation to increasing BMI more than women.[124]

The effect of age on upper airway resistance during sleep is variable across different studies. Browne and colleagues[135] and Thurnheer and associates[117] found no difference in upper airway resistance between young (<40 years) and older (>40 years) subjects. In contrast, in a group of 60 subjects without OSA, Rowley and colleagues found age to be the only independent predictor of upper airway resistance, with increased age associated with increased upper airway resistance. BMI was not a predictor of resistance.[129] More recently, however, increasing age was associated with increased upper airway resistance during sleep in a linear fashion.[136] Overall, it appears that aging is associated with increased upper airway resistance, and thus possibly increased diathesis for pharyngeal narrowing, during sleep. However, because age does not appear to be a predictor of Pcrit,[124] the significance of age-related increased upper airway resistance is unclear.

Hormonal Activity and Upper Airway Activity

There is also evidence that upper airway collapsibility can be influenced by hormonal activity, particularly leptin activity, in humans. For example, Shapiro and colleagues found in obese subjects that, although leptin levels were not associated with passive Pcrit or the severity of sleep apnea (presumably OSA), increased leptin levels were associated with an increased difference between active and passive Pcrit, independent of BMI and neck circumference.[137] Thus leptin appears to be associated with a decreased propensity to upper airway collapse.

In summary, upper airway patency during sleep is compromised by the loss of wakefulness drive of breathing (Figure 13-13). The loss of the wakefulness drive to breathe results in decreased upper airway neuromuscular activity and reflex activity, leading to decreased upper airway caliber and increased in upper airway resistance. The loss of wakefulness drive to breathe also results in increased airway compliance and collapsibility.

CLINICAL PEARL

The upper airway may be compromised and an individual put at an increased risk for OSA because of enlargement of soft tissue structures such as the tonsils, tongue, and lateral pharyngeal walls as a result of disease or obesity. Craniofacial structure, which is determined by genetics, race, and ethnicity, is an important determinant of upper airway patency; clinically significant changes can include micrognathia and retrognathia, overjet, and a high arched palate. Obesity, through a decrease in lung volume (particularly functional residual capacity), and fluid overload can each lead to changes in the intrinsic properties of the upper airway, increasing propensity to collapse. These factors, in association with sleep-related alterations in both neural control of the upper airway and central neural control of breathing, increase the propensity to upper airway obstruction or collapse in sleep in some individuals, leading to the clinical disorder of OSA.

SUMMARY

Upper airway patency is determined by multiple factors that are present during wakefulness and sleep, with sleep generally associated with compromise of these factors, leading to changes in upper airway function that contribute to upper airway obstruction. The four major determinants of upper airway patency are neuromuscular activity, craniofacial structure, tissues surrounding the upper airway, and the intrinsic properties of the airway. These determinants are modified by other factors, including age, obesity, gender, ethnicity, fluid overload, and other medical disorders, such as tonsillar hypertrophy (see Figure 13-6). During sleep, the loss of the wakefulness drive to breathing results in decreased upper airway neuromuscular activity and reflex activity, leading to decreased upper airway caliber and increased upper airway resistance (Figure 13-13). In addition, there is associated increased airway compliance and increased collapsibility, both of which are influenced by factors that determine baseline upper airway caliber, such as surrounding tissues, craniofacial structure, and the intrinsic properties of the upper airway.

This chapter has discussed the important structural aspects of upper airway structure, function, and patency. However, it is important to note that, although the upper airway narrows in humans during sleep, whether any given individual develops sufficient obstruction to develop the clinical disorder of OSA is likely an interplay between both upper airway structure and function and neural control of breathing during sleep.

Selected Readings

Genta PR, Edwards BA, Sands SA, et al. Tube Law of the Pharyngeal Airway in Sleeping Patients with Obstructive Sleep Apnea. *Sleep* 2016;**39**(2): 337–43.

Kim KT, Cho YW, Kim DE, et al. Two subtypes of positional obstructive sleep apnea: Supine-predominant and supine-isolated. *Clin Neurophysiol* 2016;**127**(1):565–70.

Kirkness JP, Schwartz AR, Schneider H, et al. Contribution of male sex, age, and obesity to mechanical instability of the upper airway during sleep. *J Appl Physiol* 2008;**104**(6):1618–24.

Malhotra A, Pillar G, Fogel RB, et al. Genioglossal but not palatal muscle activity relates closely to pharyngeal pressure. *Am J Respir Crit Care Med* 2000;**162**(3 Pt 1):1058–62.

Morrell MJ, Arabi Y, Zahn B, Badr MS. Progressive retropalatal narrowing preceding obstructive apnea. *Am J Respir Crit Care Med* 1998;**158**(6): 1974–81.

Patil SP, Schneider H, Marx JJ, et al. Neuromechanical control of upper airway patency during sleep. *J Appl Physiol* 2007;**102**(2):547–56.

Rowley JA, Sanders CS, Zahn BR, Badr MS. Gender differences in upper airway compliance during NREM sleep: role of neck circumference. *J Appl Physiol* 2002;**92**(6):2535–41.

Saboisky JP, Stashuk DW, Hamilton-Wright A, et al. Neurogenic changes in the upper airway of patients with obstructive sleep apnea. *Am J Respir Crit Care Med* 2012;**185**(3):322–9.

Sankri-Tarbichi AG, Rowley JA, Badr MS. Expiratory pharyngeal narrowing during central hypocapnic hypopnea. *Am J Respir Crit Care Med* 2009; **179**(4):313–19.

Schorr F, Kayamori F, Hirata RP, et al. Different Craniofacial Characteristics Predict Upper Airway Collapsibility in Japanese-Brazilian and White Men. *Chest* 2016;**149**(3):737–46.

Schwab RJ, Pasirstein M, Kaplan L, et al. Family aggregation of upper airway soft tissue structures in normal subjects and patients with sleep apnea. *Am J Respir Crit Care Med* 2006;**173**(4):453–63.

Schwab RJ, Pasirstein M, Pierson R, et al. Identification of upper airway anatomic risk factors for obstructive sleep apnea with volumetric magnetic resonance imaging. *Am J Respir Crit Care Med* 2003;**168**(5):522–30.

Stanchina ML, Malhotra A, Fogel RB, et al. The influence of lung volume on pharyngeal mechanics, collapsibility, and genioglossus muscle activation during sleep. *Sleep* 2003;**26**(7):851–6.

A complete reference list can be found online at ExpertConsult.com.

Chapter 14

Snoring and Pathologic Upper Airway Resistance Syndromes

Riccardo Stoohs; Avram R. Gold

Chapter Highlights

- Over the past two decades, knowledge of pathologic pharyngeal collapse during sleep has expanded from apnea and hypopnea to include even the mildest, silent inspiratory airflow limitation (IFL) during sleep. Both the clinical researcher and the sleep medicine practitioner of today must be able to recognize the mildest IFL on a polysomnogram and its clinical implications. This chapter discusses the physiologic and clinical features of IFL during sleep.

- Although habitual snoring is very common, the prevalence of isolated snoring (snoring in the absence of apnea and hypopnea, oxygen desaturations, arousals from sleep, and symptoms of obstructive sleep apnea) is unknown. Recent clinical investigation has led to uncertainty about whether such snoring can be considered benign. This chapter presents the issues involved in the diagnosis and management of isolated snoring.

- The paradigm of IFL during sleep leading to recurrent respiratory effort–related arousals is inadequate to explain the varied signs and symptoms of upper airway resistance syndrome (UARS) that have been recognized during the past decade or to distinguish between UARS patients and asymptomatic, healthy individuals whose polysomnograms are remarkably similar. This chapter discusses the evolving paradigm of UARS.

Snoring and upper airway resistance syndrome (UARS) represent obstructed breathing during sleep too mild to cause more than slight sleep fragmentation but with potential pathologic significance. In the past, the chief question to be answered was whether snoring, in the absence of obstructive sleep apnea (OSA), causes hypersomnolence, metabolic disorders, or cardiovascular disease. Currently there is growing evidence that mild inspiratory airflow limitation (IFL) during sleep, even in the absence of audible snoring or increased sleep fragmentation, may have a causative role in a variety of disabling somatic and affective disorders whose available treatment options are of limited benefit. After providing some background on the terms used in this chapter, we will first cover the physiology, recognition, and definition of IFL during sleep, the phenomenon known as increased *upper airway resistance*. We will next present the clinical manifestations of increased upper airway resistance, snoring, and UARS, attempting to organize the growing body of knowledge into a plausible pathophysiology and clinical paradigm of increased upper airway resistance in sleep.

BACKGROUND

Glossary of Terms Central to This Chapter

The terms defined below are described in detail and in context in this chapter:

Inspiratory airflow limitation. IFL describes a state of the upper airway (the pharynx) during sleep in which inspiratory airflow plateaus at a maximal level despite a continued increase in the pressure gradient between the nostrils and the hypopharynx. The failure of inspiratory airflow to increase despite the continued increase in the pressure gradient across the upper airway is caused by fluttering of the upper airway that prevents further increase in airflow. IFL can be divided into two subgroups based on whether or not it is *audible:* (1) *snoring* and (2) *silent IFL.* In this chapter, *snoring* is further divided into two subgroups: (a) *habitual snoring* and (b) *isolated snoring*

Snoring or inspiratory snoring. Audible inspiratory fluttering of the upper airway. It can occur during obstructive hypopnea when hypopnea is associated with a decrease in inspiratory airflow by 30% lasting at least 10 seconds accompanied by either an arousal from sleep or a 3% decrease in oxygen saturation. Alternatively it can occur in the absence of the above criteria for hypopnea, with higher levels of airflow, or with shorter duration or absence of arousals or oxygen desaturation. The presence of inspiratory snoring *always indicates the presence of IFL.* Although expiratory snoring exists (and will be discussed later in this chapter), the term *snoring* used without a modifier in this chapter refers to inspiratory snoring.

Habitual snoring: This term describes an observation (often a complaint) by a bed partner or roommate that a person consistently snores when asleep.

Isolated snoring: Following polysomnography, if an otherwise healthy, asymptomatic habitual snorer does not meet the current third *International Classification of Sleep Disorders*, third edition[1] (ICSD3) criteria for OSA, the patient is described as having *isolated snoring.*

Specific criteria for being "otherwise healthy" in the context of being a habitual snorer are described later in this chapter.

Silent inspiratory airflow limitation. Silent IFL is defined, and characterized by, the same *fluttering* of the upper airway that characterizes snoring; however, the frequency of the fluttering during silent IFL is, by definition, inaudible by humans.

Respiratory effort–related arousal (RERA): RERAs are transient arousals from sleep that follow a period of nonhypopneic IFL (either snoring or silent IFL) and are presumed to be caused by the inspiratory effort required to move air across a fluttering airway. As the name suggests, RERAs are *not* respiratory events per se, as are apneas and hypopneas. Whether an arousal following a period of IFL is in fact caused by the IFL cannot be definitively ascertained during clinical polysomnography; it is a presumption. To label an arousal a RERA, the authors of ICSD3 require 10 seconds of recognizable IFL preceding the arousal. A standard time requirement for IFL preceding an RERA, however, is not a feature of RERAs in the medical literature; a single flow-limited inspiration before arousal is the definition in some research.

Respiratory disturbance index (RDI): ICSD3 has replaced the apnea-hypopnea index (AHI) as a measure of the severity of OSA with the frequency of apneas, hypopneas, and RERAs. In this chapter, this new measure of the severity of OSA will be termed the RDI.

Upper airway resistance syndrome: The UARS does not exist in the ICSD3. It should be thought of as a syndrome coined by Dr. Christian Guilleminault and used by researchers who have broken away from the paradigm that hypersomnolence in patients with sleep-disordered breathing requires the presence of sleep fragmentation by apneas and hypopneas. In this chapter, UARS is defined as the symptom of either hypersomnolence or fatigue together with the presence of IFL during sleep adjudicated by polysomnography (as per the definition of IFL given previously) and an AHI of less than 5 per hour; the latter is the threshold of an OSA diagnosis in the ICSD2. In this chapter, symptoms and signs of UARS will be introduced to differentiate between UARS, OSA, and isolated snoring.

Upper Airway Resistance Versus Pharyngeal Collapse

Two terms used to describe the behavior of the upper airway (or pharynx) during sleep among snorers and patients with UARS are increased upper airway *resistance* and upper airway *collapse*. Many sleep researchers consider IFL during sleep to result from narrowing of the pharyngeal airway and increased resistance caused by the relaxation of pharyngeal dilator muscles, together with subatmospheric upper airway pressures during inspiration. As they measure increasingly negative esophageal or supraglottic pressures during inspiratory snoring, they think of upper airway *resistance* increasing. From this reasoning the clinical term *upper airway resistance syndrome* (UARS) was derived (as discussed later).

In contrast to this intuitive model of increasing upper airway resistance during sleep is the experimentally validated Starling resistor model of IFL[2] (see Chapter 13). The Starling resistor model postulates that the pharyngeal airway during sleep is a collapsible tube that will in fact collapse whenever the pressure within falls below a critical level, the pharyngeal "critical pressure" (Pcrit). It has been shown experimentally that as the severity of sleep-disordered breathing increases from isolated snoring to severe OSA, the pharyngeal Pcrit progressively increases from negative (subatmospheric) levels to positive levels.[3,4] Collapse of the pharynx, however, is not synonymous with apnea. When the pharynx collapses during sleep, one might experience either persistent apnea (no inspiratory airflow) or IFL (inspiratory airflow that has reached its maximum). When the pressure at the *upstream* end of the pharynx (the nares during inspiration) falls below Pcrit, the pharynx collapses, with resulting persistent apnea. When the pressure at the nares is above Pcrit, but the pressure at the downstream end of the pharynx (supraglottic pressure during inspiration) falls below Pcrit, as in a snorer, the pharynx also collapses. Because pharyngeal collapse leads to cessation of inspiratory airflow, pharyngeal pressure immediately equilibrates with nasal pressure opening the airway, with resumption of inspiratory airflow. The result is cyclical collapse and opening (fluttering) of the pharyngeal airway *limiting* inspiratory airflow to a fixed, maximal level (with the driving pressure fixed at nasal pressure minus Pcrit, no matter how low supraglottic pressure descends). Therefore, according to the Starling resistor model, the upper airway does not experience increased *resistance* during sleep, but a *fixed driving pressure* that limits airflow to a maximal level.

The language subsuming upper airway resistance and upper airway collapse therefore is derived from two different models of IFL. In this chapter, we will allude to *pharyngeal collapse* in the section that follows describing the polysomnographic appearance of IFL but use the term *upper airway resistance* for the remainder of this chapter, which does not require modeling of IFL.

Upper Airway Resistance Syndrome

As introduced in the glossary, we use the term UARS in this chapter, and it is found as a diagnosis in the current medical literature. However, the ICSD3[4] does not include UARS in its classification of sleep related breathing disorders but rather incorporates the polysomnographic manifestations of UARS into OSA. A brief discussion of the history of UARS will help the reader understand this dichotomy.

UARS came to public attention following the publication of a case series in 1993 by Dr. Christian Guilleminault and associates.[5] From among 48 patients with a diagnosis of idiopathic hypersomnolence, they selected 15 with the following characteristics:

- Intermittent or continuous snoring during sleep at home
- An AHI below the threshold for OSA by in-laboratory polysomnography (5/hour at Stanford University)
- More than 10 arousals per hour of sleep (a threshold they chose, attempting to limit their selected patients to those with an *increased* frequency of arousals)
- The presence of *upper airway resistive events* associated with arousals. These events were associated with reductions in airflow below the threshold to qualify as hypopnea and were identified using a pneumotachograph measurement of airflow and esophageal manometry to quantify effort.

Treatment of these 15 patients with nasal continuous positive airway pressure (CPAP) eliminated their resistive events and their associated arousals and relieved the patients' hypersomnolence (measured objectively by multiple sleep latency testing). Because the patients did not meet diagnostic criteria for OSA (their resistive events were not hypopneas), the investigators designated a new syndrome: UARS. They hypothesized that UARS is a disorder of hypersomnolence related to sleep fragmentation by upper airway resistive events too mild to meet the diagnostic criteria of hypopnea. They further hypothesized that UARS patients have increased sensitivity to the respiratory effort related to these resistive events, giving rise to repetitive arousals (compared with OSA patients who typically arouse in response to higher degrees of obstruction: i.e., apneas and hypopneas). The hypothesis that UARS patients exhibit increased sensitivity to respiratory effort during sleep led to their arousals being termed RERAs.

Almost from the start, the establishment of a new syndrome of sleep-disordered breathing based on sleep fragmentation by RERAs created controversy.[6,7] Many believed that RERAs and hypopneas were essentially the same phenomenon and that both OSA and UARS described sleep fragmentation caused by upper airway resistive events giving rise to hypersomnolence. To eliminate the need for an additional syndrome of sleep-disordered breathing based on sleep fragmentation by RERAs, the authors of ICSD3 incorporated RERAs into the diagnostic criteria for OSA, creating diagnostic thresholds for OSA based on the combined frequency of obstructive events: apneas, hypopneas, and RERAs—the RDI. Therefore, by the clinical criteria of ICSD3, UARS has been "absorbed" into OSA.

The significance of UARS, however, does not end with its *absorption* into OSA. Since first being described by Guilleminault and associates as a syndrome of sleep fragmentation leading to hypersomnolence,[5] the paradigm of UARS has evolved. Investigators have observed that the sleep of UARS patients is characterized not only by the presence of RERAs but also by electroencephalographic differences and differences in sleep architecture that distinguish it from the sleep of healthy individuals. These *qualitative* differences in the sleep of UARS patients resolve with treatments that eliminate IFL during sleep and the hypersomnolence of UARS patients. Therefore, although the ICSD3 clinical criteria for OSA will result in many patients being treated for OSA who previously were diagnosed with UARS, it is not established that these former UARS patients are hypersomnolent because of sleep fragmentation by RERAs. Consequently, UARS continues on as a syndrome being studied by researchers examining alternatives to the OSA pathophysiologic paradigm of sleep fragmentation by apneas, hypopneas, and RERAs.

In our discussion of UARS later in this chapter, we will describe more fully the clinical presentation of UARS and the findings of investigators that have led them away from a sleep fragmentation paradigm of this disorder. We will also consider the alternative pathophysiologic paradigms of UARS that continue to evolve.

Inspiratory Airflow Limitation

Classically, the term *snoring*, the audible fluttering of the pharynx during inspiration, has been used to describe IFL during sleep. The term *snoring*, however, implies that pharyngeal fluttering is present only when it can be heard by a listener (the word *snore* itself resembles the sound of snoring). Hearing, however, is an insensitive means of detecting inspiratory fluttering of the pharyngeal airway during sleep. Because using the term *snoring* may lead one to believe that IFL is

only present when audible, which is not the case, we have chosen to describe the characteristic inspiratory airflow through a fluttering upper airway during sleep as a state of *inspiratory airflow limitation* (as defined in the glossary above). The term IFL was first used by Schwartz and associates in their study of pharyngeal collapsibility during sleep in healthy humans[8] and was derived from the parallel term *expiratory airflow limitation*, used to describe expiratory airflow from the lungs of patients with asthma, chronic obstructive bronchitis, and emphysema whose bronchi flutter on expiration, limiting airflow.[9]

Recognizing Inspiratory Airflow Limitation with Physiologic Testing

With the incorporation of RERAs into the diagnostic criteria for OSA, recognizing the presence of IFL preceding an arousal and differentiating its appearance from that of non-flow-limited breathing during polysomnography is an important skill for practitioners of sleep medicine to develop. Similarly, for clinicians and polysomnographic technologists involved in titrating nasal CPAP to treat OSA, recognizing IFL during sleep is an important aspect of polysomnography to understand. In this section we begin by illustrating the appearance of IFL using airflow and supraglottic pressure tracings. We then demonstrate how IFL is recognized using the airflow and effort tracings available during clinical polysomnography.

Figure 14-1 illustrates five breaths during continuous non–rapid eye movement stage (NREM) 2 (N2) sleep at atmospheric pressure, all characterized by IFL. The individual being monitored is a 24 year-old woman with a body mass index of 19.9 kg/m^2 who does not snore audibly and has an AHI of 0.3/hour. Because Figure 14-1 has both an airflow tracing and a supraglottic pressure tracing, it precisely demonstrates the presence of IFL. Specifically, it shows that inspiratory airflow is limited to a maximal level (intersected by the vertical lines) despite the observation that the pressure gradient across the pharyngeal airway (atmospheric pressure minus supraglottic pressure) continues to increase (atmospheric pressure remains the same while supraglottic pressure continues to decrease beyond the vertical line). This defines IFL.

Figure 14-2 demonstrates both IFL and non-flow-limited inspiration in the same individual diagnosed with UARS during nasal CPAP titration. Although the left panel of the figure clearly demonstrates IFL at atmospheric pressure similar to that observed in Figure 14-1, the right panel, recorded at the therapeutic nasal CPAP level of 4 cm H$_2$O, presents airflow and supraglottic pressure tracings that parallel each other through four inspiratory cycles. The parallel tracings demonstrate that inspiratory airflow is continuously proportional to the driving pressure, 4 cm H$_2$O minus supraglottic pressure, and thus, according to the above definition of IFL, is not flow limited.

Figures 14-1 and 14-2 illustrate that, when one is provided with both an airflow signal and a supraglottic pressure signal, recognizing IFL is not difficult. It is emphasized that IFL is not defined by any specific decrease in inspiratory airflow (e.g., a 30% or 50% decrease in airflow) relative to *non*-flow-limited inspiration. Rather, IFL is defined by a specific relationship of airflow to driving pressure (nasal pressure minus supraglottic pressure). IFL can be more difficult to recognize in the absence of a supraglottic pressure signal because one is then

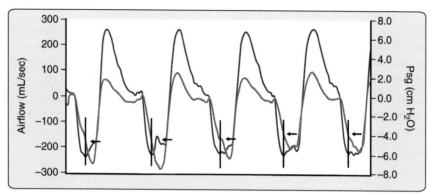

Figure 14-1 This figure illustrates inspiratory airflow limitation (IFL) in a sleeping research participant wearing a nasal mask attached to a pneumotachograph measuring airflow, with a pressure catheter placed through her nose to just above her vocal cords measuring supraglottic pressure (Psg). Airflow is the *blue tracing* with the units indicated on the left axis (inspiration is downgoing). Effort, represented by Psg, is the *yellow tracing* with the units indicated on the right axis. For each inspiration, a plateau in airflow during early inspiration is intersected by a *vertical line*. Beyond the line, there is no further increase in inspiratory airflow despite the continued decrease in Psg and a continued increase in the inspiratory pressure gradient Patm—Psg. Indeed, not only does the inspiratory airflow not increase, but also in the first four breaths it appears to decrease, a phenomenon known as *negative effort dependence* of airflow. IFL occurs when Psg decreases below this participant's pharyngeal Pcrit. The *horizontal arrows* mark the Psg at the onset of maximal flow (intersected by the *vertical line*) and suggest that this participant's pharyngeal Pcrit is approximately −4 cm H_2O, a common value for primary snorers or individuals who have upper airway resistance syndrome.[3]

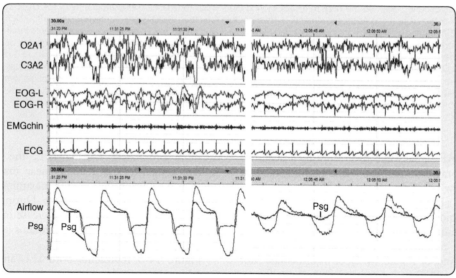

Figure 14-2 This figure demonstrates both inspiratory airflow limitation (IFL) and *non*-flow-limited inspiration in the same individual during nasal continuous positive airway pressure (CPAP) titration. The two polysomnographic tracings are obtained in stage N2 sleep, $\frac{1}{2}$ hour apart. Below the sleep monitoring channels recording electroencephalograms (O2A1, C3A2), electrooculograms (EOG-L & R), superficial electromyograms of the chin (EMGchin), and electrocardiogram (ECG) are recordings of airflow (a pneumotachograph tracing) and supraglottic pressure (Psg). The *left panel* demonstrates four breaths at atmospheric pressure, whereas the *right panel* demonstrates four breaths with nasal CPAP at 4 cm H_2O. In each panel, airflow (*black tracing*) and Psg (*blue tracing*) are superimposed. The *left panel* demonstrates the plateau of inspiratory airflow (downgoing) at a maximal level occurring as Psg continues to decrease, which defines IFL. In the *right panel*, because pharyngeal pressure and Psg do not fall much below 4 cm H_2O (the CPAP applied to the nasal mask), Psg always remains above pharyngeal Pcrit, and the airflow and pressure tracings parallel each other (airflow is always determined by the pressure gradient: 4 minus Psg).

missing driving pressure; indeed, the presence of IFL can only be *assumed* in the absence of a supraglottic pressure tracing). To enable clinicians to recognize IFL during clinical polysomnography without the recording of supraglottic pressure, researchers have investigated the possibility of identifying IFL from the airflow signal alone.

In 1998, two studies evaluated the utility of a plateau of inspiratory airflow measured as a nasal pressure signal (pressure transducer airflow [PTAF]) to identify IFL.[10,11] Hosselet and associates[10] studied more than 47,000 breaths during polysomnography in 10 symptomatic OSA patients and 4 asymptomatic individuals without OSA, classifying the shape

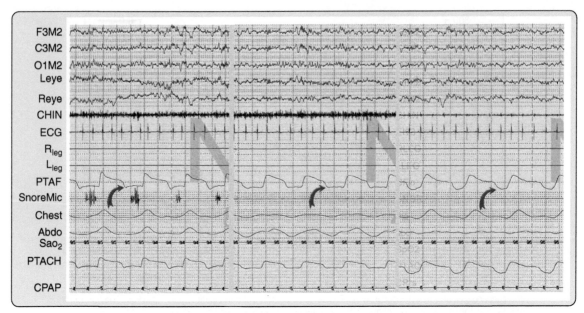

Figure 14-3 This figuure's three panels, from left to right, represent three 12-second intervals at nasal continuous positive airway pressure (CPAP) levels of 4 cm H_2O, 5 cm H_2O, and 6 cm H_2O. Below the sleep monitoring channels recording electroencephalograms (F3M2, C3M2, O1M2), electrooculograms (L & Reye), superficial electromyograms of the chin (CHIN), and right and left tibialis anterior (R & L_{leg}) and ECG are several channels recording respiratory parameters. The respiratory channels include a pressure transducer-generated airflow signal (PTAF), a microphone placed on the neck to record snoring (SnoreMic), impedance plethysmography of the chest and abdomen (Chest and Abdo; movement), oxyhemoglobin saturation (SaO_2), a pneumotachograph airflow signal (PTACH), and a pressure transducer-recorded CPAP level (CPAP). At 4 cm H_2O, the *left panel*, the patient's inspirations all demonstrate IFL with audible snoring. Inspiratory airflow (downgoing) is seen to increase rapidly and then to plateau with a prolonged time spent at maximal inspiratory airflow (highlighted by the *arrow*). At 5 cm H_2O, IFL persists without audible snoring. Inspiratory airflow, again, increases rapidly and then demonstrates a prolonged plateau at maximal flow (highlighted by the *arrow*). At 6 cm H_2O, the airflow tracing no longer demonstrates inspiratory airflow limitation. Inspiratory airflow increases to its maximum more gradually and then immediately decreases, spending only a short time at maximal airflow. Expiratory time is prolonged relative to flow-limited conditions (the two *left panels*), and inspiration is a smaller percentage of the respiratory cycle.

of each breath's PTAF signal while also recording a pneumotachograph and supraglottic pressure signal (a gold standard assessment of airflow vs. driving pressure). They used a computer algorithm to classify each PTAF inspiration as non-flow-limited (sinusoidal in shape and resembling the airflow signal in the right panel of Figure 14-2), flow-limited (having a clear plateau and resembling the airflow signal in Figure 14-1 and the left panel of Figure 14-2), or intermediate (not sinusoidal but not fulfilling their program's criteria for an inspiratory plateau). The PTAF signal clearly separated their asymptomatic controls without OSA from their OSA patients, with the former having fewer flow-limited events. In a similar study of seven habitual snorers, Clark and associates[11] found that an inspiratory airflow plateau determined by PTAF identified flow-limited inspirations with a sensitivity and specificity of approximately 80%. Thus PTAF evidence of a clear inspiratory airflow plateau is a reasonably reliable method for identifying IFL during clinical polysomnography.

The ability to recognize IFL during diagnostic polysomnography, whether in-laboratory or during out-of-center sleep testing (OCST), can also be aided by the findings of Schneider and associates: During IFL, the ratio of the inspiratory time to the time of the entire respiratory cycle (i.e., the "duty cycle") is prolonged.[12] This distinction is illustrated in Figure 14-2, where four flow-limited inspirations (left panel) take up a larger portion of the respiratory cycle time than the non-flow-limited inspirations (right panel), where expiratory time

is more prolonged. During IFL, the inspiratory airflow increases rapidly and remains near maximum throughout most of inspiration (left panel), maximizing the tidal volume under the flow-limited conditions. During the *non*-flow-limited breaths (right panel), the increase in inspiratory airflow is more gradual, and airflow remains near maximal for a shorter portion of inspiration.

Figure 14-3 represents both IFL and *non*-flow-limited breathing in a single patient with UARS undergoing nasal CPAP titration. In the absence of a supraglottic pressure signal, IFL can be recognized by the change in the airflow tracing between the two left panels recorded at CPAP levels of 4 and 5 cm H_2O demonstrating IFL, and the right panel recorded at a CPAP of 6 cm H_2O illustrating non-flow-limited airflow at therapeutic CPAP. At 4 and 5 cm H_2O, the flow-limited inspiratory airflow tracing is characterized by a rapid increase in airflow to a maximum followed by a prolonged plateau at maximal flow. At 6 cm H_2O, the non-flow-limited inspiratory airflow increases more gradually without a subsequent plateau, but a rapid decrease of airflow and a shorter ratio of inspiratory time to respiratory cycle time (exhalation is prolonged relative to flow-limited conditions). Thus, in the absence of a supraglottic pressure signal, both the shape and the relative duration of the inspiratory airflow tracing provide evidence for the presence of IFL.

Figure 14-4, a 30-second epoch of sleep from a patient with UARS, provides examples of overt IFL, more subtle IFL,

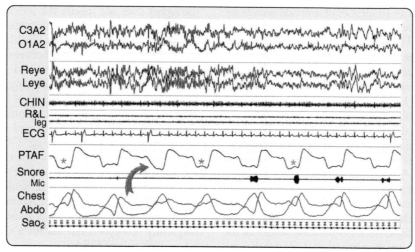

Figure 14-4 This figure demonstrates a 30-second epoch of NREM stage 2 (N2) sleep containing eight consecutive breaths representing both overt and subtle (*asterisks*) inspiratory airflow limitation and a *non*-flow-limited breath (*arrow*). The sleep parameters recorded include electroencephalograms (EEGs; C3A2, O1A2), electrooculograms (EOGs; Reye & Leye), superficial electromyogram of the chin (CHIN), superficial electromyograms of the right and left tibialis anterior (R & L$_{leg}$), and ECG. The respiratory parameters recorded are labeled similarly to those in Figure 14-3. Refer to the text for a complete characterization of the breathing.

and *non*-flow-limited breathing. Although several breaths in Figure 14-5 demonstrate the rapid increase in inspiratory airflow and long inspiratory airflow plateau of IFL, several (marked by an asterisk) demonstrate a less prolonged plateau of inspiratory airflow. The presence in these breaths, however, of a rapid increase in inspiratory airflow followed by a short plateau, as well as the accompanying snoring (recorded by microphone) for one of the breaths, can be used to identify all of these as examples of subtle IFL compared with the one *non*-flow-limited inspiration (marked by an arrow). Viewed from the perspective of respiratory cycle time, one can also appreciate that the *non*-flow-limited breath is preceded by the longest expiration and the ratio of inspiratory time to respiratory cycle time for the breath is lower than for the flow-limited breaths in the figure.

To summarize, in the absence of a supraglottic pressure catheter, IFL can be recognized, using a nasal pressure signal, as a plateau in inspiratory airflow and a prolongation of inspiratory time relative to total respiratory cycle time. Inspiratory airflow can be observed to rise rapidly to a maximum and to remain there for most of inspiration. From the figures provided, it can also be inferred that snoring, the audible manifestation of the fluttering pharyngeal airway characterizing IFL, is not as sensitive an indicator of IFL as the combined airflow and driving pressure criteria (Figures 14-1 and 14-2) or the airflow tracing alone. Figure 14-1, which in fact is a tracing of a lean female with no history of snoring, demonstrates definitive evidence of IFL determined by her airflow and supraglottic pressure recordings. In Figure 14-3, nasal CPAP of 5 cm H$_2$O resolves the patient's snoring before the airflow tracing demonstrates resolution of IFL at 6 cm H$_2$O. Figure 14-4 demonstrates five breaths clearly characterized by the airflow plateau associated with IFL, only four of which demonstrate snoring. For this reason, the presence of snoring should not be relied on to determine whether a patient with sleepiness or fatigue has sleep-disordered breathing. Even in the absence of apneas and hypopneas, silent IFL (defined in the glossary) associated with arousals (RERAs) may be

prevalent enough to establish a diagnosis of OSA when using ICSD3 criteria, or UARS, using the criteria of sleepiness or fatigue in the presence of IFL as presented in the glossary. Similarly, the absence of snoring should not be relied on to determine whether a nasal CPAP level is therapeutic (i.e., has eliminated IFL). Rather, the polysomnographer, sleep medicine physician, and polysomnographic technologist should differentiate IFL during sleep from non-flow-limited inspiration using an airflow signal generated by either a pneumotachograph or a PTAF signal and determine therapeutic nasal CPAP as the pressure that eliminates IFL (as demonstrated in Figures 14-2 and 14-3). A CPAP level that eliminates IFL will, of necessity, eliminate all apneas, hypopneas, and RERAs.

PATHOLOGIC UPPER AIRWAY RESISTANCE SYNDROMES: CLINICAL ASPECTS

Snoring

Habitual snoring, as described early in the glossary, can be observed in patients with OSA complaining of daytime sleepiness, fatigue, and insomnia. Habitual snoring may also occur in the absence of symptoms and signs of OSA and without an RDI (a frequency of apneas, hypopneas, and RERAs) adequate to establish a diagnosis of OSA in the absence of symptoms—that is, an RDI of 15 per hour. In the latter instance, according to the ICSD3, it is regarded as "isolated snoring," listed in the category of sleep-related breathing disorders. This isolated snoring was previously referred to as habitual, simple, or primary snoring in the category of other parasomnias in the ICSD2.

As already noted, snoring is a sleep-related sound caused by vibration of soft tissue in the upper airway under conditions of IFL. In most individuals with isolated snoring, the snoring is limited to inspiration, although early expiratory snoring or snoring throughout expiration can occur.[13] Whether occurring during inspiration or expiration, snoring is generated by high-frequency opening and closing (fluttering) of upper airway structures, including the tongue base and soft palate, aided by the adhesive properties of mucosal secretions. Acoustic studies have shown that the major frequency content of snoring is below 2000 Hz, with peak power below 500 Hz[14] (thus in the frequency range able to be heard by humans). Snorers experience increased total pulmonary resistance during sleep related to reduced upper airway muscle tone causing IFL and leading to increased inspiratory effort.[15]

There is, understandably, considerable variation in the prevalence figures reported for habitual snoring. Studies differ in how the study population is selected, with some determining a prevalence of isolated snoring and others including habitual snorers with OSA. Studies also differ in how snoring is assessed. *Subjective* assessment has been conducted using the report of bed partners, but clinical experience indicates that a few snorers hear their own snoring, especially during sleep-wake transitions. *Objective* measurement relies on the use of calibrated monitoring devices either during polysomnography or in a setting outside a sleep disorders center. Patients also document their own snoring using recording applications for smart devices such as cellular phones. In addition to differences in methodology regarding diagnoses and snoring assessment, differences in gender and obesity distribution between studies may affect snoring prevalence significantly. Both gender and obesity can affect upper airway resistance (alternatively, collapsibility, assessed as the pharyngeal Pcrit) either by structural changes or neuromuscular mechanisms. Therefore the variability of study design is one reason for the varied prevalence figures for habitual snoring seen in the literature.

Further complicating a determination of the prevalence of snoring is the observation that, within individual patients, the severity of subjective snoring reported by the bed partner does not correspond with either objectively assessed snoring or the subjective assessment of the sleep technician monitoring the patient.[16] Data from Somnolab Sleep Disorders Center in Dortmund, Germany show that 28% of individuals reporting habitual snoring at home fail to present significant snoring during in-laboratory polysomnographic recordings (unpublished data). This may, in part, be due to considerable night-to-night variability of snoring intensity. Interventional studies have demonstrated that time spent snoring and snoring volume within one individual can vary from night to night depending on factors such as sleeping position, medications, alcohol intake, and cumulative or acute sleep debt. Alternatively, the discrepancy observed between a bed partner's report of snoring severity and that observed during in-laboratory polysomnography could be due to allergens in the home environment altering upper airway pressure-flow relationships. Also, discrepancies between snoring reported by a bed partner and that measured during polysomnography can be observed in patients who have had a recent change in bed partner, suggesting either differences among bed partners in sensitivity to the noise or in willingness to complain.[17]

As discussed earlier, prevalence data for snoring often come from study samples containing both individuals with isolated snoring and those with OSA. The 2011 Centers for Disease Control and Prevention report on unhealthy sleep behaviors, one such study, reports a snoring prevalence of 48% based on a telephone survey.[18] The report does not indicate how many of the snorers in this survey complained of hypersomnolence or other symptoms of OSA. Furthermore,

the report does not specify the snoring severity of those individuals labeled as snorers: intermittent versus habitual. Based on data from the Sleep Heart Health Study, a sample of 5615 community-dwelling adults between the ages of 40 and 98 years, 13% of the participants had an AHI of less than 5/hour and reported *habitual* snoring (3 to 7 nights/week).[19] These data estimate a prevalence of habitual snoring without OSA of less than 15% in a community sample. Symptom data, however, are not provided and so one cannot determine a prevalence of isolated snoring. Of note, 29% of the 5615 men and women did not know whether they snored (perhaps because of absence of bed partner). Although the previous two examples illustrate the difficulty investigators have in determining the prevalence of habitual and isolated snoring, it remains clear that snoring is a common phenomenon that frequently prompts a referral for a sleep evaluation to establish a diagnosis of OSA.

When a habitual snorer presents for a sleep evaluation, polysomnography is warranted if witnessed apnea, hypersomnolence, fatigue, insomnia, somatic syndromes typically described among UARS patients (discussed in the next section), or comorbidities such as metabolic syndrome, cardiac dysrhythmia, or atrial fibrillation are present. In this case, polysomnography may lead to treatment of OSA when the ICSD3 diagnostic criteria for OSA are met. Habitual snoring in the absence of witnessed apnea, symptoms or syndromes, or comorbidities (after appropriate screening for comorbidities) does not automatically warrant a polysomnogram. Habitual snoring is a common occurrence among middle-aged, overweight men, and polysomnographic evaluations of *all* habitual snorers carries a very high cost-to-benefit ratio. A more practical approach would be to monitor asymptomatic, healthy habitual snorers over time for the development of signs and symptoms that would support obtaining polysomnography. Alternatively, OCST can be used to rule out moderate to severe OSA in asymptomatic, healthy habitual snorers in need of reassurance.

The rationale for not obtaining polysomnography in asymptomatic, healthy habitual snorers extends beyond the issue of costs, to a consideration of benefit. Specifically, even if such an individual fulfills ICSD3 criteria for OSA, the question is whether such an asymptomatic, healthy individual is in fact in need of treatment. To the contrary, cross-sectional polysomnographic data from an investigation by Pavlova and associates[20] of 163 asymptomatic, nonobese individuals screened for the absence of metabolic syndrome and cardiovascular disease (25% reporting "some" snoring) demonstrate that many such individuals have RDIs above 15/hour, fulfilling ICSD3 criteria for OSA. Indeed, the mean RDI for individuals older than 65 years was 22 per hour in Pavlova's study.[20] Similar data exist in three studies comparing inspiratory airflow dynamics during sleep between patients with somatic syndromes[21,22] and UARS[23] with those of rigorously screened healthy controls. For the three studies, 4 (11%) of 35 healthy controls (14 men and 21 women) met the ICSD3 threshold for OSA that would justify their treatment without symptoms or comorbidities (RDI ≥15/hour). Another 4 of the healthy controls had values of RDI between 10/hour and 15/hour, approximating the threshold for treatment. Thus, in the absence of data demonstrating a health risk from habitual snoring alone, a prudent approach to polysomnographic evaluation can be justified.

Before leaving the subject of whether to treat asymptomatic, habitual snorers without comorbidities, a word of caution is appropriate. In 110 overweight volunteers with snoring and mild OSA (27% smokers, 27% with hypertension, and 69% with hyperlipidemia), Lee and associates[24] demonstrated that the amount of time spent snoring was correlated with the extent of asymptomatic carotid artery stenosis independent of AHI and histories of other comorbidities. These findings suggest that in individuals predisposed to atherosclerosis (by smoking, hypertension, or hyperlipidemia), habitual snoring may be an *additional* risk factor for developing carotid artery atherosclerosis. On the other hand, data from a recently published study with a 17-year follow-up of 380 community-dwelling adults failed to document a significant relationship between objectively measured nocturnal time spent snoring and all-cause mortality from cardiovascular disease.[25] In the absence of certainty about the effects of habitual snoring, one should evaluate (beginning with noninvasive methods) an asymptomatic, habitual snorer without metabolic syndrome or atrial fibrillation for evidence of atherosclerosis before deciding that the patient is not in need of treatment and can be followed over time.

Asymptomatic, healthy individuals seeking treatment for habitual snoring or isolated snoring (following polysomnography because of reports of witnessed, or patient-perceived, apnea) will usually do so because they are concerned about the disruption of their bed partner's sleep. Any treatment that will lower the pharyngeal Pcrit, reducing the occurrence of IFL, will also have a beneficial effect on audible snoring. A wide variety of over-the-counter remedies are available for snoring, but they are of limited efficacy. A report of the American Academy of Sleep Medicine Clinical Practice Review Committee published in 2003 summarizes the absent or limited benefits of products such as nasal dilators, lubricants, oral dietary supplements, and magnetic pillows and mattresses.[26] In contrast to these ineffective treatments, any effective treatment used for OSA will be effective for asymptomatic snoring. Among these treatments, few isolated snorers choose nasal CPAP, considering it a burden to use and to maintain.

Successful or partially successful treatment of isolated snoring has been reported using lifestyle modifications. A lifestyle modification like weight reduction (by diet or bariatric surgery) can be an effective treatment for snoring because it can substantially lower pharyngeal Pcrit.[27] Because there are no "dose-response" data concerning the effect of weight loss on snoring intensity (loudness), the weight loss target should be based on factors like the pretreatment body mass index and the weight loss needed to obtain other expected health benefits. Although weight loss can effectively decrease the intensity of snoring, long-term maintenance of reduced weight is often unsatisfactory. For this reason, weight loss in combination with increased physical activity may be a more desirable approach. There is an independent, beneficial effect of physical activity on self-reported snoring in obese women.[28] Another lifestyle alteration that can decrease the intensity of snoring is avoiding alcohol consumption before going to bed. In a small group of otherwise asymptomatic snorers, Riemann and colleagues demonstrated that presleep alcohol ingestion increased the objectively measured incidence and loudness of snoring in a dose-dependent manner.[29] Other lifestyle modifications that can reduce snoring include avoiding sleep deprivation and the use of sedative-hypnotic medications.

Oral mandibular advancement appliances have been used successfully for the treatment of mild to moderate OSA and asymptomatic snoring in patients with a healthy dentition. Good results can be achieved with 50% to 75% of maximal voluntary protrusion. For patients with an insufficient number of healthy teeth, a tongue-retaining device may be a good alternative. Patients should be advised that snoring may not be completely abolished, but significant reductions in the time spent snoring and snoring intensity can be obtained.

Surgery can be performed for isolated snoring to decrease its occurrence and intensity. Surgical targets include the nasal turbinates and septum, the nasopharynx, oropharynx, tongue base, and hypopharynx. Sleep nasendoscopy with a flexible endoscope is increasingly used to perform a preoperative assessment of possible surgical targets. For this procedure, anesthesia is used to simulate sleep. At this time, the data regarding the value of nasendoscopy before surgical treatment of snoring are indeterminate. The surgical method depends on the surgeon's preference and the availability of equipment, but procedures are performed using a scalpel, radiofrequency ablation, and YAG laser. Studies assessing the efficacy of these procedures have typically shown good immediate and short-term results. However, many of these studies have relied only on subjective assessments of snoring. A study on the subjective versus the objective improvement of snoring following palatal surgery published in 1994 did not find any objective improvement in snoring despite a subjective improvement in more than 75% of the participants.[30] In a more recent study, palatal surgery for isolated snoring improved subjective (questionnaire) and objective (sound analysis of 100 supine snorers before and after surgery) evaluations of snoring. However, the objective improvement was short-lived and correlated poorly with the subjective improvement on an individual basis.[31] A recent, long-term study evaluating patients treated with palatal surgery between 1985 and 1991 found a substantial rebound of snoring even in the absence of weight gain. In addition, 38% of the patients continued to experience surgical side effects (swallowing dysfunction, altered voice, and pain) that left them dissatisfied with the decision to have palatal surgery.[32]

Surgery intended to relieve nasal obstruction alone does not produce a significant improvement of objectively assessed snoring intensity and snoring time, nor does it decrease the AHI, despite improvement in nasal resistance.[33]

The consequences of leaving isolated snoring untreated relate specifically to the concern: will untreated isolated snoring progress to OSA over time? According to a study that followed individuals with isolated snoring over 5 years with polysomnography, isolated snoring does not progress to OSA over 5 years in the absence of a significant change in body weight.[34] Thus, to date, there is no evidence that isolated snoring progresses to OSA in the intermediate term.

In summary, isolated snoring is a diagnosis of exclusion reserved for habitual snorers who are otherwise asymptomatic without metabolic syndrome and cardiovascular disease and who do not meet polysomnographic or OCST criteria for OSA. The potential for adverse long-term cardiovascular outcomes in isolated snoring remains uncertain, at this time. Treatment of isolated snoring is currently limited to attempting to improve the sleep quality of the bed partner. Available treatments include lifestyle modifications, oral appliances, and soft tissue surgery. Most available treatment options lead to short-term success but fail in the long-term.

Upper Airway Resistance Syndrome

UARS is defined as the symptom of either hypersomnolence or fatigue together with the presence of IFL during sleep by in-laboratory polysomnography and an AHI of less than 5/hour (see the glossary earlier in this chapter). As a movement away from the paradigm that hypersomnolence among patients with sleep-disordered breathing requires the presence of sleep fragmentation by apneas and hypopneas, UARS was originally accompanied by a new paradigm that sleep fragmentation by RERAs can also lead to hypersomnolence in individuals with milder resistive events[5] (discussed previously under Background). In line with this new paradigm, ICSD3 absorbs UARS into OSA by including RERAs into the severity assessment of sleep fragmentation in OSA. ICSD3 criteria for OSA now classify any patient fulfilling the previously noted UARS definition with an RDI above 5/hour as having OSA. Clearly a portion of UARS has been absorbed into OSA by the clinical criteria of ICSD3. However, there are still patients meeting the definition of UARS elaborated in the chapter with an RDI of less than 5/hour who are not included within the ICSD3 definition of OSA and are not considered, clinically, to have sleep-disordered breathing. Nevertheless, to investigators of UARS and to clinicians attempting to treat the hypersomnolence of a patient without a clear diagnosis because of too few RERAs, the recognition that sleep-disordered breathing may, in fact, exist outside the limits of ICSD3 is important and worthy of consideration. In this section, we discuss the varied clinical presentation of UARS, its polysomnographic appearance, and its evolving paradigm. To facilitate this discussion, when we refer to OSA, we will use the ICSD2 definition of OSA—an AHI of at least 5/hour—to match the definition used in the research to be presented.

Anthropometric Features and Risk Factors

Compared with patients with OSA, UARS patients are younger, leaner, and more frequently female. Published studies of UARS patients as defined by the previous criteria have established a mean age of 40 years with the average body mass index between 23 and 30 kg/m^2 (normal weight or overweight; less often, obese) and approximately 50% female.[35-37] Although craniofacial abnormalities such as a narrow, elongated face characterized by a high arched palate, reduced upper and lower intermolar distances, and a narrow anterior nasal aperture (adenoid facies) have been reported in patients with UARS, these same findings are also commonly observed in patients with OSA[38] and so cannot be considered specific for UARS. The presence of these abnormalities suggests a disturbance of facial development caused by increased nasal resistance during early childhood with mouth breathing.[39]

Signs and Symptoms

The most commonly observed polysomnographic feature of UARS patients is nonapneic, habitual snoring or silent IFL with relatively few adjudicated apneic or hypopneic events (AHI <5/hour). In clinical practice, these patients will seek medical attention for their condition because they also suffer from nonrestorative sleep, fatigue, sleepiness, or insomnia. In fact, UARS patients are more commonly referred to a sleep disorders center for their symptoms than for their snoring. Before referring these patients for cognitive behavior therapy

(CBT) for insomnia, a careful sleep-related history revealing snoring without witnessed apnea will prompt polysomnographic investigation with documentation of IFL during sleep. It is emphasized that a report of witnessed apnea does not preclude a diagnosis of UARS because about one third of UARS patients are reported to have witnessed apnea but an AHI below the threshold for OSA.[40] Similarly, the absence of audible snoring does not preclude a diagnosis of UARS because inaudible IFL is observed in about 10% of patients diagnosed with UARS.[40,41] Typically, these patients have been diagnosed with insomnia and, in the absence of a sleep-related history of habitual snoring, are referred for CBT without performing polysomnography. When CBT fails to improve their condition and a polysomnogram is performed to exclude an intrinsic sleep disorder, IFL in the absence of audible snoring can be demonstrated.

The earliest reports of UARS emphasized the importance of hypersomnolence as a diagnostic criterion distinguishing it from isolated snoring.[5,13] Before those reports, polysomnographic technology used a thermistor or thermocouple to generate a qualitative airflow signal that could not be used to recognize IFL. Thus the link between hypersomnolence and IFL could not be made, and patients with UARS often received a diagnosis of idiopathic hypersomnolence. The earliest reports of UARS substituted a pneumotachograph recording of airflow for the qualitative airflow signal together with an esophageal pressure catheter measurement of inspiratory effort to establish the presence of IFL during sleep in UARS patients.[5,13] With time and the growth of clinical experience evaluating UARS patients, the diagnostic criteria for UARS have been expanded to include complaints of hypersomnolence or fatigue.[6,7,40]

Hypersomnolence and fatigue are not synonymous. Hypersomnolence indicates increased sleep pressure expressed by short sleep latency, a state that is inconsistent with a complaint of insomnia. Fatigue, on the other hand, is generally associated with longer sleep latencies, reflecting a state of hyperarousal commonly observed in patients with insomnia. Indeed, about one third of UARS patients complain of sleep-onset insomnia, and nearly two thirds report sleep maintenance insomnia.[35] Characteristically, the complaints of fatigue and insomnia among UARS patients are associated with the complaint of nonrestorative sleep.

Interestingly, UARS patients complain of more subjective sleep disturbance than OSA patients who have much more disrupted sleep.[41a] UARS patients can also experience a variety of parasomnias. Among these are sleep-related bruxism,[40] chronic sleepwalking in children[42] and catathrenia.[43]

Currently, there is not enough evidence to conclude that UARS is an independent cardiovascular risk factor. An increased prevalence of arterial hypertension among nonapneic snorers has been reported,[44] and borderline arterial hypertension has been lowered with nasal CPAP in a small series of UARS patients.[45] Hypotension and orthostatic intolerance have also been documented in about 20% of patients with UARS.[46]

Psychiatric symptoms such as depression[36,37,47,48] and anxiety[47-49] have been demonstrated among UARS patients and have responded dramatically to treatment using nasal CPAP and rapid palatal expansion in case reports.[47,48] Conversely, failure to diagnose and treat UARS is associated with a worsening of these symptoms over time.[36]

Currently there are limited data available regarding cognitive function among patients with UARS. Using a psychomotor vigilance task, Stoohs and associates[50] have reported increased reaction times among UARS patients compared with OSA patients. Research from Broderick and associates[51] suggests that, although UARS patients perceive themselves to have impaired cognitive function compared with healthy controls, objective testing fails to demonstrate such a difference.

UARS patients also commonly present with a variety of symptoms characteristic of the functional somatic syndromes.[40] In addition to insomnia, sleepiness, and fatigue, and the affective symptoms of depression and anxiety already mentioned, UARS patients may experience headaches and functional gastrointestinal symptoms and alpha-delta sleep, all common symptoms and signs of the functional somatic syndromes.[40] These functional somatic syndrome symptoms and signs (specifically, sleep-onset insomnia, headache, irritable bowel syndrome, and alpha-delta sleep) decrease in prevalence among sleep-disordered breathing patients as the AHI increases.[40] Conversely, when patients with functional somatic syndromes undergo polysomnography, IFL during sleep is commonly observed (fibromyalgia, temporomandibular joint syndrome, Gulf War illness, and irritable bowel syndrome have been studied).[21,22,52,53] In this setting, nasal CPAP has been shown to relieve the symptoms of functional somatic syndrome patients by relieving their IFL during sleep.[53,54]

Polysomnographic Findings

Polysomnographic findings among UARS patients can be subdivided into those characterizing breathing with associated arousals and those characterizing sleep architecture (electroencephalographic frequencies, sleep staging). Concerning sleep architecture, researchers have observed findings consistent with unstable, nonrestorative sleep among UARS patients.

Polysomnographic Findings Characterizing Breathing. Breathing in UARS is, by definition, characterized by an AHI below 5/hour of sleep and periods of IFL during sleep with flows greater than 50% of waking levels (exemplified in Figures 14-2 to 14-4), terminated by arousals or changes in the background electroencephalographic rhythm associated with a return of airflow to a non-flow-limited state (i.e., RERAs).[36] Oxyhemoglobin saturation generally remains above 90% throughout sleep.[35,37] In several large studies, the mean AHI for UARS patients is consistently 2/hour, and the frequency of RERAs is between 5/hour and 20/hour.[35-37] Describing the prevalence of flow-limited breaths during sleep among UARS patients has received little attention. One large study that used a snore microphone to determine the prevalence of breaths associated with audible snoring among 424 UARS patients observed a 21 ± 23% (mean ± standard deviation) prevalence of such breaths during sleep.[37] It is likely therefore that if a study were performed that included both a snore microphone and a pressure transducer for airflow measurement to identify both snoring and inaudible IFL (as explained previously), the prevalence of such breaths would be considerably higher and not a sporadic occurrence.

The preceding description of breathing during sleep in UARS does not define the syndrome based on thresholds for IFL or RERAs. Empirically, periods of IFL during sleep in UARS may last a few breaths or be continuous for many polysomnographic epochs. The presence of IFL has not been defined by a consensus frequency of *resistive* events, but it is a characteristic of breathing during sleep that can be described in a polysomnographic report based on the sleep stages in which it occurs and an impression of the prevalence of flow-limited breaths in those sleep stages (e.g., continuous, intermittent, or uncommon; Figure 14-4 is one 30-second epoch of continuous IFL in a UARS patient). Similarly, in the UARS literature, RERAs have not been defined by a consensus length of the preceding period of IFL (as has been done in ICSD3). Rather, the duration of IFL preceding a RERA has been undefined,[5] 10 seconds[36] or one flow-limited breath,[23] depending on the study. Because the diagnosis of UARS is not dependent on thresholds for resistive events or RERAs, UARS cannot be classified as mild, moderate, or severe based on these events. Indeed, there are no published data relating the severity of hypersomnolence among UARS patients to RERA frequency or prevalence of IFL.

Polysomnographic Findings Characterizing Sleep Architecture. Polysomnography of UARS patients demonstrates findings consistent with unstable, nonrestorative sleep (the altered sleep quality referred to earlier under Background). Among these findings is alpha frequency intruding into sleep, increased sleep stage shifts, and cyclic alternating pattern (CAP).

Patients with UARS experience increased alpha frequency, a frequency observed during quiet wakefulness, within their sleep electroencephalogram.[40,55] This increased alpha frequency may be seen in stage N3 sleep, where it has been termed *alpha-delta sleep*[40,56] (Figure 14-5) or in N1 and N2 sleep[48] (Figure 14-6; also observed in Figure 14-4). It is emphasized that this alpha frequency occurs during continuous sleep and is not the consequence of an electroencephalographic arousal. Among patients with fibromyalgia and chronic fatigue syndrome, the intrusion of waking alpha frequency into the sleep electroencephalogram is hypothesized to reflect a state of *aroused*, nonrestorative sleep.[57,58] Although resolution of alpha frequency intrusion in sleep has never been described among fibromyalgia or chronic fatigue syndrome patients, such resolution has been observed among adolescent UARS patients when sleep quality improves following rapid palatal expansion[48] (Figures 14-5 and 14-6).

UARS patients also demonstrate sleep stage instability. This instability may be recognized as frequent shifting from deeper to lighter sleep stages or to wakefulness, with decreasing depth of sleep designated as the stage sequence: REM, N3, N2, N1, and wake. The frequency of sleep stage shifting in UARS patients is decreased by treatment with nasal CPAP[54] (Figure 14-7) and rapid palatal expansion,[48] which overcome upper airway resistance. The mechanism by which nasal CPAP eliminates sleep stage shifts is not simply elimination of sleep fragmentation associated with RERAs. Although shifts between stages N2, N1, and wake require an intervening arousal, stage shifts between REM, N3, and N2 do not require an arousal. Indeed the N3-to-N2 sleep stage shifts in Figure 14-7 that decrease in frequency with nasal CPAP all occur during continuous sleep (the difference between N3 and N2 being determined by the prevalence of delta waves) and do not represent the elimination of RERAs by nasal CPAP. The occurrence of frequent shifts from deeper to lighter sleep is hypothesized to be an adaptive response to a danger or *stressor*, lightening the individual's sleep and allowing for a quicker response to an emergency.[59] Increased shifts from deeper to

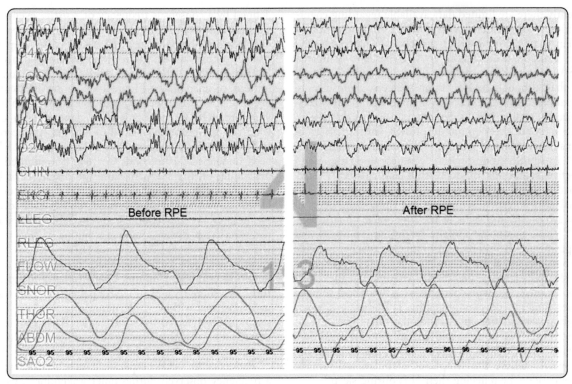

Figure 14-5 This figure demonstrates two 15-second periods of NREM stage 3 (N3) sleep recorded at the same time of night, before and after rapid palatal expansion (RPE; 13 months between studies) in a 16 year-old boy with severe chronic fatigue who was diagnosed with upper airway resistance syndrome. Recording includes four electroencephalographic channels (*purple*; C3A2, C4A1, O1A2, O2A1), left and right electrooculograms (*green*; LOC, ROC), electromyograms of the chin (CHIN) and left and right tibialis anterior muscle (LLEG, RLEG), and an electrocardiogram (EKG). Respiratory channels include pressure transducer airflow (FLOW), a snore microphone (SNOR), thoracic and abdominal wall movement (THOR, ABDO), and oxygen saturation (Sao2). Before RPE, the patient demonstrates alpha-delta sleep characterized by low-frequency, high-amplitude delta waves with superimposed prominent 7- to 11-Hz alpha waves observed best in electroencephalographic leads C3A2 and C4A1. After RPE, the alpha frequency is greatly decreased in amplitude or gone. Associated with this change, The EKG demonstrates a decrease in heart rate between studies from 72/minute before RPE to 64/minute after RPE, suggesting decreased sympathetic nervous system tone between studies.

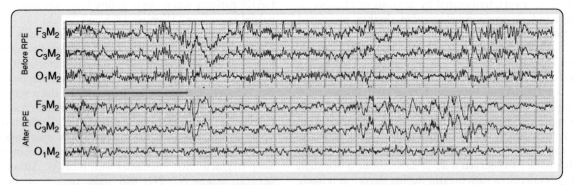

Figure 14-6 This figure demonstrates 30 seconds of stage N2 sleep recorded at the same time of night, before and after rapid palatal expansion (RPE), from an 18-year-old man with severe depression who was diagnosed with upper airway resistance syndrome. The two recordings each include three electroencephalographic channels (F_3M_2, C_3M_2, O_1M_2). As in Figure 14-5, the recording before RPE shows prominent alpha frequency (at approximately 7 Hz; seen well above the *orange line*). After RPE, the alpha frequency is greatly reduced in amplitude and the underlying theta frequency of 3 to 5 Hz is seen more clearly. (Reproduced with permission from Miller P, Iyer M, Gold AR. Treatment resistant adolescent depression with upper airway resistance syndrome treated with rapid palatal expansion: a case report. *J Med Case Rep* 2012;6[1]:415.)

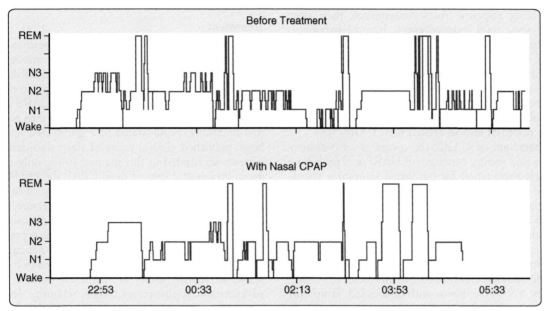

Figure 14-7 This figure demonstrates two hypnograms (plots of sleep stages against time of night with increasing depth of sleep staged as: wake, N1 [NREM stage 1], N2, N3, REM) from a 43-year-old veteran of the first Gulf War (1990–1991) who returned with complaints of moderate fatigue and severely impaired sleep quality (symptoms of Gulf War illness) and was found to have an apnea hypopnea index of 5/hour.[21] The upper hypnogram is derived from his polysomnogram before treatment, and the lower hypnogram was obtained from a polysomnogram performed (while sleeping with nasal CPAP at 9 cm H_2O) after the veteran slept with nasal CPAP nightly for 3 weeks and experienced improvement of his fatigue and sleep quality. The initial hypnogram demonstrates frequent shifts from deeper to lighter sleep stages throughout the night. The hypnogram obtained following symptomatic improvement demonstrates fewer sleep stage shifts. Frequent shifts from deeper to lighter sleep are thought to be an adaptive response to stress that enables the individual to respond more quickly to an emergency. (Reproduced with permission from Amin MM, Gold MS, Broderick JE, Gold AR. The effect of nasal continuous positive airway pressure on the symptoms of Gulf War illness. *Sleep Breath* 2011;15[3]:579–87.)

lighter sleep commonly occur in healthy people sleeping for the first night in a new location, such as a sleep laboratory.[60]

A second manifestation of sleep stage instability among UARS patients is the occurrence of CAP, which is defined by a periodic disruption of NREM sleep by electroencephalographic events that do not meet the threshold for an arousal by conventional sleep staging criteria.[61] Indeed, these electroencephalographic events constitute the changes in background rhythm associated with the return of airflow to a non-flow-limited state, referred to earlier concerning RERAs. Among UARS patients, increasing levels of these nonarousal electroencephalographic events correlate with increasing levels of sleepiness and fatigue.[61] Furthermore, the presence of CAP is a marker for increased sympathetic nervous system tone[62] commonly found under conditions of stress (see later). Therefore, CAP is one of the manifestations of unstable, nonrestorative sleep that leads to daytime sleepiness and fatigue among UARS patients.

Pathophysiology and Clinical Correlates

Hypotheses concerning the pathophysiology of UARS continue to evolve as the manifestations of the disorder and the body systems affected increase in number. The first case report of UARS patients published by Guilleminault and associates presented the disorder as one of sleep fragmentation by RERAs associated with hypersomnolence that improved with nasal CPAP treatment.[5,13] The new insight was that apneas and hypopneas associated with pronounced arousals from sleep, characteristics of OSA, were not necessary to produce hypersomnolence. Rather, the investigators hypothesized that

mildly increased upper airway resistance, with its associated increase in inspiratory effort, could, episodically, produce brief periods of alpha frequency intrusion into sleep (alpha arousals), also producing hypersomnolence. Although this paradigm of UARS (henceforth termed the *RERA paradigm*) provided an explanation for the hypersomnolence associated with UARS, it did not provide an explanation for the somatic, cognitive, and affective complaints, such as insomnia, fatigue, body pain, depression, anxiety, cognitive dysfunction, and gastrointestinal dysfunction, or for the parasomnias, such as bruxism, sleepwalking, and catathrenia, that have subsequently been associated with UARS.[40,42,43,47-49,51,63,64]

As clinical experience with UARS patients increased, investigators came to postulate that the hypersomnolence of UARS patients is not simply the consequence of sleep fragmentation but also of altered sleep quality that affects its restorative properties. The alpha frequency intrusion into sleep[40,55] and the unstable sleep stages characterized by increased shifts from deeper to lighter sleep[48,54] and CAP,[61] as described earlier, were seen as alternative responses to pharyngeal collapse during sleep that maintain a more patent pharyngeal airway while maintaining sleep continuity. In contrast, OSA patients, whose only response to pharyngeal collapse during sleep is episodic arousals terminating apneas and hypopneas, experience more sleep fragmentation.[35] Bao and Guilleminault[65] have further hypothesized that UARS evolves into OSA over time because of upper airway trauma related to snoring. According to this hypothesis, because of the effect of snoring on the upper airway, UARS patients eventually lose their increased sensitivity to pharyngeal collapse and their sleep-maintaining response. As a consequence, their sleep deepens and their mild resistive events become hypopneas and apneas terminated by arousal. This proposed *sleep quality* paradigm of UARS provides an explanation for the alpha frequency intrusion into sleep and sleep stage instability characterizing UARS patients; however, it remains focused on nonrestorative sleep leading to hypersomnolence without providing an explanation for the spectrum of somatic, cognitive, and affective disorders also associated with UARS.

A third paradigm of UARS, the *chronic stress* paradigm, builds on the *sleep quality* paradigm of UARS and provides a more complete explanation for the varied symptoms associated with the syndrome.[66] The paradigm postulates that some individuals can become sensitized to upper airway resistance as a stimulus that activates the stress response (activation of the hypothalamic-pituitary-adrenal axis and sympathetic nervous system by the brain's limbic system) as if it were an existential threat. Because upper airway resistance during sleep occurs for at least several hours daily, in these individuals, it constitutes a chronic stress with associated symptoms including sleep onset and sleep maintenance insomnia, headaches, gastrointestinal and bladder irritability, body pain, anxiety, and depression. In addition to these symptoms, so prevalent among UARS patients, chronic stress is associated with hypertension, type 2 diabetes mellitus, gonadotrophic hormone deficiency leading to sexual dysfunction (erectile dysfunction in men and polycystic ovarian syndrome in women), and growth hormone deficiency leading to diminished growth in children. These are all prominent medical conditions associated with OSA. According to such a chronic stress paradigm, the sleep fragmentation by arousals and altered sleep quality caused by alpha frequency intrusion and sleep stage instability observed among UARS patients is not a direct effect of upper airway resistance on sleep continuity, but an adaptive response of the brain to the existence of a disturbance or threat. Having sleep continuously interrupted, or having a state of vigilance maintained during sleep through alpha frequency intrusion and sleep stage instability theoretically enables the individual to respond more quickly to a danger, an apparent survival advantage.[59] This advantage, however, is accompanied by the disadvantages of parasomnias and daytime sleepiness resulting from the chronically altered sleep. The chronic stress paradigm of UARS explains not only the hypersomnolence associated with UARS but also the somatic complaints, affective disorders, cognitive dysfunction, and parasomnias observed among UARS patients. A more complete discussion of this paradigm can be found in the review by Gold.[66]

In summary, the pathophysiologic and associated clinical paradigm of UARS has evolved from sleep fragmentation by RERAs through altered sleep quality as a direct response to upper airway resistance, leading to milder resistive events than occur among OSA patients, to recent consideration of upper airway resistance, provoking chronic stress with sleep-related, somatic, cognitive, and affective consequences. The pathophysiologic paradigms of UARS will continue to evolve as new data accumulate. However, the recognition that altered sleep *quality* contributes to the hypersomnolence and fatigue of UARS patients supports the idea that UARS also exists below the RDI threshold for a diagnosis of OSA—an important possibility when one contemplates making the diagnosis of idiopathic hypersomnolence.

Treatment

The treatment of UARS uses the same treatments that have been discussed earlier for snoring. Chief among these treatments is nasal CPAP, which is highly effective and can be precisely titrated by the prescribing physician to eliminate IFL during sleep. To titrate nasal CPAP for UARS patients, one must titrate to convert IFL during sleep into non-flow-limited breathing, as illustrated in Figures 14-2 and 14-3. In a large, published clinical series of sleep-disordered breathing patients all titrated in this manner (using only nasal masks), mean therapeutic level of nasal CPAP for 22 UARS patients was found to be 7 cm H_2O with a range of 4 to 9 cm H_2O.[3] Although autotitrating positive airway pressure has not been studied specifically in UARS, the algorithms used attempt to eliminate IFL during sleep and should be acceptable for treatment of UARS as they are for OSA. For patients unable (or unwilling) to breathe with the mouth closed or to wear a nasal mask, alternative forms of treatment such as mandibular advancement appliances or tongue-retaining devices, weight loss, and surgical procedures may be considered as previously described. A growing body of literature suggests that applying positive airway pressure through an oronasal mask is not a reliable method for eliminating IFL during sleep[67,68] and anesthesia.[69] Among pediatric patients, rapid palatal expansion performed by an orthodontist has been used effectively to treat UARS (e.g., the patients in Figures 14-5 and 14-6[48]) and mild OSA.

CLINICAL PEARLS

- Silent inspiratory airflow limitation (IFL) during sleep is characterized by either an inspiratory airflow plateau or an increase in the ratio of inspiratory time to the respiratory cycle time with a prolongation of the time near maximal inspiratory airflow.
- In a patient consulting the clinician for habitual snoring that disturbs his or her bed partner, with normal alertness, no somatic or metabolic disorders, and no known cardiovascular disease, a polysomnogram will likely reveal either isolated snoring or asymptomatic OSA. Consider evaluating the results of a carotid ultrasound, looking for evidence of atherosclerosis, before foregoing specific OSA treatment in this setting.
- For patients with functional somatic syndromes complaining of insomnia, fatigue, headache, body pain, gastrointestinal or bladder irritability, anxiety and depression, with or without audible snoring, consider performing polysomnography to diagnose UARS (OSA by ICSD3 criteria) because prevention of IFL during sleep may be an effective treatment not only for fatigue and insomnia but also for somatic symptoms.

SUMMARY

Our understanding of pathologic pharyngeal collapse during sleep has progressed from recognizing obstructive apneas and hypopneas associated with arousal from sleep and oxygen desaturation (clinically, obstructive sleep apnea) to recognizing the mildest IFL without audible snoring, arousal, or oxygen desaturation. At the same time, our understanding of the consequences of pathologic pharyngeal collapse during sleep has expanded from hypersomnolence and cardiovascular and metabolic disorders to include associations with somatic syndromes, affective disorders, and carotid artery atherosclerosis independent of metabolic syndrome. Underlying this evolution is a new paradigm of *sleep related breathing disorders* (often referred to as "sleep-disordered breathing") in which pharyngeal collapse during sleep acts not only directly, causing oxygen desaturation and arousal from sleep, but also indirectly, with even the mildest IFL during sleep serving as a chronic activator of the body's stress response. In this context, one can appreciate the evolving understanding of what constitutes clinically significant sleep related breathing disorders associated with sleep-related upper airway pathophysiology.

Selected Readings

Broderick JE, Gold MS, Amin MM, et al. The association of somatic arousal with the symptoms of upper airway resistance syndrome. *Sleep Med* 2014;**15**:436–43.

de Godoy LB, Palombini LO, Guilleminault C, et al. Treatment of upper airway resistance syndrome in adults: where do we stand? *Sleep Sci* 2015;**8**(1):42–8.

Dubrovsky B, Raphael KG, Lavigne GJ, et al. Polysomnographic investigation of sleep and respiratory parameters in women with temporomandibular pain disorders. *J Clin Sleep Med* 2014;**10**:195–201.

Gold AR, Dipalo F, Gold MS, et al. Inspiratory airflow dynamics during sleep in female fibromyalgia patients. *Sleep* 2004;**27**:459–66.

Gold AR, Schwartz AR. The pharyngeal critical pressure: the whys and hows of using nasal continuous positive airway pressure diagnostically. *Chest* 1996;**110**:1077–88.

Guilleminault C, Kirisoglu C, Poyares D, et al. Upper airway resistance syndrome: a long-term outcome study. *J Psychiatr Res* 2006;**40**:273–9.

Guilleminault C, Stoohs R, Clerk A, et al. A cause of excessive daytime sleepiness: the upper airway resistance syndrome. *Chest* 1993;**104**:781–7.

Hosselet JJ, Norman RG, Ayappa I, et al. Detection of flow limitation with a nasal cannula/pressure transducer system. *Am J Respir Crit Care Med* 1998;**157**:1461–7.

Lee SA, Amis TC, Byth K, et al. Heavy snoring as a cause of carotid artery atherosclerosis. *Sleep* 2008;**31**:1207–13.

Marshall NS, Wong KK, Cullen SR, et al. Snoring is not associated with all-cause mortality, incident cardiovascular disease, or stroke in the Busselton Health Study. *Sleep* 2012;**35**:1235–40.

Schneider H, Krishnan V, Pichard LE, et al. Inspiratory duty cycle responses to flow limitation predict nocturnal hypoventilation. *Eur Respir J* 2009;**33**:1068–76.

So SJ, Lee HJ, Kang SG, et al. A comparison of personality characteristics and psychiatric symptomatology between upper airway resistance syndrome and obstructive sleep apnea syndrome. *Psychiatry Investig* 2015;**12**(2):183–9.

Stoohs RA, Knaack L, Blum HC, et al. Differences in clinical features of upper airway resistance syndrome, primary snoring, and obstructive sleep apnea/hypopnea syndrome. *Sleep Med* 2008;**9**:121–8.

A complete reference list can be found online at ExpertConsult.com.

Chapter

15

Central Sleep Apnea: Diagnosis and Management

Andrey V. Zinchuk; Robert Joseph Thomas

Chapter Highlights

- Pathologically enhanced respiratory chemoreflexes result in a spectrum of polysomnographic breathing patterns and disorders, including central sleep apnea (CSA), periodic breathing/Cheyne-Stokes breathing, high-altitude sleep apnea, and treatment emergent CSA.

- A pathologically decreased chemoreflex can result in hypercapnic CSA.

- Opiate use causes a disintegrative CSA disorder with relatively unique polysomnographic features.

- Conventional polysomnography has limitations in accurate phenotyping the sleep apneas; thus the true prevalence of various forms of central apnea syndromes is uncertain.

- Evidence suggests that about one third of those with obstructive sleep apnea have respiratory control as a key mediator of disease. Predominance of events in non–rapid eye movement sleep and persistent or enhanced

  respiratory instability during treatment with continuous positive airway pressure are key features that are readily recognized in clinical settings.

- Adaptive ventilation is a major advance in noninvasive ventilatory therapy of CSA syndromes. However, benefits in outcomes in heart failure patients are not proven, and there is potential for harm. Several other off-label approaches can be considered as primary or adjunctive therapy.

- Volume-assured positive pressure ventilation can improve oxygenation and ventilation in hypercapnic CSA and hypoventilation syndromes but may cause sleep fragmentation if pressure fluctuations are excessive.

- Residual disease during treatment is common in CSA syndromes. The long-term persistence of the residual central apnea depends on etiology and associated disorders.

The term *central sleep apnea* (CSA) describes both the pattern of an individual respiratory event and the clinical syndrome characterized by repeated episodes of apneas during sleep caused by an impaired respiratory drive system.[1,2] This is in contrast to obstructive apneas, in which respiratory drive remains active during the apnea, associated with upper airway occlusion (Figure 15-1).

Although central apneas are less frequent than obstructive, they present in ways and settings that are diverse. CSA breathing patterns can vary from the rhythmic sequences of apnea and recovery breaths in congestive heart failure (CHF) to the ataxic respiratory patterns in patients with opioid use.[3,4] Most humans exhibit central apneas during transitions into sleep, and they appear in travelers to high altitude. CSA patterns are associated with a range of medical conditions, from end-stage renal disease to multiple system atrophy and from opioid dependence to the central congenital hypoventilation syndrome.[5-9] CSA is important to recognize because of complications ranging from frequent nighttime awakenings and excessive sleepiness to adverse cardiovascular outcomes and mortality.[10-12]

Central respiratory events in sleep rarely occur in isolation, and many patients with sleep apnea appear to live on a phenotypic spectrum between the obstructive and central apneas. In heart failure and opioid-induced sleep apnea, central and obstructive apneas often coexist.[8,13] In treatment emergent CSA, alleviation of obstructive apneas with positive airway pressure (PAP) amplifies or unmasks a sensitive chemoreflex with resultant centrally mediated apneas and periodic breathing.[14] Identifying where the patient is on the obstructive-to-central spectrum and focusing on the factors responsible for this physiology are critical for accurate diagnosis of CSA and its management.

DEFINITIONS

Current definitions for central apnea and hypopnea are based on polygraphic data and are reviewed in Chapter 12 as well as the American Academy of Sleep Medicine (AASM) scoring manual.[15] A CSA syndrome is defined when five or more central apneas *and/or* central hypopneas are present per hour; that is, a central apnea-hypopnea index (CAHI) of greater than 5, with CAHI comprising more than 50% of all respiratory events.[16] For the various CSA syndromes, additional criteria related to signs and symptoms and specific etiologic entity are required.[16]

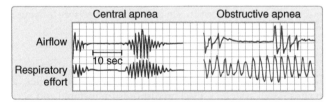

Figure 15-1 Central and obstructive sleep apnea. The relationship between airflow and respiratory effort in central and obstructive apnea. During central apnea, cessation of airflow occurs without associated ventilatory effort. Respiratory effort is present during an obstructive apnea. (From Wellman A, White DP. Central sleep apnea and periodic breathing. In: Kryger M, Dement W, editors. *Principles and Practice of Sleep Medicine*, fifth edition. Saunders: Philadelphia; 2011. p. 1140-1152.)

These diagnostic criteria can pose a challenge to investigators and clinicians alike because reliably differentiating hypopneas as central versus obstructive is difficult. Evidence of upper airway obstruction on polysomnography, including flow-limitation, does not rule out central apneas/hypopneas,[16a,16b] and esophageal manometry is rarely used in practice. Unclassified hypopneas are thus summed into the overall apnea hypopnea index (AHI), not the specific CAHI, biasing towards obstructive SDB.[16c,16d,16e] Accurately classifying SDB disorder as predominantly central or obstructive has implications for treatment.

Integrated analysis of polysomnography (PSG) features can improve identification of central hypopneas.[17] Predominance during non–rapid eye movement (NREM) rather than rapid eye movement (REM) sleep, lack of inspiratory airflow curve flattening or thoracoabdominal paradoxical breathing (chest wall moving inward with inspiration) during hypopnea, and arousal after[18] and gradual flow restoration pattern at hypopnea termination can help classify hypopneas as central.[17] Automation of hypopnea phenotyping (obstructive vs. central)[19] is possible, but accuracy in comparison to electromyography is limited (69%).

CLASSIFICATION OF CENTRAL SLEEP APNEA SYNDROMES

The *International Classification of Sleep Disorders*, third edition (ICSD3) group provides one framework for classifying CSA "syndromes"[16] (see Chapters 9 and 12). The approach in this chapter (Table 15-1) aims to demarcate physiologic and pathologic states in which CSA occurs and link mechanisms of CSA with therapies for each group. For example, it incorporates respiratory chemoreflex phenotyping based on PSG morphology or computational signal analysis. Thus "high chemosensitivity" suggests itself as a clinical category, the patterns of which could include central apneas, periodic breathing, or PAP-induced respiratory instability, signifying the need to consider chemoreflex stabilization in treatment. Our approach thus differs in some cases from the ICSD3 classification and should be considered complementary. For instance, sleep-related hypoventilation syndromes (e.g., obesity-hypoventilation syndrome [OHS]), a separate category in ICSD3, are included under the umbrella of CSA in this chapter under the hypercapnic category. Our aim is to emphasize the role impaired respiratory drive plays in the pathophysiology of these conditions and how treatment can be selected to address this impairment (e.g., bilevel ventilation with backup rate).

PATHOPHYSIOLOGY OF CENTRAL SLEEP APNEA SYNDROMES THAT AFFECT DIAGNOSIS AND TREATMENT

Pathophysiology of CSA is discussed in detail in Chapter 12, including the chemical, mechanical, and neural aspects of respiratory control; the feedback loop between the sensors and the respiratory center; the loop gain (measure of respiratory system stability) and its components (controller, plant, mixing); and other important features. Figure 15-2 summarizes the interplay between ventilatory drive (controller) and the lung's ability to excrete CO_2 (plant) in relation to normal (eupnea) and cessation (apnea) of breathing. In this section we highlight the physiologic concepts important for our approach to

Table 15-1	Pathophysiologic Classification of Central Sleep Apneas
Physiologic	**Pathologic**

• Sleep transition
• Phasic REM
	Nonhypercapnic
	  • Medical condition related
	    • Congestive heart failure
	    • Poststroke
	    • ESRD
	    • PAH
	    • Atrial fibrillation
	  • High altitude
	  • Idiopathic
	Hypercapnic
	  • Congenital central hypoventilation syndrome
	  • Primary chronic alveolar hypoventilation syndromes
	  • Other CNS disorders associated with CSA
	    • Encephalitis, tumors, strokes
	    • Anatomic abnormalities
	    • Neurodegenerative disorders
	  • Muscular and PNS disorders associated with CSA (selected examples)
	    • Muscular dystrophies
	    • Acid maltase deficiency
	    • Charcot-Marie-Tooth disease and other neuropathies
	    • Postpolio syndrome
	    • Myasthenia gravis
	Disintegrative (e.g., brainstem injury, opioid-induced)
	CSA with OSA or upper airway disorders (including treatment emergent CSA)

CNS, Central nervous system; CSA, central sleep apnea; ESRD, end-stage renal disease; OSA, obstructive sleep apnea; PAH, pulmonary arterial hypertension; PNS, peripheral nervous system; REM, rapid eye movements.

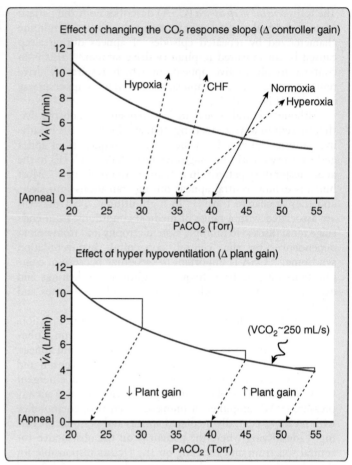

Figure 15-2 Changing plant gain (*bottom*) and controller gain (*top*) influences on CO_2 reserve. Diagrammatic representation of the steady-state relationship between alveolar ventilation and alveolar $PACO_2$ ($PaCO_2$) at a fixed resting CO_2 production (of 250 mL/min). The schematic figure shows how changing plant gain or controller gain will influence the "CO_2 reserve" or Δ $PaCO_2$ between eupnea and apnea. *Top,* Changing the background drive to breathe without changing the slope of the ΔV_A versus Δ $PaCO_2$ relationship (controller gain) above or below eupnea. For example, background hyperventilation (via metabolic acidosis or specific carotid body stimulation with almitrine) raises V_A and lowers $PaCO_2$ along the isometabolic hyperbola (decreased plant gain). This means that a greater transient increase in V_A and reduction in $PaCO_2$ is required to reach the apneic threshold than it would be under control, normocapnic conditions. The reverse is true for conditions that reduce the background drive to breathe and cause hypoventilation (e.g., metabolic alkalosis). *Bottom,* At any given level of background $PaCO_2$, changing the slope (or responsiveness) of the relationship below eupnea would alter the CO_2 reserve or the amount of reduction in $PaCO_2$ required to cause apnea. Changing the slope of the ventilatory response to CO_2 above eupnea would alter the susceptibility for transient ventilatory overshoots. Often both plant and controller gains may change together; note the reduced plant gains and increased controller gain, with hypoxia or with congestive heart failure patients. The increased controller gain dominates, and the net effect is a decreased CO_2 reserve and instability. (Modified with permission from Javaheri S, Dempsey JA. Central sleep apnea. *Compr Physiol* 2013;3[1]:141–63.)

diagnosis and treatment and discuss them in the context of specific CSA syndromes.

Pathophysiologic Changes that Lead to Central Sleep Apneas and Periodic Breathing

Interactions of three factors predispose an individual to ventilatory instability and central apneas-hypopneas during sleep[2,20]: low CO_2 reserve (CO_2 reserve = $PaCO_2$ eupneic – $PaCO_2$ apneic), abnormally high *or* low loop gain (a product of controller, plant, and mixing gains), and sleep state and stage instability.

CO_2 reserve is affected by changes in plant and controller gains. For example, CO_2 reserve is decreased in metabolic alkalosis (increased plant gain; see Figure 15-2), promoting the risk for central apneas and ventilatory instability, whereas it is increased with metabolic acidosis (decreased plant gain)[21], which is protective against central apneas (see Figure 15-2). Administration of oxygen (which reduces hypoxic stimulus to breathing) has been shown to decrease ventilation and responsiveness to $PaCO_2$ during sleep[22]. This stabilizes breathing through reduction in controller gain and increase in $PaCO_2$ reserve, whereas hypoxia leads to opposite effects (see Figure 15-2). In addition, inherent delays in the negative feedback loop controlling ventilation (mixing gain) increase loop gain.

This delayed recognition of blood gases by the controller (as in those with systolic CHF) predisposes to unstable and periodic breathing.

Transitions into and out of sleep, and between sleep stages, are inherently unstable in terms of respiratory control[5]. Brief central apneas and hypopneas occur during this time in normal individuals because of "unmasking" of the sleep apneic threshold that is very close to the wake eupneic threshold. In addition, upper airway and diaphragmatic muscle tone is reduced, with the associated increase in upper airway resistance and decreased inspiratory force, resulting in hypoventilation.[23,24] Then, as $Paco_2$ rises above the apneic threshold, rhythmic breathing is maintained.

During sleep, brief and abrupt transitions to wakefulness, termed *arousals*, can result in ventilatory instability, with level of ventilatory response and arousal threshold playing important roles. With a sudden arousal, the sleep eupneic $Paco_2$ (normally about 5 mm Hg higher than awake $Paco_2$) is detected as hypercapnic by the aroused respiratory control center. This signal to increase ventilatory drive, combined with the removal of the upper airway resistance induced by sleep, results in increased ventilatory response and reduction in $Paco_2$.[25,26] When sleep resumes, the current $Paco_2$ is considered to be hypocapnic for the sleeping brain, that is, below the apneic threshold, resulting in central apnea. Thus any process that leads to frequent sleep-wake transitions, such as sleep maintenance insomnia, sleep apnea, maladaptation to continuous positive airway pressure (CPAP), or periodic limb movement disorder, can increase the propensity to ventilatory overshoots, periodic breathing, and CSAs, especially in a setting of high chemosensitivity.[25,27-29]

Pathophysiologic Changes in Specific Central Sleep Apnea Syndromes

Nonhypercapnic Central Sleep Apnea

Disorders manifesting as nonhypercapnic (eupneic or hypocapnic) CSA have two physiologic phenomena in common: (1) normal or slightly low awake steady-state $Paco_2$, and (2) increased ventilatory responsiveness to $Paco_2$ or hypoxemia (increased loop gain). In the setting of arousals, CSAs are perpetuated owing to the so-called "inertial" effect (see Chapter 12).

Central Sleep Apnea and Periodic Breathing of Heart Failure. Heart failure is associated with Cheyne-Stokes breathing (CSB), which is seen at times during wakefulness and frequently during sleep. CSB is characterized by a crescendo-decrescendo pattern of tidal volumes with central apnea or hypopnea occurring at the nadir of the cycle (typically 60 to 90 seconds; Figure 15-3). It is in part a consequence of increased loop gain due to a heightened chemoreflex (sensitive controller)[30,31] and lack of the "normal" increase in $Paco_2$ with sleep onset (decreased CO_2 reserve).[32] These are superimposed on prolonged circulation time (increased mixing gain) resulting in cyclical ventilatory instability.[33]

Periodic breathing of shorter cycles occurs in other settings and conditions with "hyperactive" chemoreflex (as described later). Although ICSD3 defines CSB with specific cycle lengths and intervening apneas, we feel CSB represents one end of the chemoreflex activation severity spectrum, whereas at the other end of the clinical spectrum, although poorly recognized in practice, is nonapneic short cycle (≤30 seconds) periodic breathing.

Central Sleep Apnea Due to High-Altitude Periodic Breathing. In contrast to CSB in heart failure, the cycle time of periodic breathing at high altitude is short (probably owing to elimination of the mixing gain defect). The mechanism involves exposure to hypoxemia with resultant chemoreceptor-mediated hyperventilation during NREM and REM sleep. After approximately 10 minutes of hypoxia in a sleeping human, tidal volumes oscillate in a waxing and waning pattern. The oscillations increase in magnitude as hypoxia is maintained and $Paco_2$ falls further to the level of apneic threshold.[34] When that is reached, overt periodic breathing occurs with cycle times of 15 to 25 seconds (two to five large tidal volume breath clusters followed by apneas of 5 to 15 seconds).[2,35-37] There is wide variation in O_2 during this time. The predominant mechanism is increased loop gain manifested as a reduced $Paco_2$ reserve (1 to 2 mmHg) and increased chemosensitivity (see Figure 15-2).[21,38] The marked increase in arousals and decrease in slow wave sleep potentiate respiratory instability. Attesting to the key role for hypocapnia in this disorder of central apnea and periodic breathing, the breathing disorder can be improved with administration of small amounts of CO_2 (increase in $Paco_2$ reserve),[39] increasing dead space (increase in $Paco_2$ reserve),[40] and acetazolamide (reduction in plant gain and increase in $Paco_2$ reserve).[21] Patients with obstructive sleep apnea (OSA) and high loop gain have PSG features mimicking high-altitude periodic breathing, including NREM dominance and short cycle periodic breathing.

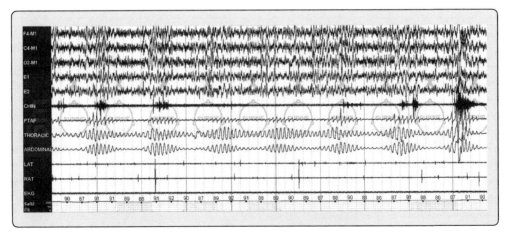

Figure 15-3 Relatively long cycle periodic breathing and Cheyne-Stokes respiration. Ten-minute screen compression, each vertical line is 30 seconds. A patient with congestive heart failure in NREM sleep. Note the symmetrical, concordant, waxing and waning flow and effort. Cycle lengths are about 45 to 50 seconds.

Primary Central Sleep Apnea. Primary (idiopathic) CSA is a rare disorder characterized by repetitive episodes of central apneas in NREM sleep, which are short and irregular (rather than periodic) and terminate with an abrupt, large breath (Figure 15-4), in contrast to what is characteristically seen in CHF. The most clearly demonstrated pathophysiology is an increased hypercapnic ventilatory response during wakefulness.[29,41] In addition, impairment of switching between expiration and inspiration has also been found in these patients.[42] It has been speculated that the long expiratory pause that typically occurs with these CSA events may be attributable to this impairment.

Other Nonhypercapnic Central Sleep Apnea Syndromes and Their Associated Medical Conditions. Common chronic medical conditions such as end-stage renal disease (ESRD), cerebrovascular accident (CVA), and pulmonary hypertension have been associated with nonhypercapnic CSA. In patients with ESRD, the central apnea index (i.e., frequency of central apneas) inversely correlates with $Paco_2$ and cardiac silhouette enlargement,[6] and ultrafiltration increases $Paco_2$ with associated decline in the CAHI by 55%.[43] These findings suggest that a similar link may be present between volume overload and the CSA-CSB of CHF.

CSB occurs in a minority of patients (~7%) after CVA.[44] Although in many cases post CVA the CSB is associated with left ventricular dysfunction and hypocapnia,[45] some authors note an increased prevalence of CSB in patients with lacunar strokes (~20%) and without left ventricular dysfunction.[46] CSB has been reported in patients with idiopathic pulmonary arterial hypertension (PAH). The postulated mechanisms include decreased stroke volume and increased mixing gain,[2] although, as in case of CVA, no PAH-specific studies have been done.

Hypercapnic Central Sleep Apnea

Hypoventilation due to a failed or failing automatic control (and effector) system is the pathophysiologic hallmark of disorders that manifest with hypercapnic CSA. They can be broadly approached as disorders of impaired central drive ("won't breathe") or impaired respiratory muscle control ("can't breathe"). In general, the former category is due to processes involving the brainstem respiratory centers (e.g.,

congenital central alveolar hypoventilation syndrome), whereas the latter is due to neuromuscular weakness disorders (e.g., amyotrophic lateral sclerosis). Most of the above disorders are associated with pathologically *low* loop gain (either because of controller or plant components) and worsening of hypoventilation and apneas during REM sleep (in contrast to hypocapnic CSA, which is NREM dominant). The latter occurs primarily because of intercostal muscle atonia during REM. Most of these conditions are classified under the sleep-related hypoventilation disorders in the ICSD3 (see Chapter 9).

Congenital Central Alveolar Hypoventilation Syndrome and Idiopathic Central Alveolar Hypoventilation. Congenital alveolar central hypoventilation syndrome (CCHS, or "Ondine's curse") is a rare disorder of respiratory control and autonomic systems, first reported by Mellins in the 1970s.[47] Small tidal volumes and monotonous respiratory rates result in hypoventilation while the wakefulness and behavioral stimuli supply the respiratory drive. With sleep onset, worsened hypoventilation, hypercapnia, and hypoxemia ensue due to the impaired automatic control system. In many cases, if not identified early, this leads to asphyxia and death.[48] Mutations of the *PHOX2B* gene are disease defining.[49] This gene encodes a transcription factor responsible for the fate of early autonomic nervous system cells, including those in the respiratory control centers.[48]

Obesity-Hypoventilation Syndrome ("Pickwickian Syndrome"). "Joe was a wonderfully fat boy, standing upright with his eyes closed." This is the first depiction of OHS, found in Charles Dickens' book, *The Posthumous Papers of the Pickwick Club*. Today's medical literature requires that obesity and awake hypoventilation ($Paco_2$ >45 mm Hg) be present (without other causes for the latter) for the diagnosis of OHS.[50] Abnormalities include progressive hypoventilation and hypoxemia during NREM sleep with further impairment in REM sleep,[51] and OSA (nearly universal in OHS[52]). Pathogenetic mechanisms are complex and insufficiently investigated, even in face of the obesity epidemic. They include ventilatory abnormalities of OSA, increased work of breathing,[53] and blunted chemosensitivity (decreased loop gain).[54-56] There is a suggestion that resistance to leptin, a hormone produced by adipocytes that normally augments ventilatory

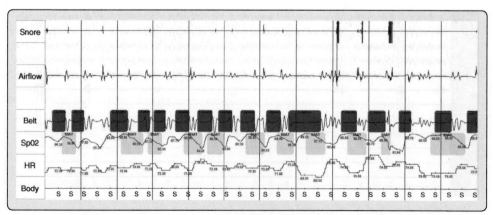

Figure 15-4 Idiopathic sleep apnea. A home sleep study on a medication-free 27-year-old nonobese man presenting with mild daytime sleepiness (Epworth Sleepiness Scale score of 9/24), nocturnal awakenings, and unrefreshing sleep. Note the short cycles (about 20 seconds) of pure central respiratory events.

response to $Paco_2$, is a possible mechanism for reduced controller gain in OHS.[57-59]

Other Central Nervous System–Related Disorders. Central neurologic processes that cause impairment of the brainstem respiratory centers, such as compression, edema, ischemia, infarct, tumor, encephalitis, and Arnold-Chiari malformations, have been associated with breathing dysrhythmias and CSA.[60-69] The specific manifestations depend on the location and the type of the insult. For instance, automatic failure of breathing control ensues following cervical cordotomy.[70] Damage to areas other than the brainstem (thalamus, basal ganglia, centrum semiovale) can lead to CSA, suggesting the importance of the descending signals for generation of the automatic breathing stimulus.[46]

Peripheral Nerve and Muscle Disorders. Neuromuscular diseases, such as muscular dystrophy, myasthenia gravis, Guillain-Barré syndrome, amyotrophic lateral sclerosis, postpolio syndrome, and Charcot-Marie-Tooth disease, can lead to awake alveolar hypoventilation, with worsening hypoventilation during sleep. This is occasionally associated with central apneas, although sleep-related hypoventilation without outright central apnea is the more prominent feature. Ventilation during sleep in patients with respiratory muscle disease often deteriorates well before awake ventilation is affected.

Disintegrative Central Sleep Apnea and Hypoventilation Associated with Opiates. Although the respiratory depressant effects of opioids are well known,[71,72] the effects of opiates on sleep are widespread and complex and affect many patients.[73] With chronic use, hypoventilation and obstructive and central apneas can occur in a single patient, fulfilling diagnostic criteria for several disorders under the ICSD3 classification. In patients with daytime hypercapnia, nocturnal hypoventilation can be profound. Two unique patterns of breathing tend to occur in patients taking chronic opioids: (1) cluster breathing characterized by cycles of deep breaths with relatively stable tidal volumes with interspersed central apneas of variable duration and (2) Biot breathing (ataxic breathing) with variable tidal volumes and rates.[2] In addition, patients taking chronic opioids with nearly pure OSA on initial PSG

evaluation can develop treatment emergent central apnea.[74] In chronic opioid use, there is also a high prevalence of obstructive events.

Of the various opioid receptors, stimulation of μ and κ receptors tends to drive respiratory depression[8] primarily in the pre-Bötzinger complex.[75,76] At low doses, tidal volumes decline,[77] whereas at higher doses, respiratory rate and rhythm generation are suppressed.[8] Morphine given to normal human subjects acutely decreases hypercapnic and hypoxic controller gain[78]; however, chronic administration results in decreased hypercapnic but increased hypoxemic chemosensitivity.[79] Mechanisms of ataxic breathing (Figure 15-5), common among those taking chronic opioids (nearly 70%) and those taking higher doses (>200 mg of morphine,[4]), have not been elucidated. Similar features could occur with injury to the carotid bodies, such as following head and neck chemoradiation (Figure 15-6).

Disordered Interplay Among Upper Airway Obstruction, Breathing Control, and Sleep-Arousal Propensity: Treatment Emergent Central Sleep Apnea ("Complex Sleep Apnea"). The $Paco_2$ reserve is labile during NREM sleep,[80] and arousals due to maladaptation to PAP can occur and drive instability.[14] Upper airway collapsibility as measured by Pcrit (pressure at which passive critical closing of the upper airway occurs) shows overlap between patients with OSA and controls.[81] Variations in Pcrit alone account for only a portion of variations in the apnea-hypopnea index (AHI)[82] or differences between those with pure OSA (100% of apneas obstructive) and predominant OSA (coexisting with CSA and mixed apneas).[83]

In some patients with OSA, central apneas and periodic breathing "emerge" during initiation of CPAP. This phenomenon is termed *treatment emergent CSA* in ICSD3[15] and is defined when there are five or more central apneas or hypopneas per hour of sleep, making up greater than 50% of all respiratory events during titration of CPAP in those fulfilling OSA criteria during diagnostic PSG. The existence of treatment emergent CSA (previously known as *complex sleep apnea*) as a unique entity has been controversial in the sleep world.[84] The original description noted a set of relatively unique features on *diagnostic* PSG and an incomplete treatment response

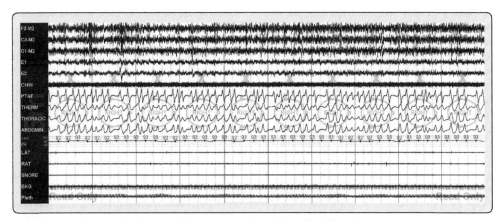

Figure 15-5 **Opiate-induced central sleep apnea and ataxic breathing.** Ten-minute screen compression; each vertical line is 30 seconds. In this methadone-treated 56-year-old woman, the most characteristic feature of opiate-related disease is the variability in expiratory duration, although tidal volumes also vary. These polysomnographic features are readily recognizable and occur in NREM sleep.

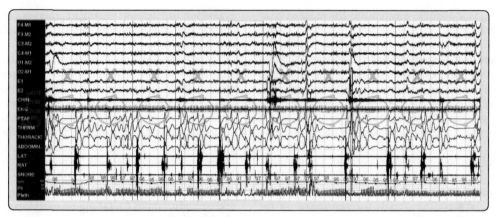

Figure 15-6 Central sleep apnea associated with head and neck chemoradiation. Ten-minute screen compression; each vertical line is 30 seconds. A 71-year-old man treated with radiation and platinum-based chemotherapy for laryngeal cancer. He presented with severe insomnia, multiple nocturnal arousals, and daytime fatigue. Note the variable-duration central apneas, mixed features, and sleep fragmentation.

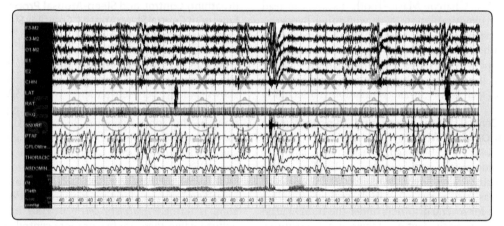

Figure 15-7 Key feature of NREM-dominant apnea. Ten-minute screen compression; each vertical line is 30 seconds. Periodic breathing with short cycles (30 seconds or less) and variable degrees of obstruction. Conventional scoring typically identifies these events as obstructive. Flow limitation is often seen, but the waxing-waning characteristic is usually evident.

that included induction of central apneas or persistent periodic breathing when CPAP was applied. The key feature is NREM-dominant central hypopneas or periodic breathing with obstruction (Figure 15-7), resolving spontaneously during REM sleep. That is, induction of central apneas was not required. However, the NREM dominance may be readily seen during positive pressure titration (Figure 15-8). A subsequent publication "defined" complex apnea, proposing the current ICSD criteria,[84] which also became the criteria used by medical insurance to qualify patients for the more expensive adaptive ventilators. The ICSD3 allows for the coexistence of periodic breathing and OSA (a "splitting" approach). The term *complex apnea* (a "lumping" approach) may have clinical utility in that a single term captures a number of ICSD categories with a common pathogenesis and identical responses to therapy. Central hypopneas are rarely scored in clinical practice, and thus reports of complex apnea or treatment-emergent sleep apnea, especially if using the ICSD3 treatment-emergent category and criteria, likely include only patients far on the spectrum of chemoreflex-driven instability than the middle ground, where a substantial minority of patients could fall. In these patients, short cycle (≤30 seconds)

periodic breathing, with features of admixed obstruction, is highly reminiscent of high-altitude periodic breathing and was part of the original description.[80] It is possible that long cycles (≥60 seconds) may be caused by subclinical (or even subechocardiographic) cardiac diastolic dysfunction, but data are lacking on cardiac function differences between patients demonstrating purely long- versus short-cycle events.

A consistent feature of patients with treatment emergent or complex sleep apnea, documented in most publications describing this phenomenon, is sleep fragmentation, which often persists despite reasonable respiration-targeted therapy. Because arousals amplify hypocapnic instability, inadequate cohesion of the NREM sleep–related network activity seems to be core pathology in some of these patients. This phenomenon is reminiscent of reports of CHF patients, in whom sleep fragmentation persists beyond that attributable to respiratory events.[85]

A pertinent question is whether the findings of the treatment emergent sleep apnea phenotype persist with continuous use of CPAP. Because central hypopneas or periodic breathing were not quantified in most studies, underestimation is probable and of uncertain degree. Lack of persistence may imply

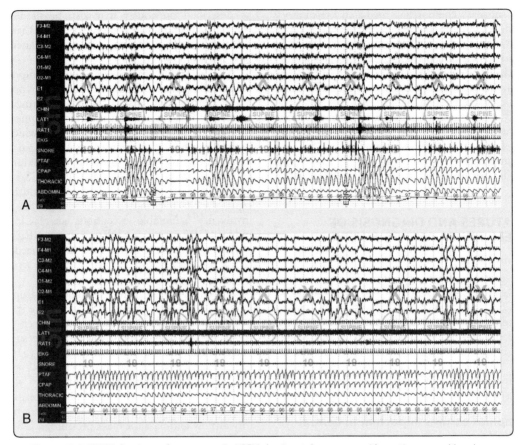

Figure 15-8 NREM-dominant sleep apnea. A, NREM-dominant sleep apnea, with continuous positive airway pressure (CPAP) during NREM sleep. Ten-minute screen compression; each vertical line is 30 seconds. Unresolved respiratory events occur across a range of CPAP pressures (5 to 19 cm) with long cycle events, some periodic breathing features, and clear obstructive features. **B,** NREM-dominant sleep apnea during REM sleep. Ten-minute screen compression; each vertical line is 30 seconds. The same subject as in **A** with spontaneous transition to REM sleep showing resolution of all abnormality. The CPAP pressures were progressively reduced to 10 cm with continued maintenance of stable breathing in REM sleep.

that it is simply a marker of the severity of OSA and dynamics of its improvement, or it may reflect an artifact of scoring approaches that ignore or misidentify central hypopneas. Some studies report resolution in 78% to 86% of patients[86,87] with 2 to 12 months of CPAP treatment, whereas others note treatment success rates of about 50%.[88] A prospective study by Cassel and colleagues,[89] who followed 675 patients with OSA with PSG at 0 and 3 months. At time zero, 12% had treatment emergent CSA, which resolved in 74% of the cases by 3 months; however, 7% of the original cohort without treatment emergent CSA were noted to have it on the 3-month study. One approach to quantifying the persistence of treatment emergent CSA is to measure residual respiratory events after several months of CPAP, using the flow data available in current generation devices. In a study (unpublished) of 217 patients after more than 6 months of therapy, the manually scored AHI_{FLOW} of 10/hour or greater was seen in 23%, and the central apnea index at the baseline sleep study was the only predictor of residual disease.

The predominant role of the CO_2 control instability in pathogenesis of treatment emergent or complex sleep apnea is supported by resolution with small increases of inhaled CO_2.[90,91] The mechanisms for improvement in chemoreflex events after prolonged use of CPAP include reduction in

controller gain and increase in $Paco_2$ reserve.[92] Stabilizing central respiratory motor output through prevention of transient hypocapnia prevents most OSA in selected patients with a high chemosensitivity and a collapsible upper airway, whereas increasing respiratory motor output through moderate hypercapnia eliminates "obstructive" apnea in most patients with a wider range of chemosensitivity and CO_2 reserve.[93] Reducing chemosensitivity through hyperoxia has a limited and unpredictable effect on OSA.[93]

EPIDEMIOLOGY OF CENTRAL SLEEP APNEA AND ITS SUBTYPES

This topic is discussed in detail in Chapter 12. The epidemiology data for CSA are largely based on standard AASM definitions of respiratory events in sleep[94] and may underestimate the prevalence of CSA. This is largely due to the inability to effectively distinguish central from obstructive hypopneas without esophageal manometry, leading to classification bias toward obstructive sleep-disordered breathing (SDB; see Definitions section).

As alternate measures for detecting centrally mediated SDB are developed and automated, CSA prevalence may rise. For example, central apneas, periodic breathing, and CSB are patterns that suggest chemoreflex-mediated respiratory control dysfunction.[95] A biomarker of heightened chemoreflex activity (narrow-band elevated low-frequency coupling [e-LFC$_{NB}$]) has been described using an electrocardiogram-based analysis of heart rate variability and heart rate–respiratory coupling. This metric quantifies the metronomic self-similar oscillations that characterize nonhypercapnic CSA and periodic breathing.[96] One third of a large, community-based patient cohort with SDB (the Sleep Heart Health Study) exhibited the e-LFC$_{NB}$, which is associated with CSA and periodic breathing.[97] This proportion is roughly in keeping with detailed phenotyping experiments performed over the years.[81,98]

CLINICAL FEATURES AND DIAGNOSIS OF CENTRAL SLEEP APNEA AND ITS SUBTYPES

Clinical Presentation

The clinical presentation of patients with CSA varies by the etiology and subtype (Table 15-2). Symptoms and signs are not specific to CSA and often overlap with those of OSA as well as the underlying conditions leading to CSA (e.g., dyspnea on awakening in heart failure patients[99]). The following sections describe the PSG characteristics important in CSA, including the differences between nonhypercapnic and hypercapnic subtypes and finally the unique features of CSA associated with specific disorders.

Polysomnographic Features Important in Central Sleep Apnea

Diagnosis of CSA syndromes generally requires a full-night recording of standard PSG with special attention to inspiratory effort, to differentiate central (no inspiratory effort throughout event) versus obstructive apneas. Although this differentiation is simple for apneas, for hypopneas it requires esophageal manometry.[100,101] Respiratory inductance plethysmography excursions are present in both central and obstructive hypopneas, and determining whether decreases in effort and flow are proportionate can be arbitrary and difficult to operationalize.[102] Alternative strategies using PSG-based algorithms have been developed but show marginal accuracy compared with esophageal manometry (68% in one study).[17] Finally, cardiopulmonary coupling signal analysis

as described previously may also be used to differentiate central predominant (chemoreflex-driven) versus obstructive SDB phenotypes[95] but has not been validated using esophageal manometry.

A consistent feature of nonhypercapnic, heightened chemoreflex-mediated central apnea is predominance of events during NREM sleep, especially during non–slow wave stages.[22,103-108] A metronomic self-similar appearance is typical, in contrast to opiate-induced CSA, in which variability of expiratory phase is characteristic. Additional features of chemoreflex modulation during sleep are noted in Table 15-3. In contrast, in many cases of hypercapnic CSA (and in OSA), the severity of SDB worsens markedly during REM sleep, especially if the motor neurons of the diaphragm are involved.[2,104] Notable exceptions are CCHS and opioid-induced CSA, in which SDB worsens in NREM sleep. Finally, objective measures of hypoventilation are needed, such as arterial, transcutaneous, or end-tidal Pco$_2$ (PETCO$_2$) to confirm hypercapnia in sleep.[15]

Propensity for sleep fragmentation and upper airway collapsibility can both worsen CSA and have specific treatment implications (see Treatment of Central Sleep Apnea). A sleep fragmentation phenotype on PSG can be suggested by prolonged sleep-wake transitional instability (>10 minutes), low sleep efficiency (<70%), persistently high N1 stage during PAP titration (>15%), and poor evolution of slow wave sleep (<1 Hz).[103] Upper airway collapsibility can be measured through the Pcrit, derived from relationships between maximal inspiratory airflow and nasal or mask pressure in OSA patients.[81,109]

Because of the challenges in diagnosing CSA without esophageal manometry, we recommend taking into account an array of the PSG features to distinguish between central and obstructive phenotypes as described previously (and in Table 15-3). Such an approach, combined with complementary measures of chemoreflex hyperactivity (e.g., cardiopulmonary coupling analysis) and identification of propensity for sleep fragmentation and airway collapsibility, can augment recognition of and treatment of CSA.

Unique Features of the Disorders

Nonhypercapnic Central Sleep Apnea

Central Sleep Apnea at High Altitude. Travelers to high altitudes often experience restlessness, frequent brief arousals, and unrefreshing sleep,[35] at least in part due to periodic breathing and CSA. Men are twice as likely to be affected as women, and at altitudes above 5000 feet it is nearly universal. PSG features are discussed in the section on Pathophysiology of Central Sleep Apnea Syndromes that Affect Diagnosis and Treatment.

Primary Central Sleep Apnea. Patients with primary CSA often present with insomnia or frequent awakenings during the night, rather than daytime sleepiness as seen in OSA.[110,111] Cycles of central apneas in idiopathic CSA are shorter (20 to 40 seconds) and not as gradual as in central sleep apnea with Cheyne-Stokes breathing (CSA-CSB) (see Pathophysiology of Central Sleep Apnea Syndromes that Affect Diagnosis and Treatment). Underlying medical conditions must be ruled out before diagnosis.

Heart Failure and Central Sleep Apnea. Clinical features, implications, and treatment of central apneas in CHF are

Table 15-2	Clinical Characteristics of Patients with Sleep Apnea		
	Central		**Obstructive**
Nonhypercapnic	Hypercapnic		
Insomnia	Daytime sleepiness Morning headache		Daytime sleepiness
Mild intermittent snoring	Snoring		Prominent snoring
Awakenings (choking, dyspnea)	Respiratory failure		Witnessed apneas, gasping
Normal body habitus	Normal or obese Polycythemia Cor pulmonale		Commonly obese Upper airway narrowing

Table 15-3 Recognition of Strong Chemoreflex Modulation of Sleep Breathing

Polysomnographic Feature	Relatively Pure Obstructive Sleep Apnea	Chemoreflex-Modulated Sleep Apnea
Periodic breathing, Cheyne-Stokes breathing	Rare	Typical (often short cycle, <30 sec in absence of CHF)
Respiratory event timing	Variable (each event tends to have different durations)	Self-similar, metronomic
Severity during sleep state	Greater severity in REM	Minimal severity in REM
Effort signal morphology	Well maintained during obstructed breath	Complete or partial loss between recovery breaths
Flow-effort relationship	Discordant: flow is reduced disproportionately to reduction in effort	Concordant: flow and effort follow each other in amplitude
Arousal timing	Early part of event termination	Crests event, often in the center of the sequence of recovery breaths
Oxygen desaturation	Irregular, progressive drops, V-shaped contour	Smooth, symmetrical, progressive drops rare

CHF, Congestive heart failure; REM, rapid eye movements.
From Thomas RJ. Alternative approaches to treatment of Central Sleep Apnea. *Sleep Med Clin* 2014;9(1):87–104.

discussed in detail in Chapters 12 and 28. In brief, age older than 60 years, male sex, and atrial fibrillation appear to be risk factors for CSA among those with CHF.[112] Patients generally present with CHF symptoms, fatigue, and weakness rather than sleepiness.[99,113-115] Symptoms and apneas improve with position changes, including lateral positioning, and are independent of the postural effects on the upper airway[116] suggesting that J-receptor activation or oxygen stores play a role in the pathogenesis of CSA-CSB. Arousals occur midcycle at the peak of the recovery.[117]

Other Medical Conditions Associated with Central Sleep Apnea. CSA is also found in patients with ESRD, CVA, PAH, and atrial fibrillation. There are no particular clinical features with high predictive value for CSA among these patients (hypocapnia may be a clue), thus diagnosis requires heightened clinical suspicion and PSG.

Patients with ESRD and CSA (concomitant obstructive and mixed apneas are common) are generally male, older, and more frequently volume overloaded.[118,119] Ultrafiltration improves $Paco_2$ and CAHI,[43] suggesting initial avenue for management of CSA in ESRD. Higher suspicion for CSA is also warranted in those with larger territory and more severe CVAs.[46,120] Patterns of CSA include CSB with long cycle times in CVA patients with left ventricular dysfunction and periodic breathing with shorter cycle lengths in those without left ventricular dysfunction.[121-123] Central apneas improve with oxygen[121] and tend to resolve as patients recover from their stroke.[124,125] In patients with PAH, older age and sleepiness (Epworth Sleepiness Scale score of >10) are predictive of SDB,[126] and CSB is the predominant CSA pattern with cycle of about 45 seconds. Presence of atrial fibrillation should raise suspicion for CSA, and vice versa.[127-130] Among community-dwelling men, increasing central apnea index correlates with increasing prevalence of atrial fibrillation, and presence of CSA-CSB is associated with odds ratio of 4.5 for atrial fibrillation, even when controlled for cardiac comorbidities, including CHF.[128]

Hypercapnic Central Sleep Apnea

Hypercapnic CSA and hypoventilation should be considered if a condition associated with them (see Table 15-1) or certain clinical features (see Table 15-3) are present. A PSG and an assessment of sleep hypoventilation through nocturnal $Paco_2$ (or surrogate) are recommended. In cases in which hypercapnic CSA and hypoventilation are discovered during a PSG obtained for another indication (e.g., OSA), a careful clinical approach to identify the underlying cause is warranted. Our initial assessment is based on locating the lesion along an anatomic pathway that could result in hypoventilation: corticobulbar tracts, brainstem, bulbospinal tracts to cervical spinal cord, anterior horn cells, lower motor neurons, neuromuscular junction, and intercostal and diaphragmatic muscles. Lung and chest wall abnormalities are generally apparent on examination and basic diagnostic studies and can help identify the underlying medical disorder (e.g., chronic obstructive pulmonary disease) in those with hypercapnic CSA and hypoventilation. Selected conditions are discussed next.

Central Congenital Alveolar Hypoventilation Syndrome. The classic feature of presentation for CCHS is mild awake and marked sleep-related alveolar hypoventilation with hypercapnia and hypoxemia (Figure 15-9). Although classically diagnosed at birth, owing to variable penetrance of the *PHOX2B* mutations (polyalanine repeat mutations [PARMs]), some patients can present as late onset in childhood or even in adulthood.[131-135] In these individuals, alveolar hypoventilation can be unmasked by administration of CNS depressants and anesthetics, recent severe pulmonary infections, or in the setting of treatment for OSA, and CCHS should be considered in those without another explanation for hypoventilation. Clinical associations that should raise suspicion for CCHS include Hirschsprung disease, tumors of neural crest origin, autonomic dysfunction, facial dysmorphology, and dermatographism.[49,136,137] The ventilatory response and sensation of dyspnea are greatly diminished or absent in children with

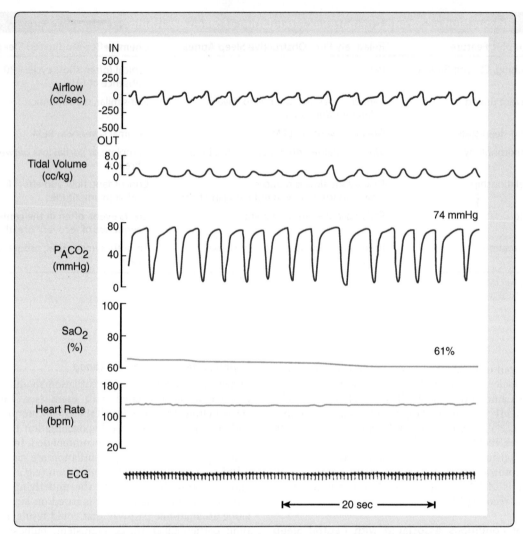

Figure 15-9 Central congenital hypoventilation. Polygraph tracing from 28-month-old girl, demonstrating typical breathing pattern during NREM sleep in congenital alveolar central hypoventilation syndrome. Note inappropriately regular (20 breaths/min), shallow breathing (tidal volumes averaging 3.5 mL/kg). Progressive hypercapnia and hypoxemia did not stimulate ventilation, arousal, or beat-to-beat heart rate variability. (Adapted with permission from Weese-Mayer et al.[9])

CCHS.[138] The respiratory pattern during sleep is characterized by markedly diminished tidal volumes and inappropriately constant respiratory rate in the face of hypercapnia and hypoxemia.[9,139] Ventilation is more stable during REM versus NREM sleep. There are variations in clinical phenotype with PARM genotype. For example, individuals with 20/25 (normal alanine repeat genotype being designated as 20/20) rarely require 24-hour ventilatory support, whereas for genotypes 20/27 to 20/33, continuous ventilatory support is needed.[140-142] Care for patients with CCHS should be provided through centers with extensive expertise in the condition.[12]

Obesity-Hypoventilation Syndrome. OHS should be suspected in an obese individual with daytime sleepiness.[143] Relative to the average OSA patient, those with OHS have a higher central fat distribution, are more likely to complain of dyspnea, and present with signs of cor pulmonale.[144-146] The diagnosis hinges on increased awake $Paco_2$ (>45 mm Hg) in the absence of other known causes of hypoventilation (e.g.,

chronic obstructive pulmonary disease, restrictive lung disease) and obesity (body mass index >30 kg/m^2). Serum bicarbonate and resting pulse oximetry can be used as simple screening tools for further testing. A bicarbonate level of 27 mEq/L or greater has 92% sensitivity for $Paco_2$ greater than 45 mm Hg (specificity of 50%[147]) among those with OSA. Rest O_2 saturation of less than 94% while breathing ambient air also suggests a need for blood gas measurement.[50,148] Up to 40% of patients with OHS continue to have persistent sleep-related O_2 desaturation despite elimination of upper airway obstruction, and hypoventilation can persist on autoadjusting PAP.[148] Hypercapnia may be more important than hypoxemia in mediating cognitive impairment individuals.[149,150] A recent study showed that although both CPAP and noninvasive ventilation improved $Paco_2$, sleep architecture, and SDB severity compared with lifestyle modification, with noninvasive ventilation, the decrease in $Paco_2$ was greater and was associated with improved 6-minute walk distance, spirometry, and some quality of life measures.[151]

Neurodegenerative Disorders. CSA and hypoventilation should be suspected in patients with neurodegenerative disorders. They are most common in multiple sclerosis (MS) and multiple system atrophy (MSA).[7] MS patients with brainstem involvement manifest with central apneas in contrast to those with nonbrainstem lesions and controls.[152] In MSA, central apneas, CSB, and apneustic breathing have all been reported.[153-155] CSA is uncommon in Alzheimer disease and Parkinson disease.[7,156-159] In amyotrophic lateral sclerosis, hypoventilation is the most common presenting feature of SDB, with nocturnal symptoms preceding daytime ventilatory failure.

Muscular and Peripheral Nervous System Disorders Associated with Central Sleep Apnea. In patients with muscular disorders, in addition to degeneration of the myocytes, impaired respiratory drive can contribute to hypoventilation. This abnormality was found in 20% of a myotonic dystrophy cohort.[160] In a recent study of 85 patients with myotonic dystrophy, 11% and 15% were found to have CSA and mixed sleep apneas, respectively, with 39% having OSA.[161] These patients were not sleepy but noted poor sleep quality as the most common symptom. The CAHI in this group correlated with slow oral swallowing time.[161,162]

Disorders affecting the diaphragm or its nerve supply (Charcot-Marie-Tooth disease and other neuropathies, myasthenia gravis, and other neuromuscular junction disorders) present predominantly with sleep-related alveolar hypoventilation.

Opiate-Induced Central Apneas and Hypoventilation (Disintegrative Central Sleep Apnea). CSA should be considered in most patients on chronic opioid therapy (COT) with symptoms of disturbed sleep. Although most extensively studied among patients taking pure opioid receptor agonists (e.g., methadone, oxycodone), recent data reveal that combinations of partial agonists and antagonists (buprenorphine and naloxone)[163] also result in significant SDB, both central and obstructive. In those with CSA, case series suggest that there is increased sleep fragmentation, increased stage 2 sleep, and decreased REM and slow wave sleep,[164] consistent with NREM predominance of central events. On PSG, patients on COT can show predominantly OSA, CSA, or mixed phenotypes. CSA in COT can present during the initial polysomnogram or emerge after treatment of predominantly obstructive disease (treatment emergent CSA).[74] There is some consistency in published reports that decreased tolerance, efficacy (high residual sleep apnea), and compliance with CPAP are present in this setting of CSA (see Treatment of Central Sleep Apnea section later). Disintegrative CSA patterns may also be seen in patients with brainstem injury such as with stroke and MS. Finally, hypoventilation is not unique to use of opioids and can be seen with anesthetics, sedatives, and muscle relaxants.

Treatment-Emergent Central Sleep Apnea. Clinical features and diagnosis of treatment emergent CSA are discussed in detail under Pathophysiology of Central Sleep Apnea Syndromes that Affect Diagnosis and Treatment above. In brief, this entity is typically recognized by the appearance of central apneas, hypopneas, and periodic breathing when continuous or nonadaptive bilevel PAP is increased to control airway obstruction in patients diagnosed with OSA.[165] The most

characteristic feature of such chemoreflex-driven respiration is not the morphology of individual events but rather is the NREM sleep dominance and the timing and morphology of the sequential events (nearly identical) in a consecutive series of events.[14,95,103]

Various techniques may be used to identify patients with heightened chemoreflex and reduced CO_2 reserve. Times series analysis of electrocardiogram, described in earlier sections, can provide a map of state sleep oscillations with e-LFC_{NB} as a marker of central apneas and periodic breathing in those with treatment emergent CSA.[95] Loop gain, along with other phenotypic traits in OSA (genioglossus muscle responsiveness, arousal threshold, and Pcrit) can be assessed using dynamic flow and pressure responses to positive pressure dial-down.[81,98] In one study[81] of OSA patients, 19% had a relatively noncollapsible upper airway similar to controls, and in these patients, loop gain was almost twice as high as in patients with a collapsible airway, despite comparable AHIs, suggesting that treatment approaches other than upper airway stabilization maybe useful in these patients (see Treatment of Central Sleep Apnea). Other methods used to quantify loop gain and predict CPAP responsiveness among those with CSA-CSB are referenced for the interested reader.[30,166-168] If confirmed, respiratory chemoreflex phenotyping may become a common clinical reality.

TREATMENT OF CENTRAL SLEEP APNEA

Positive pressure, including "enhanced" positive pressure (see later) and non–positive pressure approaches, is available for the treatment of both hypocapnic and hypercapnic CSA syndromes, including idiopathic, treatment emergent or complex, periodic breathing, hypercapnic of various etiologies, and opiate-induced CSA. All of these phenotypes, which may coexist and exhibit within-night and night-to-night dynamism, require an exact application of a multimode core therapeutic approach, including upper airway support, respiratory rhythm and drive modulation, and enhanced sleep consolidation as core approaches.[103]

Positive Pressure–Based Therapy

CPAP is a recommended initial option for CSA, based on the premise that upper airway obstruction is relevant for hypercapnic and nonhypercapnic types of CSA, a position endorsed by AASM guidelines.[169] However, there are now enough data to demonstrate that CPAP alone is poorly effective and tolerated in nonhypercapnic CSA syndromes, whereas adaptive servo ventilation (ASV) and enhanced CPAP (used with respiratory stabilization approaches that include hypocapnia minimization, sedatives, carbonic anhydrase inhibition, and oxygen) are superior treatment approaches for efficacious suppression of central apneas and periodic breathing patterns on the polysomnogram. Nonadaptive (fixed pressure) bilevel positive pressure ventilation alone is also suboptimal: this tends to exaggerate CSA and periodic breathing. Although using a backup rate with fixed bilevel positive pressure ventilation can reduce central apneas as the machine-delivered mandatory breaths substitute for lack of patient-derived respiratory effort, comparative studies with ASV show the latter to achieve superior elimination of central apneas. Nonrandomized evaluations show these devices to be about as effective as each other.[170] Because individual adaptive ventilator algorithms are substantially different, specific patient subsets may have differential responses (e.g., short vs. long cycle periodic breathing). Such individual differences in responses are currently not predictable through PSG features.

ASV devices provide expiratory support, inspiratory pressure support, and backup supportive responses guided by measures of ventilation or flow averaged over several minutes. These devices are primarily designed for patients with elevated loop gain and thus nonhypercapnic CSA but can be beneficial when hypoventilation is not the primary and sole abnormality, such as opiate-induced CSA. When used for CSA in patients with treatment emergent CSA and heart failure, central apneas are decreased in frequency, and numerous neurohumoral and cardiac function parameters are improved in heart failure patients.[171,172] Muscle sympathetic activity is reduced by adaptive ventilation but not CPAP in patients with CHF and CSA-CSB.[173] Treatment with ASV is better tolerated than CPAP and is effective in suppressing central apneas and improving oxygenation regardless of the presence of heart failure. Positive effects on sleep architecture are less impressive. The criteria for success and the respiratory event scoring criteria (often 4% desaturation association for hypopneas) can overestimate effectiveness. A randomized prospective trial of CPAP versus ASV used a success threshold of suppressing central AHI (essentially central apneas) below 10/hour of sleep as a criterion for success.[174] ASV was superior to CPAP in suppressing respiratory events, but sleep quality, sleepiness, and quality of life were not different between groups, raising the question of the best approach to quantify effectiveness beyond merely apnea suppression. Alternative indexes such as time in periodic breathing or stable breathing may provide useful efficacy information. However, in the intention-to-treat analysis, success (AHI <10/hour) at 90 days of therapy was achieved in 89.7% versus 64.5% of participants treated with ASV and CPAP.[174] The results also show how difficult it is to bring sleep and breathing back close to normal in these patients, even with optimal treatment of the CSA. Residual sleepiness in patients with CSA can be improved over auto-CPAP.[175] Similarly, opiate-induced CSA is difficult to treat with PAP, but ASV is superior to CPAP.[176] These patients do not have classic periodic breathing or metronomic central apneas and are characterized by ataxic breathing and central apneas of variable lengths. ASV devices can impose a rhythm in these conditions but can also induce patient-ventilator asynchrony and therefore need to be carefully titrated.

General Principles Regarding the Use of Adaptive Servo Ventilation Devices

All ASVs provide fixed or automatic expiratory airway support, adjustable minimal and maximal pressure support, and different options for backup rates (user specified, device algorithm estimated, or none). Volume and flow targets are used, and the sampling-averaging window extends over 3 to 4 minutes. Thus ASV devices track long-range respiratory patterns and make adjustments in the parameters to maintain the target within a prespecified range. Detection of apneic obstructive events results in expiratory pressure increases, whereas the difference between minimal and maximal allowable pressure support is the "adaptive space." The devices may be used with tight or relatively wide open user constraints depending on the preference of the physician and pressure

tolerance of the patient. Cycle lengths likely influence outcomes, and it is our observation that ASVs are less effective in patients with short cycle (≤30 seconds) periodic breathing. A subset of patients demonstrate immediate ASV intolerance and desynchrony, and this effect does not resolve with added time. Patients with prolonged sleep-wake transitional instability can have the pathology markedly amplified by an ASV. The normal fluctuations of respiration during REM sleep can inappropriately trigger the adaptive algorithms of ASVs and cause arousals, but this seems rare in clinical practice.

Recognition of Efficacy and Scoring of Respiratory Events During Adaptive Servo Ventilation Use

Scoring respiratory events during adaptive ventilation should use the pressure output signal from the ventilator. This is roughly equal and opposite to the patient's respiratory output. The flow and effort signals combine patient and ventilator contributions and give a false sense of success. See Figure 15-10 for excessive "pressure cycling," which is a response of an adaptive ventilator to ongoing periodic breathing. When pressure cycling persists, sleep fragmentation can be severe even if respiration is "improved." This pattern means than periodic breathing pathology is ongoing, necessitating the continued pressure response. When the ventilator enables stable respiration, cycling between the minimal and maximal pressure support zones is minimal. Further details on algorithms and titration strategies may be obtained from recent comprehensive reviews.[177,178] Bench testing of ASV algorithms show device-specific response characteristics, but stable breathing does not readily occur across a range of simulated central apnea patterns.[179]

ASVs are powerful devices, and if there is patient-ventilatory asynchrony, they can induce hypocapnia, excessive cycling of pressures, arousals, distorted flow patterns, and physical discomfort. Increased mortality through sudden cardiac death, and no benefits including quality of life, were reported in the Treatment of Predominant Central Sleep Apnoea by Adaptive Servo Ventilation in Patients with Heart Failure (SERVE-HF) study,[179a] which showed increased mortality with an ASV in patients with systolic heart failure (ejection fraction ≤45%) and AHI greater than 15/hour with 50% or more central events and a central AHI of 10/hour or greater. Hypocapnia, metabolic alkalosis, hemodynamic perturbations, and excessive sympathetic driving associated with excessive pressure cycling are speculative mechanisms of adverse outcomes.[180] The general consensus is that ASVs should be avoided in heart failure with reduced ejection fraction and CSA. Caution is recommended in the use of these devices in other vulnerable populations, such as patients with stroke or heart failure without reduced ejection fraction. Tracking of device data such as tidal volume stability, degree of pressure cycling, and surrogate signs of patient-ventilator asynchrony (e.g., wide variations in expiratory durations), regardless of underlying disease state, and not relying on manufacturer derived AHIs alone are prudent.

Considerations for the Treatment of Hypercapnic Central Sleep Apnea

Management of the sleep related breathing disorders of the hypoventilation syndromes is a complex process; a few key points are noted here.[181] Respiratory support may be provided by bilevel ventilation with a backup rate, volume target

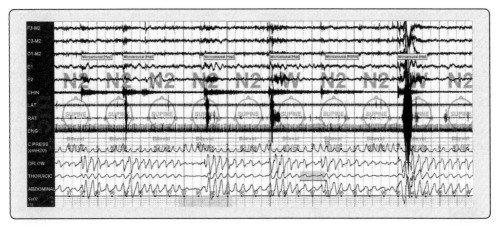

Figure 15-10 Pressure cycling during adaptive ventilation treatment. Five-minute compression snapshot; each vertical line is 30 seconds. The C-PRESS channel is the pressure output from the adaptive ventilator (Adapt SV). This 56-year-old man had predominantly central apneas, which were eliminated. However, respiratory instability, repetitive arousals, and pressure cycling continued without resolution, despite adjustments of pressure support. Persistent pressure cycling is readily recognized during home use by generating expanded night data using the device software, with attention to tidal volume and pressure traces. The device may not automatically detect respiratory events during such periods.

pressure-support ventilation, or invasive volume ventilation through a tracheostomy. These modes are also readily available on several home ventilators.

Volume-assured pressure support (VAPS) is an advance in management of hypoventilation syndromes and hypercapnic CSA. Besides expiratory, minimal, and maximal inspiratory support, backup rates, and various breath modulations such as inspiratory time and trigger and cycle sensitivity, a tidal volume target may be set. VAPS is most effective if there is hypoventilation without CSA, but it can provide benefits if used cautiously in hypercapnic CSA.

Sufficient expiratory pressure support to prevent major obstructive events is critical. REM sleep can demonstrate greater severity than NREM sleep and typically requires greater ventilation than NREM sleep. However, NREM dominance may also be seen, as in opiate-induced CSA. An autoexpiratory pressure function can aid in managing patients with markedly higher REM sleep settings. The backup rate is usually set slightly below the patient's native rate. However, if there is bradypnea (e.g., respiratory rate below 6 breaths/minute) or tachypnea (e.g., rate above 20 breaths/minute), entraining the patient to a different rate may be difficult and result in patient-ventilator desynchrony. Substantial inspiratory support (e.g., 25 cm H_2O) may be required to enable optimal ventilation.

Positive pressure ventilation therapy for hypercapnic CSA poses the specific challenge of inducing relative hypocapnia and respiratory instability and associated sleep fragmentation by overly aggressive ventilation.[182] There is a tradeoff between improving ventilation and oxygenation versus sleep quality because excessive volume targets and the associated pressure rises can induce sleep fragmentation. The rate of change in pressure support can be prescribed in these devices, providing one form of "brake" to prevent pressure-related sleep fragmentation. In the absence of PSG titration, when sleep versus wake and NREM versus REM sleep treatment requirements are not estimated, treatment may be less precise than possible. An iterative approach of two or three PSG titrations separated by a few months can result in greater precision of therapy and

sleep quality, allowing resetting of the respiratory controller. Although empirical home ventilation can be obtained under specific diagnostic conditions (such as amyotrophic lateral sclerosis) and severities based on pulmonary function tests, PSG titration with transcutaneous CO_2 monitoring can improve precision of care.

Alternative Approaches to Positive Pressure Therapy
Minimization of Hypocapnia

That CO_2 can stabilize respiration has been known for decades, and prevention of hypocapnia is a critical stabilizing factor in sleep respiratory control. However, high concentrations of CO_2 fragment sleep by inducing arousals secondary to respiratory stimulation and sympathoexcitation.[183,184] The challenge has been delivery of CO_2 in a clinically adequate, tolerated, and precise manner. Holding the CO_2 steady and just above the NREM sleep CO_2 threshold can protect the CO_2 reserve while maintaining sleep consolidation.

In a study manipulating inhaled CO_2 in OSA patients but directly relevant to CSA treatment,[93] 26 patients with OSA (AHI 42 ± 5 events/hour with 92% of apneas obstructive) were treated with O_2 supplementation, an isocapnic rebreathing system in which CO_2 was added only during hyperpnea to prevent transient hypocapnia, and a continuous rebreathing system. With isocapnic rebreathing, 14 of 26 reduced their AHI to 31% ± 6% of control ($P < .01$) (responders); 12 of 26 did not show significant change (nonresponders). The responders versus nonresponders had a greater controller gain, a smaller CO_2 reserve, but no differences in Pcrit. Hypercapnic rebreathing (+4.2 ± 1 mm Hg P_{ETCO_2}) reduced AHI to 15 ± 4 of control ($P < .001$) in 17 of 21 subjects with a wide range of CO_2 reserve. Hyperoxia (SaO_2 ~95% to 98%) reduced AHI to 36% ± 11% of control in 7 of 19 OSA patients tested. Addition of a closed volume (dead space) to exhale increases rebreathing of exhaled air and results in a rapid increase in CO_2 levels and an increased tidal volume and respiratory rate. The concept has been used in mechanical ventilation to reduce hypocapnia for several years and more recently has been successfully used to treat CSA-CSB in heart failure.[184]

Combining hypocapnia minimization with positive pressure is logical, and we have shown that keeping CO_2 above the apnea threshold with the use of enhanced expiratory rebreathing space (EERS) is an effective adjunct to PAP therapy[90]; EERS is the dead space concept applied to pressure ventilation and may be used with continuous or adaptive pressure support (Figure 15-11). There is no or a minimal increase in inspiratory CO_2 because of the positive pressure–induced washout. The physiologic target for titrations with EERS is to maintain end-tidal CO_2 (ETCO$_2$) at the low-normal range

for sleep, that is, an increase of 2 to 8 mm Hg in ETCO$_2$. CO_2 manipulation can also be done by bleeding CO_2 into the circuit by a more precisely controlled flow-independent method. Successful treatment of mixed OSA and CSA using a proprietary device, the positive airway pressure gas modulator (PAPGAM), has been reported. This device delivers precisely controlled concentrations of CO_2. In a small case series, 6 patients with an average mixed apnea AHI of 43/hour on CPAP improved, with reduction of AHI to 4.5/hour and addition of 0.5% to 1% using PAPGAM.[91] Dynamic CO_2

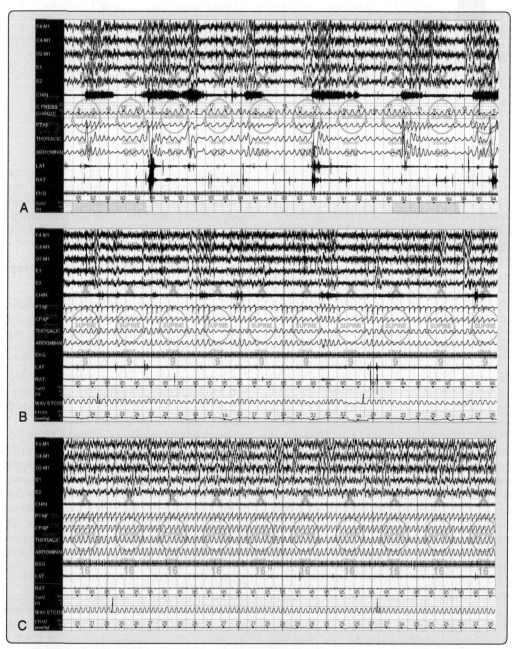

Figure 15-11   Efficacy of CO_2 manipulation for stabilizing respiration. A 72-year-old man with congestive heart failure (same patient as in Figure 15-3). *Top,* Adaptive servoventilation failure; note excessive cycling of pressure (the CPRESS channel) and the associated arousals. *Middle,* After addition of 50 mL enhanced expiratory rebreathing space (EERS), note stabilization of respiratory rhythm but residual flow limitation and mild residual periodic breathing. *Bottom,* With 100 mL EERS; note normalization of sleep and respiration. The end-tidal CO_2 (ETCO$_2$) signal plateau is slightly blunted and thus the CO_2 measured is falsely low. However, the resting wake ETCO$_2$ of this patient was 30 mm Hg, a level that can be readily seen in patients with congestive heart failure.

manipulation (delivery restricted to a specific phase of the respiratory cycle) may, in future studies, improve the stabilizing effects of CO_2.[185]

Oxygen

Nasal O_2 has a long history of use to treat CSA and periodic breathing without CSA.[186,187] Effectiveness is typically partial, and residual sleep apnea and sleep fragmentation are common. High loop gain that is not primarily driven by hypoxia may not respond to O_2 at clinically safe doses, an escape from suppression of carotid body firing. Adding oxygen to CPAP may benefit CSA and treatment emergent CSA with a reduction in responsiveness of peripheral chemoreceptors and loop gain.[188,189] A study in a U.S. veterans population showed benefit in a predominantly CSA population, but the PSG changes were delayed by as much as an hour or more.[190] Respiratory event cycles can lengthen with the use of O_2. Such a change may "reduce" the respiratory event index but not imply a true stabilization of respiration. Use of O_2 also negates use of a desaturation parameter to score hypopneas. Beneficial effects of oxygen for CSA are not limited to those with oxygen saturations below thresholds used for long-term nasal oxygen therapy (e.g., ≤88%). Use of O_2 is off-label for CSA syndromes. The limitations include the long-term cost and difficulty with reimbursement in nonhypoxic patients.

Enhancing Sleep Consolidation

Arousals from sleep have a role in sleep apnea pathophysiology.[28] Sedatives can probably be used safely in minimally nonhypercapnic hypoxic CSA and NREM-dominant apnea in general because arousals further destabilize sleep and worsen sleep apnea severity For example, eszopiclone has been shown to reduce the AHI in patients with obstructive apnea with a low arousal threshold.[191] Likely mechanisms of benefit of sedatives in nonhypercapnic CSA include reduction of arousal-induced hypocapnia and increasing the proportion of NREM sleep spent in stable breathing. Triazolam, temazepam, zolpidem, and clonazepam have all been shown to reduce periodic breathing and CSA.[192-195]

Opioid-Induced Central Sleep Apnea

CSA is commonly associated with chronic opiate use and is dose related with substantial individual differences. PSG features of opiate effects may be more common than clinical symptoms, and the impact, on health, of CSA exclusively due to opiate use remains to be defined. Decreasing the dose of opiates may help reduce the frequency of central apneas[4] and should be routinely considered within the constraints of the disorder for which it was prescribed. In many patients, however, stopping opiates entirely may not be possible. CPAP alone will rarely be effective therapy. Opiate-induced ataxic breathing is quite sensitive to CO_2 levels—with ready induction of central apnea and worsening of dysrhythmic breathing on continuous or nonadaptive bilevel positive pressure ventilation. Although these patients tend to show mild hypercapnia, with $ETCO_2$ in the high 40- to low 50-mm Hg range, using a nonvented mask and EERS as needed to hold CO_2 in the mid 40-mm Hg range (thus preventing destabilizing degrees of hypocapnia despite supporting the upper airway) can be helpful regardless of the positive pressure mode used. We have found the use of acetazolamide to be of consistent benefit. Adaptive ventilation is a double-edged sword in these patients,

being able to both enable stable breathing and markedly destabilize breathing.[176,196,197]

Carbonic Anhydrase Inhibition

Acetazolamide, a diuretic and carbonic anhydrase inhibitor, diminishes the ventilatory response of the peripheral chemoreceptors to hypoxia, decreases loop gain, and reduces the ventilatory response to arousals.[198-201] In animal models, it has been shown to lower the P_{ETCO_2} apnea threshold and widen the difference between the eupneic and P_{ETCO_2} thresholds.[21] Acetazolamide has been used in treating nonhypercapnic CSA or CSB, in patients with and without heart failure.[202] Although such results may be statistically significant, the degree of residual sleep apnea is unacceptable as sole long-term therapy. The drug may convert those with mixed OSA and CSA to mostly obstructive (the reverse of CPAP-induced CSA). Those with short cycle (≤30 seconds) periodic breathing not responding to EERS or adaptive ventilation are the best candidates. Acetazolamide has been successfully used as CPAP adjuncts at high altitude.[203,204] Zonisamide[205] and topiramate[206] have carbonic anhydrase inhibitory effects and could in theory be used in the place of acetazolamide. Acetazolamide can aid the treatment of hypercapnic CSA by reducing the propensity for worsening of respiratory instability, which pressure support ventilation can induce. The drug may have a special role in those with coexisting CSA in NREM sleep (requiring low levels of PAP) and OSA in REM sleep (requiring higher pressures that could exacerbate CSA in NREM sleep).

Other Drugs with Possible Benefits in Nonhypercapnic Central Sleep Apnea

Clonidine[207] and the 5-α reductase inhibitor finasteride[208] have been shown to improve breathing stability. Inhibition of H_2S (gaseous signal transmitted in carotid body) in a rodent model of CHF nearly normalized chemosensitivity and breathing instability, and may serve as a new therapeutic target.[209] A case report of unilateral carotid body denervation in a man with systolic heart failure and moderate CSA showed that chemosensitivity and sleep apnea severity were reduced and shifted to an obstructive phenotype 2 months after treatment, accompanied by an improvement in quality of life.[210] A recently completed trial of carotid body denervation in systolic heart failure patients may provide key risk-benefit information (ClinicalTrials.gov Identifier: NCT01653821) on pharmacologic targeting of carotid body function.

Other Treatment Options

Phrenic nerve stimulation[211,212] is an investigational approach that can improve the CAHI in heart failure patients with CSA-CSB. Sleep quality may not improve proportionately, and there is a concern that suppression of central apneas without enabling stable breathing or targeting the core pathophysiology of high loop gain may not provide long-term benefits, similar to the SERVE-HF study. A subset of CSA and treatment emergent CSA patients appear very supine position dependent, and avoidance of the supine position can markedly improve treatment efficacy.[116,213] An additional effect of body position, this time from vertical to horizontal, is on fluid redistribution from the caudal to cranial parts of the body.[214-218] The effect is rapid and is associated with increased neck circumference and hypocapnia from increased lung water in patients with central apnea. Therapeutic manipulation could include careful diuresis, a wedge pillow, or sleeping in a recliner.

CLINICAL PEARLS

- Sleep apnea caused by a pathologically activated respiratory chemoreflex results in a wide PSG spectrum of disease, with variable features of upper airway obstruction mixed with more traditionally accepted central patterns.
- Pathophysiology guides treatment. Treatment end points should aim to normalize sleep and sleep-breathing biology, not merely suppression of scored events to an arbitrary threshold.
- It is useful to consider CSA as taking hypercapnic and nonhypercapnic forms. Accurate phenotyping of sleep apnea is increasingly important because several on-label and off-label therapies, singly or in combination, have improved therapeutic options for CSA syndromes.
- Recognizing NREM sleep dominance of disease in nonhypercapnic CSA and minimizing the importance of concomitant upper airway flow limitation when identifying otherwise typical periodic breathing are applicable in clinical and research assessments. Hypercapnic CSA may be REM dominant, with the exception of opiate-induced CSA, and require ventilatory support for management. Unlike OSA, CSA is relatively difficult to treat and increases the risk for poor compliance, residual symptoms, ongoing sleep fragmentation, and high residual respiratory events despite therapy.

SUMMARY

CSA caused by pathologic activation of the respiratory chemoreflex includes idiopathic CSA, periodic breathing, high-altitude sleep apnea, and treatment emergent or complex sleep apnea. A narrow NREM sleep CO_2 reserve and propensity for arousal and sleep fragmentation are key pathophysiologic drivers. A unifying theme for nonhypercapnic CSA is predominance in NREM sleep and a metronomic appearance; cycle times, the duration of the respiratory event from peak to peak or trough to trough, can be short (≤30 seconds). Sleep fragmentation is often severe, but hypoxia is relatively moderate in nonhypercapnic CSA. The prevalence and evolution of residual CSA phenotypes with treatment remains to be accurately estimated owing to limitations of current approaches to PSG scoring; new methods need to be validated to outcomes. Non-invasive adaptive ventilation provides pressure support

approximately equal and opposite to patient-generated ventilation, with substantial differences in individual device algorithms. Off-label approaches may be considered as adjuncts to improve therapeutic efficacy, including minimization of hypocapnia with dead space adapted to PAP, acetazolamide, and sedatives to reduce the arousal threshold.

Hypercapnic CSA is associated with pathologically reduced activation of the respiratory chemoreflex and may be seen in association with hypoventilation syndromes and neurologic disorders. Disease severity can be maximal in REM sleep, although successful ventilation (and reduction in hypercapnia) may result in respiratory instability in NREM sleep owing to relative hypocapnia. Non-invasive bilevel ventilation with a backup rate and volume-assured ventilation are primary therapeutic options; acetazolamide may improve respiratory drive and reduce NREM-related instability.

Selected Readings

Abraham WT, Jagielski D, Oldenburg O, et al. Phrenic nerve stimulation for the treatment of central sleep apnea. *JACC Heart Fail* 2015;3(5):360–9.

Correa D, Farney RJ, Chung F, et al. Chronic opioid use and central sleep apnea: a review of the prevalence, mechanisms, and perioperative considerations. *Anesth Analg* 2015;120(6):1273–85.

Cowie MR, Woehrle H, Wegscheider K, et al. Adaptive servo-ventilation for central sleep apnea in systolic heart failure. *N Engl J Med* 2015;373(12):1095–105.

Dempsey JA, Smith CA, Przybylowski T, et al. The ventilatory responsiveness to CO(2) below eupnoea as a determinant of ventilatory stability in sleep. *J Physiol* 2004;560:1–11.

Dempsey JA, Xie A, Patz DS, Wang D. Physiology in medicine: obstructive sleep apnea pathogenesis and treatment—considerations beyond airway anatomy. *J Appl Physiol* 2014;116:3–12.

Eckert DJ, White DP, Jordan AS, et al. Defining phenotypic causes of obstructive sleep apnea: identification of novel therapeutic targets. *Am J Respir Crit Care Med* 2013;188:996–1004.

Eckert DJ, Younes MK. Arousal from sleep: implications for obstructive sleep apnea pathogenesis and treatment. *J Appl Physiol* 2014;116:302–13.

Gaig C, Iranzo A. Sleep-disordered breathing in neurodegenerative diseases. *Curr Neurol Neurosci Rep* 2012;12:205–17.

Javaheri S, Dempsey JA. Central sleep apnea. *Compr Physiol* 2013;3:141–63.

Priou P, d'Ortho MP, Damy T, et al. Adaptive servo-ventilation: How does it fit into the treatment of central sleep apnoea syndrome? Expert opinions. *Rev Mal Respir* 2015;32(10):1072–81.

Rao H, Thomas RJ. Complex sleep apnea. *Curr Treat Options Neurol* 2013;15:677–91.

Thomas RJ. Alternative approaches to treatment of central sleep apnea. *Sleep Med Clin* 2014;9:87–104.

Wolfe LF, Patwari PP, Mutlu GM. Sleep hypoventilation in neuromuscular and chest wall disorders. *Sleep Med Clin* 2014;9:409–23.

Xie A, Teodorescu M, Pegelow DF, et al. Effects of stabilizing or increasing respirator motor outputs on obstructive sleep apnea. *J Appl Physiol* 2013;115:22–33.

A complete reference list can be found online at ExpertConsult.com.

Obstructive Sleep Apnea: Diagnosis and Management

Harly Greenberg; Viera Lakticova; Steven M. Scharf

Chapter Highlights

- Obstructive sleep apnea (OSA) is the most common respiratory disorder of sleep, with a high prevalence that is linked to the increase in obesity.
- OSA is frequently comorbid with cardiovascular, cerebrovascular, and metabolic diseases and is commonly observed in populations with these comorbidities. The relationship of OSA with these multisystem disorders may be bidirectional.
- The pathogenesis of OSA is complex, with contributions from mechanical factors that increase collapsibility of the upper airway as well as factors that lead to instability of ventilatory control during sleep.

- Clinical assessment, in addition to various screening questionnaires, is useful to identify patients at risk for OSA. However, accurate diagnosis requires monitoring of sleep.
- In-laboratory polysomnographic testing for OSA, as well as various technologies for ambulatory or out-of-center-sleep testing, are presented. The utility and limitations of these techniques are discussed.
- Various treatment modalities for OSA are described. An individualized treatment approach that emphasizes chronic disease management that improves sleep-related health outcomes is necessary to optimize care.

DEFINITION

Obstructive sleep apnea (OSA) is a common disorder that is recognized as a major risk factor for a number of important chronic medical conditions and is responsible for poor quality of life. Ample evidence exists that patients with untreated OSA consume more health care resources than matched patients without OSA, leading to considerably increased health care use costs.[1,2] Most studies agree that treatment reduces health care use to that of matched controls. Further, estimates are that OSA remains underdiagnosed.[3]

The classic signs and symptoms of OSA include excessive daytime sleepiness (EDS), loud snoring, snorting, and gasping at night (associated with apnea termination). Physical signs commonly associated with OSA include obesity, large neck circumference, and crowding of the oropharynx (Table 16-1).

BRIEF HISTORY

Burwell and colleagues are often given credit for the first medical description of a patient with probable OSA.[4] These authors described an obese, sleepy, hypercapnic patient, demonstrating periodic breathing, who reminded them of the character Joe in the Charles Dickens 1836 novel *The Posthumous Papers of the Pickwick Club* (see also Chapter 30). However, others used this term previously to describe similar patients.[5] Although the prevailing thought was that hypoventilation, possibly owing to excess weight, contributed to somnolence,

Kuhl and associates described breathing cessations at night during polysomnography (PSG) and attributed sleepiness to the resultant sleep fragmentation.[6] As a result of these findings, the world renowned neurologist Gastaut added measurements of airflow and chest wall motion to other PSG measures to document obstruction of the upper airway (UA) at night.[7,8] The Bologna group of Lugaresi and Coccagna demonstrated large swings in arterial and pulmonary pressures during apneas, thus documenting that nocturnal breathing disorders had major adverse consequences and required treatment.[9] Following the observation of Kuhl and associates, the Bologna group reported that tracheostomy improved symptoms in a group of "pickwickian" patients.[10,11] In 1981 Sullivan and colleagues published their seminal paper demonstrating that nasally applied continuous positive airway pressure (CPAP) could alleviate UA obstruction in OSA.[12] Shortly thereafter, Rapoport and associates demonstrated that the "pickwickian syndrome" could be reversed with long-term use of nocturnal CPAP.[13] Additional therapies for the disorder, now termed *OSA*, including UA surgeries, mandibular advancement, and even stimulation of the hypoglossal nerve, have evolved and allow the physician to offer a variety of therapies tailored to the individual patient.

PHYSIOLOGIC EFFECTS

It is now well established that OSA has a number of acute physiologic effects that are thought to contribute to adverse multisystem consequences. These include intermittent hypoxia

Table 16-1	Signs and Symptoms of Obstructive Sleep Apnea

Severe snoring, snoring, gasping, or choking in sleep

Witnessed apneas in sleep

Excessive daytime sleepiness; tendency to fall asleep in inappropriate situations (e.g., while driving, attending lectures)

Lack of energy

Morning headaches

Large neck size: 17 inches in men, 16 inches in women

Crowding of the oropharynx: Mallampati score of 3 or greater, large tonsils, large tongue, elongated uvula

Facial abnormalities: retrognathia, midface deformities

Obesity (body mass index >30)

Nocturnal gastroesophageal reflux

Impotence; erectile dysfunction

Note: Male gender and postmenopausal state in women confers increased risk.

Table 16-2	Medical and Mental Health Conditions for Which There Is Evidence of Association with Obstructive Sleep Apnea*

Hypertension[155] (25% to 50% all hypertension; as high as 83% in drug-resistant hypertension)

Myocardial infarction[156] (as high as 70%)

Stroke[157] (as high as 68%)

Depression[158]

Congestive heart failure[159] (as high as 76%)

Asthma[51]

Chronic obstructive pulmonary disease[48] (as high as 50%)

Atrial fibrillation (and other dysrhythmia)[38] (49%)

Type 2 diabetes[46] (as high as 48%)

Traffic and industrial accidents[83] (as high as fivefold increase)

Overall mortality[160] (increased risk by 46%)

*Approximate risks listed where available.

(IH) occurring as a result of apneas and hypopneas, exaggerated negative swings in intrathoracic pressure (ITP), and terminal arousals. In animal models, IH leads to increased sympathoadrenal tone, a feature well demonstrated in humans with OSA.[14,15] Further, IH leads to oxidant stress in the brain[16] and in the myocardium, a finding associated with poor left ventricular function, apoptosis of myocardial cells,[17,18] and endothelial dysfunction.[19] Further, arousals associated with termination of apneas, hypopneas, and periods of inspiratory flow limitation contribute to heightened sympathetic tone.[20] In animal models, IH has been shown to be associated with release of pro-inflammatory mediators, at least partially mediated by NF-κB–related pathways.[21,22] Exaggerated swings in ITP, primarily during inspiration against an occluded airway, lead to increased venous return and stress on the right ventricle.[23] The latter appears to be primarily responsible for pulmonary hypertension, a common finding in OSA.[24] Sleepiness is thought to be, at least in part, a result of the terminal arousals and associated sleep fragmentation.

OSA is an independent major risk factor for a number of associated medical conditions (Table 16-2). Chief among these are cardiovascular disease, including hypertension, stroke, myocardial infarction, and congestive heart failure. Heightened sympathoadrenal tone, oxidant stress, and pro-inflammatory cytokines appear to be involved in the pathogenesis of these conditions.

EPIDEMIOLOGY

There are varying estimates of the prevalence of OSA, largely owing to differences in diagnostic methods, definitions of disease, and differences in age, gender, and body mass index (BMI). As reviewed by Young and colleagues in 2002, prevalence estimates range from 2% to 26% depending on gender, definition of "disease," and population studied.[25] These prevalence rates were mostly derived from epidemiologic studies performed in the 1990s. Data from the Wisconsin Sleep Cohort were used to derive the estimate that symptomatic OSA affected 2% to 4% of middle-aged adults in the United

States.[26] However, the increase in prevalence of obesity necessitated revision of these initial estimates. Using data from the National Health and Nutrition Examination Survey on BMI in U.S. populations, as well as data from the Wisconsin Sleep Cohort, Peppard and associates now estimate that among adults 30 to 70 years of age, approximately 13% of men and 6% of women have an apnea-hypopnea index (AHI) of more than 15/hour, whereas 14% of men and 5% of women have an AHI of more than 5/hour with symptoms of daytime sleepiness.[27] Both definitions meet *International Classification of Sleep Disorders,* third edition (ICSD3) criteria for OSA.[28] In the U.S. working age population, males have a twofold to threefold greater prevalence of OSA than females. A meta-analysis of community and sleep center referral–based cohorts showed that male gender is more common among patients with diagnosed OSA (odds ratio, 3.1; 95% confidence interval [CI], 2.5 to 3.8). However, among women, postmenopausal status is associated with an increased risk for OSA that equals that observed in men.[29,30] The prevalence of OSA in the United States also increases with advancing age, from about 35 to 60 years, after which there is less of an age-related increase.[31]

OSA prevalence has also been assessed in many regions of the world other than the United States and among various ethnic groups. Estimates of OSA prevalence in white European and Australian populations are similar to those observed in North America. Further, comparable OSA prevalence rates have been found in studies of Korean, Chinese, and Indian populations. Most studies have also shown similar OSA prevalence between North American white, African American, and Hispanic cohorts.[32]

PREVALENCE IN DISEASE-SPECIFIC COHORTS

Because OSA is associated with cardiac, cerebrovascular, pulmonary, metabolic, and other comorbid diseases, it is worthwhile to consider the prevalence of OSA in relevant disease specific cohorts. The pathophysiologic features of OSA, including IH, increases in sympathoadrenal tone, large swings in ITP, and sleep fragmentation, with associated increases in oxidative stress, systemic inflammation, and endothelial dysfunction, among other factors, may contribute to many of these associated comorbid conditions. It is also worthwhile to consider that the relationship of OSA with some of these diseases may be bidirectional.

One of the most studied cardiovascular comorbidities of OSA is systemic hypertension. Most observational studies have shown that up to 50% of patients with systemic hypertension have OSA.[33] Further, OSA is a common cause of "resistant" hypertension, with a prevalence of 64% in one cohort of patients with difficult-to-control hypertension.[34] Atrial fibrillation (AF) is another cardiac disorder associated with OSA. Data from the Sleep Heart Health Study (SHHS) demonstrated a higher prevalence of AF in subjects with OSA than in those without such sleep-disordered breathing (4.8% vs. 0.9%; $P = .003$).[35] Conversely, a high prevalence of OSA (32% to 49%) has been demonstrated in various cohorts of patients with AF.[36] The association between these disorders is further documented by data that demonstrate an increasing prevalence of AF with increasing severity of OSA as assessed by the nocturnal oxygen desaturation index.[37] Other studies have shown that OSA is associated with development of AF after cardiac surgery and with an increased risk for recurrence of AF after cardioversion or ablation therapy.[38] OSA is also common in congestive cardiomyopathy and may adversely affect outcomes in this disease. Eleven percent of a cohort of patients with cardiomyopathy (defined as left ventricular ejection fraction <45%) was found to have OSA, although central sleep apnea (CSA) was more frequently observed in this group.[39] In another cohort of systolic heart failure patients, 61% were found to have a sleep related breathing disorder; approximately half had OSA, whereas CSA was present in the remainder.[40] OSA is also an independent risk factor for cerebrovascular disease with a threefold to fourfold increased odds of incident stroke in moderate to severe OSA (AHI >20/hour).[41,42] In accord with this finding, the prevalence of OSA in post–cerebrovascular accident cohorts is notably high, ranging from 38% to 74%.[43,44] The relationship of these cardiovascular and cerebrovascular disorders with OSA may be bidirectional. The adverse consequences of OSA may contribute to the development of these conditions; conversely, cardiac and cerebral dysfunction may contribute to OSA by promoting pathophysiologic factors that promote apneas and hypopneas during sleep. The association of OSA with type 2 diabetes and the metabolic syndrome is also well described. Data from the SHHS, for example, demonstrated that a remarkable 58% of subjects with type 2 diabetes had an elevated AHI.[45] A study of obese adults with type 2 diabetes showed that 87 % of that cohort had OSA, with a mean AHI in the moderate range.[46]

Although some studies have suggested that the occurrence of OSA in chronic obstructive pulmonary disease (COPD) patients is not greater than expected based on the prevalence of each disease in the population,[47] others have shown an increased prevalence of COPD among OSA patients compared with matched controls.[48] A case-control study of 1497 patients with PSG-proven OSA compared with 1489 age- and gender-matched controls showed that COPD was more prevalent in the OSA group (7.6 vs. 3.7 %; $P < .0001$).[49] OSA was also found to be highly prevalent among a cohort of patients moderate to severe COPD referred for pulmonary rehabilitation.[50] Regardless of whether the concomitant prevalence of COPD and OSA is greater than can be expected by chance occurrence, the coexistence of these disorders, termed the *overlap syndrome*, is associated with more severe nocturnal hypoxemia, hypoventilation, pulmonary hypertension, comorbid obesity, and diabetes than that which is observed in isolated OSA or COPD (see Chapter 29).

Recent studies have also suggested an association between OSA and asthma.[51] Although most data regarding a possible link between these two diseases come from cross-sectional studies performed in asthma clinic cohorts, results consistently demonstrate that the prevalence of OSA is approximately double in these cohorts compared with the general population. Asthma severity, BMI, gastroesophageal reflux, and female gender have all been associated with increased OSA risk in asthma. An analysis of data from the Wisconsin Sleep Cohort showed that a diagnosis of asthma was associated with increased risk for incident OSA.[52] Whether these disorders are mechanistically linked and whether OSA treatment alters asthma outcomes remains to be investigated.

OSA is also frequently observed in patients with chronic kidney disease, with prevalence rates reported to be as high as 50% in patients with end-stage renal disease (ESRD).[53] An increasing prevalence of OSA has been associated with declining kidney function, ranging from 41% in patients with chronic kidney disease to 48% in those with ESRD.[54] The relationship between renal dysfunction and OSA may also be bidirectional. OSA might contribute to renal dysfunction by exacerbating hypertension, diabetes, endothelial dysfunction, sympathetic neural activity, systemic inflammation, and oxidative stress.[55,55a] Conversely, renal dysfunction may contribute to OSA, possibly owing to fluid overload that may increase UA edema as well as other factors. Support for the possibility of such a bidirectional relationship comes from data that demonstrate improvement in the AHI with intensive nocturnal hemodialysis in ESRD.[56] In addition, removal of fluid by ultrafiltration, without affecting uremia, was shown to improve the AHI in association with a decline in fluid volume of the neck.[57]

It is clear from these studies that OSA is frequently comorbid with several important and common diseases. Whether treatment of OSA alters disease-specific outcomes when coexistent with other major medical disorders remains a matter of ongoing investigation for most of these conditions.

RISK FACTORS

Anatomy

OSA is associated with anatomic risk factors that narrow the UA. As mentioned previously, the most widely recognized factor is central obesity, with a direct relationship observed between BMI and apnea severity. OSA is attributable to obesity in up to 58% of subjects.[58] Further, weight loss typically results in improvement in OSA. Linear regression modeling from the Wisconsin Sleep Cohort showed that in individuals with OSA, after adjustment for sex, age, and cigarette smoking, an approximate 1% increase or decrease in body weight was associated with a corresponding 3% increase or decrease in the AHI.[59] Obesity can contribute to airway narrowing by depositing adipose tissue around collapsible segments of the UA, increasing the size of the parapharyngeal fat pads and increasing fat content and volume of the base of the tongue.[60,61] Obesity may also indirectly contribute to UA collapsibility by reducing lung volume. Lower lung volume is associated with reduced tracheal caudal traction on the UA, which decreases stiffness of the lateral pharyngeal walls and promotes airway collapse.[62]

In addition to deposition of adipose tissue, overall increases in UA soft tissue volume contribute to pharyngeal narrowing and predispose the UA to collapse during sleep. Numerous imaging studies have demonstrated that the UA lumen is narrower in patients with OSA compared with control subjects. Such narrowing is largely due to an increase in volume of the surrounding soft tissues. Although the cross-sectional dimension of the OSA airway is smaller at several levels, the greatest difference compared with controls is typically in the retropalatal or velopharyngeal region.[61] Magnetic resonance imaging volumetric analyses have demonstrated increased volume of the lateral pharyngeal walls, soft palate, tongue, and parapharyngeal fat pads that compromise the airway lumen. In addition, differences in the shape and length of the UA are evident. Although the UA is normally largest in its lateral dimension, its anterior-posterior dimension is greatest in OSA; this decreases efficiency of UA dilator muscles. Further, UA length is increased in OSA, which contributes to its collapsibility.[61] In addition to soft tissues, decreased size of the maxilla, with a narrowed and high palatal arch and a small retropositioned mandible can also narrow the UA.[62,63]

Other factors that contribute to a narrow airway lumen in OSA include edema and inflammation of UA soft tissue.

Histologic studies of resected palatal tissue showed edema and lymphocytic infiltration of mucosal as well as muscular layers in OSA, possibly owing to vibratory trauma from snoring.[64] In addition, rostral shift of blood volume and edema fluid from the lower extremities when subjects with lower extremity edema assume a recumbent position during sleep has been associated with increased neck circumference, UA resistance, and increased AHI.[65]

Relationship of Upper Airway Anatomic Factors to Development of Inspiratory Flow Limitation and Obstruction

The UA can be modeled as a collapsible tube through which air flows (Figure 16-1). The propensity of the airway to collapse is determined by the elastic properties of the airway structure itself as well as activity of the UA dilator muscles. During inspiration, pressure in the pharyngeal lumen is negative relative to atmospheric pressure; otherwise air could not flow in the inspiratory direction. With increased inspiratory effort or narrowing of the pharyngeal lumen, pressure becomes more negative within the UA. This can lead to obstruction in collapsible segments of the UA if airway luminal pressure decreases to a value below what is termed the critical closing pressure (Pcrit) and the UA dilator muscles do not respond sufficiently. At this point, inspiratory flow ceases and an *obstructive apnea* occurs. Intraluminal pressure downstream (toward the thorax) of the closed segment is equal to intrathoracic pressure during no-flow conditions. Because the

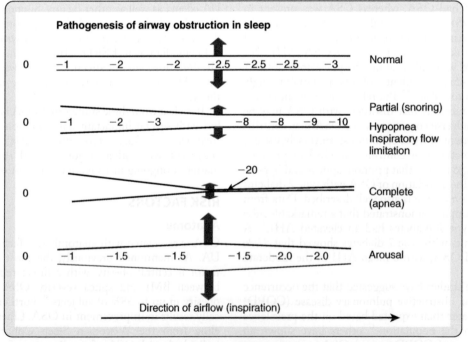

Figure 16-1 Pathogenesis of upper airway closure in OSA. The upper airway (UA) is depicted as a tube. With inspiration, there is a small gradient of pressure in the direction of flow (*upper panel*). Even though pressure is slightly negative, the airway is held open by UA dilator muscles (*orange arrow*, force represented by length of the arrow). With narrowing of the UA and some decrease in abductor force, the gradient of airway pressure is greater; flow may become limited. Vibrations in the airway produce snoring. With complete closure of the UA, no air can flow. Pressure in the airway is negative and will be equal to intrathoracic pressure (no flow condition). Closure of the UA occurs because of decreased activity of UA dilator muscles. When brainstem and other appropriate receptors sense no airflow, with hypoxia and hypercapnia, UA dilators are activated and open the airway (*bottom panel*).

patient typically generates increased inspiratory efforts against the occluded UA, exaggerated negative swings in intrathoracic pressure occur that may be quite large. If UA collapse is partial, further decreases in intraluminal pressure may not be able to overcome the increased resistance and do not result in increases in inspiratory flow, resulting in a condition of *hypopnea* or *inspiratory flow limitation* (see Chapters 5 and 14). After complete airway closure or flow limitation occurs, inspiratory flow can only be restored if UA dilator muscles respond by increasing luminal diameter, thereby decreasing resistance and restoring flow.[66]

Pcrit of the passive oropharynx varies widely among individuals. The mean value for Pcrit in a group of normal subjects has been found to be -4.35 ± 4.15 cm H_2O, whereas it was near atmospheric pressure for subjects with mild to moderate OSA (0.56 ± 1.54 cm H_2O) and above atmospheric pressure for those with severe OSA (2.23 ± 2.96 cm H_2O), although there was considerable overlap among groups.[66] For subjects with a Pcrit at or above atmospheric pressure, pharyngeal dilator muscle activity is required to maintain airway patency during wakefulness and sleep.

If anatomic and mechanical characteristics of the UA were the sole factors responsible for the occurrence of obstructive apneas and hypopneas, a strong linear relationship should exist between Pcrit and the severity of OSA as measured by AHI. However, the correlation between Pcrit and AHI is moderate at best. This indicates that factors other than mechanical or structural properties of the UA contribute to the occurrence and severity of OSA.[66,67] Primary among these nonanatomic factors is unstable or inadequate ventilatory drive during sleep to the UA dilator and ventilatory pump muscles, which can contribute to the development and perpetuation of apneas.

CLINICAL IDENTIFICATION AND ASSESSMENT

Daytime Symptoms and Functional Consequences

EDS, which is associated with persistent somnolence that may cause inappropriate or unintentional sleep episodes, is one of the most frequent symptoms of OSA, and one that adversely affects daytime function and quality of life. The presence and impact of EDS may be subtle, such as drowsiness occurring during periods of relative inactivity, or it may be more severe, with episodes of falling asleep during activities such as driving. EDS is considered to be a consequence of sleep fragmentation and has been associated with loss of vigilance. However, EDS is not universally present in all patients with OSA.[68] Further, the correlation between severity of EDS and the AHI is relatively weak.[68,69] Other factors such as nocturnal IH, autonomic dysregulation, and OSA related comorbidities such as obesity, cardiovascular disease, diabetes, and depression may also contribute to EDS.[70-73] It is worth emphasizing that the absence of a complaint of EDS does not reliably discriminate between patients with and without OSA.[74] Sleepiness may not be directly recognized by many patients who instead perceive their symptoms as fatigue. In clinical practice, EDS is often subjectively quantified using the Epworth Sleepiness Scale.[75]

EDS increases the risk for cognitive dysfunction, poor performance, injury, and motor vehicle accidents (MVAs). Despite objective evidence of EDS, some patients might not recognize impairment of performance, including driving ability, because

of sleepiness.[76] It is worth noting that the term *excessive daytime sleepiness* (EDS) is somewhat of a misnomer because excessive somnolence can be very problematic in night-shift workers, with similar adverse consequences as somnolence during the day.

OSA is also associated with reduced quality of life as measured by general and disease specific QOL scales. The Functional Outcomes of Sleep Questionnaire is a QOL assessment tool sensitive to the impact of sleep disorders and excessive sleepiness and is often used to measure the impact of OSA and its treatment.[77] Objective evidence of sleepiness, including reduced sleep latency on the Maintenance of Wakefulness Test or the Multiple Sleep Latency Test, may also be demonstrated, especially in patients with moderate to severe OSA.[78]

Deficits in Cognition, Vigilance, and Executive Function

Impairment of cognitive function may occur in OSA, possibly owing to cortical arousals, sleep fragmentation, excessive somnolence, and nocturnal IH. Deficits have also been observed in sustained attention, or vigilance, which is important for prolonged complex tasks such as driving a motor vehicle.[79-81] Further, monitoring of information, reaction time, distractibility, and processing capacity are impaired in OSA.[82] These deficits may, in part, be responsible for the twofold to sevenfold increased risk for MVAs observed in OSA.[83] Crashes, or near misses, may be caused by sleepiness, inattention, fatigue, or micro-sleep episodes that result in failure to respond rapidly and appropriately.[84,85] Some studies have found a dose-response relationship between the severity of OSA and MVA risk. However, prediction of driving risk in individual patients is not precise.[85] Deficits in cognitive function, vigilance, somnolence, and other sequelae of OSA may also contribute to poor performance in the workplace (absenteeism, presenteeism) and work-related injuries.[86]

Executive function, which encompasses cognitive processes responsible for problem solving, flexibility, decision making, and initiating appropriate responses and actions, may also be impaired in OSA. In addition, deficits in memory have been associated with OSA, although not all studies have demonstrated such an effect. The underlying mechanisms responsible for impairment in executive function and memory may be related to sleepiness and attention deficits as well as to neuronal damage from oxidant stress related to IH in the prefrontal cortex and hippocampus.[87] Improvements in memory, attention, and executive function observed after CPAP therapy for OSA have been correlated with increases in gray matter volume in these regions.[87]

Mood Disorders

A higher than expected prevalence of mood disorders has been observed in OSA. A Veterans Administration study showed that 21.8% of OSA patients had major depression, whereas 16.7% had anxiety disorder.[88] Newly diagnosed OSA patients are twice as likely to develop depression within 1 year compared with controls.[89] Conversely, investigations of patients with major depression demonstrated an increased prevalence of OSA. The association between OSA and depression is strengthened by studies which showed that CPAP therapy results in sustained improvement in depression scores, particularly in patients with moderate to severe OSA.[90,91] However, cross-sectional studies have generally not demonstrated an association of measures of apnea severity with depressive symptoms.[92]

Sleep-Related Signs and Symptoms

The classic sleep-related sign of OSA, as observed by a bed partner, is loud snoring alternating with periods of silence, associated with paradoxical movement of the chest and abdomen, terminated by a loud gasp or snort. A meta-analysis of community and sleep center cohorts with documented OSA showed that a complaint of gasping or choking during sleep was the most useful clinical predictor of OSA (likelihood ratio, 3.3; 95% CI, 2.1 to 4.6).[74] Snoring is also very common, with a prevalence of 35% in a population-based survey of persons 30 to 70 years old in Spain; importantly, an isolated complaint of snoring is not a useful predictor of OSA.[93] In contrast, the absence of snoring makes OSA less likely. Other common symptoms of OSA include awakening with a dry mouth, which may reflect mouth breathing, restless sleep, and nocturnal diaphoresis.

Nocturia may also be seen in OSA.[94] A cross-sectional analysis of the SHHS demonstrated an independent association between the AHI and prevalence of nocturia. Nocturia was also associated with disturbed sleep and with subjective complaints of daytime somnolence.[95] Increased intraabdominal pressure during obstructive apneas, confusion associated with arousals, and increased secretion of atrial natriuretic peptide are proposed mechanisms contributing to nocturia and nocturnal enuresis.[96]

Complaints of nocturnal gastroesophageal reflux (GER) are often reported in OSA. In support of an association between GER and OSA, 24-hour esophageal pH monitoring demonstrated episodes of decreased esophageal pH in 80% of OSA subjects during sleep; CPAP therapy reduced reflux events.[97] The common association of OSA with GER may be a result of large decreases in intrathoracic pressure occurring during obstructed inspiratory efforts, with increases in intraabdominal pressure, that may contribute to GER; alternatively, obesity, which increases risk for hiatal hernia, may be the primary factor leading to this association.[98]

Morning headaches are sometimes reported in OSA. The International Classification of Headache Disorders II describes OSA-related headaches as "bilateral, with a pressing quality, not accompanied by nausea, photophobia or phonophobia."[99] Headache is present on awakening and usually resolves within 30 minutes; morning headaches are eliminated with effective treatment of OSA.[99] A recent study demonstrated that 11.8% of OSA patients had morning headache. However, morning headache without OSA is also common, with a prevalence of 4.6% in this cohort.[100]

Physical Findings

As previously mentioned, obesity is the most commonly observed risk factor for OSA. Suspicion for OSA should be raised if the BMI is more than 30 kg/m^2.[101] Patients with OSA have a larger neck circumference that those without this disorder. The average neck circumference (measured at the superior border of the cricothyroid membrane in the upright position) was 43.7 ± 4.5 cm in a series of patients with OSA and 39.6 ± 4.5 cm in those without OSA ($P = .0001$).[102] A neck circumference at least 40 cm has a sensitivity of 61% and a specificity of 93% for OSA regardless of gender.[103] Neck circumference, as well as neck circumference corrected for

height, is a correlate of increased visceral fat, which is associated with OSA.

Physical examination should assess nasal patency, oropharyngeal anatomy, and craniofacial structure. Increased nasopharyngeal resistance, due to nasal septal deviation, turbinate hypertrophy, polyps, or other obstructing lesions, is associated with OSA.[104] The soft palate, uvula, base of tongue, and tonsils should be observed with attention to their size, length, and overall volume in relation to the oropharynx. A low-lying or redundant soft palate and uvula, often with edema or erythema due to vibratory trauma and inflammation from snoring, are frequently present in OSA. Both the Mallampati classification, which assesses oropharyngeal anatomy with the tongue protruded, and the Friedman classification, which is a similar assessment but without tongue protrusion, are commonly used to stage oropharyngeal crowding.[105] These scoring systems provide a numeric scale that grades the size of, and relationship among, the soft palate and uvula, lateral tonsillar pillars, and base of tongue. In addition, tonsil size should also be assessed. Anatomic crowding of the oropharynx has been shown to be related to the presence and severity of OSA, but this finding in and of itself has limited value for predicting presence of OSA (likelihood ratio range, 1.4 to 1.6).[103]

It is also important to assess craniofacial anatomy. In particular, mandibular retrognathia, or retrusion of the mandible, narrows the posterior air space and can increase the propensity for airway collapse during sleep. A high arched and narrow hard palate may also predispose to OSA. Assessment of dentition may also be useful to identify a narrowed posterior air space. In particular, the presence of *overjet*, defined as displacement of the mandibular teeth posteriorly compared with the maxillary teeth, is indicative of a small oral cavity that may result in posterior displacement of the base of the tongue, which narrows the retroglossal airway.[106]

ASSESSMENT

In-Laboratory or Full Polysomnographic Sleep Testing

The diagnosis of sleep apnea should be confirmed objectively by sleep testing. The "gold standard" test is PSG, a multichannel assessment of physiologic variables performed in a laboratory equipped with proper sensors, trained personnel, and a standardized way of recording results, with a qualified individual to interpret the study. Recorded variables usually include electroencephalogram (EEG), electromyogram (EMG) of the submentalis muscle, electrooculogram (EOG), a measure of airflow (usually sensors by the nose and mouth), a measure of respiratory effort (chest wall and abdominal movement, EMG of parasternal muscles, or changes in esophageal pressure), a measure of oxygen saturation (pulse oximetry), pulse rate, electrocardiogram (ECG), body position, EMG of legs (anterior tibialis muscle, for leg movements), and snoring (usually by microphone). Many laboratories also record continuous video imaging of the patient both for medical-legal reasons and to observe parasomnias. Table 16-3 contains a list of some of the most common variables recorded during in-laboratory PSG testing; a typical PSG epoch with recordings of these parameters is presented in Figure 16-2. More recently, efforts have been made to simplify the use of PSG for the diagnosis of sleep related breathing disorders. These systems measure fewer variables and are

Table 16-3   Commonly Recorded Parameters During In-Laboratory Polysomnography

Parameter Recorded	Purpose	Other
EEG (several channels) EMG of submentalis (other facial as indicated) EOG	Sleep staging	Usually standard 10 to 20 system for EEG—may also be used for seizure detection (EEG) if suitable montage used
Oronasal airflow Tidal swings in CO_2 measured at the mouth Respiratory effort (rib cage and abdominal movement)	Sleep-related abnormal breathing events	Nasal cannula pressure for hypopnea and flow limitation detection Thermistor for apnea detection
Pulse oximetry	O_2 saturation, pulse	Some definitions of DBEs depend on saturation, quantifies oxygenation at night
Microphone	Snoring	Some systems use perturbation in airflow
Body position sensor	Body position	
EMG: submental and pretibial	Sleep onset, REM onset, abnormal limb movements	
ECG	Rate and rhythm abnormalities	Usually precordial only; may detect rate of rhythm disturbances or changes in ST-T segments
CO_2: end-tidal, transcutaneous	Changes in alveolar ventilation	

DBE, Disordered breathing event; ECG, electrocardiogram; EEG, electroencephalogram; EMG, electromyogram; EOG, electrooculogram. Other variables often recorded during in-laboratory sleep studies include audio-videography and actigraphy.

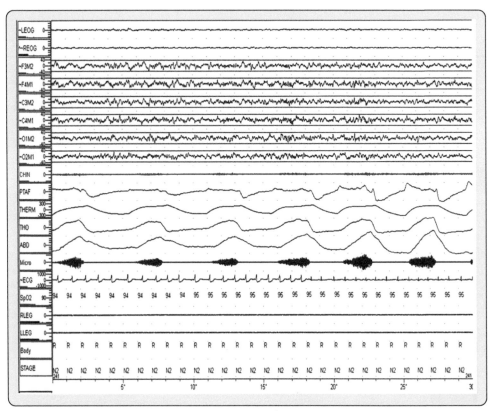

Figure 16-2 Sample montage for polysomnography. LEOG and REOG, Left and right electrooculogram; F3M2–O2M1, 6 electroencephalogram leads; Chin, electromyogram of submentalis muscle; PTAF, nasal airflow by nasal pressure; THERM, oronasal airflow estimated using a thermistor; THO and ABD, rib cage and abdominal movement by respiratory inductance plethysmograph belts; MICRO, snoring detected by a microphone taped to the neck (note the snoring); ECG, electrocardiogram; SpO2, blood oxygen obsturation of hemoglobin by pulse oximetry; RLEG and LLEG, electromyogram of the right and left legs (anterior tibialis); BODY, body position; Stage, stage of sleep (hand scored). There are timing marks at the bottom; this is a 30-second epoch.

suitable for portable or out-of-center sleep testing (OCST) under certain conditions.

Technical specifications and acceptable derivations for in-laboratory PSG testing are specified in the American Academy of Sleep Medicine (AASM) scoring manual,[107] as well as elsewhere in this volume, as are the visual rules for sleep staging, respiratory events, limb movement events, and other "events" of note. We briefly review some of the specifications for recording respiratory "events" during PSG. Airflow is usually recorded using oronasal thermistor and nasal air pressure. Nasal air pressure, measured using small cannulas in the nose, is a more accurate approximation of airflow.[108] Thermistors placed by the nose and mouth do not measure flow but indicate airflow as a change in temperature. Thus they cannot quantify flow and instead record the presence or absence of airflow. In addition, if the thermistor moves toward or away from the nose and mouth, it will record changes in the signal that do not reflect actual flow. Tidal CO_2 is also sometimes used to assess flow. It is possible to get a true quantitative measurement of airflow with a tight-fitting facemask with a pneumotachograph. However, because of discomfort, this technique is not useful on a routine basis. Further, detection of respiratory events called *respiratory event–related arousals* (RERAs; discussed later; also see Chapter 14) depends on detection of inspiratory flow limitation. As can be seen in Figure 16-3, this is not possible with thermistors or any other sensor that simply records the presence or absence of flow (e.g., tidal CO_2 monitoring). Therefore preference should be given to using nasal air pressure recording. Alternatives to

measurement of airflow include the summed chest and abdomen signal from respiratory impedance belts, use of the mask pressure signal during positive airway pressure (PAP) titrations, and various indexes of respiration derived from pulse and finger plethysmographic techniques for OCST.

The AASM scoring manual[107] recommends that the primary means for detecting apnea is absence of the oronasal thermistor signal, although alternates are suggested. The manual recommends that the primary method for identifying hypopnea should be nasal pressure, although alternates are also suggested. During PAP titrations, it is recommended to use the change in PAP mask pressure as the primary flow signal. The manual recommends the use of esophageal manometry or respiratory impedance plethysmography thoracoabdominal belts as the primary measure of respiratory effort, although belts that measure changes in resistance are also acceptable. For detection of snoring, microphones, piezoelectric sensors, or perturbations in nasal air pressure are all considered acceptable. The reader is referred to this publication for more detailed analysis.

The severity of sleep apnea is usually defined in terms of frequency of respiratory "events" (see later). This implies that counting discrete occurrences adequately characterizes the severity of disease. In general, a greater frequency of such events per hour of sleep is associated with a more severe clinical syndrome. However, this is not a tight correlation because many patients with a "severe" respiratory event index have minimal symptoms, whereas many with a "mild" index have severe sleepiness. In general, severity of OSA as estimated

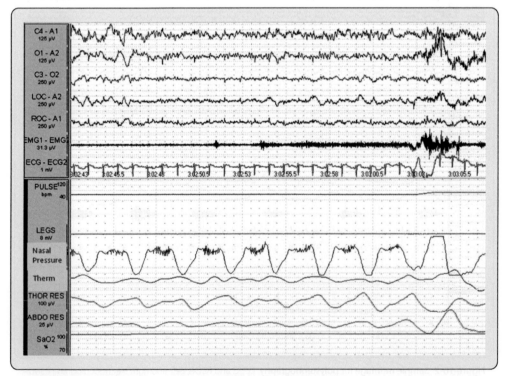

Figure 16-3 Respiratory event–related arousal (RERA). Comparison of airflow measured by oronasal thermistor (Therm) with that measured by nasal pressure (NP). For the nasal pressure signal the inspiratory direction is up, expiratory direction down. Note that with the nasal pressure transducer, inspiratory flow limitation (flattening of the signal and snoring) is readily detected. Note the arousal following this event (electroencephalogram [EEG] and electromyogram [EMG]). The first three channels are EEG, left EOG (LOC), and right EOG (ROC). EMG1-EMG; submentalis EMG; ECG, electrocardiogram; pulse is derived from the pulse oximeter; Legs, pretibial EMG.

Table 16-4 Definitions of Disordered Breathing Events in Sleep[107]

Duration	Event Type	Change in Airflow	Respiratory Effort	Associated Phenomena	Other
10-second duration measured from nadir preceding the first reduced breath to beginning of first breath approximating baseline	Obstructive apnea	Decrease ≥90%	Continues or increases throughout the entire period	NA	Oronasal thermistor (diagnostic study), PAP device (titration)
	Central apnea		Absent inspiratory effort throughout the entire period		
	Mixed apnea		Absent inspiratory effort initially with resumption in latter part of DBE		
	Hypopnea	Decrease by 30% to 90%	Continues	AASM: 3% desaturation *or* terminal arousal CMS: 4% desaturation	May score as: "Obstructive" = snoring, inspiratory flattening of flow (nasal pressure), thoracoabdominal paradox "Central" = none of above obstructive criteria
	RERA (AASM only)	Inspiratory flattening (<30%)	Increased effort	Terminal arousal	Crescendo snoring common
NA	Hypoventilation	NA	NA	NA	Increased P_{CO_2} to >55 torr for ≥10 minutes *or* ≥10 torr increased in P_{CO_2} c/w awake to >50 torr for ≥10 minutes
NA	Cheyne-Stokes breathing	NA	NA	NA	≥3 consecutive central apneas/ hypopneas separated by crescendo/ decrescendo change in airflow with cycle length >40 seconds *and* ≥5 central apneas/ hypopneas per hour sleep with crescendo/ decrescendo pattern over ≥2 hours monitoring

AASM, American Academy of Sleep Medicine; CMS, Centers for Medicare and Medicare Services; DBE, disordered breathing event; PAP, positive airway pressure; P_{CO_2} measured from arterial line, end-tidal, or transcutaneously; RERA, respiratory event–related arousal.

from accepted techniques of respiratory event indexes appears to be a reliable predictor of neurocognitive changes such as sleepiness and vigilance.

Sleep-related respiratory events have been defined in various ways. In adults, a respiratory event must last at least 10 seconds. This follows the definition of the original workers in the field who reasoned that this interval would encompass at least two breaths for the average adult.[4-11] There are other requirements for scoring specific types of sleep-related respiratory events. Table 16-4 summarizes the criteria for scoring disordered breathing events in adults as elaborated by the current version of the AASM scoring.[107] Table 16-5 lists commonly used definitions of OSA severity. The definitions are those of the Centers for Medicare and Medicaid Services.[3] Examples of PSG recordings of disordered breathing events are presented in Figure 16-3 (RERAs), Figure 16-4

Table 16-5 Severity Criteria for Obstructive Sleep Apnea*

Severity Definition	Apnea-Hypopnea Index	Coverage (CMS)
Mild	5–14	With comorbidities and symptoms[†]
Moderate	15–30	Yes
Severe	>30	Yes

*Definitions per Centers for Medicare and Medicaid Services (CMS).[3]
[†]Comorbidities that allow for coverage of "mild" disease in Medicare recipients include documentation of excessive sleepiness, impaired cognition, mood disorders, insomnia, hypertension, ischemic heart disease, history of stroke.
Note: Medicare will cover treatment for OSA when the diagnosis and severity classification were determined by home sleep testing as well as in-laboratory testing.

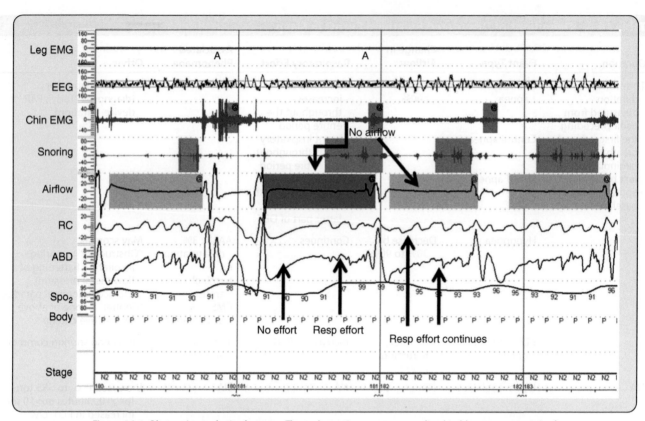

Figure 16-4 Obstructive and mixed apneas. Three obstructive apneas are outlined in blue-green, one mixed apnea in gray. Note for the obstructive apneas and the latter part of the mixed apnea, there is total cessation of airflow but chest wall movement continues. Note that the initial part of the mixed apnea shows no chest wall movement and resembles a central apnea (see Figure 16-5). Postapnea arousals are clearly seen (A). Airflow is measured by nasal air pressure. RC/ABD, Rib cage and abdominal movement by respiratory impedance pneumography; SpO_2, oxygen saturation of hemoglobin (pulse oximeter); Body, body position; Stage, stage of sleep. *Vertical lines* represent 30-second epochs.

(obstructive and mixed apneas), Figure 16-5 (central apneas), and Figure 16-6 (hypopneas).

Out-of-Center Sleep Testing

Although the previous parameters for assessing sleep-related respiratory events primarily pertain to in-laboratory, technologist attended PSG, a number of techniques have been developed to optimize the detection of sleep-related respiratory events outside of the laboratory, usually using a limited number of recording channels. Out-of-center sleep testing (OCST) offers a number of advantages compared with in-laboratory PSG. First, the initial costs are generally less than those of the state-of-the-art in-laboratory study, and primarily for this reason numerous insurance carriers require OCST for reimbursement in the initial evaluation of many patients with suspected OSA. Further, OCST offers a more rapid method of assessing the many patients with undiagnosed OSA who have limited access to, or who are reluctant to undergo, in-laboratory PSG.[109] However, Chervin and colleagues[110] performed a careful cost utility analysis, comparing in-laboratory PSG, OCST, and no testing (with treatment based on clinical characteristics). Their outcomes were based on costs per quality-adjusted life years over 5 years. These authors concluded that standard in-lab PSG provides greater quality-adjusted life years over 5 years than either OCST or no testing. Reuveni modeled costs of in-laboratory PSG

versus OCST, accounting for the published technical failure rate of OCST and the published European costs for PSG.[111] They demonstrated that there was no long-term cost saving using OCST versus in-laboratory PSG.

Recent studies have directly compared health outcomes between OCST and in-laboratory PSG in selected patients. In 2010, Skomro and colleagues performed a randomized clinical trial of OCST compared with in-laboratory PSG in diagnosis and management of OSA in patients with a high clinical suspicion for the disorder.[112] All patients were evaluated and treated by physicians facile in interpretation of sleep studies as well as in clinical identification and management of sleep disorders. Exclusion criteria included concomitant cardiopulmonary morbidities and suspicion of other sleep disorders. Clinically relevant outcomes included quality of life, CPAP treatment adherence, blood pressure, and sleep quality after 4 weeks of therapy. There were no significant differences in any of these outcomes between OCST and in-laboratory PSG.

Overall, the relative advantages and disadvantages of OCST compared with in-laboratory testing in the evaluation and management of OSA require further definition. Approximately one third of OSA patients have a concomitant sleep disorder, of which approximately two thirds require treatment.[113] Thus patients need to be evaluated by a professional skilled in the evaluation and management of sleep disorders,

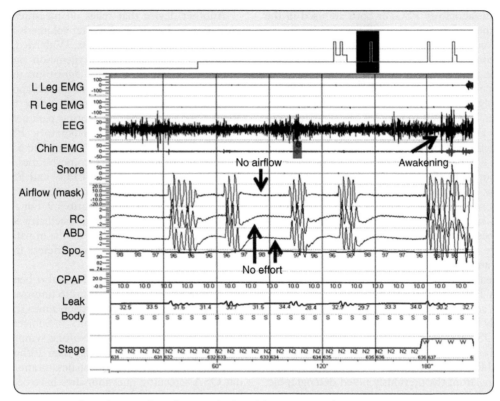

Figure 16-5 Central apneas. Central apneas developed during titration of continuous positive airway pressure (CPAP). Note absence of airflow (measured from the CPAP mask) and absence of respiratory effort (rib cage, abdominal movement measured by respiratory impedance pneumograph belts). RC, Rib cage signal; ABD, abdominal signal, snoring (absent here) measured from a microphone taped to the neck; Spo₂, oxygen saturation of hemoglobin measured from a pulse oximeter; Leak, estimation of leak from the CPAP mask; Body, body position; Stage, stage of sleep (hand scored). The *vertical lines* represent 30-second epochs. Note that after the series of central apneas, there is an arousal, and respiration resumes.

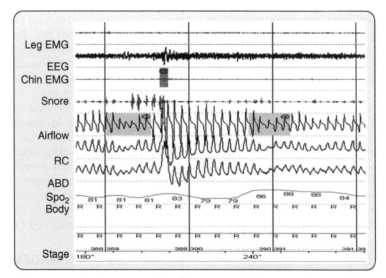

Figure 16-6 Hypopnea. In this diagnostic study airflow is measured using a nasal pressure cannula. The hypopneas are outlined in gray on the airflow signal. The first event shows a terminal arousal and 4% O₂ desaturation (the nadir of the event-associated desaturation is seen approximately 25 seconds after the arousal). The second event does not show an arousal, but there is an O₂ desaturation of 4%. The patient is in REM sleep. Body, Body position; RC/ABD, rib cage and abdominal movement by respiratory impedance pneumography; Spo₂, oxygen saturation of hemoglobin (pulse oximeter); Stage, stage of sleep. *Vertical lines* represent 30-second epochs.

whether OCST, in-laboratory PSG, or both are used in the diagnostic assessment. Incorporation of test results into a complete evaluation and management plan that encompasses all sleep-related complaints is essential. The clinician should also be aware that sleep testing is currently rated into levels of complexity. Type 1 is the classic in-laboratory full PSG as discussed previously, including measures of airflow, respiratory effort, oxygenation, EEG, EOG, and EMG to allow for sleep staging. Type 2 is an out-of-laboratory portable study essentially equivalent to the in-laboratory study (minimum of seven parameters). Type 3 is an unattended portable recording measuring at least four channels: heart rate, oxygen saturation, respiratory airflow, respiratory effort, but no sleep staging. Type 4 is an unattended portable study, measuring a minimum of three channels such as heart rate, oxygen saturation, and respiratory analysis. Appropriate documentation from a regional Medicare carrier should be consulted for details regarding coding, and the policies of specific insurance carriers should be consulted regarding requirements for allowing classical in-laboratory PSG versus portable OCST.

Even with the advent of reliable OCST, such testing still requires a relatively high level of instrumentation and analysis. Prescreening for OSA has the potential to improve sensitivity and specificity of both OCST and in-laboratory PSG, or even eliminate the need for such testing, taking into account pretest probability accruing from the previously noted demographic, physiologic, and clinical symptoms, signs, and conditions associated with OSA. A number of workers have therefore attempted to develop screening tools and techniques, some assessing physiologic parameters and some using self-administered questionnaires, with or without inclusion of key physical traits.

Early attempts at physiologic screening for OSA were based on simple pulse oximetry.[114] These devices generally relied on estimating the number of 3% or 4% drops in oxygen saturation. However, problems with validity and sensitivity remained. Newer techniques make use of the known coupling between cardiovascular (pulse, autonomic function, arterial tone) and respiratory phenomena. For example, Liu and colleagues used a sophisticated transform to analyze signals from a single ECG lead to detect breathing and sleep-related disordered breathing events.[115] Their analyses resulted in acceptable sensitivity and specificity (area under the receiver-operator curve of 0.79) for OSA screening using a single ECG electrode. An index called the *temporal variability of dominant frequency* was well correlated to AHI and could distinguish among sleep-related breathing events of various severities.

Peripheral arterial tonometry (PAT) has also been developed as an OSA screening tool. Bar and colleagues evaluated such a device (WatchPAT, Itamar Medical, Caesarea, Israel) placed on the finger that measured pulse oximetry and volume of the finger.[116] The abrupt arousals associated with termination of the obstructive events are associated with bursts of sympathetic discharge causing vasoconstriction that decreases volume of the digit. In addition to PAT and standard oximetry, the device recorded pulse rate and movement (actigraphy). The respiratory disturbance index (RDI) measured using PAT was highly correlated with RDI measured during in-laboratory PSG (the area under the receiver-operating curve was 0.82 and 0.87 for thresholds of RDI = 10/hour and RDI = 20/hour, respectively).

Another device that relies on measures of pulse, oxygen saturation and peripheral digital volume is the photoplethysmograph (PPG; Morpheus Ox, WideMed, Herzliya, Israel). Digital volume, pulse, and oxygenation signals are recorded and imputed into proprietary algorithms that generate clinically relevant respiratory waveforms and approximation of the sleep-wake state. A recent study using the AASM 2012 apnea-hypopnea detection scoring parameters validated this device against standard in-laboratory PSG.[117] A unique feature of the study was that among the 65 subjects, 19 had significant cardiopulmonary comorbidities. There was excellent correlation between the PPG- and PSG-derived AHI. For AHI of more than 5/hour, sensitivity was 80%, specificity 86%, and positive likelihood ratio 5.9. For AHI of more than 15/hour, sensitivity was 70%, specificity 91%, and positive likelihood ratio 7.83. Further, results in patients with cardiopulmonary morbidities were not different from the rest of the subjects.

Numerous questionnaires have also been designed in an attempt to use patient symptoms to improve the pretest probability for OSA. The Harvard sleep apnea screening questionnaire was one such attempt.[118] Subjects with essential hypertension were screened. No one symptom was found to be predictive of an AHI greater than 10/hour, although loud snoring was predictive of oxygen desaturation in sleep. Numerous OSA screening questionnaires have been developed that incorporate symptoms (e.g., snoring, snorting, witnessed apneas, excessive sleepiness), demographics (e.g., gender, age), physical traits (e.g., BMI, crowding of the oropharynx, neck circumference), and important c-morbidities (e.g., hypertension). Clinical prediction formulas, some requiring sophisticated calculations and even computer assistance, have been developed that assign weights to the various factors. Questionnaires that have been validated in specific populations include the Berlin Questionnaire, designed for use in primary care settings,[119] and the STOP-BANG questionnaire, designed for preoperative screening.[120] Other such instruments include the Wisconsin questionnaire[121] and the questionnaire of Haraldsson and colleagues.[122] Overall, it appears that such questionnaires have the greatest potential to screen patients at high risk for OSA. Further, validation studies indicate that the applicability of any such questionnaire is limited to the specific populations studied.

The predictive value of the clinical examination has also been assessed in an attempt to identify features on the clinical examination with the greatest value for predicting a "positive" PSG.[73] No one single symptom or sign appears sufficiently predictive of OSA, if defined as AHI greater than or equal to 10/hour, including snoring, subjective sleepiness, and morning headache. Rather, a combination of signs and symptoms, including neck circumference, habitual snoring, systemic hypertension, and bed partner report of nocturnal gasping or choking appears to optimally identify patients most likely to have sleep-study documented OSA.[123]

PRINCIPLES OF MANAGEMENT

The adverse consequences of OSA pose an enormous health and economic burden.[124,125] Effective treatment requires a patient-centered chronic disease management approach that goes beyond initial diagnosis and therapy prescription. Monitoring and enhancing adherence to therapy, providing alternative therapeutic modalities when needed, and managing comorbid sleep disorders are necessary to optimize long-term sleep-related health outcomes.

CPAP, which pressurizes the UA to prevent its collapse during sleep, remains the mainstay of therapy for OSA. Initiation and prescription of CPAP is usually accomplished by in-laboratory PSG CPAP titration, which determines CPAP pressure requirements during all stages of sleep in all sleep positions. Autotitrating positive airway pressure (APAP) devices assess inspiratory airflow and adjust positive airway pressure automatically to maintain normal inspiratory flow patterns. Data supporting noninferiority of APAP for initiation of CPAP therapy are limited.[126] Patients with comorbid cardiopulmonary disorders, especially those with obesity hypoventilation syndrome, central sleep apnea, Cheyne-Stokes breathing, or COPD, are not candidates for APAP therapy.

Multiple studies have evaluated the effect of CPAP on EDS. Most placebo-controlled studies demonstrated improvement in subjective measures of daytime somnolence, whereas data are mixed with regard to objective measures. A randomized placebo-controlled study with more than 1000 participants demonstrated that CPAP improved both subjective and objective measures of daytime sleepiness, especially in severe OSA (AHI >30/hour).[127] Similarly, clinical trials of the effects of CPAP on neurobehavioral and cognitive performance, as well as on overall quality of life, are mixed, with some studies demonstrating benefit.[128] A recent randomized placebo-controlled clinical trial evaluated the effects of CPAP on daytime sleepiness and quality of life in patients with mild to moderate OSA with a complaint of daytime somnolence, a patient type that represents a large portion of the OSA population. CPAP resulted in greater improvement in functional outcomes, including quality of life, subjective daytime sleepiness, and mood, compared with sham CPAP.[127] The optimal duration of nightly CPAP use necessary to achieve improvement in functional outcomes has also been a matter of investigation. In a multicenter effectiveness study that used both subjective and objective measures of daytime somnolence and quality of life as outcome measures, a greater percentage of patients achieved improvements in outcomes with longer nightly duration of CPAP use, up to 7 hours/night. Although the mean nightly duration of CPAP use in this trial was 4.7 ± 2.2 hours, a substantial minority of patients demonstrated benefit with a shorter duration of nightly CPAP use (even <2 hours/night), whereas some subjects exhibited residual sleepiness with more than 7 hours of use per night. Thus assessment of optimal CPAP use should rely not only on hours of nightly use but also on assessment of relevant treatment outcomes.[128]

The efficacy of CPAP is limited by suboptimal adherence. Many studies have evaluated measures to improve adherence to CPAP therapy. Technologic improvements in CPAP delivery, such as APAP, expiratory pressure reduction, heated tube humidification, and other modalities that adjust the contour of the pressure waveform, have contributed somewhat to improvements in comfort but have not solved the overall adherence problem with CPAP.[129] Other measures to enhance adherence include educational and supportive efforts, as well as cognitive behavioral therapy, that may help acclimatize patients to CPAP and encourage nightly use. A recent review indicated that these interventions can improve CPAP adherence.[130]

The identification of *treatment emergent central sleep apnea*, which is a form of sleep breathing disorder in which central apneas emerge during CPAP therapy disrupting sleep, may also limit efficacy and tolerability of CPAP. Although the pathophysiology of this form of central sleep apnea has not been fully elucidated, it may occur as a result of ventilatory instability during sleep. Cheyne-Stokes breathing, which is not well treated with CPAP, is common in patients with systolic heart failure and may contribute to failure of CPAP therapy in this population. However, while effective in reducing disordered breathing events, the newer modality of adaptive servo ventilation is no longer recommend in patients with heart failure and predominantly central sleep apnea due to an observed increase in mortality with this therapy.[132]

Mandibular advancement oral appliance therapy can be considered either as first-line therapy for mild to moderate OSA or as an alternative to CPAP. Improvement in somnolence, vigilance, and neurocognitive performance has been observed with this modality. Interestingly, the improvement in functional outcomes achieved with oral appliances is similar in magnitude to that seen with CPAP, despite persistence of mild degrees of OSA.[133,134] It is important to perform follow-up PSG to assess efficacy of the appliance because subjective reports of improvement may not reliably predict the AHI with therapy. In a study of patients with mild to severe OSA, only 65% of the cohort who had subjective symptomatic improvement with oral appliance therapy achieved an AHI of 10/hour or less on follow-up PSG. The degree of mandibular advancement was then increased in the incomplete responders. An additional 30% of the cohort achieved an AHI of 10/hour after this secondary adjustment, indicating the importance of the follow-up PSG.[135] Better predictors of response to oral appliances, as well as accurate determination of the optimal degree of mandibular advancement, may improve utility and efficacy of this modality. Remotely titratable appliances have been developed, in which the degree of mandibular advancement can be titrated during PSG, that may help identify patients who respond to this modality and accurately determine the optimal degree of mandibular advancement.[136] In addition, recent data suggest that response to oral appliance therapy may be predicted by visualization of velopharyngeal widening with mandibular advancement during awake nasopharyngoscopy.[137]

Nasal expiratory positive pressure (nEPAP) is another alternative therapy for OSA that provides positive pressure during end expiration when the cross-sectional area of the UA and dilator muscle activity are at their nadir. By increasing expiratory airflow resistance using a small valve taped to the nostrils, nEPAP is created that prevents airway collapse. In addition, increases in lung volume have been observed with nEPAP, which may reduce UA collapsibility by increasing caudal traction on the UA. Significant decreases in the AHI have been observed in efficacy trials, although tolerability and compliance remain to be fully established.[138,139]

UA surgery, including nasal septoplasty, uvulopalatopharyngoplasty (UPPP), tonsillectomy, and tongue advancement procedures, as well as maxillomandibular advancement surgery, are alternative therapeutic modalities for OSA. In addition to patient preference and consideration of medical comorbidities, UA anatomy should be evaluated when assessing suitability of a surgical approach. A clinical staging system, based on observation of the oropharynx, such as that offered by

Friedman,[105] which classifies palate position, tonsil size, and BMI, can be a useful predictor of outcome of UPPP and tonsillectomy. These authors showed that the best response is achieved when the inferior border of the palate is above the base of the tongue, with enlarged tonsils and BMI of 40 kg/m^2 or lower.

Imaging with nasopharyngoscopy can more directly assess UA anatomy than clinical observation of the oropharynx. Dynamic behavior of the UA can also be observed during a Müller maneuver. Although identification of a velopharyngeal site of collapse during a Müller maneuver was originally shown to predict response to UPPP, subsequent studies demonstrated a low predictive value.[140,141] Recently, drug-induced sleep endoscopy has been introduced in which the UA is evaluated during propofol-induced sedation in an operating room setting. The relationship of drug-induced sleep endoscopy findings to UA behavior during sleep and their relevance to UA surgical operative planning and outcomes has not been established.[142,143]

Clinical experience has shown that, although nasal surgical procedures, including septoplasty and turbinectomy, usually do not achieve resolution of OSA, they may be useful to improve tolerability of CPAP in patients with nasal obstruction. Although response to a single UA surgical procedure may be limited, a multilevel approach to the UA, including UPPP followed by genioglossal suspension or advancement with hyoid myotomy, has achieved improved success rates.[144] Modifications of current UA soft tissue surgical procedures, as well as development of new approaches, may ultimately improve outcomes. Maxillary-mandibular advancement osteotomy is also performed in the surgical management of OSA with reported high success rates. The resultant increase in volume of the UA has been correlated with reduction in the AHI. Surgical planning using three-dimensional UA imaging may also improve the success of these surgical procedures.[145,146]

Positional therapy may also be useful in selected patients in whom disordered breathing events occur predominantly during supine sleep. Avoidance of supine sleep can lead to reduction in the AHI in such cases, particularly with use of positioning devices, which are typically worn around the chest and prevent inadvertent supine sleep.[147]

Because OSA severity is sensitive to weight loss, weight reduction programs and bariatric surgery are valuable treatment modalities. Although most studies have shown that bariatric surgery is associated with resolution or improvement of OSA in most cases, it is important to recognize that OSA can persist in some cases after substantial weight loss. Because the correlation of subjective daytime sleepiness with AHI severity is relatively weak, follow-up PSG, rather than reliance on symptoms, is important to determine whether further OSA therapy is needed despite weight loss.[148,149]

Electrical stimulation of the hypoglossal nerve is a recently introduced modality that was developed in response to the observation that inadequate neural activation of the UA dilator muscles is a key factor in the pathophysiology of OSA. The stimulator can deliver phasic electrical pulses to the hypoglossal nerve at the onset of inspiration augmenting genioglossal inspiratory activity. Efficacy trials have included patients with moderate to severe OSA with BMI of less than 40 kg/m^2. Some of the studies excluded patients with concentric retropalatal collapse. Most of the trials demonstrated more than 50% improvement in the AHI, which was sustained during long-term follow-up.[150-152] Although experience remains limited, hypoglossal nerve stimulation may be a useful alternative for selected patients.

Future approaches to treatment may be developed based on identification of individual "phenotypes" of OSA. Recent studies have demonstrated interindividual differences in the pathophyphysiology of OSA. In some patients, instability of ventilatory control during sleep, measured as elevated "loop gain," is a predominant factor. Loop gain is a dimensionless value that quantifies response of the ventilatory system to decrements in ventilation such as those induced by UA obstruction. High loop gain is associated with an excessive ventilatory response to apnea (or hypopnea) that contributes to ventilatory instability and perpetuates recurrent apneas. A low arousal threshold, which destabilizes sleep, has also been shown to contribute to ventilatory instability during sleep. In other patients, inadequate activation of UA dilator muscles in response to obstruction is a predominant pathophysiologic feature. Anatomic factors, with a highly collapsible UA, indicated by a high (less negative or positive) Pcrit, is identified as the major factor contributing to OSA in other patients.[151]

Understanding OSA phenotypes may help individualize treatment. Mechanically based therapies including CPAP, mandibular advancement oral appliances, or surgical interventions are the best therapeutic options for patients in whom anatomic factors, with a highly collapsible UA, play a major role. Patients with high loop gain, or a low arousal threshold, in whom ventilatory control instability is the predominant factor, may respond to novel therapeutic measures to stabilize sleep and ventilatory control. Approaches that increase UA dilator muscle activity during sleep, such as hypoglossal nerve stimulation, may be most useful in patients that have reduced UA dilator muscle responsiveness to UA collapse. Thus thinking about OSA as a heterogeneous disorder with multiple "phenotypes" might facilitate development of new and individualized therapies.[153,154]

SUMMARY

OSA is a highly prevalent disorder and is overrepresented in populations with cardiovascular, cerebrovascular, and metabolic disease. The pathophysiologic basis of OSA is complex, with contributions from anatomic factors that narrow the UA as well as ventilatory control instability that affects neural drive to the UA and ventilatory pump muscles during sleep. The acute, repetitive physiologic perturbations during sleep that occur as a result of obstructive apneas and hypopneas include sleep fragmentation, large swings in intrathoracic pressure, increased sympathoadrenal tone, and intermittent hypoxia and reoxygenation. OSA is associated with multiple adverse systemic consequences, including excessive sleepiness, impairment of cognitive function, mood, vigilance, and performance, including driving ability. OSA is also associated with multiple cardiovascular, cerebrovascular, and metabolic disorders as well as other medical conditions. The relationship between OSA and these comorbidities may be bidirectional. Although clinical presentation can identify patients at risk for OSA, diagnosis requires objective monitoring of sleep. In-laboratory PSG testing remains the gold standard for accurate identification of OSA; however, OCST using ambulatory technology is useful in selected patients. Skilled assessment and management of this chronic disorder are necessary to ensure optimal long-term outcomes. Most studies have demonstrated improvement in daytime somnolence and quality of life with CPAP therapy for OSA. Other therapeutic modalities, including mandibular advancement oral appliances and surgical approaches to the UA, are useful alternative modalities in selected patients. Newer approaches such as hypoglossal nerve stimulation, nasal expiratory positive pressure devices, and other treatments require further investigation to establish their clinical utility. Investigational approaches that define an individual's predominant OSA phenotype may ultimately guide treatment decisions.

CLINICAL PEARL

OSA is highly prevalent, particularly in patients with comorbid cardiovascular, cerebrovascular, and metabolic disease. Because OSA independently contributes to morbidity and mortality, with multisystem consequences, clinical suspicion for OSA should be a priority for clinicians, especially in patients with these comorbidities. Clinical assessment, as well as sleep testing with in-laboratory PSG, or OCST in appropriately selected and managed patients, is necessary for accurate diagnosis. Effective treatment of OSA and any comorbid sleep disorders requires a focus on optimizing sleep-related health outcomes with a chronic disease management approach.

Selected Readings

Al Mawed S, Unruh M. Diabetic kidney disease and obstructive sleep apnea: a new frontier? *Curr Opin Pulm Med* 2016;**22**(1):80–8.

Berry RB, Brooks R, Gamaldo CE, et al. for the American Academy of Sleep Medicine. *The AASM manual for the scoring of sleep and associated events: rules, terminology and technical specifications*. Version 2.2. <www.aasmnet .org>, Darien, IL: American Academy of Sleep Medicine; 2015.

Dempsey JA, Smith CA, Blain GM, et al. Role of central/peripheral chemoreceptors and their interdependence in the pathophysiology of sleep apnea. *Adv Exp Med Biol* 2012;**758**:343–9.

Owens RL, Edwards BA, Eckert DJ, et al. An integrative model of physiological traits can be used to predict obstructive sleep apnea and response to non positive airway pressure therapy. *Sleep* 2015;**38**(6):961–70.

Peppard PE, Young T, Barnet JH, et al. Increased prevalence of sleep-disordered breathing in adults. *Am J Epidemiol* 2013;**177**(9):1006–14.

Punjabi NM, Caffo BS, Goodwin JL, et al. Sleep-disordered breathing and mortality: a prospective cohort study. *PLoS Med* 2009;**6**(8):e1000132.

Rapoport DM, Sorkin B, Garay SM, et al. Reversal of the "pickwickian syndrome" by long-term use of nocturnal nasal-airway pressure. *N Engl J Med* 1982;**307**(15):931–3.

Schwab RJ, Pasirstein M, Pierson R, et al. Identification of upper airway anatomic risk factors for obstructive sleep apnea with volumetric magnetic resonance imaging. *Am J Respir Crit Care Med* 2003;**168**(5):522–30.

Strohl KP, Brown DB, Collop N, et al. An official American Thoracic Society Clinical Practice Guideline: sleep apnea, sleepiness, and driving risk in noncommercial drivers. An update of a 1994 statement. *Am J Respir Crit Care Med* 2013;**187**(11):1259–66.

Sullivan CE, Issa FG, Berthon-Jones M, et al. Reversal of obstructive sleep apnoea by continuous positive airway pressure applied through the nares. *Lancet* 1981;**1**(8225):862–5.

Terrill PI, Edwards BA, Nemati S, et al. Quantifying the ventilatory control contribution to sleep apnoea using polysomnography. *Eur Respir J* 2015;**45**(2):408–18.

Weaver TE, Mancini C, Maislin G, et al. Continuous positive airway pressure treatment of sleepy patients with milder obstructive sleep apnea: results of the CPAP Apnea Trial North American Program (CATNAP) randomized clinical trial. *Am J Respir Crit Care Med* 2012;**186**(7):677–83.

Younes M. Contributions of upper airway mechanics and control mechanisms to severity of obstructive apnea. *Am J Respir Crit Care Med* 2003;**168**(6):645–58.

A complete reference list can be found online at ExpertConsult.com.

Obstructive Sleep Apnea: Alternative, Adjunctive, and Complementary Therapies

Susheel P. Patil; Ephraim Winocur; Luis Buenaver; Michael T. Smith

Chapter Highlights

- Medical treatments for obstructive sleep apnea (OSA) can be categorized on the basis of the pathophysiologic mechanisms (i.e., anatomic, neuromuscular, and neuroventilatory control) that the interventions generally target. Stratifying treatments by pathophysiologic target may be particularly useful in personalizing therapy for patients with OSA.

- The current and emerging medical and device therapies available for the treatment of OSA generally are indicated as alternative therapies when traditional therapies for OSA are poorly tolerated, or as adjunctive treatment to more standard therapy.

- Therapeutic interventions and strategies such as weight loss, positional therapy, hypoglossal nerve stimulation, use of expiratory nasal resistors, and oral pressure therapy can successfully treat OSA in the appropriate patient. Other approaches such as

- myofunctional therapy, nasopharyngeal stenting, high nasal flow therapy, application of compression stockings, and pharmacotherapy are not proven as efficacious treatment for OSA and currently should be considered as experimental, possibly alternative, or at times adjunctive therapies.

- Oxygen therapy alone has not been shown to improve outcomes in OSA. In fact, use of supplemental oxygen has been associated with increased duration of apneic episodes and the development of hypercapnia.

- A limited number of complementary and alternative medicine approaches also have been studied for the treatment of OSA.

- Even with otherwise effective treatment for OSA, some patients may experience persistent sleepiness despite adequate sleep time and may be appropriate candidates for adjunctive stimulant pharmacotherapy.

Obstructive sleep apnea (OSA) is a highly prevalent disorder that increases cardiovascular and metabolic disease–related morbidity and mortality, contributes to the risk of motor vehicle and occupational accidents, and reduces occupational productivity. The recurrent episodes of upper airway obstruction that characterize OSA have been attributed to both anatomic loads (e.g., retrognathia, micrognathia, excess pharyngeal muscosal tissues, large parapharyngeal fat pads) on the upper airway and impairments in neuromuscular responses.[1] Potential treatments for OSA can be considered in light of the mechanisms identified to be important in its pathogenesis (Figure 17-1).

Therapy for OSA traditionally has targeted reductions in anatomic loads on the upper airway using continuous positive airway pressure (CPAP) therapy, oral appliances, upper airway surgery, and weight reduction. However, therapeutic approaches for OSA targeting neuromuscular (e.g., muscle responsiveness) and neuroventilatory (e.g., arousal threshold, apnea threshold, and loop gain) mechanisms have also been investigated; these include electrical stimulation of the hypo-

glossal nerve, myofunctional therapy, and pharmacotherapy. Given known difficulties with adherence to conventional therapies, particularly CPAP and use of oral appliances, for OSA,[2] active investigation of alternative and adjunctive therapies continues.

This chapter presents an overview of medical and device treatments for OSA based on the pathophysiologic mechanisms (i.e., anatomic, neuromuscular, and neuroventilatory control) that the interventions target. Stratifying treatments based on pathophysiologic targets may be useful in personalizing optimal therapy for patients with OSA. Patient preference also plays an important role in therapy decisions.[3] Such treatments may be considered in three categories: primary, alternative, and adjunctive. In this chapter, *primary treatment* or *therapy* is defined as a treatment that should be considered as a first-line therapy. *Alternative treatment* or *therapy* refers to a therapy that should be considered when a primary therapy is poorly tolerated or ineffective. *Adjunctive therapy* is defined as a treatment that should be used in conjunction with a primary or alternative therapy. *Investigational treatment* or

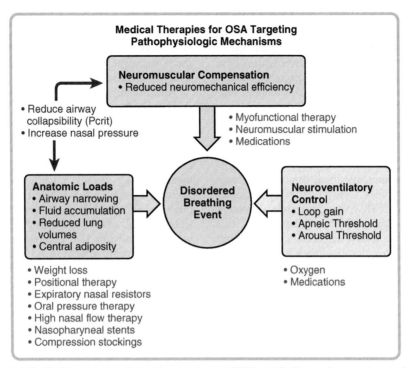

Figure 17-1 Medical therapies for obstructive sleep apnea (OSA), stratified by mechanisms targeted. Certain therapies can be considered on the basis of the pathophysiologic mechanisms targeted. OSA is thought to occur as a consequence of increases in anatomic loads on the upper airway, impairments in neuromuscular compensation, or alterations in neuroventilatory control. Traditional therapies such as continuous positive airway pressure (CPAP) use nasal pressure to overcome anatomic loads. By contrast, upper airway surgery or weight loss result in reduced airway collapsibility (Pcrit). Other therapies that may relieve anatomic loads on the upper airway include positional therapy, use of expiratory nasal resistors, oral pressure therapy, nasopharyngeal stenting, and application of compression stockings. Therapies that address impairments in neuromuscular function include myofunctional therapies, use of certain medications, and neuromuscular stimulation. Therapies that may affect neuroventilatory control include use of medications to increase the arousal threshold and supplemental oxygen, which can affect loop gain.

therapy is defined as a treatment that cannot be currently recommended except in the setting of clinical research. Another important term, *complementary and alternative medicine* (CAM) *therapy*, is used in the current literature to refer to treatments that are not part of allopathic medical treatment for OSA. Recommendations regarding whether a specific current or emerging alternative medical or device therapy for OSA should be considered primary, alternative, adjunctive, or investigational are provided, with the recognition that this is not without controversy for some treatments. Furthermore, many of the treatments discussed may be classified in more than one category, depending on the specific clinical context. Concluding the chapter is a section on management of residual excessive sleepiness in patients with otherwise adequately treated OSA and good adherence to therapy, with a focus on use of pharmacologic stimulants.

THERAPIES PRIMARILY TARGETING UPPER AIRWAY ANATOMIC LOADS

Increases in upper airway anatomic loads may be incurred through several mechanisms, including (1) airway narrowing due to complex interactions between pharyngeal soft tissues and the bony enclosure within which the upper airway resides, (2) central adiposity–mediated increases in airway collapsibility (Pcrit) through reductions in lung volume and tracheal stiffness, and (3) fluid accumulation within pharyn-

geal soft tissues. Primary treatment options targeting reduction in anatomic loads have included CPAP therapy (see Chapter 18), upper airway surgeries (Chapter 21), and oral appliance therapy (see Chapter 19). However, a number of other medical and device therapies aimed at relieving anatomic loads imposed on the upper airway have been explored, including weight loss, positional therapy, expiratory nasal resistance therapy, oral positive-pressure therapy, and use of compression stockings. These therapeutic interventions have been studied as primary, adjunctive, and alternative OSA treatments.

Medical and Surgical Weight Loss

Excess weight has long been recognized as a major risk factor for the development of OSA. The attributable risk of OSA in overweight individuals (BMI ≥ 25 kg/m^2) is estimated to be 41%.[4] Obesity-related impairments in upper airway function appear to be mediated through several mechanisms that affect upper airway anatomy. First, obesity may alter pharyngeal airspace geometry. Data from imaging studies of the human upper airway demonstrate that increases in the lateral pharyngeal fat pads are seen in patients with OSA compared with weight-matched control subjects.[5-7] Enlarged lateral pharyngeal fat pads alter the airway geometry from a horizontal elliptical orientation to an anterior-posterior orientation, which can increase susceptibility of the airway to collapse.[8,9] Second, external mass loads imposed on the upper airway increase airway collapsibility. In early studies using isolated animal upper airway preparations, application of external loads to the anterior neck and submandibular space led to elevations in Pcrit.[10] In more recent studies, investigators have demonstrated that lateral pharyngeal fat pad pressure fluctuations correlate with cyclic pharyngeal pressure changes, supporting the role of cervical fat depositions in increasing airway collapsibility.[11,12] Peripharyngeal fat deposits are clinically evident as enlarged neck circumference, with studies demonstrating a correlation between increasing neck circumference and increasing airway collapsibility.[13,14] Obesity also may indirectly impose upper airway anatomic loads through mechanical modulation of lung volumes. Central adiposity decreases functional residual capacity (FRC), reducing tracheal traction and thereby increasing upper airway collapsibility. This pathomechanism has been shown experimentally through manipulation of end-expiratory lung volumes in human volunteers, in whom reductions in lung volumes resulted in increases in Pcrit.[15,16]

Medical and surgical weight reduction has long been studied and implemented as a treatment for OSA[17-24]; however, randomized clinical trials have been published only in the past decade.[25-27] Early nonrandomized intervention studies of medical weight loss demonstrated that modest weight loss in the range of 10 to 20 kg in moderately to severely obese men with severe OSA resulted in an apnea-hypopnea index (AHI) reduction of 47% to 50%. A small subset of patients reduced their AHI below 20 (i.e., nighttime occurrence of fewer than 20/hour).[17,19]

More recent randomized, controlled studies in different patient populations have confirmed that medical weight loss decreases OSA severity. Collectively, these studies demonstrate that reductions in OSA severity with weight loss interventions are dose-dependent and sustained over a 1- to 4-year period despite a 30% to 50% weight regain. Furthermore, patients with more severe OSA at baseline demonstrate the greatest improvements in AHI,[25,26] with men tending to experience the greatest benefits.[26]

Tuomilehto and associates[27] studied obese patients with predominantly mild, positional OSA who undertook a 3-month program of a very-low-calorie diet (VLCD) and subsequent lifestyle modification. Patients in the intervention group, with a mean weight reduction of 10.7 kg at 12 months, exhibited a reduction in mean OSA severity (evidenced as occurrence of 4.0 fewer nighttime events/hour), whereas the control group subjects, with a mean weight reduction of 2.4 kg, showed no significant mean change in OSA severity (0.3/hour). Similar reductions in supine AHI were seen in the intervention and control groups (apopnea-hypopnea rate reduced by 6.5/hour and 5.9/hour, respectively). Despite the modest reduction in AHI, 61% of participants in the intervention group experienced resolution (AHI less than 5) of their OSA, compared with 32% in the control group. Improvement as evidenced by a decrease in mean OSA severity was sustained for an additional year despite a mean weight regain of 32% after termination of the supervised program.[28]

Johannson and colleagues[25] randomly assigned obese men with moderate to severe OSA either to a group managed with dietary intervention—VLCD combined with lifestyle counseling—or to a control group with no weight intervention. With a mean 18-kg weight reduction achieved after 9 weeks of intervention in the VLCD group, mean OSA sever-ity decreased, with improved AHI as evidenced by 21 fewer events/hour during nighttime sleep, with 17% demonstrating resolution of their OSA. OSA-related symptomatic improvement was sustained (mean AHI reduction by 17 events/hour) at 1 year despite a 31% weight regain.[29]

Additionally, the Sleep AHEAD (Sleep Apnea in Look AHEAD [Action for Health in Diabetes]) study investigators randomly assigned overweight and obese patients with type 2 diabetes mellitus and OSA to either an intensive lifestyle intervention (ILI) for weight loss or to diabetes support and education (DSE). At 1 year, the ILI group achieved a mean 10.8-kg weight reduction with a concomitant mean decrease in AHI of 5.4; the DSE group demonstrated an increased mean AHI of 4.2, despite no significant change in weight. OSA resolved (for an AHI of less than 5) in 36.3% of those receiving ILI, compared with 10.7% in the DSE group. The improvement in AHI persisted at 4 years despite a 50% weight regain. At year 4, 44% of participants demonstrated an improvement in OSA severity category, compared with only 18% of participants given DSE. Moreover, nearly 21% of ILI participants exhibited complete remission of OSA, to achieve an AHI below 5, compared with only 3.6% of DSE participants.[30]

Surgical weight loss, in contrast with medical weight loss, can result in more dramatic weight reduction that is more likely to be sustained over time (see also Chapter 22). Current National Institutes of Health (NIH) consensus guidelines for surgical weight loss recommend that patients with a BMI of 40 kg/m² or greater, or with a BMI of 35 kg/m² or greater associated with an obesity-related comorbid condition, including OSA, with previous unsuccessful attempts at medical weight loss, can be considered as potential candidates for surgical weight loss.[31] Bariatric surgeries can include restriction-based techniques such as laparoscopic adjustable gastric banding (LAGB) or vertical sleeve gastrectomy. More dramatic weight loss can be achieved when such techniques are combined with malabsorptive interventions such as the Roux-en-Y bypass or biliopancreatic diversion surgery (see Chapter 22).

Data regarding the effects of bariatric surgery on OSA are predominantly from uncontrolled case series or nonrandomized studies. A large meta-analysis of data for more than 20,000 patients from 134 studies that were predominantly uncontrolled case series reported outcomes from various bariatric surgical procedures. The analysis found that patients on average lost 61.2% of their excess weight, with 85.7% achieving resolution of their OSA.[32] However, resolution of OSA was adjudicated on the basis of patient self-report, rather than postoperative polysomnography, in most of these studies. A meta-analysis that examined only studies in which polysomnography was used before and after surgery reported reductions in mean OSA severity as evidenced by a decrease in AHI (apnea-hypopnea rate of 15.8 events/hour down from 54.7 events/hour) in association with a 17.9 kg/m² reduction in BMI.[33] This observation of reduction in severity but incomplete resolution of OSA was confirmed by Dixon and coworkers,[34] who conducted a randomized, controlled trial comparing LAGB with medical weight loss therapy in patients with severe OSA over a 2-year period. Patients in the LAGB group lost more weight compared with the medical weight loss group (mean weight loss of 27.8 kg versus 5.1 kg, respectively). With this weight reduction, the LAGB group had a tendency to greater reduction in OSA severity as reflected in mean AHI, although the difference was not statistically significant (apnea-hypopnea rate reduction by 25.5 events/hour versus 14.0 events/hour, respectively). In contrast with the medical weight loss studies, which demonstrated dose-dependent improvements in OSA severity with weight loss, this study demonstrated a nonlinear reduction in AHI with weight loss, with a plateau in AHI reduction after 10 kg of weight loss. Thus although some patients will experience resolution of their OSA to achieve an AHI below 5/h with surgical weight loss, the vast majority will continue to have some level of OSA that may necessitate continued treatment other than weight loss after surgery.

For several reasons, some overweight and obese patients may not experience symptomatic improvement or resolution of OSA with weight loss. Responsible factors include insufficient weight loss, persistent anatomic defects from craniofacial morphology or nasopharyngeal obstruction, or continued disturbances in neuromuscular or neuroventilatory control that contribute to increased airway collapsibility (high Pcrit). For example, obese patients who lost approximately 20% of their baseline weight demonstrated a reduction in Pcrit. However, resolution of OSA occurred only in participants for whom Pcrit fell below a threshold of −4 cm H_2O.[35]

In summary, weight loss, whether by medical therapy or surgical intervention, generally reduces OSA severity and may be curative in certain patients. Unfortunately, those subsets of patients with OSA who are most likely to benefit from these interventions have yet to be defined. Furthermore, the potential success of weight loss in mitigating OSA severity is tempered by the substantial weight regain that occurs in many if not most patients over time, particularly in the setting of medical weight loss. In addition, the risk of a major adverse outcome (e.g., perioperative death, abdominal operation, venous thromboembolism, endoscopy, extended hospitalization) with surgical weight loss interventions is approximately 4% in the first 30 days after surgery.[36] Careful consideration of the risks and benefits of surgical weight loss interventions for OSA must be individualized.

Nevertheless, given the role of obesity in the pathogenesis of OSA, medical providers should advocate weight loss in all patients with OSA who are overweight or obese. Lifestyle interventions for weight loss not only have the potential to reduce OSA severity but also may decrease morbidity and mortality from other obesity-related diseases such as metabolic syndrome, hypertension, cardiovascular disease, and diabetes mellitus.[37] Whether a weight loss program should be a primary, adjunctive, or alternative therapy depends on the patient's circumstances. For example, any overweight or obese patient treated for OSA with a primary therapy (e.g., CPAP, use of an oral appliance, upper airway surgery) should be prescribed weight loss as an adjunctive therapy. In patients with mild to moderate OSA associated with minimal daytime symptoms, weight loss could be recommended as a potentially primary therapy, provided that the patient is monitored for success with weight loss over a limited time frame. If a patient is unsuccessful with weight loss, then other primary therapies should be recommended. Patients with symptomatic OSA, however, should not be prescribed weight loss as a sole primary therapy; for example, symptoms of sleepiness may pose a safety risk and must be addressed using other traditional, primary OSA therapies. In patients who are motivated to pursue weight loss, referral to weight management programs that involve a multidisciplinary team, when available, may lead to sustained benefits over those achievable with a traditional weight loss program.[38]

Positional Therapy for Obstructive Sleep Apnea

Positional OSA typically is defined as that associated with an overall AHI less than 5, with a supine AHI that is at least twice the nonsupine AHI. The prevalence of positional OSA in affected patients overall is estimated to be approximately 56%, and it is more common among less obese patients and in those with mild to moderate OSA.[39-41] In view of the marked differences in AHI seen in these patients, positional therapy has been evaluated as a primary or alternative therapy for OSA. Many case series have demonstrated marked improvements in AHI with positional therapy in patients with positional OSA; however, randomized, controlled trial data on use of positional therapy as primary therapy are limited.[42] In one 4-week study, patients with positional OSA (mean AHI of 20.9) were randomly assigned to either a control group (lifestyle education for one session discussing exercise, weight loss, and sleep in the lateral position) or an active group (lifestyle education and the use of a tennis ball position modification device). There was a 46% versus 23% reduction in AHI in the active group versus the control group, respectively, which correlated with reduced supine sleep time in the active group. However, no difference between the groups was found for improvements in sleepiness, mood, or quality of life. Additional small randomized, controlled crossover trials have been performed comparing positional therapy with CPAP over 3 nights to 9 weeks.[43-45] In aggregate,[46] positional therapy has been less effective than CPAP in normalizing the AHI (mean posttreatment apnea-hypopnea rate of 6.2 events/hour versus 2.0 events/hour, respectively). The higher posttreatment AHI in the positional therapy groups in the data noted earlier was due to residual, nonsupine OSA, rather than to an inability to maintain the nonsupine position. Nevertheless, positional therapy improved sleep quality and quality of life measures similarly to CPAP in these studies, despite the higher posttreatment AHI.[43-45]

With most positional therapy techniques, an object is strapped to the back (tennis balls, squash balls, special vests), preventing the patient from sleeping in the supine position. This interventional strategy may disturb sleep architecture and sleep quality owing to arousals precipitated on turning from the right lateral position[47] to the left, resulting in poor long-term treatment adherence.[48] Alternative forms of positional therapy recently have been developed in attempts to improve longer-term adherence. For example, a new neck-worn device delivers a vibration when the patient moves supine, to provide feedback to the patient to shift to a non-supine position without significantly reducing total sleep time.[47,49] Other devices include sleep position trainers worn as a strap around the chest, which similarly vibrates when the supine position is detected,[50-52] and specially designed pillows to improve cervical positioning.[53] The limited data available suggest that long-term adherence to positional therapy over 6 months may be comparable to or better than that reported for CPAP[51] but may be specific to the type of positional device used. Additional randomized, controlled studies are needed to demonstrate longer-term improvements in OSA severity status and OSA-related outcomes, as well as long-term adherence, before positional therapy is considered as a primary treatment for positional OSA. Positional therapy should, however, be considered as adjunctive therapy added to primary therapies in patients with positional OSA. For example, positional therapy could be used in combination with an oral appliance to minimize the extent of mandibular advancement needed to normalize the AHI, or to improve the AHI when the appliance is already at maximum advancement and residual disordered breathing persists. Positional therapy also could be used as an adjunct to CPAP, to increase adherence by lowering the CPAP level in patients intolerant of such settings. Finally, use of positional therapy as an alternative modality in patients with positional OSA, particularly if the nonsupine AHI is near normal, could be considered when other primary therapies are not tolerated or if the patient is traveling without primary therapy appliances or devices. These decisions ideally should be guided by objective data from a sleep study, the patient's preferences, and the clinical response.

Expiratory Nasal Resistors

An expiratory nasal resistor (ENR) is a device containing a one-way valve that is superficially placed in the nares and is secured to the skin of the nose with an adhesive. The valve allows inspiration to occur unimpeded but partially closes during expiration (Figure 17-2). Closure of the valve creates expiratory nasal resistance that results in expiratory positive airway pressure (EPAP) within the pharynx, which is thought to stabilize the upper airway during subsequent inspirations.

Several mechanisms of action have been postulated for EPAP production with use of an ENR, aimed primarily at relieving mechanical loads on the upper airway.[54] First, expiratory pharyngeal airway dilation could reduce subsequent inspiratory airway narrowing. Dynamic imaging of the upper airway suggests that airway caliber is most narrow at end-expiration, when pharyngeal muscle tone is dependent on tonic muscle activity. Using fiberoptic endoscopy, investigators have reported significant expiratory narrowing of the pharyn-

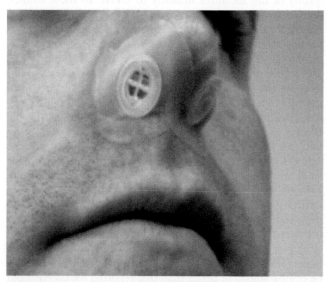

Figure 17-2 An expiratory nasal resistor. This device generates end-expiratory positive airway pressure within the pharynx. (From Walsh JK, Griffin KS, Forst EH, et al. A convenient expiratory positive airway pressure nasal device for the treatment of sleep apnea in patients non-adherent with continuous positive airway pressure. *Sleep Med* 2011;12:147-52.)

geal airspace before the development of an apnea.[55] Thus an increase in end-expiratory airway size has been hypothesized to prevent pharyngeal collapse during the subsequent inspiration. Second, similar to CPAP, ENR may increase lung volumes, thereby increasing tracheal traction and reducing upper airway collapsibility. Investigators, using MRI-based techniques to measure FRC, demonstrated that FRC increases by 47% during wakefulness in association with increases in nasal EPAP between 4 to 17 cm H_2O. The effect of ENRs on lung volumes, however, was mitigated when subjects breathed through the mouth, thus bypassing the ENR.[56] Finally, use of an ENR may improve OSA through indirect chemoresponsive mechanisms by inducing hypercapnia by means of ENR-induced hypoventilation. End-tidal CO_2 measurements have been shown to increase by approximately 2 to 6 mm Hg during ENR application with sleep.[56,57] Increases in CO_2 may then reduce airway collapsibility through recruitment of genioglossal muscle activity.[58,59]

Clinical trials of the effectiveness of ENRs have been performed[60-63] since the initial observation by Mahadevia and associates[64] that selective EPAP reduced apnea severity. Initial, uncontrolled studies demonstrated an approximately 50% reduction in AHI in patients with mild to moderate OSA, and 32% reduction in those with severe OSA.[60,61] Subsequently, a 3-month randomized, double-blinded clinical trial was conducted in patients with a new OSA diagnosis.[62] Participants were predominantly obese male patients with mild positional OSA. At 3 months, application of ENRs resulted in a 61% reduction in AHI, compared with 19% in the sham ENR group. The subgroup of patients with severe OSA also demonstrated a 61% reduction in AHI. Although improvements in sleep architecture were not observed with ENR use, decreases in subjective sleepiness based on the Epworth Sleepiness Scale (ESS) score were statistically significant. These effects appeared to be sustained with continued ENR use at 12 months in a follow-up study of a subset of adherent participants in whom ENR therapy reduced AHI by 50%, with decrease in number of events/hour to less than 10.[63] In contrast, in a study of ENR versus sham ENR therapy for 2 weeks in patients with severe OSA undergoing CPAP withdrawal, investigators demonstrated that ENR use did not lessen OSA severity.[65] Side effects reported with use of ENRs include headache, dry mouth, breathing discomfort, nasal itching, sleep maintenance insomnia, and vertigo and resulted in 7% discontinuing therapy.[62]

As indicated by the available evidence, ENR therapy should be considered an alternative therapy for the treatment of OSA in patients who are intolerant of traditional therapies such as CPAP or use of oral appliances. Patients with mild to moderate OSA, particularly positional OSA, appear to be most likely to respond, although in some situations patients with severe OSA also may respond. Patients with symptoms of nasal obstruction are less likely to tolerate ENR therapy, owing to increased nasal resistance, and are not good candidates for this therapy. Efficacy of ENR use in reducing OSA severity should be determined through objective sleep testing before long-term prescription of this therapy. For patients in whom use of ENRs has demonstrated efficacy, the ENR technique could be used as an alternative therapy during travel— for example, if the available electrical source is unreliable or if the equipment for CPAP therapy is perceived as too cumbersome. Additional research is necessary to confirm effectiveness of this therapy, including whether use of ENRs reduces excessive sleepiness and cardiovascular risk similar to that seen with CPAP or oral appliances, before ENR should be considered a primary therapy.

Oral Pressure Therapy

Oral pressure therapy (OPT) represents another alternative therapy for OSA that aims at reducing upper airway mechanical loads. The OPT system consists of a customized mouthpiece, which is worn nightly, connected by flexible tubing to a console that generates a vacuum of approximately −50 cm H_2O that is applied to the oral cavity[66-68] (Figure 17-3). The

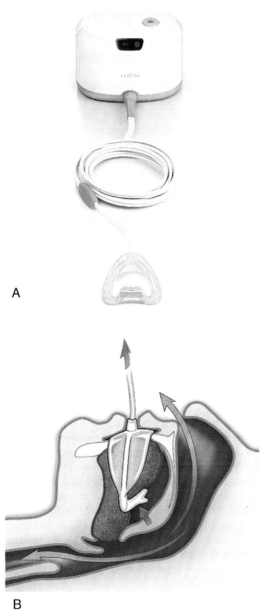

A

B

Figure 17-3 Oral positive-pressure therapy device. **A,** The device sits in the mouth and applies a gentle suction to keep the tongue and soft palate forward during breathing, while the patient lies supine. **B,** The effect of the suction pressure on tongue and palate position. (Images provided and reproduced with permission from Apnicure, Inc.)

negative pressure is isolated to the oral cavity as a consequence of the natural seal created between the soft palate and the tongue.[66] MRI studies performed during wakefulness indicate that OPT increases retropalatal airspace in the lateral and anterior-posterior dimensions through movement of the soft palate (anterior and superior) and the tongue (anterior-superior segment only). The retroglossal airspace is reduced, however, primarily owing to the resting position of the device. OPT may potentially reduce OSA severity through other mechanisms, including vacuum-mediated attenuation of airway collapse during inspiration, and through activation of upper airway negative pressure reflexes, which stabilize the upper airway through increased pharyngeal muscle activity during inspiration.[66]

Several clinical trials have been performed to assess the efficacy of OPT. Initial studies were uncontrolled and tested OPT in patients with OSA for one night compared with a baseline sleep study.[67,68] These preliminary studies demonstrated that in patients with an AHI of approximately 35, OPT reduced their AHI by 36% to 40%. AHI was reduced to less than 10 in 38% to 48% of the patients with OSA. A subsequent study performed a randomized, cross-over, first-night order study of OPT compared with control conditions, which was followed by an open-label, 4-week trial period.[69] Participants were naive to any OSA treatment, intolerant of CPAP, or actively using CPAP but electing to participate in the study. The pre-OPT mean AHI was 27.5 and was reduced by 51%, to 13.4 on OPT, which was sustained with use of OPT during sleep at the end of 4 weeks, with a mean AHI of 14.8. Thirty-two percent of patients were considered responders, defined as achieving an AHI below 10 and at least a 50% decrease in AHI from baseline. Baseline OSA severity, however, did not predict response to therapy. As in the initial studies, improvements in sleep architecture were demonstrated, characterized by reductions in stage N1 sleep, stage N1 shifts, overall sleep stage shifts, awakenings, arousal index, and by increases in stage R (rapid eye movement [REM]) sleep. In participants who were naive to any OSA treatment, improvements in subjective sleepiness and sleep-related quality of life were reported. However, participants who were actively using CPAP before the study did not demonstrate a reduction in sleepiness, presumably owing to the efficacy of CPAP in improving sleep status. Common side effects reported with OPT included oral tissue discomfort or irritation, dental discomfort, and dry mouth, with 5% of patients (n = 3) discontinuing therapy during the trial.

OPT is approved by the U.S. Food and Drug Administration (FDA) for primary treatment of OSA; in view of the limited available data, however, it should be considered an alternative therapy for OSA in patients intolerant of traditional therapies such as CPAP or use of oral appliances. Efficacy of the therapy in reducing OSA severity should be determined through sleep testing before this modality is prescribed. Randomized, controlled trials and comparative effectiveness studies need to be performed to demonstrate whether OPT decreases OSA-related morbidity similar to traditional OSA therapies.

High Flow Nasal Therapy

Several small studies have investigated the effects of high-flow-rate (20 to 30 L/minute), humidified air administered by nasal cannula for treating OSA (Figure 17-4). Such *high flow*

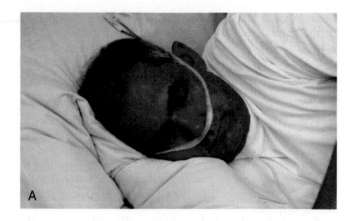

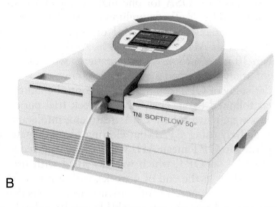

Figure 17-4 An example of a high-flow nasal therapy device. This device administers warm, humidified air by nasal cannula at high flow rates. Although the system is "open" compared with the "closed" system inherent in continuous positive airway pressure (CPAP), a positive airway pressure (PAP) of approximately 2 cm H_2O can be generated. (Images provided and reproduced with permission from TNI-Medical.)

nasal therapy (HFN) is hypothesized to improve mechanical loads on the upper airway in a manner similar to that for CPAP, by increasing end-expiratory pharyngeal pressure by approximately 2 cm H_2O.[70] In addition, HFN may prevent pharyngeal collapse through neurally mediated mechanisms. HFN reduces ventilatory drive through reductions in the inspiratory duty cycle and respiratory rate, thereby improving mean inspiratory airflow with each breath.[70,71]

In a study of 11 adult participants with mild to moderate OSA, the mean AHI was reduced by 64% (from mean of 28/h to 10/h) with HFN.[70] In 8 participants, the AHI fell below 10. HFN also has been studied in 10 patients who had experienced a recent acute ischemic stroke (mean, 4.8 days).[72] HFN in this patient population with severe OSA had more modest effects, with an AHI reduction by 24% (mean of 30.8 down from 40.4). In the largest case series of 56 patients, modest reduction in OSA severity were seen with a mean AHI reduction from 22.6 to 17.2, with similar reduction seen for separate hypopnea and apnea indices. A therapeutic response, defined by an AHI of less than 10, with a 50% reduction in AHI from baseline, was seen in 27% of patients. In a separate study using the respiratory disturbance index, patients with predominantly obstructive hypopneas, respiratory effort–related arousals, or REM-related events appeared

to be most likely to respond to HFN. By contrast, the nightly occurrence of more than 10% central apneas or more than 90% obstructive apneas predicted a poor response to HFN.[73] Although these initial results are promising, additional clinical trials are needed before HFN can be recommended as a primary or alternative therapy.

Nasopharyngeal Stents

Use of nasopharyneal stents, sometimes referred to as *nasal trumpets*, has been studied as a potential treatment for OSA since the 1970s.[74-76] Traditionally, such devices are used in the emergency setting to maintain an airway until intubation or tracheostomy can be performed. The stents are inserted into the nose and extend into the nasopharynx, protecting the airway from obstruction. If long enough, the stent may prevent obstruction of the oropharynx. The stents also prevent obstruction of the internal and external nasal valves and may decrease nasal resistance in some patients.[76] To date, no randomized, controlled trials have been performed demonstrating efficacy of nasopharyngeal stenting in improving OSA severity. A systematic review of nasopharyngeal stents identified five noncontrolled studies testing the efficacy of these devices in reducing the AHI in settings that included the sleep laboratory, the postoperative setting, and the home.[74] Overall, the AHI decreased by 49%, from a mean of 44.1 to 22.7, and the minimum oxygen saturation improved from 66.5% to 75.5%. The tolerability of nasopharyngeal stenting on a night-to-night basis, however, remains to be established. Until controlled studies are performed, use of nasopharyngeal stents cannot be recommended as a primary or alternative therapy for OSA, except on an emergent basis in the hospital setting to mitigate active airway obstruction in patients with known OSA or suspected OSA based on snoring, witnessed apneas, and oxygen desaturation in an attempt to prevent respiratory failure and the need for emergency intubation.

Venous Compression Stockings

Investigations have examined the use of compression stockings in the treatment of OSA based on the observation that fluid displacement from the legs in awake, healthy subjects without OSA results in an increased neck circumference, pharyngeal narrowing with increased pharyngeal resistance, and increased airway collapsibility.[77-79] Furthermore, increases in OSA severity correlate with the amount of fluid displaced from the legs to the neck when patients were sleeping supine.[80] Subsequently, several studies have examined the effects of venous compression stockings on OSA severity.[81,82] One randomized, crossover study recruited 12 nonobese patients with chronic venous insufficiency and OSA and assigned them in random order to 1 week of wearing compression stockings and 1 week of no stockings. Compared with control conditions, the use of stockings resulted in a 62% reduction in leg fluid volume and a 60% increase in neck circumference that was associated with a 36% reduction in AHI (from 48.4 events/hour to 31.3 events/hour).[81] More recently, the effects of compression stockings were studied in a sample of 57 patients with OSA, who were randomly assigned to a control condition or the use of compression stockings for 2 weeks. Subjects who wore compression stockings demonstrated greater reduction in overnight decrease in leg fluid volume, which correlated with a higher morning upper airway cross-sectional area and a greater AHI reduction compared with control data (reduction of 8.6 events/hour versus 0.9 event/hour, respectively).[83]

These results, although intriguing, do not support the use of compression stockings as primary therapy for the treatment of OSA. However, the use of compression stockings may have an adjunctive role in combination with primary therapies such as CPAP in treating OSA, particularly in patients who are in states of volume overload such as congestive heart failure, chronic venous stasis, or chronic kidney disease.

THERAPIES TARGETING PRIMARILY NEURAL AND NEUROMUSCULAR MECHANISMS

Pharyngeal obstruction has long been postulated to occur in part by disturbances in neuromuscular function during sleep.[84] OSA subjects have impaired dynamic responses to upper airway obstruction and have reduced tonic genioglossal muscle activity compared with age-, sex-, and BMI-matched healthy control subjects.[1,85] Furthermore, studies of motor unit potential morphology suggest signs of neurogenic remodeling of the genioglossus in persons with OSA.[86] Treatments for OSA thus aimed at relieving impairments in upper airway neuromuscular function or augmenting upper airway neuromuscular responses have been and continue to be investigated. Examples of such interventions are electrical stimulation of the hypoglossal nerve, myofunctional therapy, and pharmacotherapy, as discussed next.

Hypoglossal Nerve Stimulation

Hypoglossal nerve stimulation (HGNS) has been developed as a potential therapy for OSA, with at least one proprietary HGNS system approved by the FDA (see also Chapter 21).[87] HGNS stimulates the hypoglossal nerve, which in turn stimulates the genioglossus muscle, an upper airway dilator muscle. Early studies in animal models demonstrated the potential success of extrinsic electric stimulation of the genioglossus muscle in maintaining upper airway patency during sleep.[88-90] This initial success led to pilot human studies using submental stimulation of the genioglossus[91-93] or direct fine-wire stimulation of the genioglossus or hypoglossal nerve.[94-97] These studies, in addition to demonstrating increases in airflow during sleep in the obstructed airway (Figure 17-5), provided important lessons for the design of the most recent generation of HGNS systems. First, distal placement of electrodes along the hypoglossal nerve to provide selective stimulation of tongue protrusors, or in combination with tongue retractors, improved airway patency.[98] However, proximal nerve stimulation of tongue retractors alone led to airway obstruction.[99] Second, nerve stimulation synchronized with inspiration demonstrated the maximal benefit in airflow improvements and provided secondary benefits of extending battery life and minimizing neuromuscular fatigue.[97,99]

Several HGNS systems have now been developed using either synchronous, closed-loop stimulation or continuous, open-loop stimulation. These systems contain an implanted pulse generator similar to a cardiac pacemaker, which is connected to a respiratory sensing lead (Figure 17-6). A stimulus burst output is delivered and synchronized with inspiration to a cuff that is implanted around the hypoglossal nerve, immediately increasing inspiratory airflow. The continuous, open loop system uses an array of electrodes arranged within the electrode cuff. Stimulation is performed at a set duration,

irrespective of the respiratory cycle, in a manner targeting different nerve fibers and minimizing stimulation of the duty cycle.[100,101]

Studies testing the current generation of HGNS systems have predominantly enrolled obese, male patients with moderate to severe OSA that had difficulties "tolerating" CPAP. The studies generally have excluded patients with moderate to severe obesity and some degree of central sleep apnea (greater than 5% or 25% of the AHI events are central or mixed apneas). One system, Inspire (Inspire Medical Systems, Maple Grove, Minnesota), uses drug-induced sleep endoscopy (DISE) as an exclusion criterion based on earlier studies suggesting that concentric airway collapse during DISE predicted greater chance of therapeutic failure.[102] Despite differing eligibility criteria, the studies in aggregate have demonstrated a mean AHI reduction of 50% to 70%, from a mean baseline rate of 32 to 45 events/hour.[100,103,104] Furthermore, in the Stimulation Therapy for Apnea Reduction (STAR) trial, patients who received the HGNS system demonstrated improvements in subjective sleepiness based on ESS scores and in sleep-related quality of life as assessed by the Functional Outcomes of Sleep Questionnaire (FOSQ).[103]

Adverse events related to HGNS have been reported. Short-term surgical risks include wound infections requiring removal of hardware, hematomas, and nerve palsy. Longer-term risks associated with repetitive tongue stimulation include soft tissue abrasions, discomfort with electrical stimulation, and dry mouth.[87,103] In addition, the need for DISE may carry additional risks, such as oxygen desaturation or hypoventilation, that may necessitate bag-mask ventilation or prolonged recovery from sedation due to enhanced drug sensitivity, which warrants careful monitoring by trained professionals.

The Inspire device recently has been FDA-approved. Given that roughly one third of patients in trials of this device were considered to be nonresponders (response was defined as an AHI reduction of at least 50%, with a residual AHI below 20) and had persistent OSA, even after correct application of inclusion and exclusion criteria, additional research is needed to refine optimal patient selection criteria. Further work also is needed to determine how HGNS stimulus settings can be optimized and managed over the long term. Finally, long-term effects on OSA severity and patient safety beyond 18 months remain to be reported. At this time, HGNS should not be considered a primary therapy for OSA until results of additional studies are available. HGNS is available only through specialized centers whose personnel have undergone the appropriate training with the device manufacturer. HGNS, however, should be considered as an alternative therapy in patients with significant difficulties in adhering to or benefiting from CPAP or other primary therapies who meet the inclusion-exclusion criteria defined in the study.

Myofunctional Therapy

The term *myofunctional therapy* is used to describe oropharyngeal exercises used to improve nasal breathing, facial appearance, and mandibular growth.[105] More recently, myofunctional therapy has been studied in the treatment of OSA, using specific voice lessons, musical instruments, and oropharyngeal exercises. An early, uncontrolled study of self-reported chronic snorers found that after a single voice lesson and practice of singing daily for 20 minutes at maximum volume and control

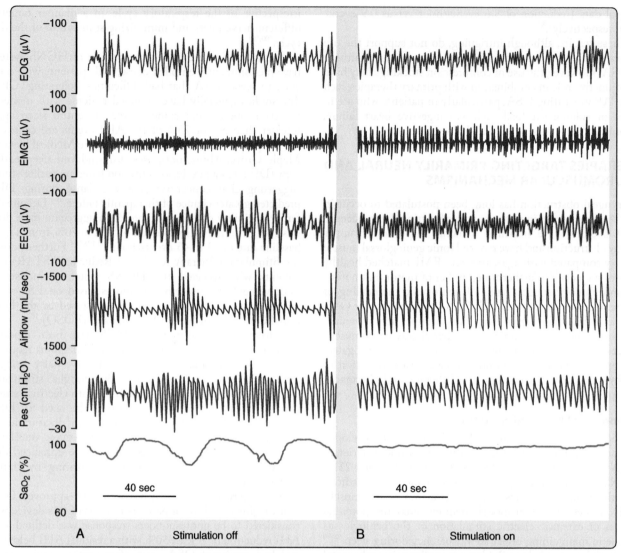

Figure 17-5 Effects of hypoglossal nerve stimulation. A, Breathing pattern during non–rapid eye movement (NREM) sleep with hypoglossal stimulation off. **B,** Breathing pattern during NREM sleep with hypoglossal stimulation on. EEG, C3-A2 electroencephalogram; EMG, electromyogram; EOG, electrooculogram; Pes, esophageal pressure; SaO₂, oxyhemoglobin saturation. (From Schwartz AR, Bennett ML, Smith PL, et al. Therapeutic electrical stimulation of the hypoglossal nerve in obstructive sleep apnea. *Arch Otolaryngol Head Neck Surg* 2001;127: 1216-23.)

reduced the duration of loud snoring after 3 months. Training included instruction in the proper use of the diaphragm and the production of sounds and scales, which cause the soft palate to rise and fall.[106] Subsequently, a cross-sectional study of orchestra musicians completing an Internet-based survey found that double-reed woodwind musicians, in comparison with those who play other wind or non-wind instruments, had a reduced prevalence of OSA risk based on the Berlin questionnaire. Although the proportion of women in the double-reed instrument group was higher, which might have explained this association, the relation persisted after adjustments for sex. Practice duration with a double-reed instrument also was associated with a reduced OSA risk score based on the Berlin questionnaire[107] In another web-based survey study of orchestra members also using the Berlin questionnaire to assess OSA risk, wind instrument players were found to have a greater odds of OSA risk; however, this was no longer

significant after adjustments for BMI.[108] Potential explanations for the discrepant findings could include that the latter study did not distinguish between wind instrument type (i.e., single-reed versus double-reed), and that double-reed instruments require both a relatively unique lip placement and a high degree of air resistance. Furthermore, statistical overadjustment for obesity by including this as a covariate may have occurred, because BMI is part of the Berlin questionnaire.

Overcoming such limitations of correlational design and the use of questionnaires to assess OSA risk, findings in at least three preliminary randomized, controlled trials provide promising support for the efficacy of oropharyngeal exercise training for OSA in selected patients. In the first of these studies, investigators performed a controlled trial and randomly assigned 25 participants with moderate OSA (with an AHI between 15 and 30)[109] either to receive digeridoo lessons,

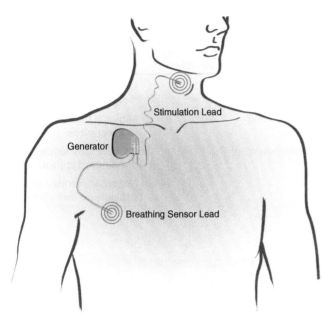

Figure 17-6 General design of a closed-system hypoglossal nerve stimulator. (Image provided and reproduced with permission of Inspire Medical Systems, Inc.)

a traditional instrument of the aboriginal Australian culture, with daily practice or to a waitlist for lessons and followed the participants for 4 months. After 4 months of playing the digeridoo for at least 5 days/week for 20 minutes per day, patients in the digeridoo group achieved an AHI reduction of 10.7, compared with 4.5 in the control group participants. Decreases in subjective daytime sleepiness as measured by the ESS also were observed in the digeridoo group.

A more recent randomized, controlled trial of speech therapy–derived oropharyngeal exercises in patients with recently diagnosed moderate OSA studied the effects of isometric and isotonic exercises of the tongue, soft palate, and lateral pharyngeal wall compared with sham exercises performed over a 3-month period. Exercises were observed weekly by a speech therapist, and participants performed exercises for 30 minutes daily for 3 months. Adherence to exercises was monitored using a diary. The investigators found that the oropharyngeal exercise group demonstrated a mean AHI reduction of 38%, compared with 6% in the sham exercise group, for a mean reduction in AHI of 8.7 events/hour versus a mean increase of 1.5 events/hour, respectively; the pretreatment mean AHI was 22.4 for both groups.[110] Significant reductions in neck circumference were found in the oropharyngeal exercise group compared with the sham group (a decrease of 1.1 cm versus a gain of 0.2 cm, respectively) and correlated with the AHI reduction. As in the didgeridoo study, significant reductions were noted in ESS score, a measure of subjective daytime sleepiness.

Myofunctional therapy also has been successfully applied to treat residual symptoms of OSA after adenotonsillectomy (AT) in children.[111] Thirty children with an AHI greater than 1 after AT were randomly assigned to either an exercise regimen targeting nasal breathing, labial seal, lip tone, and tongue posture or no treatment (control group). Children practiced three times per day for 3 months. Oropharyngeal training significantly reduced the post-AT AHI by 58%, compared with 7% for the control group. With the recognition that a majority of children who have undergone AT continue to display at least mild residual OSA symptoms, oropharyngeal training has the potential to become an important adjunctive postsurgical therapy.

These preliminary studies of oropharyngeal muscle training are promising and support continued research in this area. The studies reported to date, however, generally are small and highly selective, with inclusion of only subjects with mild to moderate OSA; thus whether similar reductions in AHI would be observed in patients with severe OSA is unknown. Furthermore, the longevity of the effects is unknown beyond the initial 3-month training period. Further elucidation of the specific types of training exercises that are most strongly associated with decreased airway collapsibility during sleep is needed. Although myofunctional therapy cannot be currently recommended as a primary therapy for OSA, it may be a useful adjunctive modality for use with other OSA therapies or as an alternative therapy in patients who refuse or otherwise cannot benefit from primary treatments for OSA.

Pharmacotherapy for Obstructive Sleep Apnea Targeting Neuromuscular Control

Selecting and studying pharmacologic targets that might successfully treat OSA in humans constitute a challenging endeavor owing to the complexity of respiratory control, the multiple neurochemical pathways that drive respiration, interactions with the sleep state, and limitations in animal models of OSA.[112,113] An ideal pharmacologic agent for the treatment of OSA would need to possess multiple properties including the ability to achieve (1) maintainance of normal airway patency and respiratory drive during both non-REM (NREM) and REM sleep and (2) mitigation of the effects of intermittent arousals and hypoxemia.[114] No such pharmacologic intervention currently exists, although various drugs have been studied in this context. Current pharmacologic approaches for the management of OSA might best be described as alternative therapy in patients for whom other primary or even alternative OSA therapies have not been of benefit. In view of the current evidence, however, such an alternative therapy approach should be considered investigational, with perhaps a few exceptions, until appropriate clinical trials have been completed. Pharmacotherapies used as adjuncts to primary treatment modalities for OSA, including PAP, oral appliance therapy (OPT), surgical treatments, and weight loss, however, also have received attention. Agents that have been evaluated include REM-suppressing agents and drugs that improve airway patency (e.g., serotoninergic, cholinergic, and cannabinoid agents). Overall, the results of these approaches for OSA treatment to date generally have been disappointing, as reviewed next (see Table 17-1 for a summary of the findings).

Serotoninergic Agents

Serotoninergic neurons are known to regulate upper airway motor output, and several studies have investigated the possible beneficial effects of serotoninergic agents in patients with OSA. Serotoninergic control of respiration, however, is complex and remains poorly understood. Whereas some serotoninergic inputs are excitatory and facilitate respiration,[115] others inhibit upper airway motor neuron function.[116] Systemically administered agents that augment or attenuate

Table 17-1   Pharmacotherapies for Obstructive Sleep Apnea

Study*	Study Design	Generic Name	Influence on Osas	Comments
Lin et al., 2012[114]	Critical review	Ventilatory stimulants Serotoninergic drugs	↔	Expert opinion
Veasey, 2003[165]	Review	Serotonin agonists and antagonists	↔	Potential future expectations
Espinoza et al., 1987	Randomized crossover, placebo-controlled study	Aminophylline	↓	Effective only for central and mixed apneas
Carley et al., 1999[117]	Animal study	Mirtazapine	↓	Not recommended owing to adverse side effects
Carley et al., 2007[118]	Randomized, double-blind, placebo-controlled, three-way crossover study			
Castillo et al., 2004	Case report			
Guilleminault and Hayes, 1983[148]	Clinical trial	Naloxone, theophylline, bromocriptine	↔	

*Complete sources for unreferenced studies follow: Castillo JL, Menendez P, Segovia L, Guilleminault C. Effectiveness of mirtazapine in the treatment of sleep apnea/hypopnea syndrome (SAHS). *Sleep Med* 2004;5(5):507-8; Espinoza H, Antic R, Thornton AT, McEvoy RD. The effects of aminophylline on sleep and sleep-disordered breathing in patients with obstructive sleep apnea syndrome. *Rev Respir Dis* 1987;136(1):80-4.
OSAS, Obstructive sleep apnea syndrome; ↓, ameliorate; ↔, no effect; ↑, exacerbate.

serotonin levels, therefore might be expected to either decrease OSA severity or exacerbate the condition, respectively.[117]

Several clinical trials have tested serotoninergic medication–based regimens for OSA. Mirtazapine, an antidepressant with both $5-HT_1$ agonist and $5-HT_3$ antagonist effects, has been more widely investigated as a medication for OSA treatment. On the basis of an animal study in which mirtazapine was found to be effective in reducing central apneas in rats,[117] investigators conducted a randomized, double-blind, placebo-controlled, threeway crossover study of mirtazapine in 12 patients with OSA.[118] The results were positive in that the daily administration of 4.5 to 15 mg of mirtazapine for 1 week reduced the AHI by approximately 50% in adult patients with OSA, from a pre-treatment mean AHI of 22.3 to an on-treatment mean of 11.4. A subsequent randomized, controlled trial, however, demonstrated no significant benefits of mirtazapine (in a dose of 7.5 to 45 mg for 2 weeks) compared with placebo in moderating OSA severity: Compared with the pre-treatment mean AHI of 24.1, on-treatment mean AHI increased to 26.7 to 39.2, depending on the dose of mirtazapine.[119] Use of this medication was associated with a mean weight gain of approximately 1 kg. Relatively common side effects of mirtazapine include both sedation and weight gain, two problems linked with OSA itself.

Subsequently, investigators compared placebo, fluoxetine (a central $5-HT_2$ agonist), odansetron (a peripheral $5-HT_3$ antagonist), and combined fluoxetine and ondansetron in a randomized, controlled 4-week trial in 35 adults with mild to severe OSA. Combined high-dose therapy with fluoxetine and ondansetron showed some efficacy: This regimen reduced the mean AHI significantly compared with baseline at days 14 and 28 for the second half of full-night polysomnography, in contrast with no significant changes in AHI with placebo.[120] However, no subsequent confirmatory trials have been performed. Common side effects reported with use of these medications include headache, constipation, dry mouth, and

hypersomnolence, although such effects were not seen during this 4-week clinical trial.

Protriptyline, a nonsedating tricyclic antidepressant, acts as a serotonin and norepinephrine reuptake inhibitor and also has been shown to have partial treatment effects in OSA at doses up to 30 mg. Mechanisms which contribute to improvements in OSA severity include reduction in REM sleep duration,[121] and increased hypoglossal and recurrent laryngeal nerve activity with increased upper airway motor tone.[122] In at least two small clinical trials, use of protriptyline for treatment of severe OSA (mean AHI range, 71 to 75) was associated with reductions in AHI by 21% to 33%,[121,123] predominantly as a consequence of reductions in apnea frequency and duration. Furthermore, subjective improvements with respect to sleepiness were reported by most patients despite significant residual disordered breathing, suggesting that protriptyline may have independent alerting effects.[121] Documentation of significant residual disordered breathing and hypoxemia, however, has diminished enthusiasm for this treatment when more effective therapies are available. Side effects of protriptyline include dry mouth, urinary hesitancy, constipation, confusion, and ataxia, all of which also may limit the use of medications of this class.[124]

Thus as a group, serotoninergic medications have modest effects on OSA severity status. In light of the availability of more effective treatments for OSA and potentially significant side effects for some of these drugs, these medications should not be used for primary therapy for OSA but rather are best considered as adjunctive therapy with other OSA treatments. Use of serotoninergic medications also could be considered an alternative therapy in patients with OSA intolerant of other forms of OSA treatment, particularly in patients in whom these medications are already planned to be used for comorbid disorders such as depression (mirtazapine or protriptyline), anorexia (mirtazapine), migraine (protriptyline), and cataplexy (protriptyline or fluoxetine). Reductions in OSA severity with these medications should not be assumed on the basis of decreased symptoms, and the patient's OSA status should be monitored by sleep testing.

Cholinergic Agents

Acetylcholine, a cholinergic neurotransmitter active primarily during REM sleep, is involved in the modulation of upper airway motor tone. Preliminary investigations of acetylcholinesterase inhibitors have been performed on the basis of findings in preclinical studies, which demonstrated that injection of physostigmine into cholinergic neurons located in the rostral ventrolateral medulla of anesthetized and vagotomized cats was followed by increased hypoglossal and phrenic nerve activity. This increased activity resulted in prolonged hypoglossal to phrenic nerve firing interval with consequent improvement in respiratory drive.[125] On the basis of such data, a double-blind, placebo-controlled trial was conducted in 12 men with moderate to severe OSA.[125] Physostigmine or placebo was injected intravenously on separate nights followed by an overnight sleep study. Comparison of sleep recordings for the physostigmine night and the placebo night demonstrated a slightly lower mean AHI (apnea-hypopnea rate of 41 events/hour and 54 events/hour, respectively), with the greatest reduction occurring during REM sleep (mean AHI of 54 versus 30, respectively).

Donepezil, a reversible inhibitor of the acetylcholinesterase enzyme often used to treat memory impairment in Alzheimer disease (AD), also has been tested as a potential agent for treatment of OSA in patients with and without AD. An initial study was performed in 23 patients with AD and mild to moderate OSA. This randomized, double-blind, placebo-controlled trial demonstrated that at 3 months, donepezil improved the mean AHI from 20.0 to 9.9 compared with placebo, for which the mean AHI did not change (23.2 versus 22.9). As would be expected with a cholinergic medication, increased REM sleep was observed in the donepezil group at 3 months.[127] Another double-blind, placebo-controlled trial of donepezil was conducted in 21 male patients with OSA but no AD. This study also found donepezil to improve mean AHI at 1 month, although the effects were more modest, with a mean AHI reduction of 23% (pretreatment mean of 42.2 versus posttreatment mean of 32.8) versus a mean AHI increase of 14% (pretreatment mean of 26.4 versus posttreatment mean of 31.0) in the placebo group.[128] This study found no differences in REM sleep between the groups. Side effects reported with donepezil included dizziness, nausea, headaches, vivid dreams, and nightmares. Although these results are promising, further confirmatory studies are needed in larger samples to determine whether donepezil has a role in the treatment of OSA. For now, there may be a role for donepezil in patients with AD with comorbid OSA, when donepezil is already being considered for memory-related conditions and other primary or alternative OSA therapies are not tolerated.

Cannabinoids

Cannabinoid agonists have recently been investigated as a candidate target for OSA therapy. Preclinical data suggest that dronabinol, a nonselective cannabinoid type 1 (CB1) and type 2 (CB2) receptor agonist, increases phasic genioglossal activity and attenuates serotonin-induced apneas in rats when injected in the nodose ganglion.[129] Dronabinol is hypothesized to inhibit afferent vagal nerve activity, which may thereby result

in disinhibition of upper airway motor neurons.[130] In an initial proof-of-concept human clinical trial,[131] participants with moderate OSA treated with CPAP were withdrawn from their CPAP regimen for 1 week. Participants were then given dronabinol in an escalated dose over 3 weeks, up to 10 mg. Pretreatment AHI was reduced by 29% from a pretreatment mean AHI of 48.8. Side effects noted during the study included somnolence and increased appetite without weight increase. Although these findings are of interest, controlled studies are needed on the potential effects of dronabinol in OSA, and this treatment should be considered investigational at present.

THERAPIES TARGETING PRIMARILY NEUROVENTILATORY MECHANISMS

Neuroventilatory mechanisms play an influential role in the expression of OSA severity. Physiologic parameters such as the arousal threshold, apnea threshold, CO_2 reserve, and circulatory time determine the subject's response to reduced ventilation from any cause whether mediated centrally (central hypoventilation) or peripherally (obstruction). Globally, these measures determine the degree of ventilatory instability (loop gain) and whether disordered breathing will be mitigated or perpetuated. Neuroventilatory mechanisms, therefore present a potential therapeutic target for OSA treatment. Examples of such interventions are oxygen therapy and pharmacotherapies and are discussed next.

Supplemental Oxygen

Many of the consequences of OSA are attributable to nocturnal hypoxemia. Studies done before the widespread use of CPAP reported that supplemental oxygen administration during sleep in patients with OSA could significantly increase oxygen saturation of hemoglobin (Sao_2) but could also lengthen apneic spells, potentially leading to hypercapnia and respiratory acidosis.[132-134] These early studies found no improvement in subjective or objective measures of daytime sleepiness with nocturnal oxygen treatment.[135] However, reduction in OSA severity with oxygen therapy alone may depend on whether the patient has stable or unstable ventilatory control (low or high loop gain, respectively). In a study of subjects with severe OSA, oxygen reduced the AHI by 53% in the high loop gain group, compared with 8% in the low loop gain group.[136] A randomized clinical trial comparing oxygen administration alone with CPAP in patients with OSA and comorbid cardiovascular disease or multiple cardiovascular risk factors found that CPAP, but not nocturnal oxygen therapy, significantly reduced 24-hour mean blood pressure.[137] Thus oxygen therapy alone during sleep is not recommended as a primary or alternative therapy for most patients with OSA.

However, subgroups of patients with OSA who might benefit from oxygen therapy are recognized. Patients with significant cardiovascular disease (e.g., coronary artery disease or cerebrovascular disease) and an only marginally elevated frequency of abnormal breathing events during sleep, but who experience severe oxyhemoglobin desaturation during those events, might benefit in terms of reduced risk of myocardial ischemia with oxygen supplementation.[138,139] The use of supplemental oxygen also could be considered as alternative therapy in patients with OSA and significant intermittent hypoxemia who are intolerant of a primary therapy such as CPAP, to minimize potential cardiovascular and metabolic risks. In the absence of any high-grade evidence, such use should be considered controversial, particularly because oxygen administration is not without risks (e.g., hypercapnia, fire risk). The clinician in this situation should consider titration of oxygen in an attended sleep study setting to document the optimal minimum oxygen dose for efficacy in patients with OSA in preventing hypoxemia and minimizing hypercapnia.

Oxygen also may be added as adjunctive therapy to PAP in patients in whom CPAP or bilevel PAP regimens are effective in treating their OSA, but in whom hypoxemia persists owing to ventilation-perfusion mismatching or hypoventilation.[140] This may occur in patients with severe obesity or a so-called overlap syndrome (see Chapter 29). Patients with OSA who require supplemental oxygen therapy during wakefulness almost always will require supplemental oxygen during sleep, even if PAP therapy maintains a patent upper airway.[141] However, it should be determined if persistent oxygen desaturation in patients on CPAP is related to hypoventilation,[10] because use of bilevel positive pressure in patients who are hyperventilating despite adequate control of OSA may obviate the need for added oxygen.

Transtracheal Oxygen Delivery

Several reports have described the use of transtracheal oxygen administration in patients with OSA who are intolerant of CPAP.[142-144] One study described the use of this modality as salvage therapy in a patient with overlap syndrome and in a patient with persistent hypoxemia despite CPAP and in-line oxygen.[145] These data are too limited to recommend this mode of oxygen delivery; accordingly, transtracheal oxygen use in OSA as either an alternative or adjunctive therapy should be considered investigational.

Pharmacotherapy for Obstructive Sleep Apnea Targeting Neuroventilatory Control

Several drugs have been studied targeting neuroventilatory control mechanisms such as a high loop gain state and a low arousal threshold. Although more often considered as potential treatments for central sleep apnea (see Chapter 15), some of these pharmacologic approaches have been examined in the setting of OSA. With the possible exception of acetazolamide, these approaches should be considered either as alternative therapies for use in patients who have demonstrated intolerance to primary therapies or as investigational therapies.

Carbonic Anhydrase Inhibitors

Acetazolamide, a carbonic anhydrase inhibitor that induces a metabolic acidosis, thereby increasing ventilation, has been studied primarily in patients with central sleep apnea secondary to high altitude exposure or heart failure, who often have unstable ventilatory control (i.e., high loop gain). Similarly, some patients with OSA also have been shown to have an elevated loop gain.[146] In one study of patients with OSA treated with CPAP, administration of acetazolamide for 7 days reduced the mean loop gain by 41% and the mean AHI by 41%.[147] However, difficulties with tolerability of acetazolamide may preclude its long-term use, because patient-reported side effects have included paresthesias, altered taste,

nocturia, and hypokalemia (when it is used in combination with a diuretic), with the need to monitor serum bicarbonate levels over time. Currently, use of acetazolamide should be considered only as alternative or adjunctive therapy for OSA.

Methylxanthines, Opioid Antagonists, and Dopamine Agonists

A randomized, crossover, placebo-controlled trial in 1987 assessed the efficacy of infusion of aminophylline, a methylxanthine derivative known to have respiratory stimulant properties, in male subjects with moderate OSA.[53] Aminophylline decreased the frequency of central and mixed apneas but did not affect the frequency or duration of obstructive apneas. Mean and minimum arterial oxygen saturation values in sleep also were unchanged, and sleep architecture was markedly disturbed.

In recognition of the effects of opiate agonists on respiratory depression, another early investigation tested multiple medications including naloxone (an opioid antagonist), theophylline, and bromocriptine mesylate (a dopamine agonist). None of these agents had any significant beneficial effects on the frequency or duration of obstructive apneic and hypopneic spells or on oxygen desaturation indices.[148] Thus none of these medications are appropriate for use as as primary agents in the treatment of OSA.

Sedatives and Hypnotics

The use of sedatives and hypnotics in the treatment of OSA appears to be counterintuitive, on the basis of concerns regarding worsening of OSA secondary to the myorelaxant and central nervous system sedative effects of many of these medications.[149] However, a low arousal threshold in a patient with OSA may result in a premature arousal before compensatory neuromuscular mechanisms have sufficient time to restore complete upper airway patency. A premature arousal when combined with an underlying state of ventilatory instability may result in persistent disordered breathing during sleep. One study[146] demonstrated that 37% of patients with OSA have a low arousal threshold, raising the possibility that increases in the arousal threshold, as may be achieved with sedative-hypnotics, may represent a therapeutic target for this population.

Initial clinical studies testing this possibility have looked at the use of eszopiclone, a nonbenzodiazepine sedative, or trazodone, an antidepressant medication with serotoninergic, antihistaminic, and antiadrenergic effects. One study randomly assigned 17 subjects with OSA with a nadir Sao_2 greater than 70% to receive one night of eszopiclone 3 mg or one night of placebo.[150] The arousal threshold, quantified by degree of nadir epiglottic pressure level associated with electroencephalogram arousal, was observed to increase by 18% in stage N2 (NREM stage 2) sleep, whereas the mean AHI was reduced by 23% (rate decrease from 31 events/hour to 24 events/hour) in the eszopiclone group compared with the placebo group. No significant difference in hypoxemia severity was seen between the two groups. In another, more rigorous study of double-blind, placebo-controlled cross-over design, however, participants with mild to moderate OSA were randomly assigned to receive either eszopiclone or placebo for two consecutive nights. No significant difference in AHI was seen between the groups.[151] Several studies have examined the use of trazodone to treat OSA.[152-154] Trazodone given at

100 mg for one night was reported to increase the arousal threshold by 32% but did not reduce the AHI[153] A subsequent study of 15 patients with severe OSA given trazodone 100 mg or placebo had conflicting results, demonstrating no significant changes in arousal threshold but mild improvements in AHI with trazodone compared with placebo (reported rate of 28.5 events/hour vs. 38.7 events/hour, respectively).[154] These data suggest that at the very least, certain sedatives and hypnotics may not exacerbate OSA and could be used in patients with comorbid insomnia when indicated. In view of the noted conflicting results, however, the use of sedatives and/or hypnotics to treat OSA, whether as adjunctive or alternative therapy, currently should be considered investigational.

Complementary and Alternative Medicine Therapy for Obstructive Sleep Apnea

The term *complementary and alternative medicine* (CAM) typically is used to refer to treatments that are not part of allopathic medical training.[155] Such treatments are not restricted to medications and typically lack a clear and compelling mechanism of action that targets known pathophysiology. In the following discussion, the concept of *CAM therapy* is differentiated from *adjunctive* and *alternative therapy* as described earlier in the chapter. CAM therapies may potentially be used as adjunctive or alternative treatments for OSA. In view of the well-established cardiovascular, cerebrovascular, and metabolic consequences of OSA and the neuromechanical nature of the disease, the role for CAM treatments, if not specifically contraindicated, is expected to be minimal. As noted earlier, however, PAP, the "gold standard" treatment for OSA, is difficult to adhere to for many patients.[2] Recent surveys suggest that a majority of patients with OSA are actively interested in CAM approaches.[156] Setting aside the general absence of well-controlled studies evaluating complementary interventions for OSA, we present a brief review of preliminary studies of acupuncture therapies, considered a form of CAM.[157,158] In general, however, other CAM-designated treatments such as use of herbal and dietary supplements and manipulative therapies (e.g., tai chi) have been studied in a very limited and uncontrolled fashion and consequently are not further discussed here. With the possible exception of acupuncture, reports of CAM treatments are of insufficient scientific quality to support their use. Placebo effects and manipulation of presleep expectancies,[159,160] which represent potential mechanisms by which some of these interventions could improve sleep parameters, have been shown to persist into and alter sleep-related physiologic measures. Indeed, some work demonstrates that REM sleep may play a role in the persistence of next-day placebo analgesia effects.[159]

Acupuncture

Most studies of CAM therapies for OSA have not used randomized, placebo-controlled experimental designs. Acupuncture is a notable exception. One single-blind study of acupuncture randomly assigned 36 patients with previously untreated OSA for 10 weeks to either an acupuncture group, a sham acupuncture group, or a control group (in which sleep hygiene and weight loss counseling was provided).[161] Weekly acupuncture significantly improved the mean AHI by approximately 50%, from a recorded rate of 19.9 events/hour to 10.1 events/hour, compared with the sham acupuncture or

control group, for which mean AHI was unchanged or significantly worsened, respectively.[161] The acupuncture group also demonstrated improvement in subjective measures of sleepiness based on the ESS and in some quality of life domains based on the short form 36 health survey questionnaire (SF-36). A more recent randomized, controlled study by the same group of investigators compared manual acupuncture and electroacupuncture for one session with no treatment (control condition) in 40 patients with previously untreated, moderate OSA. Both manual acupuncture and 10-Hz electroacupuncture administered just before sleep significantly reduced the mean AHI by approximately 50% (apnea-hypopnea rate for manual acupuncture: 21.9 events/hour reduced to 11.2 events/hour; rate for 10-Hz electroacupuncture: 20.6 events/hour reduced to 10.0 events/hour), compared with 2-Hz electroacupuncture and no treatment (control condition) (both groups: no significant change in mean AHI).[162]

A randomized, controlled trial of auricular plaster therapy, a form of acupuncture administered only to the ear, compared this treatment against vitamin C supplementation in the control group.[163] Forty-five participants with severe OSA were randomly assigned to receive either auricular acupuncture three to five times per day or vitamin C three times daily for 10 days. Patients in the auricular acupuncture group demonstrated modest, but statistically significant, improvement in the mean AHI (pretreatment apnea-hypopnea rate of 72.4 events/hour versus posttreatment rate of 59.2 events/hour), in contrast with the control group (pretreatment rate of 73.5 events/hour versus posttreatment rate of 72.0 events/hour).

Although the mechanisms by which acupuncture may modulate OSA severity, and the longevity of such effects, are unknown, these preliminary studies are promising and merit further research. Acupuncture should not replace established primary treatments in current use, but if this modality is added, it should be performed using published protocols by professionals trained in this discipline to promote standardization of effects.

PHARMACOLOGIC MANAGEMENT OF "RESIDUAL" EXCESSIVE DAYTIME SLEEPINESS WITH ADEQUATELY TREATED OBSTRUCTIVE SLEEP APNEA

Even with objectively documented successful treatment of OSA, including acceptable adherence to therapy, it has been estimated that as many as 10% of patients with OSA continue to report significant excessive daytime sleepiness (EDS).[164] The significance of EDS cannot be overstated in view of its role in contributing to motor vehicle accidents, impaired psychological functioning, and reduced work performance.[45] The cause of such "residual" EDS, however, can be difficult to definitively ascertain. Data from mouse models suggest that intermittent hypoxia may result in irreversible oxidative injury to brain centers associated with sleep.[165]

As part of the clinical management of patients with appropriately treated OSA but persistent EDS, other contributing factors and conditions such as insufficient sleep time, insomnia, medication-related side effects, or other comorbid sleep disorders should be carefully ruled out. Successful treatment of OSA should be documented by objective measures of adherence to therapy and a normal AHI with the prescribed

CPAP regimen as confirmed by a sleep study. Objective documentation of EDS with a Multiple Sleep Latency Test (MSLT) or Maintenance of Wakefulness Test (MWT) could be considered, although this is not a requirement for most third party payers, and such testing typically is performed when the possibility of a primary CNS hypersomnolence disorder such as narcolepsy is a concern. If EDS persists despite adequate OSA treatment, nonsympathomimetic stimulants (e.g., caffeine) can be used, as well as psychostimulant medications (i.e., nonamphetamine or amphetamine derivatives). Such regimens should be considered as part of an overall management strategy to improve daytime alertness.[166]

Traditionally, amphetamine-class medications have been used to treat residual EDS in patients with OSA, on the basis of data for subjects with narcolepsy and sleep-restricted persons. The potential for harmful cardiovascular consequences and potential negative mood- and sleep-related effects with this class of medications has led to investigational use of pharmacologic agents other than amphetamines, for which these effects seem less likely to occur. Comparative effectiveness studies of different stimulants in the treatment of residual EDS in patients with OSA are needed because many of the amphetamine derivatives are considerably less expensive than the nonamphetamine medications. The use of these medications is not discussed further here owing to the absence of data regarding their use in the treatment of residual EDS in patients with OSA.

Modafinil and armodafinil, the R-isomer of modafinil, are nonamphetamines currently FDA-approved for the treatment of residual hypersomnolence in patients with OSA considered to be otherwise adequately treated with PAP.[167] The wake-promoting effects of the medication are incompletely understood but are reported to be due primarily to dopaminergic-mediated pathways.[168] Several relatively large randomized, placebo-controlled clinical trials have demonstrated that modafinil[148,149,169,170] and armodafinil[167,171-174] can safely reduce EDS, as indicated by subjective and objective measures,[175] and can improve quality of life in patients with OSA adequately treated with CPAP.[176,177] For example, an initial 4-week randomized, double-blind, placebo-controlled, parallel group study[169] of modafinil versus placebo reported normalization of the ESS score in 51% of the modafinil group versus 27% in the placebo group. Although the mean sleep latency on an MSLT was decreased in the modafinil group compared with the placebo group, normalization of the mean sleep latency (to less than 10 minutes) was similar in both groups (29% versus 25%, respectively). A subsequent randomized, controlled trial[170] performed over 12 weeks evaluated the effects of placebo versus modafinil at a 200-mg or 400-mg dose. Improvements in ESS scores and mean sleep latency on the MWT were reported, with similar improvements for the 200-mg and 400-mg modafinil dose groups. Improvements in sleep-related quality of life and global function as assessed by the FOSQ and Clinical Global Impression of Change questionnaires were observed to a similar degree in both modafinil groups compared with placebo. No change in CPAP adherence was reported in these two studies.[169,170] However, in a separate 12-week open label continuation of modafinil from the initial study,[169] mean CPAP use was observed to decline from 6.3 hours/night to 5.9 hours/night,[178] suggesting that such agents may in fact reduce adherence to CPAP. Accordingly, clinicians should continually remind their patients to be adherent to CPAP, to maximize the wake-promoting effects of both therapies.

A similar literature base is available regarding the efficacy of armodafinil for residual EDS in patients with treated OSA.[167,171-174] Armodafinil has a duration of action that is 10% to 15% longer than that of modafinil. Data from a pooled analysis[172] of two 12-week multicenter, double-blind, placebo-controlled, parallel group clinical studies[176,179] found that adjunctive treatment with armodafinil in CPAP-adherent participants with OSA coupled with residual EDS significantly improved wakefulness, long-term memory, and ability to engage in activities of daily living. Armodafinil also reduced patient-reported fatigue, evaluated separately from sleepiness, and was well tolerated in terms of side effects.[172] Treatment with armodafinil showed no effect on subsequent CPAP adherence, but active monitoring of CPAP adherence by the clinician is advocated in this setting.[174] A multicenter, flexible-dose, open-label study found that armodafinil remained effective for more than 12 months in patients with residual EDS and treated OSA.[173]

The most commonly reported adverse events in the studies that were associated with both medications included headache (occurring in approximately 15% to 20% of subjects), nausea (in 10% to 20%), insomnia (in 5% to 10%), and anxiety (in 5% to 15%). Up to 15% of patients in one study discontinued medications owing to such adverse events. A rare but serious adverse event that clinicians should be aware of is the occurrence of serious rashes, including Stevens-Johnson syndrome and toxic epidermal necrolysis, which typically occur within 5 weeks of the initiation of therapy but in rare cases may appear later than that. Rare cases of multiorgan hypersensitivity manifesting as fever, rash, and organ system dysfunction have been reported with modafinil and armodafinil, as well as anaphylactoid reaction with armodafinil. Modafinil and armodafinil may decrease the effectiveness of hormonal birth control systems, so women should be advised of this possibility, with consideration given to use of nonhormonal contraceptive approaches.

In summary, the use of pharmacologic stimulants in patients with OSA should be considered as adjunctive therapy for the management of residual EDS in patients with OSA adequately treated with CPAP, with documentation of acceptable adherence to CPAP, and after exclusion of other causes of EDS. More controversial is whether stimulants should be considered as an alternative therapy for patients with EDS due to OSA who are intolerant of treatments for their OSA. At least two studies suggest that use of modafinil during a 2-day CPAP withdrawal period or for 2 weeks in patients with mild to moderate untreated OSA resulted in significant improvements in driving performance in a driving simulator, decrease in subjective sleepiness, and better scores for attention and vigilance on the psychomotor vigilance test.[180,181] In patients in high-risk situations in which alertness and performance are critical (e.g., professional drivers, military personnel) and those for whom use of primary PAP therapy is interrupted (such as with an unreliable electrical source during travel), there may be a role for stimulants as sole treatment for brief periods. However, continued reinforcement of adherence to the patient's prescribed OSA treatment, as well as monitoring for medication side effects, is necessary to avoid potential long-term adverse effects of stimulants.

CLINICAL PEARLS

- Despite the efficacy of traditional primary treatments such as CPAP, oral appliance therapy, and upper airway surgery for OSA, patient factors such as suboptimal adherence or poor tolerance of a therapy may lead to incomplete treatment.
- In such situations, alternative therapies should be considered, either alone or as adjunctive treatment with other OSA treatment options (e.g., use of positional therapy with supplemental oxygen in a patient with positional OSA and persistent hypoxemia).
- In patients with OSA and residual sleepiness, adjunctive pharmacologic stimulant therapy can be considered, but only after ensuring that OSA treatment and sleep time are adequate, and that no other sleep disorders are present that may explain the residual sleepiness.

SUMMARY

In light of the fact that traditional primary treatment modalities for OSA, including CPAP, use of oral mandibular advancement devices, and upper airway surgery, often have poor adherence rates and/or insufficient long-term outcomes (e.g., upper airway surgery for OSA), adjunctive and alternative treatment options for OSA should be considered in nonadherent patients and those who are otherwise not fully benefiting from primary and adjunctive therapies. Furthermore, OSA treatments can be individualized in accordance with the known pathophysiologic basis for OSA in a particular patient, and with the patient's personal preferences. Treatment measures such as weight loss, positional therapy, HGNS, ENRs, and OPT have been studied and shown to successfully treat OSA in appropriate, sometimes selected patients. Other potential therapies such as myofunctional therapy, nasopharyngeal stenting, highnasal-flow therapy, use of compression stockings, and pharmacotherapies do not have proven efficacy and should currently be considered as adjunctive or investigational therapy, rather than primary therapy, for OSA. Oxygen therapy alone has not been shown to improve outcomes in OSA, although treatment of severe hypoxemia with supplemental O_2 alone or in combination with PAP can be considered a reasonable adjunctive or alternative treatment option in some patients, including those who cannot maintain adherence to or benefit from primary therapies, or who need supplemental O_2 with PAP to adequately ameliorate sleep-related hypoxemia. Promising preliminary data are available for the use of acupuncture, a form of CAM therapy for OSA, as an adjunctive or alternative therapy, but this modality requires further investigation before it can be recommended for use in OSA. Even with effective treatment for OSA, some patients may experience persistent sleepiness despite adequate sleep time and may be appropriate candidates for adjunctive stimulant therapy. In view of the difficulties that some patients experience with primary therapies for OSA, continued investigation into alterative and adjunctive OSA treatment options can be expected.

Selected Readings

Berry RB, Kryger MH, Massie CA. A novel nasal expiratory positive airway pressure (EPAP) device for the treatment of obstructive sleep apnea: a randomized controlled trial. *Sleep* 2011;**34**:479–85.

Billings KR, Maddalozzo J. Complementary and integrative treatments: managing obstructive sleep apnea. *Otolaryngol Clin North Am* 2013;**46**:383–8.

Campbell T, Pengo MF, Steier J. Patients' preference of established and emerging treatment options for obstructive sleep apnoea. *J Thorac Dis* 2015;**7**(5):938–42.

Colrain IM, Black J, Siegel LC, et al. A multicenter evaluation of oral pressure therapy for the treatment of obstructive sleep apnea. *Sleep Med* 2013;**14**:830–7.

Foster GD, Borradaile KE, Sanders MH, et al. A randomized study on the effect of weight loss on obstructive sleep apnea among obese patients with type 2 diabetes: the Sleep AHEAD study. *Arch Intern Med* 2009;**169**:1619–26.

Freire AO, Sugai GC, Chrispin FS, et al. Treatment of moderate obstructive sleep apnea syndrome with acupuncture: a randomised, placebo-controlled pilot trial. *Sleep Med* 2007;**8**:43–50.

Gottlieb DJ, Punjabi NM, Mehra R, et al. CPAP versus oxygen in obstructive sleep apnea. *N Engl J Med* 2014;**370**(24):2276–85.

Greenburg DL, Lettieri CJ, Eliasson AH. Effects of surgical weight loss on measures of obstructive sleep apnea: a meta-analysis. *Am J Med* 2009;**122**:535–42.

Guimaraes KC, Drager LF, Genta PR, et al. Effects of oropharyngeal exercises on patients with moderate obstructive sleep apnea syndrome. *Am J Respir Crit Care Med* 2009;**179**:962–6.

Lin CM, Huang YS, Guilleminault C. Pharmacotherapy of obstructive sleep apnea. *Expert Opin Pharmacother* 2012;**13**:841–57.

McGinley BM, Patil SP, Kirkness JP, et al. A nasal cannula can be used to treat obstructive sleep apnea. *Am J Respir Crit Care Med* 2007;**176**:194–200.

Puhan MA, Suarez A, Lo CC, et al. Didgeridoo playing as alternative treatment for obstructive sleep apnoea syndrome: randomised controlled trial. *BMJ* 2006;**332**:266–70.

Sukhal S, Khalid M, Tulaimat A. Effect of wakefulness-promoting agents on sleepiness in patients with sleep apnea treated with CPAP: a meta-analysis. *J Clin Sleep Med* 2015;**11**(10):1179–86.

Tuomilehto HP, Seppa JM, Partinen MM, et al. Lifestyle intervention with weight reduction: first-line treatment in mild obstructive sleep apnea. *Am J Respir Crit Care Med* 2009;**179**:320–7.

White LH, Lyons OD, Yadollahi A, et al. Effect of below-the-knee compression stockings on severity of obstructive sleep apnea. *Sleep Med* 2015;**16**:258–64.

Woodson BT, Soose RJ, Gillespie MB, et al; STAR Trial Investigators. Three-year outcomes of hypoglossal cranial nerve stimulation for obstructive sleep apnea: the STAR trial. *Otolaryngol Head Neck Surg* 2016. [In press].

A complete reference list can be found online at ExpertConsult.com.

Obstructive Sleep Apnea: Positive Airway Pressure Therapy

Neil Freedman

Chapter Highlights

- Continuous positive airway pressure (CPAP) therapy is indicated for patients with moderate to severe obstructive sleep apnea (OSA) with or without symptoms and for patients with mild OSA with associated symptoms or comorbid illnesses.

- CPAP consistently improves or resolves respiratory events across the spectrum of disease severity and improves symptoms of daytime sleepiness, especially for patients with moderate to severe OSA. Improvements in blood pressure are relatively small, with reductions in blood pressure tending to be greatest in patients with untreated hypertension and in those with better compliance with therapy. Improvements in other outcomes are inconsistent across the spectrum of disease severity.

- Compliance with positive airway pressure (PAP) therapy is far from perfect. Systematic education through several approaches, with or without behavioral therapy, have been the only interventions that have been associated with consistent improvements in compliance with PAP therapy. The roles of other interventions, including heated humidification, prescription hypnotics, telemedicine, and sleep specialist care, for most patients with OSA are not clear.

- Advanced PAP technologies, including bilevel PAP and expiratory pressure relief devices, have not been associated with better compliance or improvements in other important outcomes compared with standard CPAP therapy. The roles for bilevel PAP and devices with expiratory pressure relief technology in the management of most patients with OSA are not clear.

- Autotitrated positive airway pressure (APAP) used in an unattended setting, either to determine a fixed CPAP pressure or as a primary treatment, is reasonable therapy for most patients with uncomplicated moderate to severe OSA syndrome. APAP therapy has been shown to result in similar compliance and improvements in other important outcomes compared with conventionally titrated CPAP therapy. In appropriate OSA patients, an ambulatory approach using portable testing and APAP therapy should lead to reductions in the cost of management of OSA while not adversely affecting patient outcomes.

Treatment with positive airway pressure (PAP) remains the primary therapy for most patients with obstructive sleep apnea (OSA), especially those with moderate to severe OSA. This chapter reviews various forms of PAP therapy for the treatment of OSA, highlighting the indications for treatment, methods for determining an effective pressure prescription, treatment outcomes, and methods that may improve compliance with therapy. The initial part of the chapter focuses on continuous positive airway pressure (CPAP) therapy, and the later portion of the chapter emphasizes the technologic advancements in the delivery of PAP therapy, including autotitrating positive airway pressure (APAP), bilevel PAP, and expiratory pressure reduction (EPR) technologies.[1]

CONTINUOUS POSITIVE AIRWAY PRESSURE TREATMENT

CPAP therapy was initially described as a treatment for OSA by Sullivan and colleagues in 1981.[1a] Since its initial description, CPAP has become the predominant therapy for the treatment of patients with OSA because it has been demonstrated to resolve sleep-disordered breathing events and improve several clinical outcomes.[2,3] Treatment with CPAP is typically indicated for patients with moderate to severe OSA by apnea-hypopnea index (AHI) of 15 or more events/hour with or without associated symptoms or comorbid diseases and for patients with mild OSA (AHI ≥5 to ≤14 events/hour) with associated symptoms or comorbid diseases (Box 18-1).

CPAP is conventionally delivered through a nasal mask at a fixed pressure that remains constant throughout the respiratory cycle. The proposed mechanism of action of CPAP therapy is that it acts as a pneumatic splint that maintains the patency of the upper airway in a dose-dependent fashion. It does not exert its effects by increasing upper airway muscle activity[4] and acts only as a treatment, and not a cure, for the disorder. Several studies have demonstrated that withdrawing CPAP therapy in patients with OSA across the spectrum of disease severity results in the recurrence of OSA and associated daytime symptoms in most patients within 1 day to several days.[5-7]

Box 18-1 TYPICAL INDICATIONS FOR CONTINUOUS POSITIVE AIRWAY PRESSURE THERAPY FOR OBSTRUCTIVE SLEEP APNEA

- Moderate to severe obstructive sleep apnea (≥15 events per hour of sleep) with or without associated symptoms or comorbid diseases
- Mild obstructive sleep apnea (≥5 to ≤14 events per hour of sleep) with symptoms or associated comorbid diseases:
  - Symptoms: excessive daytime sleepiness, impaired cognition, mood disorders, or insomnia
  - Comorbid diseases: hypertension, ischemic heart disease, or history of stroke

Table 18-1 Adequacy of Continuous Positive Airway Pressure Titration Definitions

Optimal	Reduces the RDI <5 for at least a 15-minute duration and should include supine REM sleep at the selected pressure that is not continually interrupted by spontaneous arousals or awakenings
Good	Reduces the RDI ≤10 or by 50% if the baseline RDI <15 and should include supine REM sleep that is not continually interrupted by spontaneous arousals or awakenings at the selected pressure
Adequate	Does not reduce the RDI ≤10 but reduces the RDI by 75% from baseline (especially in severe OSA patients), or in which the titration grading criteria for optimal or good are met with the exception that supine REM sleep did not occur at the selected pressure
Inadequate	Does not meet any one of the above grading criteria

RDI, respiratory disturbance index, which accounts for apneas, hypopneas, and respiratory effort–related arousals.
Adapted from Kushida CA, Chediak A, Berry RB, et al. Clinical guidelines for the manual titration of positive airway pressure in patients with obstructive sleep apnea. *J Clin Sleep Med* 2008;4:157–71.

Determining the Optimal Setting

The optimal CPAP settings for home use may be defined as the minimal pressure required to resolve all apneas, hypopneas, snoring, and arousals related to these events in all stages of sleep and in all sleep positions.[2,8-10] Simply, the optimal CPAP setting should resolve all sleep-disordered breathing in supine rapid eye movement (REM) sleep to account for the effects of gravity and changes in muscle tone that may occur in different sleep stages and positions.[8] The optimal pressure should also maintain oxygen saturation at or above 90% and should minimize mask leak, allowing and maintaining only mask leak that that is appropriate for the given pressure. The most current American Academy of Sleep Medicine (AASM) Practice Parameters recommend a full night of CPAP titration based on the criteria outlined previously.[9,10] A repeat CPAP titration need only be performed if symptoms of OSA reappear despite compliance with CPAP therapy, if a patient sustains a significant weight loss either through diet or bariatric surgery, or if CPAP compliance and benefits remain suboptimum by current standards.

A "split-night" sleep study, in which the initial portion of the study is used to objectively document an individual's sleep related breathing disorder followed by a CPAP titration during the second portion of the night, may be indicated in certain situations.[8-10] A split-night sleep study may be considered when the following criteria have been met: (1) an AHI of 40 or more events/hour is recorded during the initial 2 hours of the polysomnography (PSG) study and (2) at least 3 hours remain during the PSG study to conduct an adequate CPAP titration. A second full night of CPAP titration should be considered if an optimal CPAP pressure setting could not be achieved during the second portion of the split-night study. Split-night studies can also be considered for individuals who demonstrate less severe OSA, with an AHI of 20 to 40 events/hour, during the initial 2 hours of a sleep study, although data suggest that CPAP titrations in this subgroup of patients may be less accurate when performed in the split-night protocol setting. Although split-night studies potentially reduce waiting times to initiate home CPAP therapy, especially in areas with long sleep laboratory waiting times, a significant portion of patients with OSA may undergo suboptimal CPAP titrations using this format.[11]

The use of home sleep testing (HST) is currently not recommended for the titration of CPAP or other PAP therapies because there are few data on the reliability of HST for this indication. Given the absence of data regarding HST for CPAP titration, the Centers for Medicare and Medicaid Services and commercial insurance companies in the United States typically will not reimburse providers who use HST for this indication.

Although there are current recommendations to help guide clinicians on how to manually titrate CPAP therapy in an attended laboratory-based setting, these recommendations largely serve as guidelines because they are principally based on the consensus of expert opinion and not on randomized trials demonstrating their superiority over other methods of manual titration.[8] The AASM guidelines classify the adequacy of a CPAP titration as delineated in Table 18-1. The AASM guidelines currently recommend considering a repeat titration study for patients who do not achieve an optimal or good PAP titration.

There are actually few data on the quality or efficacy of CPAP titrations, as defined by the AASM clinical guidelines, in clinical practice. Specifically, few data exist on how often patients actually achieve an optimal PAP titration, despite having their PAP pressures determined in an attended setting. Furthermore, there are few data examining the outcomes of patients who are initiated on CPAP therapy after undergoing PAP titrations that are less than optimum. Many of the randomized controlled trials evaluating the effect of CPAP on various outcomes have shown a mean residual AHI or respiratory disturbance index (RDI) of 5 or greater, indicating that more than 50% of these patients underwent CPAP titrations that did not achieve optimal results. Of the limited existing data from clinical settings, approximately only 50% to 60% of patients with OSA achieve an "optimal" titration and up to 30% to 40% achieve only an "adequate" or "inadequate" titration.[12,13] Thus many patients on CPAP therapy, even those who undergo attended in-laboratory titrations, may currently be treated with suboptimal pressures settings. More data are needed to better define the optimal clinical and physiologic benchmarks for the various levels of PAP titration adequacy as well as to determine the outcomes and proper management for patients who do not achieve optimal or good PAP titrations during an in-laboratory titration study. The important point is that the clinician should not assume that a given patient is on an adequate CPAP setting simply because the patient's CPAP pressure was determined during an in-laboratory titration study.

Although current recommendations warrant that CPAP titrations occur during a full overnight in-laboratory PSG study, some data suggest that a fixed-pressure CPAP can be successfully initiated in an unattended home setting using various approaches.[14-21] Specifically, several studies confirm that CPAP therapy initiated in an unattended home setting (without HST or PSG monitoring to confirm the efficacy of treatment) can be successful in many patients with uncomplicated OSA (OSA without associated chronic obstructive pulmonary disease [COPD], congestive heart failure [CHF], or hypoventilation syndromes) when CPAP settings are determined by a clinical prediction formula,[20] by CPAP self-adjusted to resolve snoring and daytime symptoms,[17,18] or APAP therapy[14-16,21] (Table 18-2).

It is important to note that all of these methods typically offer only a starting pressure for initiating CPAP therapy. As observed in several of the study protocols, many patients may require pressure adjustments based on symptoms and problems with therapy. Because results from several studies continue to support the efficacy of PAP titrations in unattended nonlaboratory settings for patients with uncomplicated OSA, specifically with the use of APAP devices, PAP therapy may potentially be initiated in the home for many patients with uncomplicated OSA. It is possible that in the future, in-laboratory attended CPAP titrations may be reserved for patients with OSA and concomitant cardiac or respiratory disease, those with obesity hypoventilation syndrome, and those who are having difficulty with CPAP initiated in an unattended setting. If such an approach to CPAP treatment comes to fruition, patients with OSA may benefit by realizing shorter waiting times for CPAP therapy, and health care dollars should be saved by reducing the need for unnecessary PSG studies.[15,16,18,19,22]

Benefits of Therapy

It is the perception of many non–sleep practitioners and the lay public that CPAP treatment consistently resolves or improves several important outcomes, including sleep architecture, daytime sleepiness, neurocognitive function, mood, quality of life, and cardiovascular disease in all patients with OSA. When titrated appropriately, CPAP therapy has been demonstrated to resolve most sleep breathing disorder across the spectrum of disease severity and has been demonstrated to be superior to placebo, conservative management, and positional therapy with regard to this outcome.[9,23] Randomized controlled trials have also shown CPAP therapy to be superior to placebo at increasing the percentage of time and total time in stages N3 (non–rapid eye movement [NREM] sleep stage 3) and REM sleep. The effects of CPAP on other sleep parameters, including stages N1 and N2 sleep, total sleep time, and the arousal index, have been inconsistent across studies.[9,23]

Effect on Daytime Sleepiness

Several randomized controlled studies have shown that CPAP therapy significantly improves or resolves subjective symptoms of daytime sleepiness in OSA patients who suffer from this complaint, predominantly in those who suffer from severe OSA (AHI >30 events/hour).[18,21,24-31] The minimal and optimal amounts of nocturnal use necessary to improve symptoms of daytime sleepiness are, however, not well defined because even partial nocturnal use (as little as 2 hours per night) has been associated with significant improvements in daytime symptoms in some patients.[32,33] Although the minimal amount of time required on a nightly basis to improve symptoms of daytime sleepiness is not well established, it is clear that CPAP therapy is required for a least a portion of each night because symptoms of daytime sleepiness reappear when CPAP therapy is discontinued for as little as one to two nights.[6,34,35] Reoccurrence of daytime symptoms on CPAP withdrawal has been observed across the spectrum of OSA severity. As mentioned previously, a specific threshold for nightly use of CPAP, in terms of improvements in symptoms of daytime sleepiness, does not exist and is likely dependent on the individual.[32,33] In general, greater adherence to CPAP therapy on a nightly basis has been associated with greater improvements in symptoms of daytime sleepiness.

The data regarding the effects of CPAP on more objective measures of daytime sleepiness are more inconclusive across the spectrum of disease severity.[23,24] A large meta-analysis of randomized controlled trials comparing CPAP therapy with placebo or conservative management demonstrated only a small, although statistically significant, improvement in the mean sleep latency as measured on either the Multiple Sleep Latency Test (MSLT) or Maintenance of Wakefulness Test (MWT). Across all studies, the mean sleep latency improved by 0.93 minutes ($P = .04$). Whether this small improvement in objective sleepiness is clinically significant is unclear.

Although most patients with daytime sleepiness related to OSA will achieve significant improvements in symptoms after CPAP therapy has been instituted, this is not the case for all patients. There remains a subgroup of OSA patients who continue to suffer from symptoms of residual daytime

Table 18-2	Clinical Prediction Formulas Used to Determine an Effective Continuous Positive Airway Pressure Setting
Study	**Clinical Prediction Formula**
Miljeteig & Hoffstein, 1993[166]	P(eff) = 0.13 (BMI) + 0.16 (NC) + 0.04 (RDI) – 5.12
Lin et al, 2003[167]	P(eff) = 0.52 + 0.174 (BMI) + 0.042 (AHI)
Stradling, 2004[168]	P(eff) = 2.1 + 0.048 (ODI) + 0.128 (NC)
Hukins, 2005[169]	BMI < 30 = 8 cm H_2O BMI 30–35 = 10 cm H_2O BMI > 35 = 12 cm H_2O
Loredo, 2007[170]	P(eff) = 30.8 + RDI (0.03) – nadir SaO₂ (0.05) – mean SaO₂ (0.2)

AHI, Apnea-hypopnea index; BMI, body mass index; NC, neck circumference; ODI, oxygen desaturation index; P(eff), effective continuous positive airway pressure; RDI, respiratory disturbance index.

sleepiness despite adequate compliance with CPAP therapy,[32,33,36,37] although the actual prevalence of residual daytime sleepiness in CPAP-compliant patients remains undefined. Prospective observational data have demonstrated that as many as 20% to 30% of patients who are compliant with CPAP therapy for 7 hours or longer per night may still complain of subjective sleepiness (Epworth Sleepiness Scale score of >10) after 3 months of treatment.[32,33] In addition, many patients also may not achieve a normal level of objective alertness (as defined by the MSLT or MWT) or associated functional outcomes (as defined by the Functional Outcomes of Sleep Questionnaire [FOSQ]), despite seemingly adequate nightly use of CPAP therapy. The mechanisms responsible for this syndrome of residual daytime sleepiness also remain unclear but may in part be related to the oxidative injury effects of long-term intermittent hypoxemia on the sleep-wake cycle–promoting regions in the brain.[38]

Effect on Neurocognitive Function, Mood, and Quality of Life

Numerous studies have assessed the effects of OSA on neurocognitive functioning, mood, and quality of life.[9,30,39-50] Most randomized controlled studies demonstrate inconsistent improvements in several neurobehavioral performance parameters across the spectrum of disease severity.[23,30,31,35,39-41,51] For example, large-scale randomized controlled trials have demonstrated mild, transient improvements in several measures of executive function in patients with severe OSA, but similar improvements have not been consistently demonstrated in patients with less severe disease.[31] The data regarding the therapeutic effects of CPAP treatment on mood and quality of life are also variable and inconsistent, with many randomized trials demonstrating no clear benefits of CPAP therapy compared with placebo or conservative treatments in these parameters.[23]

One reason for the inconsistent improvements in neurocognitive function demonstrated with CPAP therapy is that the impact of OSA on neurocognitive function for most patients with OSA may be relatively small across the spectrum of disease severity. The Apnea Positive Pressure Long-Term Efficacy Study (APPLES) trial demonstrated that most patients with OSA did not have significant neurocognitive deficits and that the degree of deficit was only weakly associated with the degree of oxygen desaturation and not associated with the AHI.[52] Another possible explanation for the inconsistent effect of CPAP in improving outcomes associated with neurocognition, mood, and quality of life is the use of multiple, different measures of function to assess similar parameters. For example, there is nearly universal use of the Epworth Sleepiness Scale when assessing improvements in subjective sleepiness, yet there are multiple tests that are used across several studies to assess for improvements in mood, neurocognitive function, and quality of life. Further research is required to better define the role of CPAP therapy in alleviating these symptoms and deficits in susceptible OSA patients.

Despite the inconsistent data regarding improvements in neurocognitive function with CPAP use, several observational studies support a significant reduction in the incidence of motor vehicle accidents in patients with OSA following the initiation of CPAP therapy.[53] Although the actual time course to improved driving performance in real-life situations is not clear, driving simulator performance can improve in as little as two to seven nights of therapy. Similar to other aspects of neurobehavioral performance that may be adversely affected by OSA, many patients with OSA may continue to demonstrate impaired driving simulator performance despite several months of high adherence to CPAP therapy.[54] The explanation for this last finding is not completely clear, although it is likely that many patients may still not be adhering to PAP therapy enough on a nightly basis or achieving enough sleep on a regular basis to normalize their driving skills. Unfortunately, there is no specific threshold of CPAP use or duration of treatment that can accurately predict a given individual's fitness to safely drive a vehicle. Because the severity of OSA alone is not a reliable predictor of motor vehicle accident risk, the clinician must take into account several factors, including improvements in subjective symptoms and compliance with therapy, before determining a driver's ability to safely operate a motor vehicle.

Effect on Cardiovascular Disease

Although untreated OSA has been associated with an increased risk for hypertension and other cardiovascular diseases in certain populations, the literature and outcomes data supporting the beneficial effects of CPAP on cardiovascular outcomes have been inconsistent.[9,23,55,56] Several randomized clinical trials and meta-analyses have assessed the effects of CPAP on blood pressure.[57-59] Overall, CPAP treatment appears to attenuate the adverse effects of untreated OSA on daytime and nocturnal systolic and diastolic blood pressure and on 24-hour mean blood pressure. These data demonstrate that, compared with placebo, sham CPAP, or supportive therapy alone, CPAP treatment is associated with small (−1.8 to −3.0 mm Hg) but statistically significant improvements in diurnal mean arterial systolic and diastolic blood pressures. When considering pooled data, improvements in systolic and diastolic blood pressures have been observed both during the daytime (2.2 ± 0.7 mm Hg and 1.9 ± 0.6 mm Hg, respectively) and nighttime (3.8 ± 0.8 mm Hg and 1.8 ± 0.6 mm Hg, respectively).[57] In general, improvements in blood pressure with CPAP therapy have been associated with greater severity of baseline OSA (higher AHI), the presence of subjective daytime sleepiness, younger age, and greater adherence with CPAP use on a nightly basis.

One of the main limitations of the current studies evaluating the effect of CPAP use on blood pressure in patients with OSAS is that, although these studies evaluated blood pressure as an outcome measure, several of the studies either did not include patients with hypertension or included patients with hypertension who were already adequately controlled on antihypertensive medications. More robust reductions and clinical improvements in blood pressure with CPAP therapy have been observed when evaluating data from studies that included patients with uncontrolled hypertension.[60] In patients with uncontrolled hypertension at baseline, the use of CPAP has been associated with significantly greater reductions in awake systolic and diastolic blood pressure (7.1 mm Hg and 4.3 mm Hg, respectively) compared with placebo or sham PAP therapy. These improvements have been observed even after controlling for several potential confounders, including severity of disease, daytime sleepiness, patient demographics, use of antihypertensive medications, CPAP adherence, and duration of CPAP therapy.

Few studies have compared the effects of CPAP and antihypertensive medication on blood pressure reduction in patients with OSA and hypertension. In one randomized controlled trial, medical treatment with valsartan (160 mg daily) alone without CPAP therapy reduced several parameters of blood pressure significantly more than CPAP therapy alone over an 8-week period.[61] Specifically, valsartan therapy demonstrated superior reductions in 24-hour mean arterial pressure (-2.1 ± 4.9 mm Hg with CPAP vs. 9.1 ± 7.2 mm Hg with valsartan; $P < .001$) as well as mean arterial blood pressures during the daytime and throughout the night compared with CPAP therapy. The addition of CPAP therapy to antihypertensive medication does appear to improve blood pressure control in some patients with resistant hypertension and moderate to severe OSA.[62] Based on limited data, the addition of CPAP therapy to a regimen of several antihypertensive medications improved 24-hour mean blood pressure (3.1 mm Hg; 95% confidence interval [CI], 0.6 to 5.6; $P = .02$) and 24-hour diastolic blood pressure (3.2 mm Hg; 95% CI, 1.0 to 5.4; $P = .005$), but did not result in a significant improvement in 24-hour systolic blood pressure (3.1 mm Hg; 95% CI, -0.6 to 6.7; $P = .10$) compared with the control group. In addition, CPAP therapy resulted in a greater proportion of patients demonstrating a normal nocturnal "dip" in blood pressure compared with controls (35.9% vs. 21.6%; adjusted odds ratio [OR], 2.4; 95% CI, 1.2 to 5.1; $P = .02$). Similar to other studies, there was a significant dose-response effect, with greater nightly CPAP use being associated with greater improvements in 24-hour mean blood pressure, systolic blood pressure, and diastolic blood pressure. Although reductions in nocturnal blood have been observed more consistently in his patient population, improvements in daytime blood pressure with CPAP therapy have been less consistent.[63]

As noted previously, the presence of subjective daytime sleepiness has generally been associated with a more robust improvement in blood pressure with CPAP therapy. There is some bias in these data because most of the studies that have evaluated various outcomes have in fact predominantly assessed patients with OSA and such associated daytime sleepiness. Because more than half of all patients with OSA, including those with severe disease (AHI $\geq$30 events/hour) do not have associated daytime sleepiness, it would be important to determine whether treating patients with OSA who do not complain of subjective sleepiness improves blood pressure or reduces the incidence of hypertension and other cardiovascular morbidities. One large randomized controlled trial assessing CPAP therapy compared with conservative therapy in patients with moderate to severe OSA without daytime sleepiness found that CPAP therapy did not result in a statistically significant reduction in incident hypertension or cardiovascular events (nonfatal myocardial infarction or stroke, transient ischemic attack, congestive heart failure, or cardiovascular death) over a period of 4 years of follow-up.[64] When the data were stratified by CPAP adherence, however, patients using prescribed CPAP therapy for more than 4 hours per night did demonstrate a small but statistically significant ($P = 0.04$) reduction in the incidence of hypertension over the 4-year study period. Thus the benefit of treating patients with moderate to severe OSA who do not have symptoms of daytime sleepiness or cardiovascular disease remains to be better defined regarding the risk for future cardiovascular morbidity and mortality. In fact, however, the role of CPAP

therapy in reducing the incidence of hypertension and other cardiovascular morbidity in OSA patients even with daytime sleepiness is also unclear because there are no large-scale long-term prospective data addressing this at this time.

The role of CPAP therapy in resolving or reducing the occurrence or reoccurrence of cardiac arrhythmias is uncertain. Several observational studies have demonstrated an association between OSA and atrial fibrillation as well as a higher risk for recurrence of atrial fibrillation after electrical cardioversion or catheter ablation therapy. These studies also have shown an association between increased adherence with CPAP therapy and a lower reoccurrence rate of atrial fibrillation after these procedures.[65-68] Because all of the current data regarding CPAP therapy and atrial fibrillation are based on observational studies, the role of CPAP as an adjunct treatment to improve atrial arrhythmia control remains uncertain. Although there may be an increased risk for ventricular arrhythmias (tachycardia and fibrillation) in some patients with untreated OSA, there are limited data on the effect of PAP therapy for reducing the incidence and prevalence of these events.[69] Thus the role of PAP therapy in reducing ventricular arrhythmias in patients with OSA is not clear.

There are several possible explanations for why CPAP therapy has not been demonstrated to result in more consistent and greater improvements in blood pressure and other cardiovascular outcomes in patients with OSA. First, most of the literature assessing the effects of CPAP on blood pressure has been based on small trials of relatively short duration ($\leq$3 months). This duration of treatment, even in patients with underlying hypertension, may not be a long enough treatment time to improve blood pressure. Second, as mentioned previously, although several of the studies used blood pressure as an outcome measure, many of the studies enrolled patients without hypertension at baseline. Thus one would not necessarily expect to observe a change in blood pressure if hypertension was not present at the initiation of the studies. Also, most of the patients who had hypertension at enrollment were on antihypertensive medications during most of the studies, which is likely to attenuate the effect of CPAP on blood pressure decreases. Third, although improvements in blood pressure tend to be associated with better CPAP adherence, overall adherence in most studies have typically averaged between 4 and 5 hours per night. Thus inadequate nighttime CPAP use may limit the beneficial effect of therapy on blood pressure in those with and without hypertension. Fourth, even though OSA is found to be an independent risk factor for hypertension in many populations, hypertension is typically associated with several comorbid conditions that are also related to OSA. Thus treating OSA without treating the other comorbid conditions may not result in significant improvements in blood pressure or other cardiovascular outcomes. Fifth, it is possible that many patients with longstanding hypertension have fixed disease that CPAP therapy may not improve. Sixth, many studies use different definitions for hypopneas (i.e., associated with a 4 percentage-point oxygen saturation, 3 percentage-point oxygen desaturation, or 3 percentage-point oxygen desaturation with or without an associated electroencephalogram arousal), and it is difficult to compare such studies because changing the definition of the hypopneas also changes the definition of OSA as well as the severity of disease for many patients. Finally, not all untreated OSA patients are necessarily at similar risk for the development of hypertension.

Thus trials that are unable to stratify patients deemed to be at higher risk for hypertension may only demonstrate mean results across a given population. When, and if, biomarkers are discovered that may identify patients at higher risk for hypertension and other cardiovascular diseases, therapies such as CPAP may be targeted to at-risk populations that would be deemed to derive greater benefits from therapy.

Aside from the one randomized controlled trial evaluating the effects of CPAP on incident hypertension and cardiovascular disease in patients with moderate to severe OSA without daytime sleepiness, there are currently limited long-term randomized controlled data evaluating the effect of CPAP on any cardiovascular outcomes, including mortality. The most convincing long-term data regarding the potential beneficial effects of CPAP therapy on cardiovascular outcomes comes from Marin and colleagues,[70] who followed a large group of male OSA patients with a spectrum of OSA severity and associated daytime sleepiness in a prospective observational study over a period of 10 years. Their results demonstrated two important findings: (1) Compared with normal nonsnoring controls, patients with untreated severe OSA (defined as an AHI >30 events/hour) had a significantly increased incidence of both fatal and nonfatal cardiovascular events; and (2) CPAP treatment (>4 hours/night) in patients with severe OSA (AHI ≥30 events/hour) reduced the incidence of adverse cardiovascular outcomes and improved survival, demonstrating outcomes similar to normal controls. Similar improvements in outcomes with CPAP therapy were not observed in OSA patients with less severe disease because untreated mild to moderate OSA was not observed to be associated with increased risk for cardiovascular morbidity or mortality in this study. Another observational study also demonstrated improvements in cardiovascular mortality across a spectrum of OSA severity, although the data are limited by absence of a control group.[71]

Given the inconclusive nature of CPAP therapy on cardiovascular outcomes in general, the AASM Practice Parameters recommend CPAP therapy only as an adjunctive therapy to lower blood pressure in hypertensive patients with OSA.[9] Several other authorities and professional societies have recommended that further supporting data are required to better determine the role of CPAP therapy on improving cardiovascular outcomes before making recommendations for its use in various populations.[55,56]

Effect on Mild Obstructive Sleep Apnea

Most of the literature assessing the effects of CPAP on various outcomes has predominantly evaluated OSA patients with moderate to severe disease. Although approximately 28% of patients with mild disease (AHI = 5 to 14 events/hour) complain of subjective daytime sleepiness,[72] it remains unclear whether treating this group of patients with CPAP therapy improves their daytime symptoms. Results from the CPAP Apnea Trial North American Program (CATNAP) demonstrated that CPAP therapy significantly improved daytime symptoms as measured by the FOSQ compared with sham CPAP therapy in patients with mild to moderate OSA over an 8-week period of follow-up.[73] APPLES was a large multicenter randomized controlled trial comparing the neurocognitive effects of therapeutic CPAP with sham CPAP across the spectrum of OSA severity.[31] As expected, subjective daytime sleepiness and objective alertness as assessed by the

MWT was improved by CPAP therapy at 6 months, but significant improvements in both of these parameters were only observed in patients with severe OSA (AHI ≥30 events/hour). In patients with moderate disease (AHI = 15 to 29 events/hour), improvements in subjective sleepiness, but not objective alertness, were observed after 6 months of therapy. In patients with mild disease, there were no significant improvements in objective alertness or subjective sleepiness after 2 and 6 months of CPAP therapy. Thus the role of CPAP therapy for this indication in patients with mild disease remains unclear based on the current data. It appears reasonable to initiate CPAP therapy in patients with daytime symptoms, but the decision to continue chronic therapy in this patients group should be based on a response to therapy. For patients with mild disease without daytime symptoms, it is not clear that treating these patients is beneficial or should be recommended based on the current data.

Effect on REM-Predominant Obstructive Sleep Apnea

The prevalence of REM sleep–related or REM-predominant OSA is unclear, in part because of the absence of a standard definition for this entity. This OSA variant tends to be more common in women, although it may affect adult patients of both genders across the age spectrum.[12,74] The association of this OSA variant with daytime or nighttime symptoms is not clear, but it appears that a subgroup of patients are affected. For patients who demonstrate this type of OSA and complain of daytime symptoms or nighttime sleep disturbance, it is unclear whether treatment with CPAP consistently improves daytime or nighttime symptoms. Limited observational data of CPAP therapy in symptomatic patients with such REM-predominant OSA have demonstrated significant improvements in daytime sleepiness, fatigue, and the FOSQ. These improvements with CPAP therapy were similar to those in patients with OSA not limited to REM sleep.[12] However, there are no randomized controlled data assessing any outcomes in this subgroup of patients, including cardiovascular disease outcomes.

Effect on Obstructive Sleep Apnea and Comorbid Diseases

CHF is a common disease with an estimated prevalence of concomitant OSA of approximately 33%. Two small randomized controlled trials demonstrated a beneficial effect of CPAP therapy on left ventricular ejection fraction (LVEF) in patients with concomitant OSA and CHF with systolic dysfunction.[75,76] Compared with optimal medical management alone, CHF patients with moderate to severe OSA showed left LVEF improvements of 5% to 9% over 1 to 3 months.[75,76] Since these earlier studies, several additional randomized controlled studies have assessed the effects of CPAP therapy on LVEF in CHF patients with and without systolic dysfunction.[77] Overall, CPAP therapy has shown statistically significant improvements in LVEF in patients with OSA and concomitant systolic dysfunction, with an average improvement in LVEF across studies of approximately 5%. In patients with diastolic CHF and concomitant OSA, CPAP therapy has not been associated with significant improvements in LVEF (1%). For patients with CHF and systolic dysfunction, one would expect this degree of improvement in LVEF to be associated with improvements in other outcomes based on trials of medical therapies for CHF. However, it is uncertain whether the improvements in LVEF in patients with OSA and concomitant CHF translate into improvements in other important outcomes, such as reductions in hospitalizations and mortality. Most of the studies evaluating this patient population have been limited by small sample sizes and relatively short durations of follow-up (typically 12 weeks or less). Currently, two large randomized trials are evaluating the role of advanced PAP therapies in this population to determine whether PAP treatment can be used to enhance these important outcomes. Until these studies are completed, the role of CPAP therapy in patients with CHF and OSA to improve important outcomes beyond LVEF remains unclear. Patients with severe heart failure may also have concomitant central and obstructive sleep apnea. An interim analysis of this therapy suggests that advanced PAP therapies (such as adaptive servo ventilation) may have a negative effect on cardiovascular mortality in heart failure patients with predominantly Cheyne-Stokes breathing and a left ventricular ejection fraction of 45% or less (see Chapter 28).[78]

The *overlap syndrome* refers to the coexistence of OSA with COPD (see Chapter 29). The prevalence of OSA in patients with COPD appears to be similar to that of the general population. Prospective observational and retrospective studies have shown that untreated OSA in this patient group is associated with an increased risk for death and severe COPD exacerbations leading to hospitalizations compared with groups of COPD patients without concomitant OSA.[79,80] Observational data have shown that CPAP therapy in OSA patients with COPD has been associated with significant reductions in both acute exacerbations of COPD requiring hospitalizations and death, with outcomes similar to COPD patients without OSA. Increased adherence to CPAP therapy has been independently associated with reduced mortality in this patient population, whereas decreased CPAP adherence and increased age have been independently associated with increased mortality.[80] Observational data suggest that adherence to CPAP therapy for as little as 2 hours per night has been associated with a reduction in mortality in this group of patients. Given the current observational data, it is reasonable to recommend CPAP therapy in patients with the overlap syndrome, although given the absence of randomized controlled data in this patient population, the role of CPAP therapy to reduce exacerbations or improve mortality remains undefined.

The role of CPAP therapy in improving important outcomes associated with diabetes mellitus (short-term and long-term glucose control) in patients with concomitant OSA is unclear because most of the trials evaluating the use of CPAP in this patient population have yielded inconsistent results.[81,82] The role of CPAP as an adjunct therapy to improve weight loss is also uncertain, and adequate treatment of OSA has not been observed to result in enhanced weight loss in most studies.[83]

Comparison with Other Obstructive Sleep Apnea Treatments

Oral appliances (nonadjustable mandibular advancement devices and tongue-retaining devices) are typically recommended for patients with mild to moderate OSA as well as for patients with severe disease who fail or do not tolerate CPAP therapy. In general, CPAP therapy results in greater improvements in the AHI and degree of oxygen desaturation

compared with oral appliance treatment. Despite these findings, improvements in daytime sleepiness tend to be similar between the two therapies. This may be related to greater overall compliance with oral appliance therapy compared with CPAP.[84,85] Comparisons of CPAP with oral appliance therapy for improvements in blood pressure are difficult. Although most of the pooled data suggest a favorable effect of oral appliance therapy on many parameters of blood pressure, most of the studies have been observational, with few head-to-head comparisons between the two treatments.[86,87] Thus based on the current data, it is difficult to draw conclusions or make recommendations between the two therapies concerning the outcome of blood pressure control.

Oxygen Therapy

The risk for cardiovascular disease related to untreated OSA is dependent on numerous factors, including the severity of disease, as defined by the AHI, and the degree of associated oxygen desaturation. Several small studies have shown that nocturnal oxygen therapy alone can in fact improve both the AHI and degree of oxygen desaturation, although such therapy may be associated with a prolongation of apneas and hypopneas. CPAP, however, has been associated with greater improvements in the AHI compared with nocturnal oxygen therapy alone.[88] Further, a short-term (12 weeks) randomized controlled trial has shown that CPAP results in greater reductions in 24-hour mean arterial blood pressure compared with nocturnal oxygen (2 liters/minute) or supportive therapy without CPAP in patients with moderate to severe OSA and cardiovascular disease or multiple cardiovascular risk factors. Similar to other studies, decreases in blood pressure with CPAP therapy were relatively small compared with baseline or the control group (−2.4 mm Hg).[89] Oxygen therapy alone was not associated with any changes in blood pressure compared with baseline or the control group over the study period.

Outcomes Summary

CPAP consistently improves or resolves OSA events across the spectrum of OSA severity and improves symptoms of daytime sleepiness predominantly in patients with moderate to severe OSA. Improvements in other outcomes are inconsistent. Treatment with CPAP has been associated with small reductions in blood pressure, with greater reductions being observed in patients with poorly controlled or resistant hypertension. The role of CPAP therapy in reducing long-term cardiovascular risk or mortality in OSA is uncertain based on the current data. Finally, the role of CPAP in patients without daytime symptoms, cardiovascular disease, or cardiovascular risk factors across the spectrum of OSA severity is undefined.

ADHERENCE AND PROBLEMS WITH CONTINUOUS POSITIVE AIRWAY PRESSURE TREATMENT

In a perfect world, all patients with OSA would use their CPAP therapy all night, every night. Unfortunately, just like many therapies associated with other chronic diseases, adherence with CPAP therapy for OSA is far from perfect. Although there are no formal definitions of what constitutes adherence with CPAP therapy, most studies have arbitrarily defined adherence as use of CPAP greater than or equal to 4 hours per night for 70% of the observed nights.[90] Using this definition, subjective adherence ranges between 65% and 90%, whereas objective measures of CPAP adherence have demonstrated use in the range of 40% to 83%.[91] Most studies have shown that patients usually overestimate their CPAP use by approximately 1 hour per night, a pattern that is observed in both new and long-term OSA patients.[90,92]

Short-term follow-up of OSA patients demonstrates that CPAP use patterns typically fall into two groups: (1) use of CPAP on more than 90% of the nights, with an average use time of greater than 6 hours per night, and (2) use of CPAP intermittently, with an average use of less than $3\frac{1}{2}$ hours per night.[93] Early follow-up for patients newly initiated on CPAP therapy is important because these patterns of use can typically be identified within the first several days to several months of CPAP therapy.[86-89] Long-term objective follow-up has demonstrated that approximately 68% of OSA patients continue to use their CPAP therapy after 5 years.[92]

Some studies have suggested certain parameters that may predict greater short- and long-term adherence to therapy. Improved adherence has been associated with symptoms of subjective sleepiness (Epworth Sleepiness Scale score of >10), severity of OSA (AHI >30 events/hour), and average nightly adherence within the first 3 months of therapy. Reduced short- and long-term adherence has been observed in patients reporting problems during their initial night with CPAP therapy in the sleep laboratory.[92,94] Interestingly, although one might expect higher levels of CPAP pressure to predict poorer adherence, neither high nor low CPAP pressures have been shown to reliably predict CPAP use. Several studies have also associated African American race and lower socioeconomic status with poorer adherence with CPAP therapy, even in patients with standardized access to care and treatment.[95-97] The reasons for this last observation are not clear.

Role of Objective Adherence Monitoring and Limitations with Current Technology

Unfortunately, when taken together, most studies have not been able to identify factors that consistently predict short- or long-term adherence with CPAP therapy.[26,90,98-101] Because adherence with PAP therapy tends to be suboptimal, subjective adherence tends to overestimate objective PAP use, there are no consistent early predictors of PAP adherence, and PAP adherence patterns tend to be determined early in most patients, professional societies currently recommend, and many payer policies require, objective adherence data review to document adherence with therapy and identify problems that can be addressed.[3] Although most randomized controlled trials have used objective adherence data to monitor outcomes related to PAP therapy, the overall effect of assessing objective compliance data for all patients on PAP therapy is uncertain.

Most of the PAP manufacturers have developed sophisticated online software programs for monitoring several parameters of PAP therapy, including nightly adherence, efficacy of therapy (residual AHI), and problems with mask fit (primarily amount of air leak). Although there are several potential advantages to these programs, the technologies also have several potential limitations. To improve the effect of these technologies on meaningful patient outcomes, several improvements will be required, including (1) standardization of respiratory event and leak definitions among manufacturers as well as validation of the device outputs compared with

PSG; (2) improved access of PAP adherence data for frontline providers, including determining ways to more easily integrate PAP adherence data into the various electronic medical record software programs; and (3) education of non–sleep specialists on interpretation of the available adherence information.

Interventions to Promote Adherence

Typical problems that may lead to reduced adherence with CPAP therapy include claustrophobia, nasal congestion, and poor mask fit, leading to leaks and skin irritation. Several interventions have been proposed and instituted in an attempt to improve adherence with CPAP therapy (Table 18-3).

The most consistent intervention that has been associated with improved CPAP adherence in most PAP-naïve patients is systematic education. Several approaches, including provider and home-based education of the patient and spouse, supportive care at therapy initiation or follow-up, phone calls, home-based videos, and daylong educational programs, have been associated with improved adherence, although no one intervention has been demonstrated to be consistently beneficial in all patient groups. In general, increased intensity of patient education or frequency of health provider contact have been associated with improved CPAP adherence.[9,23] Overall, these educational interventions tend to improve CPAP adherence by approximately 35 to 50 minutes per night,[102] although the effects of these interventions on other important outcomes such as daytime sleepiness, quality of life, and cardiovascular disease and risk are unclear. Several behavioral approaches have also been associated with improved adherence. In general, these behavioral approaches, including motivational interviewing and cognitive behavioral therapy delivered in individual or group settings, have been associated with an average improvement in adherence of 1.5 hours per night. The overall effect of these behavioral approaches on CPAP adherence is not well defined because the data supporting these approaches are of lower quality than the data supporting the previously discussed educational interventions.

The data evaluating the effects of heated humidification on adherence to CPAP therapy remain controversial. Although there are some studies that demonstrate that the addition of heated humidification can improve adherence to CPAP therapy, there are several studies demonstrating no improvement in adherence with this intervention.[9,103-106] Patients who tend to benefit the most from the addition of heated humidification are those with symptoms of nasal congestion or rhinitis. Limited data evaluating the role of heated tubing have shown no improvements in adherence in patients with and without nasopharyngeal complaints.[107] The role of nasal steroids with or without heated humidification therapy, especially in unselected CPAP-naïve patients with OSA, remains unclear because many studies have demonstrated little benefit of this intervention in improving CPAP use.[106,108]

CPAP delivery interfaces, or masks, come in several shapes and sizes, including nasal masks, full-face (oronasal) masks that cover both the nose and the mouth, nasal pillows that fit into the nostrils, and oral interfaces that fit into the mouth. Some studies have observed a negative effect of oronasal masks on CPAP compliance, whereas other studies have not confirmed these findings.[109] Oronasal masks may be better for patients with chronic nasal congestion or obstruction, for those patients who are predominantly mouth breathers, and

Table 18-3 Effects of Interventions on Positive Airway Pressure Adherence

Intervention	Effect on PAP Adherence	Comments
Education and supportive care	Beneficial	Various approaches helpful, including phone calls, office and home visits, and individual and group sessions Best intervention, or combination, unclear
Behavioral therapies	Beneficial	Various therapies helpful, including motivational interviewing and CBT Most interventions studied in addition to education Best intervention, or combination, unclear
Heated humidification	Beneficial	Some data support improved adherence Most helpful for patients with nasal congestion or rhinitis Addition of nasal steroids not helpful
Advanced PAP (bilevel, EPR, and APAP)	No benefit	Not associated with improved compliance BiFlex may be the exception in CPAP noncompliant patients
Mask type	Unclear	Best mask type unclear Changing masks may alter effective PAP pressure
Hypnotics	Unclear	Eszopiclone may improve PAP titration efficacy and 6-month compliance Data do not support other hypnotics
Telemedicine	Unclear	Limited data suggest benefit, whereas other data do not support approach
Adherence monitoring	Unclear	Objective adherence monitoring recommended, but no clear data that the intervention itself improves compliance
Sleep specialist care	Unclear	Observational studies support approach RCTs show no advantage in uncomplicated OSA

APAP, Autotitrated positive airway pressure; CBT, cognitive behavioral therapy; EPR, expiratory pressure relief; OSA obstructive sleep apnea; PAP, positive airway pressure; RCT, randomized controlled trial.

for patients requiring higher CPAP pressures when mask leak is an issue. Nasal pillows have typically not been recommended for CPAP settings of more than 12 cm H_2O owing to the potential for interface leak, although more recent data show that select patients may do well with a nasal pillows interface even with higher PAP settings.[110] Overall, although proper mask fit may be crucial to the initial and ongoing acceptance of CPAP therapy, the optimal form and type of CPAP delivery interface remain unclear.[111,112] In general, the best interface for a given patient (which tends to correlate to the best adherence with therapy) is the one that the patient is most comfortable wearing.

Changing interfaces after a problem has developed has not been shown to consistently improve long-term adherence in various studies, although from a clinician's standpoint attention to mask complaints and changing masks when problems arise can improve adherence in select patients. The provider should be aware that changing the mask type from nasal to oronasal or vice versa might change the necessary effective treatment pressure that was initially identified during an in-laboratory titration.[113] Thus for patients on fixed PAP therapy, the clinician should consider the need to adjust the pressure or to have the patient perform an in-laboratory PAP titration if problems that could result in reduced adherence with therapy persist after a mask change has been instituted.

Because many patients may complain of sleep disruption or difficulty initiating sleep during the first few days to weeks of CPAP therapy, several studies have evaluated the use of prescription hypnotics to improve adherence to CPAP treatment either in the sleep laboratory during a PAP titration study or during the first few weeks of therapy. Although some studies have demonstrated that, in newly diagnosed patients

with severe OSA, treatment with eszopiclone 3 mg before an overnight titration study or during the first 14 days of PAP therapy has been associated with improved quality of CPAP titrations (greater proportion of patients with optimal or good titrations) or improved adherence to CPAP therapy over the first 6 months of treatment, respectively, these results are not typical of most of the literature regarding the use of hypnotics as adjunctive therapies to improve adherence to PAP therapy.[13,114] When compared with placebo or usual care, other randomized controlled studies have demonstrated no significant benefits, but no significant adverse effects of other hypnotic therapies (zaleplon or zolpidem), on CPAP adherence.[115,116] As with most studies, the data evaluating the effects of hypnotics on CPAP adherence have looked at relatively short-term adherence in specialized centers of care. The ability to generalize these data to a typical clinical population and office setting is uncertain based on the current literature, and care should be used when applying this approach to a given patient or population. Given the limited data in patients with OSA, the use of short-term or chronic hypnotics should generally be avoided in patients with OSA.

Role of the Sleep Specialist in Improving Adherence

Several retrospective and observational studies have shown that sleep specialist consultation, before an in-laboratory sleep study or during the initiation and follow-up of CPAP therapy, has been associated with improved CPAP adherence and other important outcomes, such as patient satisfaction and timeliness of care.[91,117] Alternatively, three randomized controlled trials in symptomatic patients with a high clinical suspicion of uncomplicated moderate to severe OSA demonstrated that management by either a specially trained nurse, nurse–primary care physician team, or primary care physician resulted in outcomes (CPAP adherence and improvements in daytime sleepiness) that were similar to management by sleep specialists.[118-120] In addition to similar CPAP adherence, all of these studies demonstrated a significant cost savings in the non–sleep specialist group. Thus the data supporting the role of the sleep specialist in the treatment and overall management of all patients with uncomplicated moderate to severe OSA is not well defined based on the current literature. More research is necessary to better determine which groups of patients with OSA may receive the most benefit from sleep specialist management of CPAP therapy.

Current recommendations, based predominantly on expert opinion, suggest that patients should have initial office follow-up during the first few weeks of prescribed CPAP therapy. Thereafter patients using CPAP should be followed on an annual basis and as needed to troubleshoot problems as they arise.[9,23] Centers for Medicare and Medicaid Services has defined its own rules regulating how and when patients on CPAP should have office follow-up, and commercial payers have also adopted their own policies on CPAP follow-up and adherence monitoring. Based on the current outcomes literature, the optimal method or schedule for short- or long-term follow-up is not clear. Clinicians must determine appropriate follow-up based on a given patient's response to therapy as well as payer policies that may guide requirements to continue treatment.

Technology to Improve Adherence

In addition to technologic advancements in the delivery of PAP therapy that are discussed later in this chapter, several applications of technology have been employed in an attempt to improve PAP adherence. Interventions include the use of online PAP adherence monitoring software as described earlier, telemedicine, and patient interactive technologies. As noted previously, most patients overestimate their compliance with therapy and thus objective monitoring of CPAP therapy has been recommended by the AASM.[3,9] Although the literature supports the concept that CPAP use can be reliably determined by CPAP tracking systems, the role of objectively measuring PAP adherence and its effect on improving adherence in all patients are uncertain.[121] Limited data suggest that online monitoring of PAP adherence and the use of a telemedicine management strategy may be associated with improved adherence, although more data are required to better define the role of this approach.[122] Finally, although several PAP device manufacturers have developed software (smartphone and computer-based applications) aimed at improving patient involvement with their CPAP therapy, there are currently no randomized trials that have objectively evaluated the effect of this approach on adherence or, in fact, any outcomes.

TECHNOLOGIC ADVANCEMENTS IN THE DELIVERY OF POSITIVE AIRWAY PRESSURE THERAPY FOR OBSTRUCTIVE SLEEP APNEA

Although CPAP remains the mainstay of therapy for OSA, there are several other methods of delivering PAP therapy. This section of the chapter focuses on technologic advancements in the delivery of positive pressure therapy, including bilevel PAP, EPR devices, and APAP.

Bilevel Positive Airway Pressure Therapy

The potential benefits of bilevel PAP in treating patients with OSA were first described in 1990.[123] As opposed to CPAP, which delivers a fixed pressure throughout the respiratory cycle, bilevel PAP therapy allows the independent adjustment of the expiratory positive airway pressure (EPAP) and the inspiratory positive airway pressure (IPAP). In its initial description, bilevel PAP therapy demonstrated that obstructive events could be eliminated at a lower EPAP compared with conventional CPAP pressures.[123] Bilevel PAP is typically titrated during an attended in-laboratory sleep study. As is the case for CPAP titrations, the current guideline recommendations for bilevel PAP titration strategies are based on consensus opinion.[8] Although intuitively one would predict that bilevel PAP would increase adherence by reducing expiratory pressure–related discomfort and side effects, there are in fact no objective outcomes studies that show that bilevel PAP improves adherence and daytime sleepiness compared with CPAP in patients with uncomplicated OSA.[9,23,124]

Newer bilevel PAP systems have been introduced by several companies. The BiFlex device (Respironics, Murrysville, Pa.) differs from conventional bilevel systems in two major respects. First, the inspiratory pressure is reduced slightly near the end of inspiration, and the expiratory pressure is slightly reduced near the beginning of expiration. Second, the amount of pressure relief change of the EPAP during expiration is proportional to patient effort. Although the data regarding the use of traditional bilevel and BiFlex therapies do not demonstrate any advantages over CPAP therapy in patients with newly diagnosed OSA, one study has demonstrated a potential role for BiFlex therapy in patients who are noncompliant with CPAP therapy.[125] Ballard and colleagues studied a large group of OSA patient who were noncompliant with CPAP therapy despite significant education, attention to proper mask fitting, and the addition of heated humidification. After 3 months of therapy, those patients randomized to BiFlex therapy demonstrated significantly better nightly adherence ($P = .03$) compared with those who were randomized to continuing on standard CPAP therapy. Importantly, because BiFlex technology provides PAP through its own unique algorithm, these findings are specific to the BiFlex devices and cannot be generalized to other non-bilevel PAP therapies.

Overall, bilevel PAP therapy remains a reasonable option for CPAP-intolerant patients, patients with OSA with concurrent respiratory disease (e.g., COPD), and patients with obesity hypoventilation syndrome.[2,9,23] The role of bilevel PAP therapy, and its variants, in otherwise uncomplicated OSA remains unclear.[3,126]

Expiratory Pressure Relief Systems

A common complaint in many patients with OSA using CPAP is the uncomfortable feeling of exhaling against positive pressure. This consequence is one potential barrier to the long-term acceptance of CPAP therapy. Several PAP manufacturers have developed EPR systems in an attempt to remedy this potential problem. EPR device technologies allow pressure relief during exhalation with the goal of making CPAP therapy more comfortable. EPR technologies briefly reduce the CPAP pressure, between 1 and 3 cm H_2O, during exhalation and then return the pressure to its set CPAP setting before the initiation of inspiration. Certain EPR technologies monitor the patient's airflow during exhalation and reduce the expiratory pressure in response to the airflow and patient effort. The amount of pressure relief varies on a breath-by-breath basis, depending on the actual patient's airflow, and is also dictated by the patient's preference setting on the device.

Although several PAP manufacturers have developed EPR devices for the marketplace, only the Philips Respironics (Respironics, Murrysville, PA) technology (C-Flex) has been evaluated in the peer-reviewed literature.[120-128] Several randomized controlled trials have evaluated the role of C-Flex technology compared with standard CPAP therapy in patients with uncomplicated, predominantly moderate to severe OSA. Overall, the use of such C-Flex technology at fixed pressure relief settings between 1 and 3 cm H_2O has not been associated with improved adherence in either parallel or crossover trials.[129] In addition, improvements in other commonly measured outcomes (subjective sleepiness, objective alertness, vigilance, or residual OSA) were similar to, but not better than, standard CPAP therapy. C-Flex therapy has not been shown to offer significant benefits in that subgroup of patients who require CPAP pressures of 9 cm H_2O or greater. Based on these data, the routine use of C-Flex technology is not recommended as a method to improve compliance or other major outcomes compared with fixed CPAP therapy. Further randomized controlled trials are necessary to determine whether this technology offers any objective advantages over fixed CPAP therapy in select groups of patients.

Autotitrating Positive Airway Pressure

APAP (also known as auto-, automated, autoadjusting, or automatic positive airway pressure) incorporates the ability of the PAP device to detect and respond to changes in upper airway flow and resistance in real time.[130] This section focuses on the literature related to APAP in the treatment of patients with previously diagnosed OSA because there is currently little evidence to support the use of APAP technology for the diagnosis of OSA.[131]

Currently available APAP devices use proprietary algorithms to noninvasively detect and respond to variations in patterns of upper airway inspiratory flow or resistance. Most APAP machines monitor a combination of changes in inspiratory flow patterns, including inspiratory flow limitation, snoring (indirectly measured through mask pressure vibration), reductions of airflow (hypopnea), and absence of flow (apneas), using a pneumotachograph, nasal pressure monitors, or alterations in compressor speed. Most units detect flow limitation through proprietary algorithms using flow-versus-time profiles to determine a flattening index. The other less commonly used technology uses the forced oscillation technique method, which is an alternative method that detects changes in patterns of upper airway resistance or impedance.[132-134] Because the forced oscillation technique method measures changes in upper airway resistance that are independent of patient activity and ventilatory effort, this technology has the potential advantage of better differentiating central apneas from obstructive apneas or mask leak. There are currently no peer-reviewed data to substantiate efficacy of such detection, or clinical outcomes, with such technology.

When upper airway flow or impedance changes have been detected, the APAP devices use proprietary algorithms to automatically increase the pressure until the flow or resistance has been normalized. After a therapeutic pressure has been achieved, the APAP devices typically reduce pressure until flow limitation or increases in airway resistance resume. Most devices have a therapeutic pressure range between 4 and 20 cm H_2O, giving the clinician the ability to adjust the upper and lower pressure limits based on the clinical conditions and the patient's response to therapy. This should be differentiated from bilevel PAP or autobilevel PAP (discussed later), in which a separate IPAP and EPAP are set with changes in pressure across each respiratory cycle. Similar to CPAP, expiratory relief and other pressure delivery modifications are available for APAP technologies, although these additional pressure modifications have not be shown to consistently improve several APAP-related outcomes, including in-laboratory titration success, PAP adherence, or daytime sleepiness.[135-137] Because pressures changes occur throughout the sleep period, some have postulated that APAP devices may actually increase sleep fragmentation.[138] This concern has not been substantiated in studies evaluating changes in sleep structure or in clinical trials that have measured subjective sleepiness as a main outcome. Specifically, the frequency of microarousals and sleep fragmentation induced by APAP devices appears to be small,[139] and clinical outcomes related to subjective sleepiness also show no significant differences compared with conventional CPAP therapy.[18,140-143]

Currently available APAP machines have several potential limitations. Most flow- and pressure-based APAP devices are somewhat limited in their ability to distinguish between central and obstructive apneas as well as large mask leaks.[144-147] These flow patterns are "interpreted" by these types of devices as an absence of flow, which in the cases of central apneas and leaks may erroneously lead to increases in pressure and worsening of the central events or leaks. Newer APAP algorithms appear to be better at differentiating obstructive from central events as well as compensating for large mask leaks. Also, the ability of the APAP devices to respond to sustained hypoventilation in the absence of upper airway obstruction is unclear because most APAP studies have excluded patients at high risk for hypoventilation, including patients with obesity hypoventilation syndrome or chronic respiratory diseases. Given these potential limitations in technology, as well as the exclusion of patients with many comorbid diseases from the randomized trials comparing APAP to in-laboratory titrated CPAP therapy, the current AASM Practice Parameters regarding the use of APAP recommend that APAP devices only be used for patients with uncomplicated moderate to severe OSA.[131,148,149] APAP devices typically should *not* be used in the patients with comorbid medical conditions that could potentially affect their respiratory patterns (complicated OSA), including patients with CHF, patients with lung diseases such as COPD; and patients expected to have nocturnal arterial oxyhemoglobin desaturation due to conditions other than OSA (e.g., obesity hypoventilation syndrome and other hypoventilation syndromes). Patients who do not snore (either because of palatal surgery or naturally) should not be titrated with an APAP device that relies on vibration or sound in the device's algorithm.[131,148,149] Finally, APAP devices are not recommended for split-night titrations given the lack of data to support such a practice.

There have been several randomized controlled trials that have compared APAP technology to conventionally titrated CPAP therapy for the treatment of uncomplicated OSA.[18,19,126,134,140-143,150-159] Compared with standard fixed CPAP therapy, APAP devices as a group are almost always associated with a reduction in mean pressure across a night of therapy in the range of 2 to 2.5 cm H_2O, although peak pressures through the night tend to be higher than fixed CPAP therapy. Aside from these differences, APAP and standard CPAP are similar with regard to improvements in several outcomes, including objective adherence, ability to eliminate respiratory events, and subjective daytime sleepiness as measured by the Epworth Sleepiness Scale.[160] There are few data regarding improvements in blood pressure with APAP therapy and no long-term data regarding any cardiovascular outcomes. These findings have been consistently demonstrated for APAP therapy used as a primary chronic therapy and for APAP used for a short therapeutic trial to determine a fixed CPAP setting for ongoing CPAP therapy.

Most of the literature concerning APAP technology as a treatment for OSA has evaluated patients with uncomplicated predominantly moderate to severe OSA (AHI ≥15 events/hour), and therefore the results and recommendations that have been reviewed predominantly apply to this group of patients. The data comparing efficacy of APAP versus attended in-laboratory titrated CPAP in patients with mild OSA (AHI = 5 to 14 events/hour) are more limited.[159,160] Based on the available information, there appear to be similar improvements in important outcomes, including resolution of sleep-disordered breathing and daytime sleepiness and adherence with therapy between APAP and CPAP, even in patients with more mild disease, although it is difficult to make reliable recommendations concerning the use of APAP for this subgroup of patients.

Although the use of APAP as a therapy with or without changing the patient to a fixed CPAP device has also been well described, the optimal method for determining treatment success is controversial. Most of the newer PAP devices calculate several parameters, including device use time, an AHI, and leak data. Compliance with PAP therapy can be reliably determined using the various PAP tracking systems, but the validity of the PAP-calculated AHI data are not as easy to interpret because the various PAP manufacturers define respiratory events differently from each other and differently from the standard scoring definitions used by the AASM. In general, most studies comparing the APAP-calculated AHI to a PSG-determined AHI show that the PAP-calculated AHI tends to overestimate the AHI, especially at the lower end of the AHI spectrum.[161,162] In general, PAP-calculated AHIs of less than 10 events/hour tend to correlate with adequately treated sleep-disordered breathing events and have been associated with improved outcomes in randomized controlled trials.[121] This is especially true when these findings are associated with the resolution of nighttime snoring and daytime symptoms. Because the various proprietary APAP algorithms are far from perfect for detecting and resolving all sleep-disordered breathing events, the clinician should consider an in-laboratory attended PAP titration study when a patient is having difficulty with unattended APAP therapy or when residual daytime symptoms persist even if the APAP-calculated parameters suggest adequately treated OSA syndrome.[163]

Autobilevel Therapy for Obstructive Sleep Apnea

Autobilevel therapy has also been developed that, using proprietary algorithms, automatically adjusts both the EPAP and IPAP in response to sleep-disordered breathing events. Limited data indicate that, compared with CPAP, autobilevel therapy results in similar compliance and other important outcomes in patients who have had poor initial experiences with CPAP therapy.[164,165] There is currently no peer-reviewed literature evaluating outcomes with autobilevel therapy for OSA in PAP-naïve patients. Thus unlike non-autobilevel PAP therapy, no recommendations can be made for autobilevel PAP therapy for treating patients with OSA.

In summary, APAP technologies appear to be as effective as conventional fixed CPAP therapy when used for treatment in attended and unattended settings in patients with moderate to severe uncomplicated OSA.[131] Although APAP technologies as a group reduce the mean treatment pressure across the night, they appear to result in similar objective adherence and improvements in other important clinical outcomes compared with in-laboratory titrated CPAP therapy. Although APAP therapy has demonstrated some shortcomings in the peer-reviewed literature, the technology is rapidly advancing. The main benefits of APAP technology in the future will likely be the ability to provide more rapid treatment to patients with uncomplicated OSA and possibly the saving of health care dollars by eliminating some attended in-laboratory sleep studies that are typically required for CPAP titrations.[18,19,141]

CLINICAL PEARLS

- CPAP is the first-line therapy for patients with moderate to severe OSA, especially for those with daytime symptoms.
- CPAP therapy consistently resolves sleep-disordered breathing events and improves symptoms of daytime sleepiness in symptomatic patients, especially for patients with moderate to severe disease. There are inconsistent data concerning the benefits of CPAP therapy with regard to neurocognitive function, mood, quality of life, and cardiovascular outcomes across the spectrum of disease severity. The data regarding the benefits of CPAP therapy in patients with more mild disease are even more controversial, especially in those without daytime symptoms or underlying cardiovascular disease.
- The role of CPAP therapy for patients without associated daytime symptoms across the spectrum of OSA severity is unclear based on the current data. Most randomized controlled trials in this patient group have failed to demonstrate improvements in important outcomes, including blood pressure control, cardiovascular morbidity and mortality, neurocognitive function, and quality of life.
- Adherence with CPAP therapy is suboptimal for many patients, although improvements in adherence have been consistently associated with systematic education with and without behavioral therapy. The roles of other interventions, including heated humidification, hypnotics, and telemedicine, to improve adherence to CPAP therapy are unclear based on limited or inconsistent outcomes data from observational and randomized controlled trials.
- The roles of advanced PAP technologies, including EPR and bilevel PAP pressure devices, are not clear because they have typically not been associated with improved adherence, daytime sleepiness, or quality of life in patients with OSA.
- APAP used in an unattended setting, either to determine a fixed CPAP setting or as a primary treatment, is reasonable therapy for patients with moderate to severe OSA without underlying comorbidities. Most of the data on APAP therapy have been limited to patients with daytime sleepiness; thus the role of APAP therapy in patients without associated daytime sleepiness is not clear.

SUMMARY

CPAP therapy remains the mainstay of treatment of patients with moderate to severe OSA, especially those patients with daytime sleepiness. The role of PAP therapy in patients with OSA in the absence of daytime sleepiness is not clear. Despite its potential to improve several clinical outcomes including daytime sleepiness, neurocognitive dysfunction, quality of life, and blood pressure, long-term adherence with therapy remains suboptimum. Newer technologies such as APAP have the potential to improve the treatment of OSA, with most data demonstrating that this technology is as effective as in-laboratory titrated CPAP in patients with uncomplicated moderate to severe OSA. Although the role of APAP in the treatment of OSA is still not well defined, it has the potential to improve the delivery of PAP therapy by replacing laboratory-based PAP titrations in patients with uncomplicated OSA, thus reducing the current sleep laboratory waiting times and potentially reducing health care spending on in-laboratory studies. Other technologic advancements such as EPR and bilevel PAP devices are supported by limited data and appear to offer no advantages over conventionally titrated CPAP therapy in most patients with OSA.

Selected Readings

Barbe F, Duran-Cantolla J, Sanchez-de-la-Torre M, et al. Effect of continuous positive airway pressure on the incidence of hypertension and cardiovascular events in nonsleepy patients with obstructive sleep apnea: a randomized controlled trial. *JAMA* 2012;**307**(20):2161–8.

Billings ME, Auckley D, Benca R, et al. Race and residential socioeconomics as predictors of CPAP adherence. *Sleep* 2011;**34**(12):1653–8.

Chai-Coetzer CL, Antic NA, Rowland LS, et al. Primary care vs specialist sleep center management of obstructive sleep apnea and daytime sleepiness and quality of life: a randomized trial. *JAMA* 2013;**309**(10): 997–1004.

Fava C, Dorigoni S, Dalle Vedove F, et al. Effect of CPAP on blood pressure in patients with OSA/hypopnea a systematic review and meta-analysis. *Chest* 2014;**145**(4):762–71.

Gagnadoux F, Le Vaillant M, Paris A, et al. Relationship Between OSA Clinical Phenotypes and CPAP Treatment Outcomes. *Chest* 2016;**149**(1): 288–90.

Holmqvist F, Guan N, Zhu Z, et al. Impact of obstructive sleep apnea and continuous positive airway pressure therapy on outcomes in patients with atrial fibrillation: results from the Outcomes Registry for Better Informed Treatment of Atrial Fibrillation (ORBIT-AF). *Am Heart J* 2015;**169**(5): 647–54.

Ip S, D'Ambrosio C, Patel K, et al. Auto-titrating versus fixed continuous positive airway pressure for the treatment of obstructive sleep apnea: a systematic review with meta-analyses. *Syst Rev* 2012;**1**:20.

Johnson KG, Johnson DC. Treatment of sleep-disordered breathing with positive airway pressure devices: technology update. *Med Devices (Auckl)* 2015;**8**:425–37.

Lettieri CJ, Shah AA, Holley AB, et al. Effects of a short course of eszopiclone on continuous positive airway pressure adherence: a randomized trial. *Ann Intern Med* 2009;**151**(10):696–702.

Marin J, Carrizo S, Vincente E, Agusti A. Long-term cardiovascular outcomes in men with obstructive sleep apnoea-hypopnea with or without treatment with continuous positive airway pressure: an observational study. *Lancet* 2005;**365**(9464):1046–53.

Marin JM, Soriano JB, Carrizo SJ, et al. Outcomes in patients with chronic obstructive pulmonary disease and obstructive sleep apnea: the overlap syndrome. *Am J Respir Crit Care Med* 2010;**182**(3):325–31.

Parthasarathy S, Subramanian S, Quan SF. A multicenter prospective comparative effectiveness study of the effect of physician certification and center accreditation on patient-centered outcomes in obstructive sleep apnea. *J Clin Sleep Med* 2014;**10**(3):243–9.

Phillips CL, Grunstein RR, Darendeliler MA, et al. Health outcomes of continuous positive airway pressure versus oral appliance treatment for obstructive sleep apnea: a randomized controlled trial. *Am J Respir Crit Care Med* 2013;**187**(8):879–87.

Sanchez-de-la-Torre M, Nadal N, Cortijo A, et al. Role of primary care in the follow-up of patients with obstructive sleep apnoea undergoing CPAP treatment: a randomised controlled trial. *Thorax* 2015;**70**(4): 346–52.

Schwab RJ, Badr SM, Epstein LJ, et al. An official American Thoracic Society statement: continuous positive airway pressure adherence tracking systems. The optimal monitoring strategies and outcome measures in adults. *Am J Respir Crit Care Med* 2013;**188**(5):613–20.

Sun H, Shi J, Li M, Chen X. Impact of continuous positive airway pressure treatment on left ventricular ejection fraction in patients with obstructive sleep apnea: a meta-analysis of randomized controlled trials. *PLoS ONE* 2013;**8**(5):e62298.

Weaver TE, Mancini C, Maislin G, et al. Continuous positive airway pressure treatment of sleepy patients with milder obstructive sleep apnea: results of the CPAP Apnea Trial North American Program (CATNAP) randomized clinical trial. *Am J Respir Crit Care Med* 2012;**186**(7):677–83.

Wozniak DR, Lasserson TJ, Smith I. Educational, supportive and behavioural interventions to improve usage of continuous positive airway pressure machines in adults with obstructive sleep apnoea. *Cochrane Database Syst Rev* 2014;(1):CD007736.

A complete reference list can be found online at ExpertConsult.com.

Obstructive Sleep Apnea: Oral Appliance Therapy

Chapter

19

Christopher J. Lettieri; Fernanda R. Almeida; Peter Anthony Cistulli; Maria Clotilde Carra

Chapter Highlights

- Oral appliances are an accepted and reliable treatment option for patients with snoring and obstructive sleep apnea–hypopnea syndrome (OSAHS). They are currently indicated for patients with mild to moderate OSAHS; however, they have been shown to be effective in patients with more severe disease. Oral appliances are most effective in younger, thinner patients with mild to moderate OSAHS. They are less likely to be effective in obese patients.

- In general, and especially for more severe disease, custom-made titratable devices offer superior treatment and a greater likelihood for successful therapy than other types of oral devices. Successful therapy is more likely to be achieved by performing an at-home progressive titration using a custom-made titratable device. This may be further enhanced by the application of adjunctive means to monitor the therapeutic response.

- Oral appliances are not as effective as positive airway pressure devices for reducing the apnea-hypopnea index and other sleep measures. However, short- and long-term improvements in daytime somnolence, quality of life, neurocognitive function, and cardiovascular outcomes (primarily blood pressure) appear to be similar with both treatments.

- Oral appliances are generally well tolerated, and serious side effects or adverse consequences resulting in discontinuation of therapy are uncommon. Malocclusion is the most common long-term effect. However, this typically does not lead to discontinuation of therapy and may be mitigated by simple exercises each morning after removal of the device.

- Concomitant sleep bruxism (SB) with OSAHS is common. Although the true etiologic nature of these disorders is not fully understood, there appears to be a modest causal relationship. Patients with SB and symptoms of OSAHS should be assessed for underlying sleep-disordered breathing as common SB occlusal splint therapies may, in some cases, worsen obstructive events if they are not recognized.

- Oral appliances appear to provide adequate therapy for both OSAHS and SB alone or in comorbidity.

Currently, positive airway pressure (PAP) remains the most accepted, common, and efficacious management tool for obstructive sleep apnea–hypopnea syndrome (OSAHS). In this chapter, we use the word *treatment*, although we recognize that most devices or appliances do manage sleep-disordered breathing (SDB), in the whole spectrum from snoring to severe OSAHS, whereas some residual apnea and hypopnea, oxygen desaturation, high blood pressure, inflammation, sleepiness, and cognitive alterations, although improved, may persist over time. However, given the ongoing challenges related to the acceptance of and adherence to PAP therapy, there remains an increasing need for reliable and effective treatment alternatives (e.g., appliance, nerve stimulation, sleep positioning devices). Oral appliances (OAs) of various designs are a solid alternative used to manage OSAHS, sleep bruxism (SB), and both when they are concomitant.

The main objective of this chapter is to describe the use of oral appliances for OSAHS, with special attention to sleep bruxism which may be present in apnea patients. Other medical management tools for OSAHS are described in more detail in Chapters 17 and 18, and surgical management is reviewed in Chapters 20 to 22.

WHY USE ORAL APPLIANCES FOR SLEEP-DISORDERED BREATHING AND OBSTRUCTIVE SLEEP APNEA–HYPOPNEA SYNDROME?

OAs offer effective therapy for many patients with simple (primary) snoring and OSAHS and have become a proven, validated, and accepted treatment option. With the release of numerous clinical trials and published practice parameters establishing their efficacy and the expanded availability of

201

these devices, OAs have become an increasingly common treatment modality for patients with SDB.

OAs offer several advantages over PAP. They are generally well tolerated in most individuals, and published reports have consistently shown that therapeutic adherence and patient preferences are as good as if not superior to those with PAP.[1,2] In addition, these devices do not require a ready and reliable source of electricity and may be easier to use, especially during travel or for people who live in an area with restricted access to electricity (e.g., sailors, fishermen, humanitarian workers, military). OAs may be useful in patients non-adherent to PAP.[2a]

As published in the American Academy of Sleep Medicine's "Practice Parameters for the Treatment of Snoring and Obstructive Sleep Apnea with Oral Appliances: An Update for 2005," these devices are recommended as primary therapy for patients with snoring and mild to moderate OSAHS or as a reasonable treatment alternative in patients who prefer these devices to PAP or are intolerant of other therapies.[3] A long awaited update to these Practice Parameters was published by the American Academy of Sleep Medicine in 2015.[3a]

The route to the current best accepted practices encompasses the role of the physician and dentist[4] in the proper selection of the patient and device and the need for an interdisciplinary approach to the appropriate application and ongoing care of OA therapy.

TYPES OF ORAL APPLIANCES FOR SLEEP-DISORDERED BREATHING AND SLEEP BRUXISM

For SDB and OSAHS management, two broad OA types in common clinical use are mandibular repositioning appliances and tongue-repositioning devices. Mandibular repositioning appliances, also known as mandibular advancement splints (MAS) or mandibular advancement devices, are the focus of this chapter as they are more widely used in clinical practice and have a greater evidence base. Numerous design types are available, but these devices generally fall into either one-piece (monobloc) or two-piece (duobloc) configurations. They can differ substantially in size, type of material, degree of customization to the patient's dentition, and coupling mechanisms. In addition, the amount of occlusal coverage, adjustability of mandibular advancement, degree of mandibular mobility permitted (vertical and lateral), and allowance for oral respiration also vary between the different available devices.

This chapter focuses on customized OAs for managing OSAHS. Although prefabricated MAS exist, many of which are available over the counter, there is a paucity of outcome measures validating their clinical use. Whereas these devices may offer a reasonable and cost-effective treatment, particularly for simple snoring, the existing data show limited efficacy and lower acceptance rates compared with customized OAs.[5,6] As such, prefabricated devices are not recommended for clinical use in patients with OSAHS.

Two-piece OAs have become more commonly used in clinical practice and consist of removable upper and lower plates that are coupled together to promote advancement of the mandible and to mitigate subluxation during sleep. There are a variety of modes of coupling between the upper and lower plates, including elastic or plastic connectors, metal pins and tube connectors, hook connectors, acrylic extensions, and magnets. Duobloc splints offer advantages over

monobloc devices by allowing adjustability, which facilitates achievement of the most comfortable and efficient position of the mandible and greater degree of lower jaw movements. OAs that permit lateral jaw movement or opening and closing while maintaining mandibular advancement may offer additional advantages by reducing the risk of complications and improving the patient's comfort and acceptance. Because the patient's tolerance to the amount of protrusion increases over time, splints capable of incremental advancement seem to have a clear practical advantage. These adjustable devices also facilitate improved efficacy as they can be titrated to a more optimal setting needed to ablate obstructive events. Although prefabricated appliances ("off the shelf") are commercially available, their efficacy and potential role as a "trial" device have been called into question.[6] The best retention, comfort, and efficacy are achieved with custom-made, titratable OAs. Further comparisons between the different available types of OAs and potential advantages in the management of patients with SDB are discussed later in this chapter.

The most frequently used OA for SB management (i.e., preventing grinding sound and tooth wear and possibly reducing pain) is the occlusal splint (a one-piece monobloc) that can be custom made to fit either the upper or lower jaw. The efficacy in the short term is recognized, but in patients with OSAHS, it is to be used with caution because, as described later, it may exacerbate their condition. In some subgroups of patients, in their lifetime course, it is possible that SB and OSAHS coexist. Although some association was found, as described later, it is premature to conclude that SB causes SDB or the reverse, that SDB causes SB; association is not causality.

ORAL APPLIANCE MECHANISM OF ACTION

Current evidence suggests that OSAHS pathogenesis reflects reduced upper airway size and altered upper airway muscle activity, resulting in diminished patency and airflow obstruction (see Sections 3 and 14 in this volume for more information). Although it has been thought that the primary mechanism of action of OAs arises from the anterior movement of the tongue and consequent increase in the anteroposterior dimensions of the oropharynx, it appears that this is an overly simplistic view. Many studies using a range of imaging modalities, including computed tomography, magnetic resonance imaging, and nasoendoscopy, suggest that OAs induce more complex anatomic changes.[7-10] An increase in airway volume appears to result, in large part, by an increase in cross-sectional area of the velopharynx, in both the lateral and anteroposterior dimensions, and increases in the lateral dimension of the oropharynx. Figure 19-1[10] illustrates the effects of an OA and tongue-stabilizing device on the upper airway. These changes are thought to be mediated through the palatoglossal and palatopharyngeal arches, which link the muscles of the tongue, soft palate, lateral pharyngeal walls, and mandibular attachments. Interindividual variability in the airway configurational changes that occur with mandibular advancement may reflect variations in anatomy, and this is likely to have major relevance to the variable clinical response associated with this treatment modality.

Anatomic imbalance has been proposed as an underlying mechanism in the pathogenesis of OSAHS.[11] In this model,

Baseline   MAS   TSD

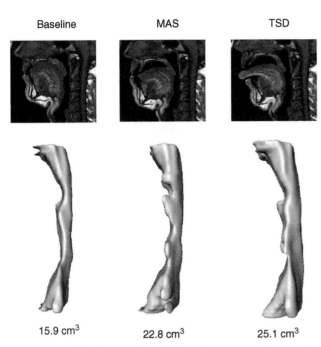

15.9 cm³   22.8 cm³   25.1 cm³

Figure 19-1 Modes of action of mandibular advancement splint (MAS) and tongue-stabilizing device (TSD). Magnetic resonance imaging representation of the increase in upper airway volume while patients have the appliance in place. (From Sutherland K, Deane SA, Chan AS, et al. Comparative effects of two oral appliances on upper airway structure in obstructive sleep apnea. *Sleep* 2011;34:469–77.)

excess tissue within the bony enclosure must be present to generate sufficient tissue pressure to collapse the airway lumen. This extraluminal tissue pressure occurs in the context of either an excess of soft tissue within a normal bony enclosure size or a normal amount of tissue compressed into a reduced bony enclosure. Mandibular advancement delivered by OAs effectively enlarges the bony enclosure and appears to improve anatomic balance.[12]

The effects of OAs on upper airway neuromuscular pathways have not been well studied to date. Whereas some studies indicate that these devices stimulate genioglossus muscle activity,[13,14] studies using inactive "sham" OAs have shown little change in SDB.[15,16] This suggests that mechanical advancement of the mandible is the primary mechanism of action of these devices. This mechanical effect results in greater airway stability, which is evidenced by a reduced upper airway closing pressure during sleep.[17] This effect was demonstrated in a study of anesthetized OSAHS patients by Kato et al,[18] who observed dose-dependent reductions in closing pressure of all pharyngeal segments with progressive mandibular advancement.

CLINICAL OUTCOMES AND MEASURES OF SUCCESS

Since the last published guidelines on the use of OAs in the treatment of OSAHS,[15,16,18-23] there has been a substantial increase in the quantity and quality of clinical trials evaluating the efficacy and effectiveness of OA therapy[2,24-27] (see Figure 19-2). Several trials, including prospective designs using placebo arms and sham comparisons, have produced a high

level of evidence and have allowed stronger treatment recommendations. In addition, trials assessing the treatment response between OAs and other primary therapies for OSAHS focusing on clinically important outcomes help further the understanding of appropriate patient selection and the expected therapeutic effect. In short, OAs have been shown to have a good level of efficacy in improving polysomnographic measures, daytime somnolence, quality of life, cardiovascular outcomes, and neurocognitive function for patients with both simple (primary) snoring and OSAHS.

Snoring

Several placebo-controlled trials have found that OAs reduce both subjective and objective measures of snoring frequency and intensity among nonapneic patients with habitual (primary) snoring.[17,19,22,23,28,29] OAs have also been shown to improve quality of life measures in nonapneic snorers. In one trial, the use of OAs produced a mean improvement in Functional Outcomes of Sleep Questionnaire (FOSQ) scores by 3.21 (95% confidence interval, 2.82–3.60; $P < .001$) among patients with habitual snoring.[29]

Polysomnographic Variables and Reduction of the Apnea-Hypopnea Index

OAs have been well established as an effective treatment in the management of OSAHS. There is strong evidence from randomized, controlled trials that these devices produce a significant reduction in the apnea-hypopnea index (AHI) across the full spectrum of OSAHS severities. Abolition of obstructive events to an AHI less than 5 events/hour is achieved in 36% to 70% of patients.[15,16,26,30-32] With use of an AHI threshold of less than 10/hour, OAs provide successful therapy in 30% to 86%.[2,18,30] The likelihood of successful treatment is progressively greater with lower severities of disease. Table 19-1 illustrates success rates with OA therapy according to different disease severity at baseline.

Daytime Somnolence and Quality of Life Measures

OAs have been shown to improve daytime sleepiness and quality of life in patients with OSAHS. In one trial, improvements in daytime somnolence were significantly better with customized OAs compared with nontherapeutic devices.[33] Specifically, the Epworth Sleepiness Scale (ESS) score decreased from 14.7 ± 5.1 to 5.1 ± 1.9 ($P < .05$) in those receiving OA therapy compared with 16.3 ± 2.5 to only 13.6 ± 6.7 ($P = NS$) in the nontherapeutic group. Similarly, in a long-term follow-up study, OAs produced a decrease in ESS from 13.9 ± 1.3 to 9.3 ± 1.2.[28] OAs have also been shown to improve objective measures of sleepiness. In a placebo-controlled trial, 4 weeks of OA therapy led to an additional improvement in the mean sleep latency on the Multiple Sleep Latency Test of 1.2 minutes compared with an inactive control oral device.[28] Two additional trials evaluating objective measures of wakefulness found that the improvements in Maintenance of Wakefulness Test were similar between both PAP and OA therapy.[1,34] Across numerous published studies, the improvement in both subjective and objective measures of somnolence achieved with OAs appears to be similar to that reported with PAP therapy. However, as with PAP, whereas OAs are shown to improve daytime somnolence, residual sleepiness may persist despite otherwise adequate therapy.

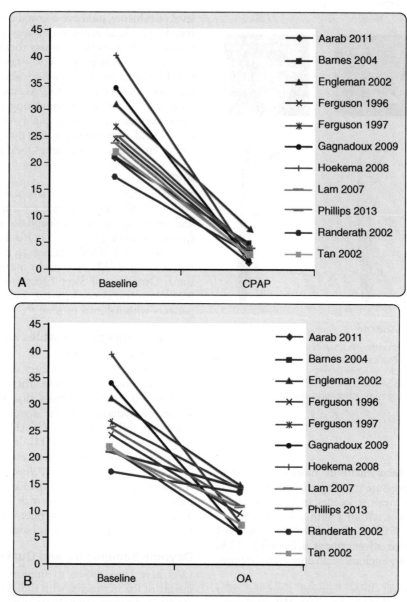

Figure 19-2 Average decrease in apnea-hypopnea index (AHI) from published randomized controlled trials. CPAP, Continuous positive airway pressure; OA, oral appliance.

Compared with no treatment or nontherapeutic (sham) therapy, OAs have also been shown to significantly improve quality of life measures in patients with OSAHS. In one trial, overall FOSQ scores improved by 27.1% from baseline (P < .001; effect size, 0.90) in those using a customized OA compared with a −1.7% decline in those using a nontherapeutic sham device.[33] In a randomized, controlled trial comparing OA therapy with a placebo tablet, mandibular advancement produced superior improvements in quality of life as measured by the FOSQ and 36-Item Short Form Health Survey overall health score.[1] The magnitude of improvement was similar to that found with PAP.

Cardiovascular Outcomes
Several studies have addressed the impact of OA therapy on measures of systolic blood pressure.[1,2,29,32,35-39] Overall, OAs were found to lower the systolic, diastolic, and mean blood pressure (Table 19-2). Further, the results from three randomized trials suggest that OAs are as effective as PAP in reducing blood pressure measures.[1,2,32] These studies are largely limited to custom-made, titratable devices. One small, randomized, controlled trial of 36 patients using nontitratable OAs failed to observe significant changes in either the systolic or diastolic blood pressure.[35]

OAs have also been shown to produce significant improvements in endothelial function and markers of oxidative stress similar to those observed with PAP therapy.[1,2,27,32,40] However, as with PAP therapy, the available data suggest that OAs produce only modest reductions in blood pressure recordings and other cardiovascular end points.

Whereas blood pressure and other markers of cardiovascular health have shown small but significant improvements, two studies evaluating cardiovascular morbidity and mortality noted a marked cardiovascular risk reduction with OA therapy.[41,42] In a study of patients with mild to moderate OSAHS receiving either OA or PAP therapy, there was a marked cardiovascular risk reduction of at least 38%.[42] Recently, a study focused on severe sleep apnea patients described no difference in the cardiovascular death rate of those receiving either treatment.[41]

Despite the limited literature and the presence of residual apneas with OA therapy, the current studies available have shown continuous PAP (CPAP) and OA to be equally effective in the reduction of cardiovascular events.

Neurocognitive Outcomes

OA therapy has been shown to improve neuropsychological functioning. In a trial comparing OAs, PAP, and a tablet placebo for mild to moderate OSAHS, OA therapy improved

tension-anxiety, divided attention, and executive functioning compared with placebo.[1] However, PAP was superior to OAs in improving psychomotor speed and mood. Similarly, treatment with an OA was found to significantly improve attention, vigilance, and motor speed, as measured by the distraction–working memory test and continuous performance.[43] In contrast, other trials have failed to demonstrate improved neurocognitive function after OA therapy despite improvements in other measured end points.[1,34,44]

Despite the similarity to PAP, the existing literature shows mixed results with only modest improvements in neurocognitive measures for patients undergoing OA therapy.

OUTCOME COMPARISON BETWEEN TYPES OF ORAL APPLIANCES AND POSITIVE AIRWAY PRESSURE THERAPY

Fixed versus Adjustable Appliances

Customized, individually fabricated MAS are either fixed (nonadjustable) or titratable (adjustable). Nonadjustable devices are monobloc or single-piece appliances in which the degree of mandibular advancement is permanently fixed. Titratable appliances (adjustable or duobloc) allow adjustments in the degree of mandibular protrusion to optimize treatment efficacy. This is an important distinction both in selection of the most effective treatment and in understanding the published literature. Published studies using fixed or single-jaw position appliances may underestimate the impact of OA therapy compared with titratable appliances.[1,25,27,34,45] Titratable or adjustable appliances allow progressive protrusion of the mandible, and the amount of anteroposterior mandibular movement varies considerably among patients. Previous studies have shown that OA efficacy is related to the amount of mandibular advancement.[18,46,47] Determining the optimal degree of mandibular advancement is the most important step in using OA therapy successfully.[48,49] As an

Table 19-1	Success Rates with Oral Appliance Therapy according to Different Disease Severity at Baseline		
OSA Severity at Baseline	Mild	Moderate	Severe
Success			
Study A	62.3%	50.8%	39.9%
Study B	56.6%	48.1%	21.2%
Partial success			
Study A	13%	25%	24.3%
Study B			
Failure			
Study A	30.4%	26.9%	54.5%
Study B			

The results are expressed in percentage from two trials using custom-made titratable oral appliances: Study A, Holley et al[60] and Study B, Phillips et al.[2] Success is described as an apnea-hypopnea index (AHI) <5 with oral appliance therapy; partial success is at least 50% reduction in AHI but AHI >5; and failure represents <50% reduction in AHI.

Table 19-2	Impact of Oral Appliance Therapy on Blood Pressure Measurements in Different Clinical Trials					
Author	Mean ΔSBP	Mean ΔDBP	Mean Δ24-h SBP	Mean Δ24-h DBP	Mean ΔNight SBP	Mean ΔNight DBP
Gauthier[149]	−4.3	−10.1				
Trzepizur[32]	−8.8	2				
Andren[36] (3 months)	−14.3	−8.6				
Andren[36] (3 years)	−15.5	−10.3				
Yoshida[39]	−4.5	−2.9				
Gotsopoulos[37]	−4.9	−3.7	−2.3	−1.5	0.5	0.6
Barnes[1]			0.2	0		−2.2
Otsuka[38]	−3.1	−4.2	−4.5	−4.9	−4.7	−4.4
Zhang[151]	−2.1		−2.2	−0.6	−4	−2.7
Lam[27]	−1.2	−2.8				−2.1*
Phillips[2]	0.2	−0.5	0	−0.2	−0.4	−0.2
Phillips[2] (hypertension patients only)	−2.5	−2.4	−2.9	−2.1	−3.4	−1.9

Measurements are in millimeters of mercury. Some studies have only clinical blood pressure, whereas some also describe 24-hour blood pressure. A negative change (Δ) in blood pressure refers to a reduction of the blood pressure.
*Refers to a nighttime clinical blood pressure, not 24-hour assessment.
SBP, Systolic blood pressure; DPB, diastolic blood pressure.

analogy, titration of OAs is similar to PAP. The amount of pressure (or degree of mandibular advancement) required for each patient cannot be predetermined on the basis of OSAHS severity or patient-specific characteristics. Objective assessment of the treatment response at progressive increases in the delivered pressure (or advancement) is needed to determine the optimal treatment for each individual patient to optimize the ablation of obstructive events. A systematic review of different types of MAS concluded that there is no one MAS design feature that influences treatment efficacy, although efficacy does depend on the degree of mandibular protrusion and whether the device is a fixed or titratable appliance.[50] The comparison of the efficacy rates between fixed and titratable appliances has demonstrated titratable devices to be superior in their ability to reduce the AHI for patients at all levels of OSAHS severity.[51] Although fixed devices were frequently effective in patients with mild sleep apnea, they had high failure rates in those with moderate or severe disease. These studies reinforce that in future meta-analysis of treatment outcomes, fixed single-jaw positioners should not be evaluated together with titratable devices as these therapies have different treatment outcomes.

Oral Appliances versus Positive Airway Pressure Therapy

Several published randomized controlled trials and crossover studies have compared the efficacy of OAs to PAP in the treatment of OSAHS.[52] As seen in Table 19-3, although both PAP and OAs led to improvements in objective sleep measurements such as AHI, arousal index, and minimum arterial oxygen saturation, the magnitude of improvement in AHI is significantly greater with PAP. Although statistically superior, these differences are not necessarily clinically significant. OAs decrease both subjective and objective measurements of snoring in the majority of the patients.[15,31,53] This reduction is less robust than with PAP, which frequently uses the elimination of snoring as an objective assessment of treatment efficacy. Subjective and objective measurements of sleepiness are similarly improved with both forms of therapy.

Both OAs and PAP have been shown to be superior to placebo or no treatment in improving quality of life measures.[24] With a disease-specific questionnaire, the FOSQ, both treatments similarly improved quality of life. Direct comparative studies (randomized controlled trials) demonstrated that both OAs and PAP are effective in improving quality of life, with each treatment providing certain advantages in specific subcategories.[2] Whether this reflects a true difference between the effects of each treatment or is a product of differing study designs and data collection is uncertain. Regardless, it appears that both forms of therapy are similarly effective, and both are highly dependent on the patient's compliance. Given that adherence with OAs is typically superior to that with PAP, outcomes in clinical practice may favor these devices over PAP, particularly for mild and moderate OSAHS.

Whereas both OAs and PAP significantly reduce the AHI, PAP has been consistently shown to be superior in this measured outcome. Table 19-3 shows the results of randomized controlled trials and their average reduction in AHI. However, there is equivalence in overall health outcomes with both therapies. This may reflect that the greater efficacy of PAP is offset by inferior compliance relative to OAs, resulting in similar effectiveness. In other words, higher adherence rates with OAs likely translate into a similar mean disease alleviation and consequently similar effectiveness compared with PAP.[54] These findings strongly challenge current practice parameters recommending that OA treatment should be considered only in patients with mild to moderate OSAHS or in those who have failed to respond to or refuse PAP treatment. Long-term comparative effectiveness studies of these two treatment modalities are clearly needed.

PATIENT AND DEVICE SELECTION

Proper selection of the patient and device can increase the likelihood of success, improve the therapeutic effect, and enhance outcomes. There are multiple factors that should be considered in determining which patients are ideal candidates for OA therapy. Similarly, there are multiple different types, designs, and brands of OA devices, each with its inherent advantages and limitations. Understanding these factors can aid clinicians in making appropriate treatment decisions.

Indications and Contraindications

The American Academy of Sleep Medicine's Practice Parameters on OAs in the treatment of SDB advocate the use of these devices in patients with mild to moderate OSAHS who prefer this form of treatment to PAP or who do not respond to or are unable to tolerate PAP.[3] Since these guidelines were published, the evidence base supporting the use of OA therapy has grown considerably and suggests that clinicians should use custom-made titratable OAs as first-line therapy or as an alternative to PAP as an effective and reliable means to improve physiologic sleep measures, daytime sleepiness, and quality of life in adult patients with OSAHS.

Selection of appropriate patients for OA therapy, based on the likelihood of successful treatment, remains a somewhat elusive goal at present. Whereas considerable research has attempted to identify the factors that predict a good response, the clinical utility of such approaches remains to be proven. In general, younger, thinner patients with positional OSAHS and an overall lower AHI appear to be the preferred candidates for OA therapy. However, in the absence of clear selection criteria, the clinician should rely on clinical judgment and the patient's preference when choosing the appropriate therapeutic approach.

Dentists experienced in dental sleep medicine have a prominent role in determining whether a patient is an ideal candidate for OA therapy. Patients require a sufficient number and location of healthy teeth to retain the device and to promote mandibular advancement. Specifically, patients require a minimum of eight teeth in the upper jaw and in the lower jaw, with at least two teeth in each quadrant.[55] In addition, the patient should have the ability to protrude the mandible forward to achieve a therapeutic result.

Not all patients are suitable candidates for the use of OAs because of associated medical or dental conditions and factors. In general, PAP affords a more prompt initiation of therapy. A major clinical limitation of OA therapy is in circumstances in which there is an imperative to commence more immediate treatment as there are inherent delays to attaining optimal therapy with use of these devices. This includes situations involving severe symptomatic OSAHS (e.g., concern about driving risk or profound daytime impairments) and coexistent

Table 19-3 Summary of the Outcomes of Randomized Controlled Trials Comparing Oral Appliances with Continuous Positive Airway Pressure

Study	Design	No. of Subjects (% Male) [Withdrawals]	Inclusion	Oral Appliance	Treatment [Washout] Duration	Baseline AHI	Treatment AHI		OA vs. CPAP		
							CPAP	OA	AHI	ESS	Patient Preference
Aarab, 2010[27]	Parallel (placebo group included)	57 (74%) (20 OA/18 CPAP) [7]	AHI 5–45 + ESS ≥ 10	Customized, two-piece, set 25%, 50%, or 75% advancement, depending on sleep study results at each level	24 weeks	CPAP: 20.9 ± 9.8 OA: 22.1 ± 10.8	1.4 ± 13.1	5.8 ± 14.9	↔ (P = .092)	↔	N/A—parallel groups
Barnes, 2004[58]	Crossover (placebo group included)	80 (79%) [24]	AHI 5–30	Customized 4-week titration to maximum comfortable advancement	3 × 12 weeks [2 weeks]	21.5 ± 1.6^	4.8 ± 0.5^	14.0 ± 1.1^	CPAP	↔	CPAP
Engleman, 2002[54]	Crossover	48 (75%) [3]	AHI ≥ 5/h + ≥2 symptoms (including ESS ≥ 8)	Customized, one-piece, 80% maximal protrusion, two deigns: (a) complete occlusal coverage or (b) no occlusal coverage, assigned randomly	2 × 8 weeks [not reported]	31 ± 26	8 ± 6	15 ± 16	CPAP	CPAP	↔
Ferguson, 1996[60]	Crossover	25 (89%) [2]	AHI 15–50 + OSA symptoms	Snore-Guard (Hays & Meade Inc), maximum comfortable advancement	2 × 16 weeks [2 weeks]	24.5 ± 8.8	3.6 ± 1.7	9.7 ± 7.3	CPAP	N/A	OA
Ferguson, 1997[50]	Crossover	20 (95%) [4]	AHI 15–55 + OSA symptoms	Customized, two-piece appliance titration starting at 70% maximum advancement over 3 months	2 × 16 weeks [2 weeks]	26.8 ± 11.9	4.0 ± 2.2	14.2 ± 14.7	CPAP	↔	OA
Gagnadoux, 2009[55]	Crossover	59 (78%) [3]	AHI 10–60 + ≥2 symptoms, BMI ≥ 35 kg/m²	AMC (Artech Medical), two-piece, advancement determined by single-night titration	2 × 8 weeks [1 week]	34 ± 13	2 (1–8)#	6 (3–14)#	CPAP	↔	OA
Hoekema, 2008[56]	Parallel	103 (51 OA/52 CPAP) [4]	AHI ≥ 5	Thornton Adjustable Positioner type 1, titratable	8–12 weeks	CPAP: 40.3 ± 27.6 OA: 39.4 ± 30.8	2.4 ± 4.2	7.8 ± 14.4	CPAP	↔	N/A—parallel groups
Lam, 2007[61]	Parallel (placebo group included)	101 (79%) (34 OA/34 CPAP) [10]	AHI ≥ 5–40 + ESS > 9 if AHI 5–20	Customized, nonadjustable set to maximum comfortable advancement	10 weeks (83% referred for concurrent weight loss program)	CPAP: 23.8 ± 1.9^ OA: 20.9 ± 1.7^	2.8 ± 1.1^	10.6 ± 1.7^	CPAP	CPAP	N/A—parallel groups
Phillips, 2013[57]	Crossover	108 (81%) [18]	AHI ≥ 10 + ≥2 symptoms	Customized two-piece appliance (SomnoMed), titrated to maximum comfortable limit in acclimatization period before study	2 × 4 weeks [2 weeks]	25.6 ± 12.3	4.5 ± 6.6	11.1 ± 12.1	CPAP	↔	OA
Randerath, 2002[62]	Crossover	20 (80%)	AHI 5–30 + OSA symptoms	IST; Hinz (Herne, Germany) two piece, nontitratable, set to two-thirds of maximum advancement	2 × 6 weeks [not reported]	17.5 ± 7.7	3.2 ± 2.9	13.8 ± 11.1	CPAP	N/A	N/A
Tan, 2002[63]	Crossover	21 (83%) [3]	AHI 5–50	One-piece, 75% maximum advancement and Silensor (Erkodent Gmbh) two-piece, titratable	2 × 8 weeks [2 weeks]	22.2 ± 9.6	3.1 ± 2.8	8.0 ± 10.9	↔	↔	N/A

AHI, Apnea-hypopnea index; CPAP, continuous positive airway pressure; OA, oral appliance; ESS, Epworth Sleepiness Scale; OSA, obstructive sleep apnea; BMI, body mass index; N/A, not applicable, not measured in study.
Data are presented as mean ± standard deviation, unless denoted; ↔ equivalent between treatments; ^ mean ± standard error of mean; #median (interquartile range).
From Sutherland K, Vanderveken OM, Tsuda H, et al. Oral appliance treatment for obstructive sleep apnea: an update. *J Clin Sleep Med* 2014;10:215–27.

medical comorbidities, such as ischemic heart disease. Moreover, this treatment modality has no known role in treating central sleep apnea or hypoventilation states. In addition, some case reports have shown worsening of OSAHS severity in some patients using OAs.[22,56] This, together with the known potential for a placebo response, highlights the need for objective verification of treatment outcome using in-laboratory or home sleep testing with an OA in place at its prescribed, therapeutic position.[15,16] Patients with temporomandibular joint (TMJ) problems may require concomitant use of exercises to be able to adhere to OA therapy.[57] Long-term use of OAs results in few or no TMJ problems.[58] The presence of periodontal disease may promote excessive tooth movement or worsening of dental caries with an OA. These factors tend to limit the scope and application of this form of therapy; it is therefore highly important that a dentist with expertise in sleep medicine assess dental and TMJ health before initiation of therapy.

Predictors of Successful Oral Appliance Therapy

An important and currently unresolved issue limiting the role of OAs for the treatment of OSAHS is the inability to reliably predict an effective response to treatment. Ultimately, the response to therapy is likely to be related to multiple patient factors, device features, and clinical expertise of the treating provider. Patient factors, including anthropomorphic and polysomnographic variables, have been the subject of numerous studies. Clinical features reported to be associated with better outcomes and greater likelihood of success include younger age, lower body mass index, supine-dependent OSAHS, lower AHI, smaller oropharynx, less overjet, shorter soft palate, and smaller neck circumference.[59] In general, it is considered that a good response is more likely in mild to moderate OSAHS, although benefit in severe OSAHS has been reported.[2,60,61] Cephalometric measures, such as a shorter soft palate, longer maxilla, and decreased distance between mandibular plane and hyoid bone, either in isolation or in combination with other anthropomorphic and polysomnographic variables, are thought to provide some predictive power regarding successful therapy with OAs.[16,61]

Physiologic studies indicate that retroglossal rather than velopharyngeal collapse during sleep is highly predictive of OA success.[62] Physiologic measurements during wakefulness, including nasal resistance and flow-volume loops, have been reported to differ between OA responders and nonresponders.[63,64] However, upper airway imaging during wakefulness may aid in predicting the treatment response. Upper airway magnetic resonance imaging studies suggest that, although baseline airway and soft tissue anatomic characteristics may not differ between responders and nonresponders, the changes consequent to mandibular advancement do differ such that increases in airway volume are reasonably predictive of a favorable outcome.[65] Furthermore, computational modeling techniques further add to the information that can be derived from sophisticated imaging and appear to enhance these predictions.[66] Whereas such studies are helpful in understanding fundamental mechanisms of airway collapse during sleep and the mechanism of OA therapy, the clinical utility of such approaches is limited by cost and accessibility. Nasoendoscopy offers a more clinically accessible imaging modality. Studies during both wakefulness and drug-induced sleep[67,68] have established the predictive potential of this technique. Lateral widening of the velopharynx during awake endoscopy in the supine position is associated with a higher response rate with OAs.[67] Drug-induced sleep endoscopy (DISE) has shown good sensitivity for predicting treatment success by allowing visualization of the magnitude and patterns of pharyngeal collapse and identifying patients with greater improvements in pharyngeal patency with mandibular advancement.[69] See Chapters 20 and 21 for more information about DISE.

Remotely controlled mandibular positioning devices offer a relatively novel approach to identifying individuals who will or will not respond to OA therapy.[70-72] During a single-night titration procedure, these devices use hydraulic or electronic means to incrementally advance the mandible during sleep to determine both the treatment responsiveness and the required degree of advancement to ablate obstructive events. In addition, this may help establish tolerability for OA devices before costly acquisition. A prospective study using a commercially available system demonstrated that it is feasible both to predict treatment outcome and to determine the required "dose" of mandibular advancement during a single-night titration polysomnographic study.[71]

Appliance Selection

It is the sleep dentist's role to determine the most appropriate type of appliance based on specific clinical features to ensure that the patient is provided the most efficacious and cost-effective therapy. Given the wide variability in the reported efficacy across different studies, there is a strong suggestion that OA design has an important influence on treatment outcomes. Duobloc OAs, consisting of upper and lower plates, offer the advantage of a greater degree of mandibular movement (vertical and lateral) and adjustability (advancement), permitting attainment of the most comfortable and efficient position of the mandible. It is generally considered that the best retention is achieved with OAs that are customized and individually fabricated from the patient's dental impressions.[73]

Associated dental conditions, such as bruxism, may influence the choice of appliance design. As discussed later in this chapter, sleep bruxism/tooth grinding is common in patients with OSAHS,[74] although the causal relationship between the two conditions is unclear.[31] Patients who experience jaw discomfort after wearing a rigid monobloc oral appliance may benefit from using an appliance that allows lateral and vertical jaw movement.

Another important consideration is the vertical dimension of the OA. Minimum vertical opening depends on the amount of overbite. There are conflicting data on the effect of the degree of bite opening induced by OAs on treatment outcomes, although most patients appear to prefer minimal interocclusal openings.[75] In mouth-breathing patients, the selected OA design should have an anterior opening to permit comfortable breathing. In the case of edentulous patients wearing partial dentures, the splint design selected for that patient should adapt to the remaining natural dental structures when the dentures are removed. Whereas tongue-repositioning devices have a limited role in the treatment of OSAHS, they may play a role in individuals with insufficient teeth who fail to respond to or are not tolerant of other therapies.

A number of studies comparing the efficacy of different OA designs have emerged recently.[28,76,77] A retrospective analysis of 805 patients using either an adjustable OA or a fixed device found a higher treatment response rate for adjustable devices (56.8% vs. 47.0%).[77] Two crossover studies have compared two-piece adjustable appliances with different advancement mechanisms and found similar improvements in AHI, symptoms, and side effects.[28,76] One study assessing the addition of tongue protrusion using an anterior tongue bulb on an existing OA device showed further reductions in AHI compared with mandibular advancement alone.[78] These studies suggest that appliance design features are relevant to treatment efficacy, patient tolerance, and use and highlight the need for further research to differentiate the advantages of different OA designs and to aid in the appropriate appliance selection in clinical practice.

OPTIMIZATION OF TREATMENT

Although similar in concept, the optimization of OA treatment is different from that of PAP, which can be performed either during polysomnography or with an automatic/autotitrating PAP platform. One of the main differences is that patients may not be able initially to tolerate the degree of mandibular advancement required to completely relieve obstructive events and may require several months of progressive mandibular advancement to achieve a therapeutic position.[18,46,47,79] Several studies have evaluated whether titration of mandibular advancement during polysomnography could be used to optimize OA treatment, similar to PAP titrations.[47,70,80,81] These protocols have mixed results and only a fair sensitivity in predicting the amount of mandibular advancement needed for successful OA therapy. A remotely controlled mandibular positioner[80] using a success criterion of less than 10 events/hour and 50% improvement with a 4% oxygen desaturation criterion showed a positive and negative prediction value for subsequent successful OA therapy of 94% and 83%, respectively. These studies are promising, but non–industry-supported studies are required to further assess the prediction of treatment outcome with this tool.

The use of a systematic, home-based titration in which patients incrementally advance their devices until subjective improvements in sleep quality and daytime symptoms are achieved is significantly more likely to render more effective OA therapy. Studies have shown that, although 55% of patients achieve successful self-titration at home, another 32% can reach success with further polysomnography-guided titration.[48,82] Similarly, the use of home oximetry during titration does help titrate OAs.[49,82] Interestingly, 25% of the patients required additional mandibular advancement because of an abnormal oxygen desaturation index despite resolution of symptoms, whereas 20% of patients required further titration because of persistent symptoms despite a normal oxygen desaturation index.

Similar to PAP, appropriate OA titration is vital to achieve optimum therapeutic efficacy. Successful therapy requires both a dentist with experience in OA treatment to ensure proper adjustments of these devices and a sleep physician who should conduct follow-up evaluations and sleep testing to confirm that effective treatment is achieved. The dentist should observe patients on a yearly basis and may advance/titrate the appliance further if symptoms recur. If maximum mandibular advancement is reached and symptoms are still present, the patient should be referred to the referring physician for further evaluation and consideration of adjunctive or alternative therapies.

The other concept of optimization of treatment is the combination of treatment modalities. One study included patients who were unable to tolerate CPAP because high pressure was required to abolish the apneas. The combination of CPAP with an OA, not interconnected but used simultaneously, resulted in a CPAP pressure reduction of about 2 cm H_2O.[83] Another form of combination is to use the treatments interchangeably. Interestingly, when patients have the opportunity to use either treatment on a regular basis, patients tend to fluctuate between therapies. When patients compared the sleepiness while receiving CPAP only, they showed a significant decrease in their ESS score when they were able to use both treatments. One could hypothesize that patients were less likely to occasionally drop treatment, and therefore the long-term effects on sleepiness were further consolidated.[84] The combination of positional therapy with OA therapy has also been shown to improve clinical outcomes.[85]

Optimization of OA treatment, as described here, is indeed important and can be related to proper titration of the appliance and also the ability to offer combination therapies.

SIDE EFFECTS AND COMPLICATIONS

The primary reasons for discontinuation of OA treatment are an insufficient reduction of snoring, the persistence of apneic events, and the development of treatment-related side effects.[21] The most common reasons that patients completely discontinue OA therapy are device discomfort/cumbersome and limited perceived efficacy, and about 45% of nonadherence occurs within the first 6 months of therapy.[53]

Most side effects caused by OA are typically mild and transient. The most frequently reported events are excessive salivation, dry mouth, mouth or teeth discomfort, muscle tenderness, and jaw stiffness. Device adjustment can decrease short-term side effects by reducing pressure on the anterior teeth and excessive mandibular advancement. The clinical importance of short-term OA side effects has been compared with PAP published observations. By use of the same visual analog scale to categorize side effects of either OA or PAP, the two treatment modalities had a similar side effect score.[25] More persistent and severe side effects, including TMJ dysfunction and dental crown damage, are uncommon.[21] OAs in the titrated position appear to be innocuous to the TMJ in OSAHS patients.[53] Whereas existing TMJ disorders were typically considered a contraindication to OAs, a study of patients with known or prior TMJ dysfunction found that these patients can become eligible for OA therapy after simple physiotherapy exercises.[57,86] Transient and nonserious TMJ pain occurs more frequently with OAs than with PAP, but the risk for development of impairment of the temporomandibular complex is infrequent with long-term MAS use. Therefore pain related to the initial use of OAs is typically transient and not associated with a significant risk of long-term complications or functional limitations.

Long-term side effects of OA therapy are related to a significant impact on the occlusion. Changes in dentition are not restricted to OA therapy as the use of nasal masks can also alter the craniofacial structures.[58,87] However, these changes are more prominent in OA users compared with PAP users. Changes observed in craniofacial structures were mainly related to significant dentoalveolar changes (tooth movements).[88-90] There are important concerns about the timing and continuation of dental changes during a long-term period.[91] Importantly, overbite changes were observed to decrease less with time, whereas overjet continuously changed at a constant rate of 0.2 mm per year of OA use. Interestingly, on evaluation of various studies of different appliance designs, such as Herbst, Mobloc, Klearway, SomnoMed, and TAP, it has been shown that the amount of change was related to the duration of therapy and not the type of appliance that was used.[86,89-93]

Although changes in dental occlusion do occur, these are generally not a significant cause of treatment discontinuation. The patient's perceptions do not typically correlate with objective measurements, and occlusal changes often go unnoticed[90]; also, most individuals developed new occlusal contacts resulting from the development of a new occlusal equilibrium over time.[94] In addition, several reports have consistently found that patients perceive dental side effects to be less important than the benefits of improved daytime sleepiness and other sleep apnea symptoms. Therefore despite the presence of irreversible long-term occlusal changes, OA therapy should be considered a lifelong treatment for patients with OSAHS.

ADHERENCE AND PATIENT PERCEPTIONS

Adherence is defined by the World Health Organization as "the extent to which a person's behavior—taking medications, following a diet, and/or executing lifestyle changes—corresponds with agreed recommendations from a healthcare provider."[95] Numerous factors affect treatment adherence, including social and economic factors, health care system/team, characteristics of the disease, disease therapies, and patient-related factors. The consequences of a nontailored treatment with poor patient adherence are related to poor health outcomes and increased health care costs. As stated before, OSAHS is a chronic disease, and treatment with either PAP or OAs requires cooperation of the patient.

Treatment preference has been correlated to the degree of effectiveness, the impact of treatment on quality of life improvements, and the perceived severity of side effects.[96] Treatment expectations, lifestyle and personality of the patient, marital status, perceived stigma related to the treatment, and cost of treatment may also have an impact on a patient's preferences.[97] It is therefore important to include patients in the decision-making process regarding their treatment choices to promote better acceptance of and adherence with therapy as well as to identify potential barriers of one treatment option over another.

Treatment adherence with OAs appears to be dependent on the type of the appliance, disease severity, and patient supervision.[98,99] For example, adherence rates are greater with custom-made MAS than with tongue-retaining or "boil and bite" type appliances.[100,101] Studies have shown that about 75% of patients remained adherent after 12 months of treatment, which may decrease to 50% after 5 years.[102-105] Table 19-4 summarizes adherence rates in recent studies.[106]

Table 19-4   Adherence Rates of Oral Appliance Therapy in Selected Studies that Evaluated Use after a Minimum of 1 Year

Author	Interval (Months)	No. of Patients	Compliance Rate WCS/BCS
McGown,[99] 2001	22	166	42/56
Dort,[98] 2004	22	110	40/57
Marklund,[103] 2004	12	630	75/76
Almeida,[53] 2005	68	544	30/64
Marklund,[90] 2006	60	450	56/56
Gindre,[150] 2008	17	66	82/82

BCS, Best case scenario, relates to the percentage of patients who responded to the questionnaire only; WCS, worst case scenario, relates to an analysis interpretation of patients who did not return the questionnaires as compliance failures.
From Fleetham J, Almeida FR. Oral appliances. In: McNicholas WT, Bonsignore MR, editors. *European respiratory monograph.* Sheffield, UK: European Respiratory Society Journals; 2010. p. 267–85.

Adherence with OAs is consistently greater than that seen with PAP.[1] Whereas the existing literature strongly suggests that adherence with OAs is superior to that with PAP, most studies are based on subjective reports.[2,25] Recently, devices that provide a means to objectively monitor OA use have been developed.[54] Three microsensors are currently available that can be integrated into OAs: TheraMon (IFT Handels-und Entwicklungsgesellschaft GmbH, Handelsagentur Gschladt, Hargelsberg, Austria), AIR AID SLEEP (AIR AID GmbH & Co KG, Frankfurt, Germany), and Denti-Trac (Braebon Medical Corporation, Kanata, Canada). All three microsensors provide reliability and accurate wear time and can be incorporated into OAs fabricated from different materials.[107]

SLEEP BRUXISM IN PATIENTS WITH OBSTRUCTIVE SLEEP APNEA–HYPOPNEA SYNDROME

Sleep bruxism (SB) is classified as a sleep-related movement disorder in the *International Classification of Sleep Disorders.*[108] This is usually treated by dental practitioners.

During sleep, individuals with SB will engage in jaw movements described as tooth clenching and grinding, but on the basis of electromyographic recordings of masseter and temporalis, this has been described as rhythmic masticatory muscle activity (RMMA) to facilitate the recognition of and further refine the specificity of the SB clinical diagnosis.[29,108]

Although the etiology of SB remains unclear, 50% to 80% of SB episodes are associated with sleep arousals in otherwise healthy subjects.[109-114] Sleep arousal precedes the onset of RMMA-SB, and it is characterized by a rise in sympathetic cardiac activation, blood pressure, muscle tone, and breathing amplitude.[111,114-116] Clearly, there is not a single cause for SB, and the role of stress, anxiety, breathing, and cardiac reactivity in relation to wake and sleep hyperarousal is a current question of interest.

SB has been frequently observed with other sleep conditions, such as snoring, upper airway resistance syndrome, and obstructive sleep apnea.[73,113,117-121] It has been estimated that up to 50% of both adults and children with OSAHS may have comorbid SB; in such cases, it is named *secondary SB*.[73,122,123] In addition, a positive correlation between the severity of OSAHS and the frequency of tooth grinding and clenching has been established.[117,124] A questionnaire-based epidemiologic study by Ohayon et al[120] suggested that OSAHS is a low but significant risk factor for SB (odds ratio, 1.8; 95% confidence interval, 1.2–2.6). All this evidence is derived from questionnaires and lacks power to explain a causative relationship.

A recent population-based community sleep study, which investigated more than 1000 adults using polysomnography, observed no difference in the AHI between individuals with and without SB.[109] This is not surprising; the prevalence of SB, which decreases with age, and the rise in the prevalence of SDB prevent such an association. Furthermore, a recent polysomnographic study failed to show a clear temporal association between RMMA-SB and OSAHS. In one study of OSAHS patients, the majority of SB events were temporally related to apneas and hypopneas, occurring between 0 and 30 seconds after the event. However, 25% of SB episodes showed an opposite temporal relationship (i.e., the SB event occurred before the obstructive event), and 20% had no time correlation with obstructive events.[125] Furthermore, it is possible that SB resulted in some cases from unrecognized or unmeasured respiratory effort–related events. Regardless, this study did demonstrate a significant association of SB in those with SDB and identified a potential dependent relationship between the two conditions in the majority of events.

Given the limited and conflicting existing evidence, the nature of the relationship between SDB and SB remains controversial.

Some authors have suggested that SB-related masticatory muscle activities have a role in reinstating upper airway patency after an episode of respiratory obstruction during sleep.[114,116,125-127] On the basis of this suggestion, it would appear that SB occurs secondary to obstructive events and is a consequence of an OSAHS-related phenomenon similar to sleep arousal or oxygen desaturation. If this is true, treatments of OSAHS would be expected to improve SB.[117,124,128] Indeed, some clinical studies have shown a decrease in SB activity after treatment of OSAHS using different modalities, including adenotonsillectomy, OA, and PAP.[126,129-131] However, as described before, the temporal association between OSAHS events and the masticatory muscle activity has not been confirmed in most of the available studies.[73,125,128,132] Alternatively, SB has been described as masticatory movements required to lubricate the oropharyngeal structures during sleep, which may be particularly dry in snorers and OSAHS patients.[133,134] However, in all cases, the role of sleep arousal and related autonomic sympathetic activation has to be taken into account while investigating the potential relationship between OSAHS and SB.[113,114,116,117,125,132]

The Impact of Bruxism Therapies on the Upper Airway

Management strategies for SB include dental (i.e., OAs and guards), cognitive-behavioral, and pharmacologic approaches.[114] These approaches typically aim to reduce the detrimental consequences of sleep bruxism on the teeth (e.g., tooth wear) and dental restorations/prosthesis (e.g., fracture) and to reduce accompanying orofacial complaints (e.g., pain, headache). However, these treatment options largely mitigate the consequences of SB and do not address the SB events or potential underlying etiology or role of comorbidities such as OSAHS.

To protect dental surfaces and to relax the masticatory muscles, various designs and types of OAs are used. The soft vinyl mouth guards or hard acrylic occlusal splints have been extensively used in the management of SB.[114,135-139] These devices are more frequently designed to cover maxillary dentition, and patients are instructed to use them during sleep. The exact mechanism of action is still under debate, and there is no evidence to support their role in halting SB. Their main effect is to protect teeth against damage. Moreover, the lack of well-designed randomized controlled clinical trials and long-term studies makes it difficult to assess their true effectiveness on SB and oropharyngeal functions during sleep.[137] The majority of studies show a decrease in the RMMA-SB index by 40% to 50% during the initial period of treatment (2 to 6 weeks), regardless of the specific design of the occlusal splint.[136,138-140] However, the effect appears to be transitory, with values typically returning to pretreatment levels after a short time, and the outcomes are highly variable between subjects. Indeed, some studies have also reported no effect on or even an increase in electromyographic activities during sleep when an occlusal splint is worn, especially with soft mouth guard designs.[139,141,142]

The Use of Oral Appliances in Patients with Sleep Bruxism and Obstructive Sleep Apnea–Hypopnea Syndrome

Although occlusal splints have been thought to be a safe and conservative option for management of SB, few studies have investigated the effects of OAs designed to treat SB in patients who may have concomitant OSAHS. A pilot study of 10 patients with OSAHS found that a maxillary occlusal splint increased the AHI by more than 50% in half of the patients, likely by reducing the intraoral space and changing the tongue position during sleep.[143] Another group reproduced the direction taken by the pilot study, a risk for exacerbation of breathing in OSAHS patients but with a milder effect due to different morphologic patient characteristics.[144] Although there is a paucity of data, the potential adverse influence of maxillary occlusal splints on snoring and the respiratory disturbance index cannot be ignored, and clinicians should be cautious and consider the potential medical and dental complications of occlusal splints, especially when SB and OSAHS occur in the same patient. Given the potential association between SB and OSAHS in some patients and the potential negative effects of traditional SB therapies with SDB, it is imperative to assess risk of SDB in SB patients with OSAHS mild symptoms to select appropriate treatment options. In general, when SB is concomitant with OSAHS or when SDB is suspected, a mandibular advancement appliance would be preferable.

Some clinical studies have shown a decrease in RMMA-SB activity by using mandibular advancement devices in the absence of OSAHS.[126,145,146] These duobloc titratable OAs appear to be effective in decreasing SB and have been shown to reduce up to 70% of bruxism events in otherwise healthy young adult subjects.[126,145,146] Duobloc OAs also appeared to relieve morning headaches and snoring concomitant with SB.[126,147] In an experimental study among adolescents, SB-related symptoms were significantly mitigated and sleep structure and quality were preserved by the use of mandibular advancement OAs during sleep.[126] In general, OAs are well tolerated by SB patients, especially if some range of jaw movements is permitted.[126,145-147] The use of mandibular advancement OAs for the treatment of SB seems promising but probably for cases with SDB symptoms. Intuitively, OAs seem ideally suited to treatment of patients with concomitant SB and OSAHS. However, data on the utility of these devices in patients with both conditions are lacking, and the long-term effectiveness of OAs in patients with both SB and OSAHS has not been established.

FUTURE DIRECTIONS

OA therapy has emerged as the main alternative to PAP in the treatment of OSAHS. There is now a strong evidence base demonstrating the benefits of this therapy for improving physiologic sleep measures, daytime sleepiness, and quality of life in OSAHS patients across the spectrum of disease severity. The existing literature suggests that the superior treatment efficacy of PAP is mitigated by inferior compliance relative to OA therapy, resulting in similar health outcomes. Long-term comparative effectiveness studies, using patient-centered and clinically important outcome measures, are required to verify this. The advent of objective compliance monitors for OA therapy is critical to such studies.[148] Cost-effectiveness studies are also warranted to appropriately inform and direct clinical care. In addition, prospective validation studies are required to evaluate predictors of treatment outcome, and more research is needed to determine optimal titration protocols to increase the effectiveness of OA and to decrease the time taken to attain optimal treatment.

Future studies are needed to compare the effectiveness of different types of appliances and different design features (e.g., the amount of vertical opening). Likewise, these studies ideally would help differentiate which patients should receive custom-made, titratable devices and identify those who could be appropriately managed with less expensive, fixed devices. Ongoing refinements and standardization of appliance design may eventually lead to improved outcomes and will be enhanced by a better understanding of the mechanisms of action of OAs.

Snoring and SDB are chronic and progressive conditions, raising the possibility that early intervention of snoring may retard the development of OSAHS. OA therapy would appear to have a major role in such a preventive approach, and further work is warranted to evaluate this possibility.

OSAHS is increasingly recognized as a heterogeneous disorder with multiple pathophysiologic causes. Currently, PAP represents a "one size fits all" solution by preventing upper airway collapse. However, new concepts in OSAHS pathogenesis and phenotypes have recently emerged and could help the field move toward a future "personalized medicine" approach in which treatment is tailored to the patient. Finally, the use of OAs for SDB in the presence of comorbidities, such as SB, headache, pain, gastroesophageal reflux, and opioid use, needs to be better delineated.

SUMMARY

OAs, occlusal splint on single dental arch, can be used to prevent SB consequences on the teeth and pain, but in the presence of OSAHS, they may be contraindicated. Use of OAs with mandibular advancement is the ideal approach to manage OSAHS, conversely to occlusal splint. The putative mechanism is associated with increase in the anterior-posterior diameter of the upper airway space by advancing the oropharyngeal anatomic trio: the mandible, tongue, and soft palate. OAs with such advancement properties also add one important feature: they prevent posterior retrusion of the mandible during sleep, reducing the upper airway collapse. However, there appears to be a more robust and complex mechanism of improved airway patency and stability of upper airway muscle activity provided by these devices.

Although OAs provide reliable and effective treatment for most individuals with OSAHS, especially those with mild and moderate disease, there is a growing body of literature supporting that OAs are effective across a larger range of OSAHS severity. Nowadays, OAs for OSAHS should be considered an additional first-line treatment option. However, as with most appliances, success with OAs is not optimal. Even with titratable devices, a residual AHI is expected in more than 50% of individuals, and much work is expected to achieve higher success on most relevant outcomes, such as optimal sleep continuity, and reversal of signs and symptoms, such as sleepiness, cognitive alteration, blood pressure, and inflammatory reaction linked to SDB.

We recognize that OAs are not as effective as PAP in reducing the AHI, but they perform equally well compared with other measured variables, plus the OAs are more likely to be preferred by patients with better measures of adherence. Treatment with OAs provides a unique opportunity for interdisciplinary collaboration. Diagnosis and follow-up are performed by sleep medicine physicians; OA selection and follow-up are performed by dental sleep medicine professionals. OAs for either SB or OSAHS cannot be made for patients with gum infection, periodontal disease, or jaw pain without dental supervision. OAs may also induce orthognathic and dental changes in some patients that only a dentist can monitor and manage.

Selected Readings

Balasubramaniam R, Klasser GD, Cistulli PA, Lavigne GJ. Link between sleep bruxism, sleep disordered breathing and temporomandibular disorders: an evidence-based review. *J Dent Sleep Med* 2014;**1**:27–37.

Barnes M, McEvoy RD, Banks S, et al. Efficacy of positive airway pressure and oral appliance in mild to moderate obstructive sleep apnea. *Am J Respir Crit Care Med* 2004;**170**:656–64.

Chan ASL, Cistulli PA. Oral appliance treatment of obstructive sleep apnea: an update. *Curr Opin Pulm Med* 2009;**15**:591–6.

Dieltjens M, Verbruggen AE, Braem MJ, et al. Determinants of objective compliance during oral appliance therapy in patients with sleep-related disordered breathing: a prospective clinical trial. *JAMA Otolaryngol Head Neck Surg* 2015;**24**:894–900.

Gjerde K, Lehmann S, Berge ME, et al. Oral appliance treatment in moderate and severe obstructive sleep apnoea patients non-adherent to CPAP. *J Oral Rehabil* 2016;**43**(4):249–58.

Krishnan V, Collop NA, Scherr SC. An evaluation of a titration strategy for prescription of oral appliances for obstructive sleep apnea. *Chest* 2008;**133**:1135–41.

Kushida CA, Morgenthaler TI, Littner MR, et al. Practice parameters for the treatment of snoring and obstructive sleep apnea with oral appliances: an update for 2005. *Sleep* 2006;**29**:240–3.

Marklund M, et al. Oral appliance therapy in patients with daytime sleepiness and snoring or mild to moderate sleep apnea: a randomized clinical trial. *JAMA Intern Med* 2015;**175**(8):1278–85.

Phillips CL, Grunstein RR, Darendeliler MA, et al. Health outcomes of continuous positive airway pressure versus oral appliance treatment for obstructive sleep apnea: a randomized controlled trial. *Am J Respir Crit Care Med* 2013;**187**:879–87.

Ramar K, Dort LC, Katz SG, et al. Clinical practice guideline for the treatment of obstructive sleep apnea and snoring with oral appliance therapy: an update for 2015. *J Clin Sleep Med* 2015;**11**(7):773–827.

A complete reference list can be found online at ExpertConsult.com.

Obstructive Sleep Apnea: Anesthesia for Upper Airway Surgery

David R. Hillman; Peter R. Eastwood; Olivier M. Vanderveken

Chapter Highlights

- This chapter presents an overview of anesthetic considerations relating to upper airway surgery for patients with obstructive sleep apnea.
- Insightful anesthetic management of such cases requires an appreciation of the similarities and differences between the sleep and anesthetic states in relationship to their effects on upper airway and breathing function and on the arousal responses that help protect against disturbance of these essential physiologic functions.
- These issues are discussed in regard to both sedation for preoperative evaluation for obstructive sleep apnea surgery and perioperative management when surgery is undertaken.

Upper airway surgery is an undertaking that requires particularly close cooperation between surgeon and anesthesiologist. Patients presenting for these procedures do so because of compromised upper airway structure or function. In some circumstances, upper airway obstruction is the presenting complaint, as may occur with tumors in the upper airway. In others, the potential for obstruction may be great, as is the case for patients with obstructive sleep apnea (OSA). Managing such airways is challenging in the perioperative period. In anesthesiology terms, they are known as "difficult." A *difficult airway* has been defined by the American Society of Anesthesiologists as one that causes a conventionally trained anesthesiologist difficulty with face mask ventilation delivered to the upper airway, difficulty with tracheal intubation, or both.[1] Patients with OSA are vulnerable in both of these respects. In addition, they are, of course, at increased risk for upper airway obstruction whenever they are asleep or sedated. Whereas the sleeping patient is naturally protected from prolonged asphyxia by a capacity to arouse and reactivate effective breathing function, mild sedation compromises arousal mechanisms, and deep sedation or anesthesia abolishes these responses.[2] Patients with OSA are therefore particularly vulnerable throughout the perioperative period because of their airway compromise, compounded by the effects of anesthetic, opioid, and other sedative drugs and the risk of postoperative hemorrhage or edema associated with upper airway surgery.

In keeping with the orientation of this book toward sleep disorders, the focus of this chapter is on anesthetic considerations relating to upper airway surgery for OSA. Surgery frequently is undertaken to treat OSA in children, in whom tonsillar and adenoidal hypertrophy is a common cause.[3] Upper airway surgery also is regularly undertaken in adults for treatment of OSA, with several specific indications: removal of certain obstructing lesions in the upper airway; correction of abnormalities of the facial skeleton; unacceptability of nonsurgical treatments such as continuous positive airway pressure (CPAP) therapy and oral appliance therapy; and the need to relieve nasal obstruction to allow use of nasal masks for more comfortable, less intrusive delivery of CPAP than that offered by face masks.[4] A variety of procedures are available including nasal, palatal, and tongue base surgery; adenotonsillectomy (if hypertrophy is present); and a variety of orthognathic procedures.[5,6] The choice between them requires careful preoperative evaluation, often involving upper airway endoscopy and radiography including cephalometry, conventional computed tomography (CT), and, increasingly, three-dimensional studies using cone beam CT scans.[7]

Insightful anesthetic management of such cases requires an appreciation of the similarities and differences between the sleep and anesthetic states in relationship to their effect on upper airway and breathing function and on arousal responses that act to protect against disturbance in these functions. One facet of these shared considerations is illustrated by the use of anesthesia to simulate sleep-like conditions during drug-induced sedation endoscopy (DISE), sometimes termed *drug-induced sleep endoscopy*—a test to evaluate suitability for and type of OSA-related surgery, as described further on. More broadly, anesthetic management of patients with OSA presenting for upper airway surgical procedures must take into account several important factors: the shared influences of sedation, anesthesia, and sleep on upper airway behavior; how surgery can affect this behavior; the potential influences of OSA comorbid conditions including obesity and heart disease; and the early postoperative challenges associated with emergence from anesthesia, pain and its management, and the possibility of airway compromise from edema or hemorrhage.

Children present particular difficulties because of their small airway size and lung volumes relative to body size, predisposing them to upper airway obstruction and to rapid desaturation under such circumstances. Congenital problems associated with airway compromise, such as Down syndrome, also regularly manifest in childhood, further highlighting the challenges that confront pediatric anesthesiologists.[8] Relatively recently, DISE has been introduced into preoperative evaluation of pediatric patients with OSA, adding to these challenges.[9,10]

PREOPERATIVE EVALUATION OF PATIENTS PRESENTING FOR OBSTRUCTIVE SLEEP APNEA SURGERY

Preoperative evaluation of patients presenting for general anesthesia of any kind should include consideration of the possibility of OSA, in view of its prevalence and the associated perioperative risks.[11] Patients presenting for OSA surgery, however, usually have already had their OSA well characterized by a diagnostic home or laboratory-based sleep study. Often a trial of CPAP to treat the problem may be under way, or CPAP therapy may be a more-or-less established management component. Emergent or subsequent problems with compliance arising from difficulty in accepting or tolerating CPAP, usually because of its intrusive nature, are well documented as a common reason why adults patients with OSA present for upper airway surgery.[12] Other patients may elect nasal surgery to allow easier application of CPAP delivered by means of a nasal mask; otherwise, a more cumbersome face mask is the required interface when there is nasal obstruction.

Often, upper airway surgery for OSA is preceded by a surgeon-initiated investigation to determine the primary site of obstruction (velo-, oro-, or hypopharyngeal) and the nature of the obstructive process (lateral, anteroposterior, or concentric narrowing). This assessment allows the surgeon to determine the best procedure to counteract the problems identified by it.

Apart from radiographic imaging (such as cephalometry and CT scans), such evaluations usually involve endoscopic visualization of the upper airway under conditions conducive to obstruction. Early methods involved the performance of Mueller maneuvers (inspiratory effort against an obstruction—the opposite of the Valsalva manuever) during awake endoscopy or with the patient under mild sedation.[13] However, this approach is far removed from sleep-like conditions, in which the upper airway muscles are relaxed and obstruction occurs without exaggeratedly negative intraluminal pressures, so it has limited validity as an assessment of site and nature of upper airway collapse during sleep.[14]

Drug-Induced Sedation Endoscopy

To better simulate the conditions of sleep, DISE has evolved as a test to help determine suitability for surgery and the type of surgical procedure to be undertaken.[15,16] This procedure directly involves anesthesiologists because drugs are administered (usually intravenous propofol with or without midazolam) to produce sedation and sleep-like muscle relaxation, which induces snoring and upper airway obstruction (partial or complete) in predisposed patients. A recent European position paper on DISE provides an overview of the possible protocols for sedation during DISE, the indications for the procedure, and how the findings might be reported.[17]

Of note, with use of mild (wakeful) sedation, the upper airway muscles remain quite active, and sleep-like conditions cannot be assumed.[18] It is only if sleep itself supervenes or if sedation is deepened to a level at which consciousness is lost through a direct drug effect that behavior of the relaxed upper airway is observed. Indeed, a steplike reduction in phasic genioglossus muscle activity, a major upper airway dilating force, is seen at the transition to unconsciousness at sleep onset and with anesthetic induction.[18,19]

Observations made under the relaxed conditions of DISE will help determine suitability for non-CPAP treatment such as upper airway and skeletal surgery and for oral appliance therapy, as well as guiding the choice of surgical procedure to be undertaken. Resolution of pharyngeal collapse at all levels of the upper airway is necessary to achieve successful treatment in the individual patient. Indeed, it has been demonstrated that multilevel collapse is present in a majority of patients with OSA, and that the prevalence of complete collapse and multilevel collapse increases with increasing OSA severity and overweight and obesity.[20,21]

The use of DISE is based on the concept that upper airway behavior during drug-induced unconsciousness is similar to that in natural sleep, with similar reductions in muscle activation, respiratory drive, and reflex gains at transition to unconsciousness in each state.[18,19] The results of a study evaluating polysomnography with or without propofol administered by continuous target-controlled intravenous infusion demonstrated that, although propofol significantly changes sleep macroarchitecture, the main respiratory parameters, apnea-hypopnea index and mean arterial oxygen saturation remain unaffected.[22]

However, a critical difference that is highly relevant to the considerations that follow (and to recovery after the DISE procedure) is that with sleep, the capacity for spontaneous arousal is preserved, whereas with drug-induced unconsciousness, a dose-dependent depression of arousal responses prevails. This depression persists until physiologic drug elimination allows return of consciousness, so the anesthetized patient is highly vulnerable to asphyxia if upper airway obstruction occurs and is not detected by and dealt with by attending medical or nursing staff.

ANESTHESIA FOR SURGERY TO TREAT OBSTRUCTIVE SLEEP APNEA

Patients with OSA present the anesthesiologist with many challenges. The problems they experience during sleep signify the presence of a narrow airway predisposed to obstruction when the upper airway (and other) muscles relax with onset of anesthesia. Obesity and presence of other comorbid conditions (such as hypertension—systemic and pulmonary, cardiovascular disease, cerebrovascular disease, metabolic syndrome, atrial fibrillation, or heart failure) may be contributing factors. If sufficiently severe, obesity also may predispose the patient to atelectasis under anesthesia and to hypoventilation if spontaneous ventilation is preserved.[23,24]

A reduction in functional residual capacity (FRC) is another phenomenon that occurs with the muscle relaxation (in this case of chest wall muscles) that accompanies onset of anesthesia (and of sleep). The decrease can be profound in the morbidly obese, with FRC dropping to near residual volume.[24] This reduction in FRC is associated with atelectasis in the dependent parts of the lung with consequent shunt and hypoxemia. The loss of lung volume also is a significant contributor (along with upper airway muscle relaxation) to the

Table 20-1 Obstructive Sleep Apnea (OSA) and Perioperative Risk*

Risk Factor	Potential Perioperative Consequences	Identification of Risk	Reducing Risk
OSA	Upper airway obstruction with asphyxiation if unrecognized and untreated	Clinical evaluation Screening tools (e.g., STOP-Bang) Sleep study when indicated	Early identification Preparation for potential difficulties with airway management (including intubation) Techniques to minimize postoperative sedation Perioperative use of CPAP therapy Intensive monitoring until sentient and arousal responses unimpaired Referral for definitive diagnosis and treatment when OSA is first suspected perioperatively
OSA-predisposing factors Obesity Familial Craniofacial Mandibular retrusion Maxillary hypoplasia Other indicators of difficult intubation	OSA-related problems (above) Difficult tracheal intubation Difficult airway management Delayed extubation/ reintubation Atelectasis, hypoventilation when patient is morbidly obese	Clinical evaluation Endoscopy Cephalometry Upper airway imaging (CT, MRI)	Awareness of predisposition and associated risks Monitoring for these risks Preparation for potential risks, including availability of appropriate equipment to manage them Techniques to minimize postoperative sedation
OSA comorbid conditions Hypertension Cardiovascular/ cerebrovascular disease Metabolic syndrome Depression	Worsening of comorbid condition Delayed recovery	Clinical evaluation Biochemical testing when indicated	Optimize control preoperatively Careful perioperative management

*See text for further details.
CPAP, Continuous positive airway pressure; CT, computed tomography; MRI, magnetic resonance imaging.

increased airway collapsibility observed during ansthesia, because of associated loss of longitudinal traction on the upper airway.[25] Conveniently, CPAP counteracts both problems, providing a pneumatic splint to the upper airway and increasing FRC, helping prevent or recruit atelectatic lung, and offsetting the negative influence of volume loss on upper airway patency.

When hypoventilation is a prominent feature, bilevel ventilatory assistance is a preferred form of positive airway pressure therapy for obese patients, because it combines a background level of pressure to provide the benefits of CPAP with inspiratory pressure support to counteract the inadequate inspiratory flow.[26]

OSA is not restricted to the obese, however, and other pathogenetic factors are involved that are relevant to anesthesia. These include facial skeletal characteristics such as retrognathia and maxillary hypoplasia.[27] Such anatomic configurations, perhaps more than obesity itself, can present substantial challenges to the anesthesiologist. Potential problems include difficulty in performing endotracheal intubation and/or in maintaining airway patency during mask ventilation. Patients presenting such problems are said to have a "difficult airway." The presence of a difficult airway under anesthesia is an indicator of vulnerability to OSA.[28] Conversely, OSA is a risk factor for difficult intubation and/or difficulty with airway maintenance during the anesthetic

procedure.[29] Hence the anesthesiologist should approach patients with OSA prepared for a difficult intubation. It is likely that in the assessment of such patients, other factors indicating this possibility will be present, such as oropharyngeal crowding with high Mallampati scores, retrognathia with reduced thyromental distances and/or increased mandibular angulation, or increased neck circumference.[28] Increased neck circumference is a risk factor for OSA that is independent of obesity, although it reflects central fat deposition. Patients with large muscular necks also are at increased risk for OSA and may present additional airway management difficulties under anesthesia.[30] Apart from clinical evaluation, the anesthesiologist also should take advantage of the various radiographic and endoscopic preoperative investigations undertaken by the surgical team to assess upper airway structure and function in preparation for surgery (as outlined previously), to develop greater insights into the challenges ahead (Table 20-1).

Tracheal Intubation

Although some upper airway surgery procedures relevant to OSA can be done using local anesthesia (such as minor nasal surgery undertaken to improve the prospects of successful nasal CPAP delivery in patients with OSA along with nasal obstruction), most cases require general anesthesia. In such cases, the patient is almost always tracheally intubated. The presence of an endotracheal tube allows the anesthesiologist to step back from immediate proximity to the head, to allow surgical access, while ensuring airway patency and, in addition, ensuring protection of the lower airway from aspiration of blood and other material during the course of the procedure. The principal challenges in dealing with patients with obstruction-prone upper airways lie in placing the tracheal tube at the start of the procedure and in ensuring airway patency after removal of the tube on completion of anesthesia.

Airway Patency after Extubation

Several measures are required to ensure airway patency after extubation. First, apart from adequate reversal of any neuromuscular blockade if such drugs have been used, it is prudent to ensure that the patient has regained consciousness before extubation. Early return of consciousness requires the choice of appropriate anesthetic drugs and titration of doses to facilitate this outcome. Second, extubation in the lateral posture should be considered when practicable, with the patient maintained in this position during sleep for the postoperative period in the hospital. Third, CPAP or other positive airway pressure therapies should be readily available and used during sleep or sedation in patients with threatened or actual upper airway obstructive episodes. This is not a problem with CPAP-compliant patients, who expect the continuation of such therapy. It is more problematic in noncompliant patients, which is a good reason for preoperative induction of CPAP therapy when possible. Although the nose is the favored route of administration of CPAP for a majority of users, a face mask may be required perioperatively, particularly in the presence of edema or other conditions causing nasal obstruction. In the case of nasal surgery, nasal packs should be avoided when possible. Furthermore, an important caveat is that CPAP therapy may be needed in the early postoperative period despite the fact that the aim of surgery was to restore airway patency. This is because edema, secretions, blood, and clots can temporarily worsen airway patency. Although CPAP is a mainstay, use of other devices to improve airway patency, such as mandibular advancement devices, may have a perioperative role. Available literature to guide the perioperative use of these other devices is limited at present, however.

Early Postoperative Care

Finally, the patient must be closely monitored while he or she remains at increased risk. Clinical care thus requires a higher nurse-to-patient ratio than in the general ward and continuous monitoring of oxygenation (oximetry) and ventilation (capnography, oronasal airflow). Such facilities are available in the postanesthetic care unit and other high-dependency areas. Oxygen therapy should be used with caution because it can conceal obstructive events, potentially leading to their prolongation. It is for this reason that monitoring oronasal airflow, either directly or with capnography, adds value to oximetry monitoring.[31] Attending staff members must be expert in the use of CPAP and noninvasive ventilation. Discharge of the patient from such an environment demands return of consciousness and subsequent unimpeded arousal responses to threatened airway compromise. To ensure this outcome, it is highly desirable to avoid opioids and other drugs with sedative potential whenever possible. Alternative analgesic techniques include use of nonsteroidal anti-inflammatory drugs and acetaminophen and analgesic-sparing strategies such as use of corticosteroids. There also is a place for use of topical anesthesia and nerve blocks in the perioperative setting.[32]

Postoperative edema and secretions can temporarily compromise airways in which procedures have been undertaken to ultimately improve patency. Hemorrhage also is a risk, particularly in the early postoperative period.

Postoperative Sleep

Owing to the aforementioned considerations, the perioperative period is one of vulnerability. Added to these potential airway and ventilatory impairments is the disruption to sleep that occurs during the first few days postoperatively. Such sleep impairment increases the risk of postoperative delirium. Furthermore, as this early sleep disruption settles, a night or two of rapid eye movement (REM) sleep rebound may follow, with an increased proportion of sleep spent in the REM stage. This is of relevance because REM is the stage of sleep during which muscle activation and respiratory drive are most depressed and, consequently, the risk of upper airway obstruction and hypoventilation is greatest.[33]

Discharge Requirements

The ideal circumstances for discharge of these patients from high-dependency care and from the hospital are achieved with the following clinical objectives: return of consciousness with no plan for subsequent use of opioids or sedatives that may impair arousal responses; resolution of edema and of the particular risk of hemorrhage; and, when indicated, ability to self-administer CPAP, with willingness to use it when asleep. In some settings, these conditions may be met in the early postoperative period, depending on the nature of the procedure and the anesthetic technique used. If so, and if any comorbid conditions are well controlled, same-day discharge from the hospital after surgery is possible.

These recommendations are consistent with current published guidelines for perioperative care of patients with OSA.[32,34] It must be recognized, however, that this is an evolving area, and such guidelines currently are based largely on expert opinion. An evidence base developed from careful study and analysis of methods to improve perioperative outcomes is slowly accumulating and can be expected to eventually result in well-supported recommendations. Much work in this area remains to be done.

CONCLUSIONS

Anesthesia for upper airway surgery to treat OSA is challenging. The surgery often is undertaken in patients who have been unable or unwilling to tolerate CPAP therapy or in those who have surgically correctable upper airway or craniofacial abnormalities. Sometimes it is undertaken to improve CPAP compliance by relieving nasal obstruction. Anesthetic management requires careful preparation, allowing for the possibility of difficult intubation, and careful management of extubation and emergence to ensure maintenance of airway patency particularly in the period that precedes full return of consciousness and ability to promptly arouse from subsequent sleep in response to hypopneic or apneic events.

CLINICAL PEARLS

- The similar effects of anesthesia and of sleep in reducing muscle activation and ventilatory drive mean that vulnerability to upper airway obstruction in one state indicates high risk of problems in the other.
- The anatomic features (e.g., retrognathia) that predispose to airway obstruction also increase difficulties with tracheal intubation and mask ventilation performed with the patient under anesthesia.
- A key difference between the states is suppression of the arousal responses that protect the sleeping patient by anesthetic agents, with increased risk of asphyxia in those with obstruction-prone airways, such as patients with OSA. Postoperative use of opioid and sedative drugs may extend these risks beyond the immediate postoperative period, and caution with use of these agents is mandatory.
- Postoperative edema further compounds potential problems for patients who have undergone surgery for OSA.
- Close perioperative and postoperative monitoring and management must take these matters into account.

SUMMARY

Anesthesia for upper airway surgery to treat OSA is challenging. Often such surgery is undertaken in patients who have been unable or unwilling to tolerate CPAP therapy. Sometimes it is undertaken to improve CPAP compliance by relieving nasal obstruction. Preoperative surgical evaluation often entails DISE to assess suitability for and determine the optimal type of surgery. This procedure requires an appreciation of the relationships between drug-induced sedation and sleep in terms of muscle relaxation, ventilatory depression, and reflex suppression to ensure that airway behavior is observed under sleep-like conditions. Anesthetic management for the upper airway surgery requires careful preparation, allowing for the possibility of difficult intubation, and careful management of extubation and monitoring of emergence to ensure maintenance of airway patency, particularly in the period that precedes full return of consciousness and the capability for prompt arousal from subsequent sleep in response to hypopneic or apneic events.

Selected Readings

Brown KA. Outcome, risk, and error and the child with obstructive sleep apnea. *Paediatr Anaesth* 2011;**21**:771–80.

Chung F, Subramanyam R, Liao P, et al. High STOP-Bang score indicates a high probability of obstructive sleep apnoea. *Br J Anaesth* 2012;**108**:768–75.

De Vito A, Carrasco Llatas M, Vanni A, et al. European position paper on drug-induced sedation endoscopy (DISE). *Sleep Breath* 2014;**18**(3):453–65.

Ehsan Z, Mahmoud M, Shott SR, et al. The effects of Anesthesia and opioids on the upper airway: A systematic review. *Laryngoscope* 2016;**126**(1):270–84.

Hillman DR, Walsh JH, Maddison KJ, et al. Evolution of changes in upper airway collapsibility during slow induction of anesthesia with propofol. *Anesthesiology* 2009;**111**:63–71.

Hiremath AS, Hillman DR, James AL, et al. Relationship between difficult tracheal intubation and obstructive sleep apnoea. *Br J Anaesth* 1998;**80**:606–11.

Lee CH, Kim DK, Kim SY, et al. Changes in site of obstruction in obstructive sleep apnea patients according to sleep position: a DISE study. *Laryngoscope* 2015;**125**(1):248–54.

Pelosi P, Croci M, Ravagnan I, et al. The effects of body mass on lung volumes, respiratory mechanics, and gas exchange during general anesthesia. *Anesth Analg* 1998;**87**:654–60.

Practice guidelines for the perioperative management of patients with obstructive sleep apnea: an updated report by the American Society of Anesthesiologists Task Force on Perioperative Management of patients with obstructive sleep apnea. *Anesthesiology* 2014;**120**(2):268–86.

Rosenberg J, Wildschiodtz G, Pedersen MH, et al. Late postoperative nocturnal episodic hypoxaemia and associated sleep pattern. *Br J Anaesth* 1994;**72**:145–50.

Vroegop AV, Vanderveken OM, Boudewyns AN, et al. Drug-induced sleep endoscopy in sleep-disordered breathing: report on 1,249 cases. *Laryngoscope* 2014;**124**:797–802.

A complete reference list can be found online at ExpertConsult.com.

Upper Airway Surgery to Treat Obstructive Sleep Apnea

Olivier M. Vanderveken; Aarnoud Hoekema; Edward M. Weaver

Chapter Highlights

- Management with continuous positive airway pressure (CPAP) remains the treatment of choice for moderate to severe obstructive sleep apnea (OSA). Some patients cannot or will not accept CPAP therapy, or CPAP may not be effective in certain cases, so use of other therapies may be indicated.

- Objective sleep testing is always required before the decision for surgical treatment, to identify those patients at risk for complications of OSA, to guide selection of appropriate management,

and to provide a baseline to establish the efficacy of treatment.

- Surgical treatments for OSA fall into the following categories: surgical upper airway modifications including tongue suspension techniques, upper airway neurostimulation therapy, tracheostomy, skeletal modifications, and bariatric surgery.

- Objective sleep testing is always required after surgical treatment, to document efficacy.

OVERVIEW AND BACKGROUND

Management with continuous positive airway pressure (CPAP) remains the treatment of choice for moderate to severe obstructive sleep apnea (OSA).[1] Adequate CPAP treatment improves blood pressure to combat hypertension and reduces the risk of nonfatal and fatal cardiovascular events, and successful CPAP treatment has been shown to prolong survival.[2-5]

The clinical effectiveness of CPAP often is hampered and limited by important patient-specific factors: low rate of acceptance, poor tolerance, and suboptimal adherence.[6] Therefore many patients with OSA remain inadequately treated owing to inconsistent CPAP adherence,[6,7] with consequent reduced clinical effectiveness of therapy.[5,6,8-12] When the response to CPAP is considered inadequate as indicated by both symptom evaluation and objective monitoring data, despite intensive efforts to improve adherence to the CPAP regimen including trials of combination therapies, non-CPAP alternatives for the management of OSA need to be considered.[13,14] At this stage, proper and careful selection of the right patient for the right treatment option(s) is of utmost importance.[13]

The focus of this chapter is on upper airway surgery to treat OSA. Sometimes surgery is most helpful to facilitate CPAP or oral appliance therapy, such as with surgical correction of nasal obstruction. Alternatively, surgical management may be indicated in place of these other therapies—for example, when factors including unfavorable anatomy or patient intolerance preclude their use. It is important to recognize that often multimodality therapy is the best strategy, and surgery can be combined with any and all other OSA treatments including CPAP and non-CPAP approaches when indicated.[15]

Surgical modifications for treating OSA fall into five main categories: upper airway bypass procedure, surgical upper airway modifications including tongue suspension techniques, upper airway neurostimulation therapy, skeletal modifications, and bariatric surgery. Anesthetic issues are reviewed in Chapter 20.

Objective sleep testing is required before initiation of surgical treatment, to identify those patients at risk for complications of OSA, to guide selection of appropriate management, and to provide a baseline to establish the physiologic efficacy of subsequent treatment.[14] Follow-up sleep studies are routinely indicated to monitor the response to surgery for OSA.

PREOPERATIVE EVALUATION

The comprehensive diagnostic workup of the patient with OSA should include a complete medical and thorough sleep history. Previous OSA treatments and their clinical and polysomnographic results also should be evaluated and documented in this workup, as described in Section II and the other chapters in Section III of this volume. Before proceeding with surgery, the medical workup should identify complicating factors that can increase the medical, anesthetic, and surgical risk of the surgical procedure. A thorough upper airway examination should be performed, including assessment of the anatomy and functional status of the nose, mouth, pharynx, larynx, and related structures (e.g., craniofacial, dental, and airway structures). The OSA examination often includes upper airway endoscopy to visualize all of the levels of the pharynx, larynx, and related structures—the palate, tongue base, the lateral pharyngeal walls, the vallecula, the pyriform sinuses, the larynx, and the epiglottis. The diagnostic pretreatment assessment needs to include a baseline sleep study. The polysomnographic recording should be recent enough that it represents the current status of the OSA and ideally consists of a full-night diagnostic study.

The option of surgical interventions for OSA is based in part on the demonstration that the upper airway is significantly smaller in patients with OSA than in normal subjects, especially at the retropalatal and retroglossal levels.[16,17] The upper airway is described as a structure with a rigid support in its proximal (laryngeal) and distal (nasal) segments, with a collapsible portion in between. This collapsible anatomic portion extends from the soft palate to the epiglottis, with the size of its lumen subject to the influence of surrounding anatomy, presence of fat tissue, pressures gradients, tissue laxity, and dilator muscle activity. The potential loss of upper airway patency during sleep in patients with OSA is therefore usually localized to this so-called *collapsible segment* (Figure 21-1).

In the early days of OSA therapy, tracheostomy, or "upper airway bypass surgery," offered the only effective management, and it often was used in patients with profound OSA.[18] Tracheostomy, however, does not address the collapse directly in the vulnerable segment of the upper airway but instead successfully bypasses the obstruction, thereby moderating OSA. Tracheostomy is thus a highly effective treatment for OSA. On the other hand, tracheostomy is a physically and socially invasive procedure that may substantially reduce perceived quality of life.[18] The more commonly used upper airway surgical procedures nowadays have greater acceptance but are less effective.[19]

The decision process to select the appropriate upper airway surgical procedures for any specific patient are determined by the site(s), the degree, and the pattern of upper airway obstruction[13] (Figure 21-2). Indeed, most upper airway surgical approaches, apart from surgical treatments with a global effect (i.e., tracheostomy bypass, bariatric surgery, and maxillomandibular advancement [MMA]) (Table 21-1), ideally strive to intervene at the specific anatomic region(s) that become obstructed during sleep. In addition to the history, examina-

tion, and in-office awake upper airway endoscopy, a variety of other modalities may be used to assess sites, degree, and pattern of obstruction. Pharyngeal pressure measurements, imaging and endoscopic techniques can be used to gain insight into the pathogenesis of this disease, as well as to identify appropriate therapeutic options.[20-23] Imaging techniques available for the preoperative evaluation include

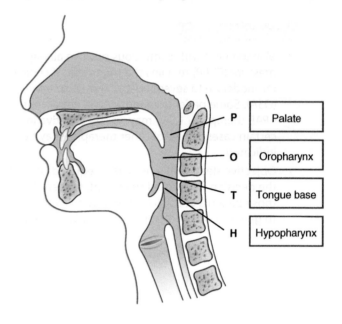

Figure 21-1 Sagittal cross section of the upper airway with the different levels prone to upper airway collapse during sleep within the "collapsible segment": the velopharynx with the palate as the most relevant structure; the oropharynx, including both the palatine tonsils and the lateral oropharyngeal walls; the level of the tongue base, including the lingual tonsils; and the hypopharynx, including the epiglottis and the hypopharyngeal lateral walls. The upper airway has rigid support in its proximal and distal segments but has a collapsible portion, the so-called *collapsible segment* extending from the soft palate to the epiglottis, with the size of its lumen subject to the influence of surrounding pressures and the activity of dilator muscles.

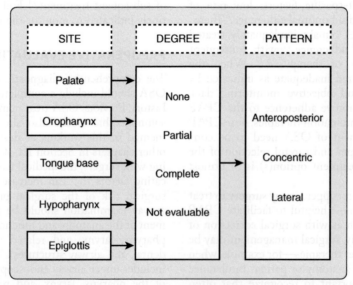

Figure 21-2 Scoring form for drug-induced sedation endoscopy (DISE): Reporting of the assessment of the site, the corresponding degree, and pattern of upper airway collapse. (From Vroegop AV, Vanderveken OM, Wouters K, et al. Observer variation in drug-induced sleep endoscopy: experienced versus nonexperienced ear, nose, and throat surgeons. *Sleep* 2013;36:947–53.)

Table 21-1	Treatment Options Other than Continuous Positive Airway Pressure (CPAP) for Patients with Obstructive Sleep Apnea
Category	Intervention/Procedure
General measures	Avoidance of sedatives Avoidance of alcohol Sleep hygiene Weight loss in case of overweight or obesity Avoidance of supine position during sleep in case of positional sleep apnea

Specific therapeutic options	Oral appliance therapy
	Surgery
	    Surgical upper airway modifications
	    Upper airway neurostimulation
	    Skeletal modifications including maxillomandibular advancement
	    Upper airway bypass: tracheostomy
	    Bariatric surgery

Table 21-2	Sample List* of Site-Specific Surgical Upper Airway Modifications for Treatment for Obstructive Sleep Apnea
Site-Specific Category	Procedures
Nasal surgery	Septoplasty, septorhinoplasty Turbinate reduction Nasal valve surgery

Pharyngeal procedures	Adenoidectomy, tonsillectomy, lingual tonsillectomy
	Uvulopalatopharyngoplasty (UPPP) and variations (e.g., expansion sphincter pharyngoplasty, many others)
	Tongue base reduction
	    Radiofrequency tongue reduction
	    Transoral robotic surgery
	    Coblation ablation or excision
	    CO_2 laser excision
	Epiglottoplasty
	Genioglossus advancement
	Hyoid suspension
	Tongue suspension

*Not exhaustive.

radiography, fluoroscopy, conventional computed tomography (CT), magnetic resonance imaging (MRI), and three-dimensional studies of the upper airway using cone beam CT (CBCT) scans.[24-28] In addition, cephalometric analysis can be performed.[28-30,30a] More recently, computational models of the upper airway based on CT or MRI have been introduced to simulate the effects of upper airway manipulations and to predict success of various treatment options.[17,31-34]

The different techniques available for investigation of the upper airway all have their specific advantages and limitations.[20] Differences among the various techniques include aspects on invasiveness, exposure to radiation, costs related to the examination, and potential side effects.[20,22,35] In addition, a crucial question of whether the upper airway behaves differently during wakefulness versus during natural sleep remains unanswered to date.[36] Inasmuch as OSA occurs exclusively during sleep, it would be ideal to evaluate the upper airway during a full night of natural sleep; such investigation during natural sleep, however, is of limited feasibility, owing to the associated sleep disruption and the labor-intensive nature of such studies.

The technique of drug-induced sedation endoscopy (DISE), first described as "sleep nasendoscopy" by Croft and Pringle in 1991, has emerged as an alternative method to dynamically investigate the upper airway before non-CPAP treatment selection in patients with OSA.[13,36-38] Drugs typically used for DISE include propofol, midazolam, dexmedetomidine, and/or ketamine.[36,39] In a comparison of DISE with awake endoscopy, identical findings were observed in only 25% of the cases.[40] In this particular study reporting on 250 patients with OSA, the discrepancies between awake endoscopy and DISE involved the oropharynx in 33%, the hypopharynx in 50%, and the larynx (e.g., epiglottis) in 33% of the patients.[40] These findings have important implications for surgical treatment choices, especially with operations involving the tongue base.[41]

Recent studies indicate that both inter- and intra-rater reliability of DISE are reasonably good but that experience in performing DISE is needed in order to obtain reliable observations.[42-44] Much investigation, standardization, and optimization of DISE techniques are needed regarding factors such as method of sedation, depth of sedation, patient position, use of airway anaesthetics, duration of observation, and others.[36] In the literature, no consensus exists on a standard DISE classification system or quantification of degrees of collapse or obstruction; in Figure 21-2, a generic scoring form is depicted.[44]

Several studies confirm that the most frequent site of upper airway obstruction in patients with OSA is the palatal level[23,38,45]; however, a majority of patients with OSA have other sites of obstruction as well (multilevel collapse).[23,27] The probability of multilevel collapse increases with increasing OSA severity and with an increased level of overweight or obesity.[23] Logically, resolution of pharyngeal collapse at all levels involved in the upper airway collapse during sleep will be necessary to achieve successful management in the individual patient with OSA undergoing surgery.

Surgical Upper Airway Modifications

A schematic overview of several different site-specific techniques available for surgically modifying the upper airway in patients with OSA is provided in Table 21-2.

Nasal Surgery

Depending on the anatomic or functional abnormalities at the level of the septum, turbinates, and nasal valves, nasal surgery can be indicated to correct nasal obstruction. However, nasal surgery including septoplasty, septorhinoplasty, turbinate reduction, and nasal valve surgery usually is insufficient to treat OSA and cannot be recommended as a stand-alone procedure for the management of OSA in most patients.[46] On the other hand, nasal surgery might be performed in patients with nasal obstruction that experience problems with the use of CPAP or oral appliance therapy because of these nasal complaints in order to improve adherence to treatment.[47] Successful nasal surgery may also be associated with a reduction in therapeutic CPAP pressure required to alleviate OSA.[48,49] Accordingly, a recent systematic review with meta-analysis of the existing literature on the relationship between nasal surgery and its effect on therapeutic CPAP pressure has been performed by Camacho et al.[50] The authors concluded that, indeed, isolated nasal surgery in patients with OSA associated with nasal obstruction reduces therapeutic CPAP pressures and that the data consistently suggest that isolated nasal surgery in these selected patients also increases CPAP use.[50]

Pharyngeal Surgery

The most commonly used surgical treatments for OSA are aimed at the pharyngeal airway where collapse and obstruction occur. It is important to recognize that an isolated single-level pharyngeal procedure would not be expected to solve multilevel obstruction. In cases of multilevel obstruction, isolated procedures might have a partial treatment effect or be one part of a multilevel treatment plan (e.g., staged surgery or multiple procedures). Adenotonsillar hypertrophy is the most common cause of OSA in children but a rare cause of OSA in adults.[46] As a consequence, adenotonsillectomy is the first-line therapy for nonobese children with OSA. In adult patients with OSA, (adeno)tonsillectomy can be recommended in the presence of (adeno)tonsillar hypertrophy with an expected reduction in sleep respiratory disturbances and improvement in architecture.[50a]

Uvulopalatopharyngoplasty (UPPP) is the most commonly performed pharyngeal surgical procedure for the treatment of OSA.[51] The classical UPPP procedure consists of partial excision and closure of the soft palate, uvula, and pharyngeal pillars, as well as tonsillectomy, if not previously performed[51] (Figure 21-3). A pooled data analysis of the literature (predominantly case series) published in 1996 revealed that UPPP had an overall success rate (i.e., reduction of AHI by more than 50%, with less than 20 events per hour of sleep, or reduction of apnea index by more than 50%, with less than 10 events per hour of sleep) of only 41% in unselected patients with OSA, but selecting patients with appropriate anatomy had an important impact on polysomnography outcomes.[18] When DISE is added to the diagnostic workup and preoperative evaluation for patient selection, it has been demonstrated that the success rate of UPPP increases over that for historical control data.[52] Recently, a randomized controlled trial comparing a modified UPPP with surgery delay showed a major reduction in OSA severity in the UPPP group compared with the control group (mean AHI reduction of 60%, versus 11%).[53] More important, UPPP improves clinical outcomes such as mortality risk, cardiovascular disease risk, motor vehicle crash risk, symptoms, and quality of life.[4,9,10,54-58]

The many variations of UPPP published in the literature aim to improve effectiveness, reduce surgical morbidity, and target specific patterns of collapse or obstruction. Examples are the uvulopalatal flap (UPF) technique, expansion sphincter pharyngoplasty, transpalatal advancement pharyngoplasty, and lateral pharyngoplasty.[59-61] The advantage of the UPF is that it is a potentially reversible flap that can be taken down if necessary to reduce the risk of nasopharyngeal incompetence; the technique comes with less postoperative side effects as there are no sutures and scar along the free edge of the palate[60] (Figure 21-4). The expansion sphincter pharyngoplasty (ESP) addresses lateral oropharyngeal or velopharyngeal collapse[62] (Figure 21-5). The early results with ESP are promising, and minimal complications have been reported with the procedure.[62] Transpalatal advancement pharyngoplasty is aimed at addressing anterior-posterior narrowing of the velopharynx, especially in concert with a long hard palate and vertically oriented soft palate.[59] The technical details and the wide array of UPPP variations are beyond the scope of this discussion.

Laser-assisted uvuloplasty (LAUP) is an office-based surgical procedure that progressively shortens and tightens the uvula and palate through a series of CO_2 laser incisions and vaporizations. This technique has not demonstrated consistent effect or benefit on OSA severity or symptoms or on quality of life measures and therefore also in accordance with the practice parameters of the American Academy of Sleep Medicine (AASM), LAUP is not recommended for the management of OSA.[46,63]

Radiofrequency ablation (RFA) can be used to reduce or stiffen soft tissues. RFA of the palate is considered to be a minimally invasive surgical outpatient clinic procedure that decreases socially disturbing snoring as reported by the partner

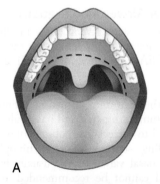
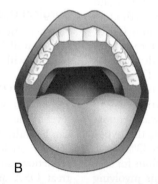
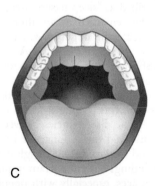

A   B   C

Figure 21-3 Classical uvulopalatopharyngoplasty technique. **A,** Redundant soft palate and pharyngeal pillar mucosa are outlined. **B,** Tonsils, pharyngeal pillar mucosa, uvula, and soft palate have been excised. The extent of soft palate excision is determined by placing traction on the uvula and noting the position of the mucosal crease. **C,** Mucosal flaps of the lateral pharyngeal wall and palatal muscle are advanced and closed with absorbable suture. (From Troell RJ, Strom CG. Surgical therapy for snoring. *Fed Pract* 1997;14:29–52.)

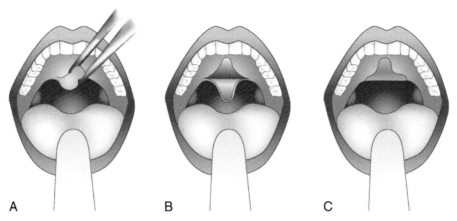

Figure 21-4 Uvulopalatal flap (UPF) technique. **A,** Uvula is reflected to identify mucosal crease of muscular sling. **B,** Knife removes mucosa on proposed flap site. **C,** Wound is closed with a half-buried suture of braided 3-0 Vicryl at the tip of the uvula and simple interrupted sutures along the mucosal closure. (From Troell RJ, Strom CG. Surgical therapy for snoring. *Fed Pract* 1997;14:29–52.)

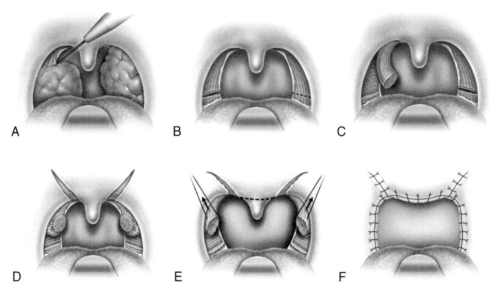

Figure 21-5 Expansion sphincter pharyngoplasty (ESP) technique. **A,** Tonsillectomy is performed. **B,** Horizontal incision made to divide the middle part of the palatopharyngeus muscle. **C,** The palatopharyngeus muscle is mobilized, although not completely, with care taken to leave its fascia attachments to the deeper horizontal constrictor muscles. **D,** Superolateral incision made on the soft palate, revealing the arching fibers of the palatini muscles. **E,** Vicryl sutures are used to hitch up the palatopharyngeus muscle to the soft palate muscles superolaterally. **F,** Closure of the palatal incisions. (From Pang KP, Woodson BT. Expansion sphincter pharyngoplasty: a new technique for the treatment of obstructive sleep apnea. *Otolaryngol Head Neck Surg* 2007;137:110–14.)

of the patient. RFA of the palate has minimal effect on OSA severity, however, so it is not recommended as a single-stage procedure for the management of OSA.[46,64-67]

Taken together, the available evidence on pharyngeal procedures that address the palatal level suggests that UPPP and its variations can be applied in well-selected patients, whereas both LAUP and RFA of the palate are not recommended for the management of OSA.[52,53,57,63,64]

RFA tongue reduction is a minimally invasive technique for decreasing tongue volume when tongue hypertrophy contributes to the OSA.[68] When combined with RFA of the palate in patients with mild to moderate OSA, the procedure had a significant effect on airway volume, apnea index, and

quality of life in a randomized sham placebo-controlled trial.[69] However, the magnitude of treatment effect is modest, especially in patients who are obese or have more severe OSA.[70,71] Consequently, RFA tongue reduction usually is performed as a valuable adjunctive surgical procedure, and not a primary procedure, in the management of OSA.[72,73]

In patients with OSA primarily related to hypertrophy of the tongue base, various techniques of partial glossectomy have led to significant reduction in OSA severity. The original studies describing partial glossectomy for OSA used laser techniques.[74,75] More recently, investigators have obtained good success, with less patient morbidity, using an irrigating, suctioning bipolar device instead of the laser.[76-79,79a] Tongue

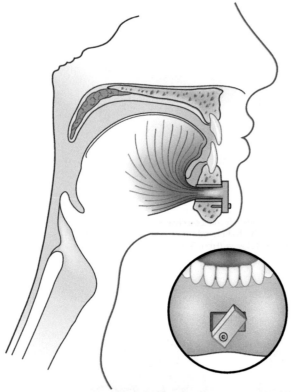

Figure 21-6 Genioglossus advancement. In this procedure, the tongue is placed under anterior traction by performing a limited mandibular osteotomy, with subsequent advancement of the genial tubercle–genioglossus muscle complex. After removal of the buccal cortex and medullary bone, the lingual cortex of the advanced bony segment including the genial tubercle is fixated in its new anterior position (*inset*). (From Riley RW, Powell NB, Guilleminault C. Obstructive sleep apnea and the hyoid: a revised surgical procedure. *Otolaryngol Head Neck Surg* 1994;111:717–21.)

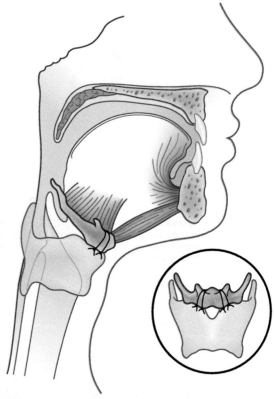

Figure 21-7 Modified hyoid myotomy and suspension (HMS) procedure. The hyoid bone is isolated, the inferior body is dissected clean, and the major portion of the suprahyoid musculature remains intact. The hyoid is advanced over the thyroid lamina and immobilized with sutures placed through the superior aspect of the thyroid cartilage (*inset*). (From Riley RW, Powell NB, Guilleminault C. Obstructive sleep apnea and the hyoid: a revised surgical procedure. *Otolaryngol Head Neck Surg* 1994;111:717–21.)

reduction achieved using transoral robotic surgery (TORS) techniques also has been proved to be feasible, low-risk, and well tolerated.[80-82] As with most surgical upper airway modification techniques, it has been shown that the preoperative BMI predicts treatment success using TORS for OSA management.[83]

Another treatment approach to manage tongue obstruction is to advance or stabilize the tongue using various techniques. Genioglossus advancement uses the forward placement of the geniotubercle to place sufficient tension on the tongue, preventing it from collapsing (Figure 21-6). Hyoid suspension or hyoidthyropexia for the treatment of OSA consists of securing the hyoid arch anteroinferiorly to the thyroid lamina, with or without hyoid myotomy (Figure 21-7). Alternatively, the hyoid bone can be suspended from the mandible using any of various methods. Genioglossus advancement and hyoid suspension are rarely performed in isolation, so assessment of isolated effectiveness is difficult. Suture-based tongue suspension procedures aim to tether the tongue to the mandible by means of sutures, ribbons, or barbs.[84] Adjustable tongue advancement, effected through placement of a tissue anchor in the tongue base and an adjustment spool at the mandible, and of a tetherline to suspend the tongue, was reported to be feasible and well tolerated, but further research is needed on the efficacy of this novel procedure.[85,86] Tongue suspension should be considered in patients with OSA who demonstrate

tongue base obstruction. As a stand-alone procedure, its success rate is only 36.6%,[84] possibly related to the multilevel obstruction common in OSA. In addition, tongue suspension is effective and safe as part of a multilevel surgical approach for patients with OSA.[84]

Various case series have shown mixed results with the various hypopharyngeal procedures, but most demonstrate at least partial effectiveness.[84,87-89] As a result, consensus is lacking regarding which procedure is best used to address hypopharyngeal obstruction in OSA, because individual anatomy and obstruction patterns are indications for different types of procedures. For example, tongue hypertrophy might best be treated with tongue reduction (e.g., partial glossectomy), whereas tongue collapse might be more readily treated with tongue advancement or stabilization (e.g., genioglossus advancement, hyoid suspension, tongue suspension). The previously described surgical procedures are site-directed to specific areas of the upper airway. Often these procedures are combined in various ways to address multilevel obstruction. Other surgical procedures also have a multilevel effect on the airway and are indicated in specific circumstances. As described next, neuromuscular upper airway stimulation therapy, especially with electrical stimulation of the hypoglossal nerve, is a new multilevel treatment that activates pharyngeal airway dilator muscles to enlarge the lower pharynx and indirectly can stabilize the upper pharynx.[90-92] MMA, also described further on, has a multilevel effect by enlarging the anteroposterior dimensions of the upper and lower pharynx and stabilizing lateral wall collapse.[93]

Upper Airway Neurostimulation Therapy

Direct electrical stimulation of the hypoglossal nerve, which innervates the intrinsic and extrinsic muscles of the tongue, during sleep, to restore or maintain upper airway patency, is an experimental therapy for OSA with a history of 20 years of research and development.[90,94-98] From a pathophysiologic standpoint, selective stimulation of the hypoglossal nerve during sleep may provide an interesting approach to management of OSA based on the restoration or improvement of upper airway dilator muscle activity during sleep.[90,91]

The feasibility of and therapeutic potential for chronic hypoglossal nerve stimulation using a first-generation system (Inspire 1, Medtronic, Inc., Minneapolis, Minnesota) in patients with OSA were investigated in a multicenter study.[97] Eight patients with OSA received this first-generation, fully implantable pulse generator (IPG) triggered by a pressure sensor, located at the sternum, detecting respiratory effort. Electrical stimulation was sent from the IPG to the hypoglossal nerve by way of a stimulation lead containing a half-open cuff around the nerve.[97] Throughout the entire study, unilateral hypoglossal nerve stimulation decreased the severity of OSA. After a minimum follow-up period of 6 months, all patients tolerated long-term stimulation, and no adverse effects were noted.[97]

On the basis of this first experience, the safety and therapeutic feasibility as well as the efficacy of three different second-generation hypoglossal nerve stimulation devices have been explored in recent clinical studies. Three types of systems were analyzed in these studies: the HGNS (Hypoglossal Nerve Stimulation) system (Apnex Medical, Inc., St. Paul, Minnesota), the Aura6000 system (ImThera Medical, Inc., San Diego, California), and the Inspire II Upper Airway Stimulation (UAS) device (Inspire Medical Systems, Inc.,

Maple Grove, Minnesota). Early results of these studies have been published and confirm the safety and feasibility of the second-generation implantable systems for upper airway neurostimulation therapy for OSDB.[94,95,98] The primary component in all three systems is an IPG. Furthermore, the main difference between the three systems is that with the Aura6000 system, the stimulation onto the body of the proximal hypoglossal nerve from the multielectrode lead is continuous, obviating the need for respiration-sensing leads, whereas with the two other systems, the HGNS system and the Inspire II UAS device, the hypoglossal nerve stimulation will be intermittent and synchronized with the signal of the respiration-sensing leads that measure the respiratory cycle.[94,95,98] Among other differences, during the surgical technique for the Inspire II UAS system, the cuff section of the stimulation lead needs to be placed on the medial division of the distal hypoglossal nerve, thereby aiming at selective stimulation of the protrusor muscles of the tongue only.[90,92] Subsequently, appropriate placement of the stimulation lead needs to be confirmed by observing tongue protrusion during stimulation and by electromyographic monitoring during surgery.[90] The identification of patients with OSA who are more likely to benefit from upper airway neurostimulation therapy has been an important part of the research agenda.[98,99] Recent data suggest that responders to this therapy have a body mass index (BMI) of 32 kg/m² or less and AHI of 50 or below (i.e., fewer than 50 events per hour of sleep).[98] In addition, the absence of complete concentric collapse at the level of the palate as documented during DISE may predict therapeutic success with implanted upper airway neurostimulation therapy (Figure 21-8).[98,99] Therefore DISE can be recommended as a patient selection tool for use of implanted upper airway stimulation therapy for OSA.[99]

Although the early experience with stimulation is promising, the study results have been mixed. A prospective randomized trial of upper airway neurostimulation used the HGNS system, but the trial was discontinued in 2013 because the

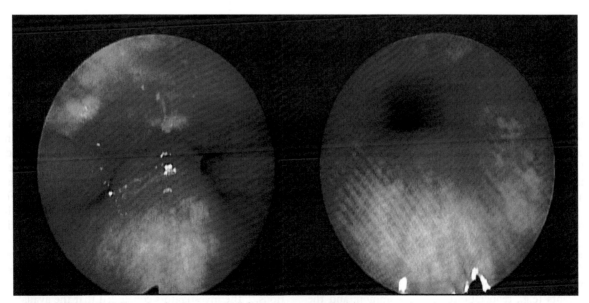

Figure 21-8 Example of anteroposterior (*left*) versus concentric (*right*) collapse at the palatal level during drug-induced sedation endoscopy (DISE). (From Vanderveken OM, Maurer JT, Hohenhorst W, et al. Evaluation of drug-induced sleep endoscopy as a patient selection tool for implanted upper airway stimulation for obstructive sleep apnea. *J Clin Sleep Med* 2013;9:433–8.)

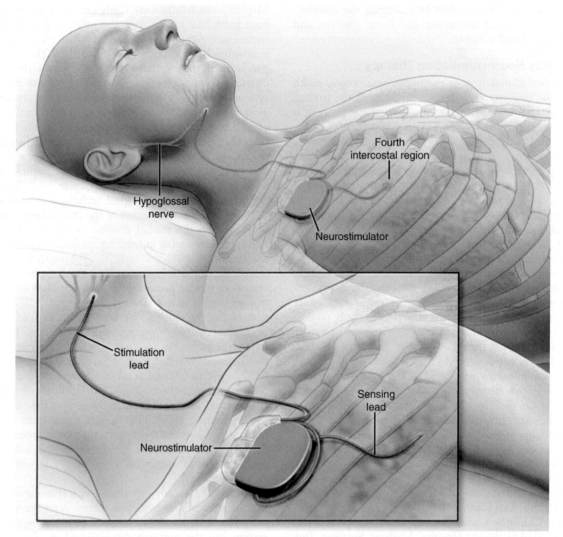

Figure 21-9 Upper airway stimulation using Inspire 2 implant (Inspire Medical Systems). The neurostimulator delivers electrical stimulating pulses to the protruding branches of the hypoglossal nerve through the stimulation lead; the stimulating pulses are synchronized with ventilation detected by the sensing lead. (From Strollo PJ Jr, Soose RJ, Maurer JT, et al. Upper-airway stimulation for obstructive sleep apnea. *N Engl J Med* 2014;370:139–49.)

interim analysis showed that it was unlikely to meet the primary efficacy end point. Apnex Medical, the producer of HGNS and the trial's sponsor, ceased its activity in 2013 because of the nonviable results of that trial (available at ClinicalTrials.gov—https://clinicaltrials.gov/ct2/show/NCT01446601).

More recently, a large multicenter, prospective case series assessed the safety and effectiveness of upper airway neurostimulation therapy using the Inspire II UAS device (Figure 21-9) in 126 well-selected patients with OSA.[90] The results of this pivotal study demonstrated that hypoglossal nerve stimulation led to significant improvements in polysomnographic parameters in 66% of patients, with associated improvements in sleepiness, snoring, and quality of life, in this sample.[90] Unfortunately, exploratory analysis did not yield predictors of failure in the 34% of nonresponders. Serious adverse events (e.g., reoperation) were uncommon, and the side effects, such as tongue irritation, were not bothersome or else resolved in most patients.[90] In a minority of patients, a tooth guard was needed to permit healing of tongue soreness

or abrasion related to the overnight tongue protrusion induced by the stimulation.[90] In addition, the results of a randomized, 1-week therapy-withdrawal trial among a subset of responders showed that continuation of stimulation was necessary to maintain the effect (i.e., withdrawal of stimulation led to worsening OSA almost to pretreatment levels).[90] A randomized withdrawal trial in responders, however, should not be confused with a prospective randomized trial like the HGNS trial. The promising results of this multicenter case series assessing the Inspire II UAS device led the U.S. Food and Drug Administration (FDA) to approve the Inspire UAS device for treatment of selected patients with moderate to severe OSA.

The results of a recent systematic review and metaanalysis of the literature indicate that hypoglossal nerve stimulation for OSA is reported to carry low risk of serious complications.[91] The investigators concluded that the available data in literature show high rates of therapy adherence and stable outcome results over 12 months of follow-up in selected patients with OSA.[91,96] Endoscopic findings in a subset of

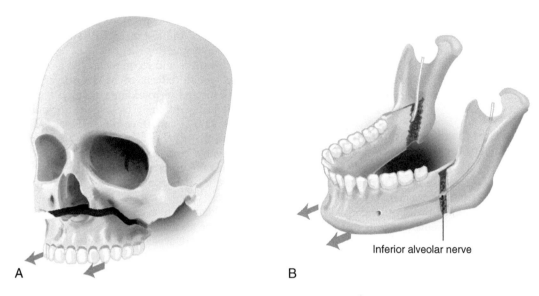

A   B

Figure 21-10 Maxillomandibular advancement (MMA) surgery for obstructive sleep apnea syndrome provides enlargement of the upper airway by means of a Le Fort I advancement osteotomy of the maxilla **(A)** and a bilateral sagittal split advancement osteotomy of the mandible **(B)**. (From Rosenberg AJ, Damen GW, Schreuder KE, Leverstein H. [Obstructive sleep-apnoea syndrome: good results with maxillo-mandibular osteotomy after failure of conservative therapy]. *Ned Tijdschr Geneeskd* 2005;149:1223–6.)

patients who underwent upper airway neurostimulation therapy using the Inspire II UAS device revealed that responders had greater retropalatal enlargement with stimulation than nonresponders, and that the neurostimulation increased both the retropalatal and retrolingual cross-sectional areas.[100] This observation of multilevel enlargement induced by upper airway neurostimulation therapy may explain the sustained reductions in OSA severity in two thirds of the selected patients receiving UAS therapy.[90,100] It is important to reiterate that patient selection appears to be critical, and even among carefully selected patients (e.g., BMI of less than 32 kg/m^2, no complete circumferential velopharyngeal collapse, and other criteria), the nonresponder rate is still significant, with no clear predictors.[96] Further research is ongoing and will be necessary to elucidate the optimal roles for this exciting therapy.

SKELETAL MODIFICATIONS

Orthognathic surgery for the treatment of OSA was first described when mandibular advancement surgery was reported to reverse the symptoms of sleep apnea.[101] In 1986, Riley and coworkers were the first to describe the combination of advancement of both maxilla and mandible to improve airway patency in patients with OSA.[102] Although trial-based evidence is still scarce, MMA currently is regarded as a highly effective and safe surgical modality for treatment of OSA.[93] MMA surgery in patients with OSA consists of a bilateral sagittal split osteotomy (BSSO) of the mandible with advancement and a Le Fort I osteotomy of the maxilla with advancement (Figure 21-10). In patients with OSA, MMA surgery generally requires a minimum advancement of the mandible by 10 mm to achieve optimal effectiveness.[103,104] As a consequence of the skeletal advancement, several upper airway muscles and ligaments are repositioned anteriorly,

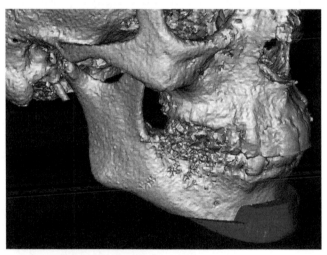

Inferior alveolar nerve

Figure 21-11 Modified genioplasty. In this procedure, the tongue is put under anterior traction by performing a trapezoid-shaped osteotomy with advancement of the chin (*purple*) and the genial tubercle–genioglossus muscle complex.

including the anterior belly of the digastric, mylohyoid, genioglossus, and geniohyoid muscles. The advancement of the maxilla pulls the soft tissue of the palate forward, tightens the palatoglossal and palatopharyngeal muscles, and increases tongue support. Moreover, adding the maxillary advancement also increases the amount of mandibular advancement that can be accomplished with surgery. To achieve additional improvements in oro- and hypopharyngeal airway patency, MMA surgery can be combined with a genioglossus advancement or a modified genioplasty[105,106] (Figure 21-11; see also Figure 21-6). To decrease the cervical fat mass, as appropriate, and to further improve airway patency, cervicomental liposuction may be added to the surgical plan in selected cases.[106]

MMA results in structural enlargement of the nasoorohypo-pharyngeal airway and enhanced tension and decreased collapsibility of the pharyngeal airway. When these surgical techniques are applied only for OSA and not for dentofacial abnormalities per se, the procedure is referred to as *telegnathic surgery* instead of *orthognathic surgery*. Post-surgery patients will usually require orthodonctic therapy to restore an acceptable bite.

General Outcomes of Maxillomandibular Advancement Surgery for Obstructive Sleep Apnea

OSA management after MMA surgery generally is successful in a high proportion of patients. A recent metaanalysis of data for 627 patients from 22 studies demonstrated that the median rate of surgical success, defined by a postoperative AHI less than 20 (i.e., fewer than 20 events per hour of sleep), with greater than 50% reduction overall, is 86%.[93] Surgical cure, defined more stringently by a postoperative AHI less than 5, was observed in 43% of patients in this metaanalysis. After a mean follow-up period of 5 months, a statistically and clinically significant reduction in the mean AHI, from 63.9 to 9.5, has been observed.[93] Although the number of studies evaluating long-term outcomes of MMA surgery is still limited, long-term results appear to be relatively stable over follow-up periods exceeding 2 to 5 years.[103,104,107-109] In addition, several studies found statistically and clinically significant improvements in blood pressure after MMA surgery in patients with OSA.[110,111] Finally, evidence for the medium- to long-term stability of the mandibular or maxillary advancement with MMA surgery in patients with OSA has been corroborated by several cephalometric studies.[104,112-114]

In evaluations of subjective outcomes after MMA surgery for OSA, most patients report improvements in snoring, wit-nessed apneas, excessive daytime sleepiness and quality of life, morning headaches, memory loss, and impaired concentration.[93,110,115,116] In most cases, CPAP can be discontinued after MMA surgery, with patients overall reporting that treatment was worthwhile and recommendable to others.[115]

The specific effects of MMA surgery on upper airway dimensions and surrounding structures have been extensively studied using different techniques, including cephalometry (Figure 21-12) and three-dimensional CT studies (Figures 21-13 to 21-15).[30a,116-118] On the other hand, up to this date, the available data are insufficient to support a relationship between OSA improvements such as reductions in AHI and changes in the upper airway and its surrounding bony structures.[117]

Simultaneous advancement of the maxilla and mandible changes the skeletal framework of the face, thereby resulting in a possible rejuvenation of the middle and lower third of the face. This concept of a "reverse face lift," with positive effects on facial aesthetics, after MMA surgery in patients with OSA is observed in a majority of cases (Figure 21-16). One study found that at 6 months after surgery, 50% of patients reported a younger and 36% reported a more attractive facial appearance.[105,107] Of note, however, 9% of patients in this study reported a less attractive facial appearance after surgery. Conversely, in another study, patients with OSA indicated that they were not bothered by their appearance after MMA surgery.[119] Although patients seeking treatment for OSA generally do not desire an aesthetic facial improvement, it is mandatory to communicate the anticipated facial changes before surgery. Indeed, although 50% of patients undergoing MMA are satisfied with the aesthetic result after the surgery, 30% are indifferent to their postoperative appearance, whereas up to 13% and 5% are disappointed and unsatisfied,

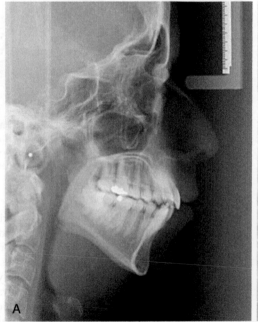 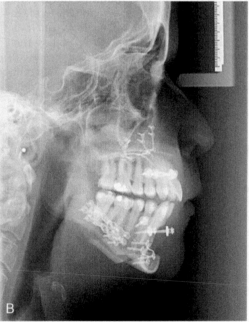

Figure 21-12 Two-dimensional airway changes after maxillomandibular advancement surgery. Preoperative **(A)** and postoperative **(B)** lateral cephalometric radiographs indicating the sagittal changes in upper airway space after maxillomandibular advancement surgery combined with a modified genioplasty and cervicomental liposuction in a patient with severe obstructive sleep apnea syndrome. (From Doff MH, Jansma J, Schepers RH, Hoekema A. Maxillomandibular advancement surgery as alternative to continuous positive airway pressure in morbidly severe obstructive sleep apnea: a case report. *Cranio* 2013;31:246–51.)

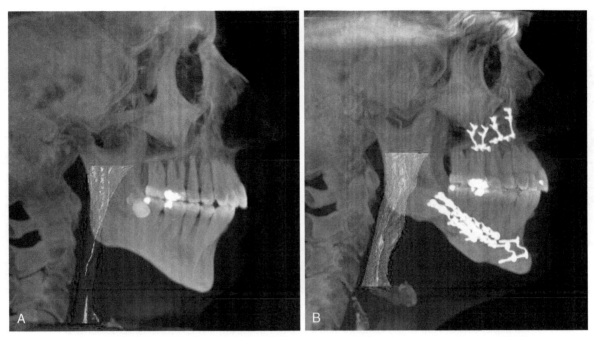

Figure 21-13 Three-dimensional airway changes after maxillomandibular advancement surgery. In *purple* the preoperative **(A)** and in *green* the postoperative **(B)** cone beam computed tomography (CBCT) three-dimensional reconstruction of the upper airway indicating changes in upper airway space after maxillomandibular advancement surgery combined with a modified genioplasty and cervicomental liposuction in a patient with severe obstructive sleep apnea syndrome.

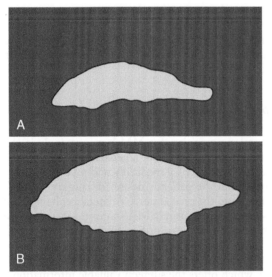

Figure 21-14 Velopharyngeal airway changes after maxillomandibular advancement surgery. Enlargement of the minimal cross-sectional area of the velopharyngeal airway before **(A)** and after **(B)** maxillomandibular advancement surgery combined with a modified genioplasty and cervicomental liposuction in a patient with severe obstructive sleep apnea syndrome. (From Doff MH, Jansma J, Schepers RH, Hoekema A. Maxillomandibular advancement surgery as alternative to continuous positive airway pressure in morbidly severe obstructive sleep apnea: a case report. *Cranio* 2013 31:246–51.)

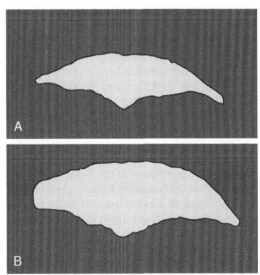

Figure 21-15 Oropharyngeal airway changes after maxillomandibular advancement surgery.Enlargement of the minimal cross-sectional area of the oropharyngeal airway before **(A)** and after **(B)** maxillomandibular advancement surgery combined with a modified genioplasty and cervicomental liposuction in a patient with severe obstructive sleep apnea syndrome. (From Doff MH, Jansma J, Schepers RH, Hoekema A. Maxillomandibular advancement surgery as alternative to continuous positive airway pressure in morbidly severe obstructive sleep apnea: a case report. *Cranio* 2013;31:246–51.)

respectively.[120] A surgical technique involving a so-called *counterclockwise rotation* of the occlusal plane, which previously has been used in correcting severe "bird-face" deformity, may be used both to achieve aesthetic goals and to fulfill the main objective in the treatment of patients with OSA—an optimal increase in airway patency.[121]

Major complications associated with MMA surgery in patients with OSA are rarely reported.[93] Individual and non-fatal cases of postoperative cardiac arrest or dysrhythmia have been reported.[122] One study described a case of a life-threatening airway obstruction after extubation that required reintubation.[123] However, no immediate postoperative deaths

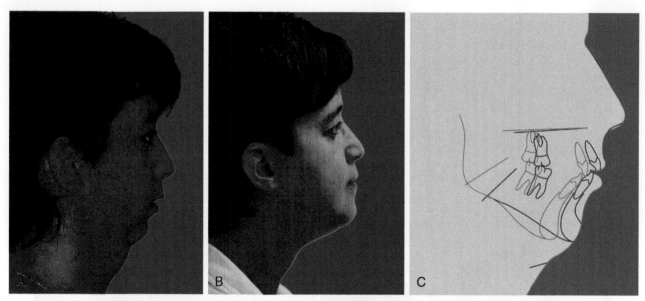

Figure 21-16 Effects on facial aesthetics of maxillomandibular advancement surgery. Preoperative **(A)** and post-operative **(B)** photographs illustrating the rejuvenation of the middle and lower thirds of the face after maxillo-mandibular advancement surgery combined with a modified genioplasty and cervicomental liposuction in a patient with severe obstructive sleep apnea syndrome. The effect on the patient's profile of profound advancement of the lower third of the face can be appreciated when the pre- and postsurgical cephalometric radiographs are superimposed **(C)**. (From Doff MH, Jansma J, Schepers RH, Hoekema A. Maxillomandibular advancement surgery as alternative to continuous positive airway pressure in morbidly severe obstructive sleep apnea: a case report. *Cranio* 2013;31:246–51.)

have been reported after this type of surgery in patients with OSA.[93] (See also Chapters 20 and 22.)

Minor complication rate has been reported to be approximately 3%.[93] Minor complications include hemorrhage or local infections that generally are cured with either antibiotics or surgical drainage. The presence of postoperative malocclusions or facial paresthesia is not included in this minor complication rate. Facial paresthesia is present in almost all patients after surgery, but resolution has been reported in approximately 85% of patients at the 1-year follow-up evaluation.[93] By contrast, some studies indicate that one half of the patients treated report a persistence of facial paresthesia.[120] Although malocclusions may be seen in up to 44% of patients, they generally can be resolved with (prosthetic) dental treatment or equilibration of the dental occlusion.[122] However, when patients are orthodontically prepared for MMA surgery, malocclusions generally pose no long-term problem with postoperative orthodontics. Some studies report a trend for poor bone healing and increased foreign body reactions after MMA surgery in patients with OSA.[124]

At 3.5 days, average hospital stay is slightly longer after MMA surgery in patients with OSA than in "conventional" orthognathic patients.[93] Most patients with OSA are able to return to full-time work within 2 to 10 weeks after their surgery.[110,125]

The most relevant patient characteristics and clinical factors predictive of a favorable outcome after MMA surgery in patients with OSA include younger age, lower preoperative BMI, and less severe OSA.[93] Moreover, an increased postoperative posterior airway space, determined from lateral cephalometric radiographs, appears to be the only relevant cephalometric variable of predictive value for a successful outcome of MMA surgery.[93] In addition, the amount of advancement of the maxilla appears to correlate with the degree of reduction in AHI.[93,116]

Preoperative Evaluation for Maxillomandibular Advancement

In general, prerequisites for MMA surgery include clinically "significant" OSA that is not amenable to conservative management (e.g., CPAP), a medically and psychologically stable condition, and the patient's desire for surgery and informed consent before the procedure.[126] A lateral cephalometric head film is mandatory to plan MMA surgery, as well as a preoperative polysomnographic recording. Surgery also may be planned using three-dimensional imaging techniques such as (cone beam) CT. Subsequently, virtual surgical planning can be conducted, which offers the surgeon valuable information on the anticipated skeletal, airway, and facial aesthetic changes (Figure 21-17).[127] Fiberoptic nasopharyngoscopy also is recommended before surgery. This imaging procedure can further help identify nasal, retropalatal, or tongue base pathology that may affect the outcome of MMA surgery (e.g., lingual tonsillar hypertrophy).

Finally, the response to an oral appliance also may be used to select suitable candidates for MMA surgery.[128] Patients demonstrating a substantial reduction in baseline AHI (i.e., to less than 50%) with oral appliance therapy appear to be especially good candidates for MMA surgery.[128] Despite the variety of treatment protocols, a precise treatment algorithm for choosing MMA surgery in OSA management has yet to be established, and the decision depends in large measure on patient's preference.

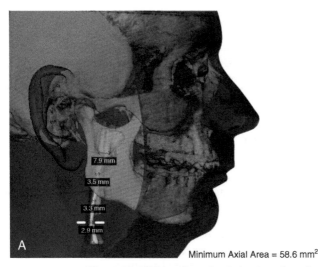
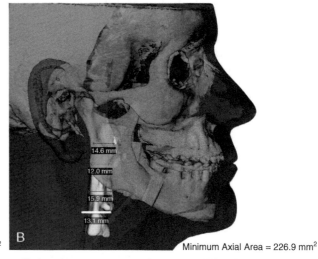

Figure 21-17 Three-dimensional planning of maxillomandibular advancement surgery. Preoperative **(A)** and postoperative **(B)** "morphs" illustrating the anticipated skeletal, airway and facial aesthetic changes after maxillomandibular advancement surgery with a genioplasty in a patient with sleep-disordered breathing. (Courtesy D. Brock; 3D Systems, Inc., Rock Hill, S.C.)

Postoperative Management after Maxillomandibular Advancement

Medical surgical management of the postsurgical patient with OSA is more complicated than with conventional orthognathic patients, despite the profound and immediate postsurgical improvement in pharyngeal airway patency. If recovery is sufficient, discharge is up to the surgeon and patient but requires proper pain control and capability of oral intake. Because younger patients tend to recover more quickly, discharge usually is earlier in this patient category.

Follow-up evaluation depends on the surgeon's individual protocol and the specific patient characteristics. Of note, postoperative edema usually is maximal 72 hours after surgery. Frequent postoperative follow-up visits are recommended until full recovery has been achieved. A polysomnographic follow-up study at 6 months or later after MMA is recommended.[129] As with all other surgical options for OSA treatment, it should be stressed to the patient that weight loss is an important part of the pre- and posttreatment OSA management, because even modest weight change will affect the outcome.

Upper Airway Bypass: Tracheostomy

Tracheostomy remains an important treatment option for OSA even though it is used by only a small minority of patients. The tracheostomy provides an alternative airway that bypasses the upper airway obstruction, and it is highly effective for controlling the OSA.[25] It becomes an important treatment option in patients with severe OSA and serious comorbid illnesses that render other surgical treatments too risky.

Tracheostomy has several important advantages. The surgery is relatively simple and short compared to what would otherwise typically be required to address severe OSA. The major treatment effect is immediate. Patients function normally with eating and speaking by capping the tracheostomy cannula during waking hours and then simply uncap the cannula for sleep. A tracheostomy is reversible in case it is

somehow intolerable to the patient, which is unlike almost every other surgical treatment of OSA. Patients typically become very skillful with management of the tracheostomy cannula. Specific disadvantages of a tracheostomy have been recognized. The cannula requires daily maintenance with cleaning and/or changes, although this process is simple. Some patients are self-conscious about the visible cannula. The stoma can accumulate granulation tissue or scar tissue that may require intermittent procedures to clear. Local infections can occur, requiring antibiotics or topical stoma treatment. Cannula dislodgement can be problematic in rare cases, and even life-threatening if the cannula dislodges from the the normal stoma position into the trachea. In addition, patients must avoid submerging the neck under water lest water aspiration occur, even if the cannula is capped.

Bariatric Surgery

Bariatric surgery is indicated in morbidly obese patients (BMI of 40 kg/m^2 or greater) with OSA in whom significant weight loss cannot be achieved through conservative measures such as hypocaloric diet and exercise training[46] (see also Chapter 22). In case of significant obesity-related comorbidity such as hypertension or diabetes, bariatric surgery should be considered starting from BMI of 35 kg/m^2 or greater. It has been clearly demonstrated that the surgical weight loss induced by bariatric surgery can result in significant decrease in OSA severity.[130,131] However, OSA of considerable degree can persist in some patients even after substantial weight loss.[130,132,133] Therefore a follow-up sleep study is recommended after bariatric surgery to check for residual OSA, especially in patients with low minimum SaO$_2$ levels and high supine AHI preoperatively.[130,131] If necessary, retitration of CPAP settings may be scheduled, which may lead to higher treatment compliance afterward.[131] CPAP optimization and vigilance may be necessary to treat residual OSA when present and to help maintain weight loss, because there are limited data to suggest an association between postoperative CPAP use and weight loss outcomes.[133]

Combination Therapy Including Multilevel Surgery

To reach the therapeutic target, preferably an alleviation of the disease, it may be necessary to prescribe two or more therapies, with adjunctive modalities used as needed to supplement the primary treatment options.[14] In the management of OSA, however, combining treatment options has been somewhat undervalued. A combination approach is especially appropriate in this setting because as described earlier in the chapter and elsewhere in this book, no single therapy (surgical or nonsurgical) is universally effective. Many of the surgical treatments are site-specific, so combinations of procedures may be necessary to address all sites of obstruction.

Concerning the nonsurgical treatment options for OSA, several possible combinations have been reported, such as combining oral appliance therapy with sleep positioning therapy (SPT) or the combination of CPAP with oral appliance therapy (see Chapters 17, 18, and 19).[134-136] In addition, positional therapy may also be an adjunctive treatment in patients on CPAP who require high pressure levels in the supine position to improve adherence to the CPAP regimen.[46] The addition of oral appliance therapy has been shown to be an effective mode of combination therapy to control OSA after UPPP failure.[137] The combination of positional therapy and surgical upper airway modifications can result in a significant decrease in OSA severity in patients in whom surgery converted non-positional OSA into positional OSA.[138,139] Similarly, the combination of two or more surgical techniques, performed either simultaneously or staged, or so-called *multilevel surgery*, can be regarded as combination therapy for OSA. For example, combining UPPP (or anatomically directed variants) with hypopharyngeal procedures results in a significant decrease in OSA severity, a significant improvement in daytime sleepiness, and a high degree of patient satisfaction, with an acceptable complication rate.[140,141,142,143] With currently available upper airway surgery protocols to address all relevant areas of obstruction can achieve clinical outcomes (e.g., reduction in symptoms and improvement in quality of life) comparable to CPAP therapy.[144]

CLINICAL PEARLS

- CPAP remains the standard modality to treat OSA. The clinical effectiveness of CPAP treatment, however, often is limited by poor patient (and partner) acceptance, leading to suboptimal adherence. Consequently, an urgent need for non-CPAP treatment options is well recognized.
- To move away from a "trial and error" empirical clinical paradigm, there has been increasing interest in drug-induced sedation endoscopy (DISE), as part of the therapeutic decision-making process regarding upper airway surgery.
- Many surgical options are available, and each has its indications. Nasal airway surgery complements most other surgical and nonsurgical treatments when the nose is obstructed. Site-directed upper airway procedures can be very effective, when combined appropriately, for addressing many combinations of obstruction. Upper airway neurostimulation appears promising for selected patients with multilevel soft tissue collapse and possibly in patients with particularly collapsible tissue (as opposed to structural abnormalities). MMA is an especially useful option in patients with malocclusion, which can be addressed simultaneously, or with facial skeletal compromise. Tracheostomy is an important option for patients with severe comorbid illnesses who cannot tolerate CPAP or more extensive surgery. Bariatric surgery can allow weight loss for significant clinical improvement in patients presenting with severe obesity associated with OSA or other obesity-related comorbidity.

SUMMARY

OSA has major socioeconomic consequences and should be approached as a chronic disease requiring long-term, multidisciplinary management. Although CPAP is overall the most successful treatment for moderate to severe OSA when used properly and consistently, its clinical effectiveness often is limited by poor patient and partner acceptance, which leads to suboptimal adherence. Because many patients with OSA remain inadequately treated owing to inconsistent levels of adherence to CPAP, and because mild OSA deserves treatment in those with problematic symptoms, there is a genuine need for non-CPAP treatment options (Table 21-1). Additionally, it may be necessary to combine two or more of the available treatment options to achieve a successful outcome targeting disease alleviation.

The spectrum of OSA is quite diverse in terms of nature and severity, so the selection of the right treatment regimen for each individual patient will be of utmost importance. Among the different techniques that can be used for the preoperative upper airway assessment, DISE is increasingly performed for dynamic upper airway evaluation to select the proper non-CPAP treatment for patients with OSA.

Surgical treatment of upper airway abnormalities, craniofacial deformations, or obesity may be applied in selected patients with OSA. In general, sleep surgery procedures are directed at specific collapsible upper airway structures, so preoperative upper airway investigation may add to proper selection of a specific surgical procedure for an individual patient. Taking into account that in a majority of patients with OSA, a multilevel collapse is observed within the upper airway, the treatment plan should aim at resolution of the anatomic compromise at all levels involved in the obstructions occurring during sleep.

The results of upper airway neurostimulation therapy in carefully selected patients with OSA are promising. Its safety, combined with associated high rates of therapy adherence and sustained reductions in OSA severity, should sustain further effectiveness research in this particular area.

MMA surgery plays an important role in the correction of OSA that is refractory to noninvasive therapies. MMA surgery in patients with OSA generally is more complex than "conventional" orthognathic surgery because OSA patients require large advancements, are usually older, and often have other comorbidities. With proper precautions, however, it is a safe and highly effective treatment modality for OSA. MMA surgery probably is the most effective surgical intervention besides tracheostomy in patients who are skeletally compromised (e.g., retrognathia or bimaxillary retrusion). These patients should therefore be informed about MMA surgery as one of the primary treatment modalities.

Tracheostomy remains an important treatment option for patients with severe OSA and serious comorbid conditions that might limit the other surgical treatment options. Bariatric surgery is a valuable treatment option to treat obesity-related OSA and other obesity-related diseases and conditions in patients who are unable to lose sufficient weight by conservative measures.

Finally, combining different treatment options for the alleviation of OSA is undervalued and underinvestigated. Further research on the possible combinations is strongly needed, because no single treatment can adequately manage all patients with OSA.

Selected Readings

De Vito A, Carrasco Llatas M, Vanni A, et al. European position paper on drug-induced sedation endoscopy (DISE). *Sleep Breath* 2014;**18**:453–65.

Deacon NL, Jen R, Li Y, Malhotra A. Treatment of Obstructive Sleep Apnea. Prospects for Personalized Combined Modality Therapy. *Ann Am Thorac Soc.* 2016;**13**(1):101–8.

Denolf PL, Vanderveken OM, Marklund ME, Braem MJ. The status of cephalometry in the prediction of non-CPAP treatment outcome in obstructive sleep apnea patients. *Sleep Med Rev* 2015;**27**:56–73.

Epstein LJ, Kristo D, Strollo PJ Jr, et al. Clinical guideline for the evaluation, management and long-term care of obstructive sleep apnea in adults. *J Clin Sleep Med* 2009;**5**:263–76.

Murphey AW, Baker AB, Soose RJ, et al. Upper airway stimulation for obstructive sleep apnea: The surgical learning curve. *Laryngoscope* 2016;**126**(2):501–6.

Murphey AW, Kandl JA, Nguyen SA, et al. The effect of glossectomy for obstructive sleep apnea: A systematic review and meta-analysis. *Head Neck* 2015;**153**:334–42.

Murphey AW, Kandl JA, Nguyen SA, et al. The effect of glossectomy for obstructive sleep apnea: a systematic review and meta-analysis. *Otolaryngol Head Neck Surg* 2015;**153**:334–42.

Senchak AJ, McKinlay AJ, Acevedo J, et al. The effect of tonsillectomy alone in adult obstructive sleep apnea. *Otolaryngol Head Neck Surg* 2015;**152**:969.

Strollo PJ Jr, Soose RJ, Maurer JT, et al. Upper-airway stimulation for obstructive sleep apnea. *N Engl J Med* 2014;**370**:139–49.

Thaler ER, Rassekh CH, Lee JM, et al. Outcomes for multilevel surgery for sleep apnea: Obstructive sleep apnea, transoral robotic surgery, and uvulopalatopharyngoplasty. *Laryngoscope* 2016;**126**(1):266–9.

Vanderveken OM. Combination therapy for obstructive sleep apnea in order to achieve complete disease alleviation: from taboo to new standard of care? *J Dental Sleep Med* 2015;**2**:7–8.

Weaver EM, Woodson BT, Yueh B, et al. Studying Life Effects & Effectiveness of Palatopharyngoplasty (SLEEP) study: subjective outcomes of isolated uvulopalatopharyngoplasty. *Otolaryngol Head Neck Surg* 2011;**144**:623–31.

Woodson BT, Soose RJ, Gillespie MB, et al. Three-Year Outcomes of Cranial Nerve Stimulation for Obstructive Sleep Apnea: The STAR Trial. *Otolaryngol Head Neck Surg* 2016;**154**(1):181–8.

Zaghi S, Holty JE, Certal V, et al. Maxillomandibular Advancement for Treatment of Obstructive Sleep Apnea: A Meta-analysis. *JAMA Otolaryngol Head Neck Surg* 2016;**142**(1):58–66.

A complete reference list can be found online at ExpertConsult.com.

Obstructive Sleep Apnea, Obesity, and Bariatric Surgery

Eric J. Olson; Anita P. Courcoulas

Chapter Highlights

- Excessive body weight is a growing global health issue. In the United States, two of every three adults weigh more than their ideal body weight. Obesity (defined as a body mass index of 30 kg/m² or greater) predicts increased morbidity and mortality. One of the health conditions that obesity has a significant impact on is obstructive sleep apnea.

- Inconsistent results from dietary, behavioral, and pharmacologic weight loss therapies have led to increasing interest in bariatric surgery, which encompasses a variety of abdominal operations that restrict caloric intake, absorption, or both. The global total number of bariatric procedures performed annually is estimated at more than 300,000.

- Familiarity with the principles and applications of bariatric surgery is emerging as an appropriate requirement for sleep medicine practitioners, in view of the frequency with which coexistent obesity and sleep-related breathing disorders, obstructive sleep apnea and obesity-hypoventilation syndrome, are encountered in clinical practice. The sleep specialist has an important role in a comprehensive perioperative bariatric care program.

DEFINITIONS AND OVERVIEW

The increasing proportion of people who weigh more than their ideal body weight is a worldwide health concern, with significant medical, psychological, and economic ramifications. In adults, overweight and obesity traditionally have been defined by the *body mass index* (BMI), which is the quotient of the weight in kilograms divided by the height in meters squared. Table 22-1 depicts the National Heart, Lung, and Blood Institute's weight classification system for adults, in which *overweight* is defined as a BMI of 25 to 29.9 kg/m² and *obese* is defined as a BMI of 30 kg/m² or more.[1] Excess abdominal fat, defined by a waist circumference of greater than 40 inches (102 cm) in men and greater than 35 inches (88 cm) in women, is an independent predictor of risk for type 2 diabetes mellitus, dyslipidemia, hypertension, and cardiovascular disease in adults with a BMI between 25 and 34.9 kg/m².[1] Overweight and obesity are a result of a complex interplay of genetic and sociocultural forces that lead to long-term positive energy balance.[2] Obesity is associated with myriad complications, including obstructive sleep apnea (OSA).

Obesity is one of the most important risk factors for OSA.[3] Excessive body weight may increase propensity for upper airway narrowing during sleep by altering the function and the geometry of the pharynx.[3] In addition, obesity may alter ventilatory control and respiratory muscle function, leading to obesity hypoventilation syndrome (OHS), which is characterized by the combination of obesity, chronic hypercapnia in the absence of another identifiable cause, and usually some component of sleep-related breathing disorder, most commonly OSA (see Chapter 30).[4] Treatment for OSA includes continuous positive airway pressure (CPAP), oral appliances, upper airway surgeries, and risk factor modifications, including weight loss.

For patients desiring to lose weight, initial interventions include dietary modifications to reduce energy intake, enhanced physical activity to increase energy expenditure, and behavioral therapies to overcome barriers to compliance.[1] Pharmacotherapy may be considered for patients with a BMI of 30 kg/m² or more, or for those with a BMI of 27 kg/m² or more and obesity-related disease who fail to achieve their weight loss targets after 6 months of diet and lifestyle changes.[1]

Surgical therapy for obesity, or *bariatric surgery*, is indicated for morbidly obese persons for whom other attempts at nonsurgical approaches to weight control have failed. Some bariatric surgery procedures restrict food intake, and others induce malabsorption or maldigestion.[5] The number of bariatric procedures being performed has increased dramatically as a result of the rise in prevalence of severe obesity and refinement of operative techniques.

This chapter considers the epidemiology of overweight and obesity, potential mechanisms linking overweight and obesity with OSA, indications for bariatric surgery, technical aspects of common bariatric procedures, perioperative management of patients with OSA, and outcomes of bariatric surgery, including its impact on OSA.

EPIDEMIOLOGY

Epidemiology of Overweight and Obesity

According to the latest National Health and Nutrition Examination Survey (NHANES), for the year 2011 to 2012, 68.5% of U.S. adults were either overweight or obese, 34.9% were obese, and 6.4% had class 3 obesity, which translates to a total of approximately 15 million adults with a BMI of 40 kg/m² or greater.[6] Among U.S. youth, 31.8% were either overweight or obese and 16.9% were obese.[6] Between 1980 and 2007, the prevalence of obesity doubled, and the prevalence of class 3

Table 22-1	Classification of Overweight and Obesity by Body Mass Index
Category	**Body Mass Index (kg/m²)**
Underweight	<18.5
Normal	18.5–24.9
Overweight	25–29.9
Obesity	
Class 1	30–34.9
Class 2	35–39.9
Class 3 (extreme)	≥40

From North American Association for the Study of Obesity and the National Heart, Lung, and Blood Institute. *The practical guide: identification, evaluation, and treatment of overweight and obesity in adults.* NIH publication 00-4084. Bethesda (Md.): National Institutes of Health; 2000. <http://www.cdc.gov/nccdphp/dnpa/obesity/defining.htm>.

obesity nearly quadrupled.[7] Figure 22-1 shows the prevalence of adult obesity in 2014 per state and territory in the United States.[8] Obesity prevalence also has roughly doubled among Canadian adults, although the overall prevalence of adult obesity in Canada (approximately 25%) remains lower than in the United States.[9] Obesity rates in the United States are highest among non-Hispanic black adults (47.8%), followed by Hispanic Americans (42.5%) and then non-Hispanic whites (32.6%) and Asian Americans (10.8%).[6] Obesity prevalence in Native Americans is similar to that in non-Hispanic blacks.[10] Data from the Framingham Heart Study attribute a reduction in life expectancy of 7.1 years in nonsmoking women and 5.9 years in nonsmoking men at age 40 to obesity,[11] with the increased mortality resulting primarily from cardiovascular disease.[12]

Epidemiologic Association between Overweight/Obesity and Obstructive Sleep Apnea

Cross-sectional analyses of clinical and population samples have demonstrated notable colocalization of OSA and

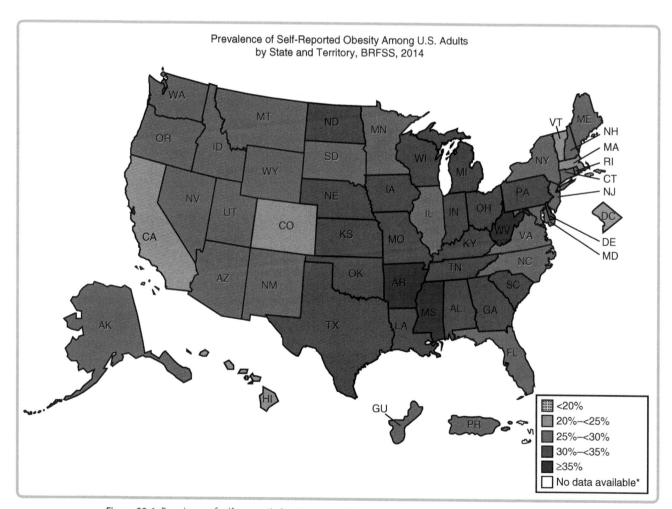

Figure 22-1 Prevalence of self-reported obesity among adults in the United States by state and territory per the Behavioral Risk Factor Surveillance System (BRFSS), 2014. No state has an obesity prevalence of less than 20%. Eighteen states have an obesity prevalence between 30% and less than 35%, and 2 states have an obesity prevalence of 35% or greater. The South has the highest prevalence of obesity, followed by the Midwest, the Northeast, and the West. (From Centers for Disease Control and Prevention. Obesity prevalence maps, 2016. <http://www.cdc.gov/obesity/data/prevalence-maps.html.> Accessed February 1, 2016.)

obesity.[3] OSA has been found in 50% to 80% of obese patients seen in clinical settings,[3] and from 60% to 90% of adults with OSA may be overweight.[13] In the Wisconsin Sleep Cohort, an increase of 1 standard deviation (5.7 kg/m^2) was associated with a fourfold risk of an apnea-hypopnea index (AHI) of 5 events/hour or greater.[14] Furthermore, the Sleep Heart Health Study reported a dose-dependent relationship between increasing BMI and OSA: The prevalence of an AHI of 15 or higher was 10% in the lowest BMI quartile (16 to 24 kg/m^2), as opposed to 32% in the highest quartile (32 to 59 kg/m^2).[15]

Longitudinal population and clinical samples also indicate that weight and AHI change congruently. In the Wisconsin Sleep Cohort, each 1% increase (or decrease) in weight was associated with a 3% increase (or decrease) in AHI, and in patients with mild OSA (AHI of 5 to 15) at baseline, a 10% weight gain led to a sixfold risk for developing moderate to severe OSA (AHI of 15 or higher).[16] In the Sleep Heart Health Study, parallel changes in weight and AHI were similarly found over a 5-year follow-up period, but AHI increased more with weight gain than it decreased with weight loss.[17] Men tend to suffer a greater increase in AHI with weight gain than women,[17] whereas BMI has a greater effect on AHI in postmenopausal women than in premenopausal women.[3] Increasing age may attenuate the association of BMI and AHI.[15]

PATHOGENESIS

Mechanism Linking Obesity to Obstructive Sleep Apnea Risk

Upper airway anatomic and neuromuscular factors may be influenced by parapharyngeal fat accumulation in several ways.[18] In obesity, upper airway size may be compressed by the deposition of adipose tissue, especially in the lateral pharyngeal fat pads, intraluminal structures (tongue, soft palate, uvula), and neck.[19-23] During wakefulness, increased pharyngeal dilator muscle activity provides compensation; the state-dependent attenuation of pharyngeal muscle activity with sleep, by contrast, leaves the upper airway vulnerable to collapse.[24] Accrual of fat around the upper airway may alter soft tissue properties, thereby heightening the propensity to collapse by increasing upper airway compliance,[25,26] or may change upper airway geometry,[3] with a consequent decrease in the ability of pharyngeal muscles to dilate the airway.[27]

Obesity, a chronic inflammatory state itself, may contribute to increasing upper airway tissue inflammation,[28] or upper airway neuropathic damage through the pathophysiologic changes of diabetes mellitus.[29] Abdominal viscera fat accumulation in patients with OSA also is of likely pathogenetic importance, as highlighted by population surveys reporting a twofold to threefold increase in prevalence of symptomatic OSA in men compared with women,[14,30] with a central distribution of fat involving the neck, trunk, and abdominal viscera typical in men, versus fat deposition in the lower body and extremities characteristically seen in women. The interaction of hormonal changes and accompanying increases in central fat deposition may contribute to the increased prevalence of OSA in postmenopausal women.[3] Central obesity–induced reduction in lung volume[31] decreases "tracheal tug," a caudally directed, pharyngeal-stabilizing, lung volume–dependent traction force directed along the trachea.[32] The reduction in lung volumes coupled with globally increased

oxygen demand also may promote the oxygen desaturation that accompanies obstructive apneas and hypopneas.

An evolving discussion in sleep medicine concerns the existence of a bidirectional relationship between obesity and OSA. The intermittent hypoxia, sympathetic activation, and sleep fragmentation caused by repeated episodes of obstructive apnea and hypopnea produce metabolic alterations that provide biologically plausible means by which OSA also may exacerbate overweight and obesity (see Chapter 24). The pathogenetic interactions between obesity and OSA, however, are complex and not fully explored, leaving the subject open for active research.[13]

BARIATRIC SURGERY FOR MEDICALLY COMPLICATED OBESITY

Bariatric surgery has emerged in the context of the rising prevalence of severe obesity, heightened concern about associated comorbid medical conditions, and the limited success of traditional weight loss approaches of diet, exercise, and behavior modification. Although the number of bariatric procedures performed had been increasing for many years, only 1% of clinically eligible patients are being treated for medically complicated obesity in this manner.[33] Lack of access to bariatric surgery probably results from many as-yet poorly studied factors, including lack of insurance coverage, poor understanding of the procedures and their effects, and prohibitive costs—facility costs alone for bariatric surgery, for example, range from $10,000 to $15,000 per case.[34]

Patient Selection

Guidelines originally issued by the National Institutes of Health[35] and recently reaffirmed by the American Association of Clinical Endocrinologists, The Obesity Society, and the American Society for Metabolic and Bariatric Surgery (AACE-TOS-ASMBS)[36] state that bariatric surgery is a treatment option for severely obese patients who failed to achieve weight loss on a structured and monitored exercise and diet program and who have a BMI of 40 kg/m^2 or greater, or a BMI of 35 kg/m^2 or greater in conjunction with one or more obesity-related severe comorbid conditions.[1] Such obesity-associated comorbid conditions include diabetes mellitus, arterial hypertension, dyslipidemia, coronary artery disease, pseudotumor cerebri, asthma, venous stasis, severe urinary incontinence, debilitating arthritis, gastroesophageal reflux disease, nonalcoholic fatty liver disease, and OSA.[36] The most recent AACE-TOS-ASMBS clinical practice guidelines also state that bariatric surgery may be offered to patients with a lower BMI of 30 to 34.9 kg/m^2 along with diabetes mellitus or metabolic syndrome, with the acknowledgment that current evidence to support this expansion of potential bariatric surgery candidates is based on limited and short-term data demonstrating benefit and is not universally accepted.[36]

Patients preparing to undergo bariatric surgery must complete nutritional and psychological evaluation screening to rule out untreated depression, substance abuse, or a history of untreated eating disorders. The potential bariatric surgery recipient must demonstrate a complete understanding of the risks and benefits of the operation as a weight loss "tool," recognize the necessity after surgery to limit portion size and food types, and agree to follow a postoperative vitamin supplementation regimen. Patients should be deemed ineligible

Table 22-2	Patient Selection Criteria for Bariatric Surgery
Factor	**Criteria**
Weight (adults)	BMI of 40 kg/m² or greater, with no comorbid conditions BMI of 35 kg/m² or greater with obesity-associated comorbidity
Weight loss history	Failure of previous nonsurgical attempts at weight reduction, including nonprofessional programs (e.g., Weight Watchers)
Commitment	Expectation that patient will adhere to postoperative care Follow-up visits with physician(s) and team members Recommended medical management, including use of dietary supplements Instructions regarding any recommended procedures or tests
Exclusion	Reversible endocrine or other disorders that can cause obesity Current drug or alcohol use Uncontrolled, severe psychiatric illness Lack of comprehension of risks, benefits, expected outcomes, alternatives, and lifestyle changes required with bariatric surgery

From Mechanick JI, Youdim A, Jones DB, et al. Clinical practice guidelines for the perioperative nutritional, metabolic, and nonsurgical support of the bariatric surgery patient—2013 update: cosponsored by American Association of Clinical Endocrinologists, The Obesity Society, and American Society for Metabolic and Bariatric Surgery. *Obesity* 2013;21:S1–27.

for surgery if they cannot understand or will not commit to the dietary changes and lifestyle modifications necessary to complement the procedure. In addition, poor surgical or anesthetic risk status (as with advanced congestive heart failure or suboptimally controlled angina), older age (greater than 50 years), reversible endocrine or other disorders that might cause obesity, and active addiction behaviors are contraindications to bariatric surgery. Selection criteria for bariatric surgery are summarized in Table 22-2.[36]

Rationale for Patient Assessment for Obstructive Sleep Apnea before Bariatric Surgery

High OSA prevalence has been reported among patients being considered for bariatric surgery. In a large series of consecutive patients undergoing bariatric surgery ($n = 342$) in whom preoperative polysomnography was performed regardless of suspicion for OSA, the prevalence of OSA (defined as an AHI of 5 or higher) was 77%; 19% had moderate (AHI of 15 to 30) and 27% had severe OSA (AHI higher than 30).[37] In bariatric surgery candidates, many potential reasons to consider the possibility of OSA preoperatively have been documented: Concurrent OSA may complicate the intubation and/or increase the difficulty of mask ventilation in obese patients. Commonly used perioperative drugs have inhibitory influences on central ventilatory drive, protective upper airway reflexes, and arousal mechanisms, which may further jeopardize the airway of the severely obese patient with known

OSA. Upper airway edema associated with endotracheal intubation and forced supine positioning also can acutely aggravate OSA risk after bariatric surgery. Spells of desaturation associated with postoperative obstructive apneic episodes or hypoventilation may be exaggerated by the interaction of obesity-related reduction in pulmonary functional residual capacity with factors in the postoperative milieu. OSA may increase risk for and/or destabilize comorbid conditions in the obese patient, such as hypertension, atrial fibrillation, heart failure, and diabetes mellitus, and these conditions may require attention preoperatively or adversely affect the postoperative course. Therefore close collaboration among the sleep specialist, the anesthesiologist, the bariatric surgeon, and the patient is crucial for proper planning to mitigate OSA-related complications perioperatively.

Preoperative Assessment for Bariatric Surgery in the Patient without Known Obstructive Sleep Apnea

The AACE-TOS-ASMBS clinical practice guidelines[36] stipulate that the possibility of OSA should be considered in *all* bariatric surgery candidates. However, uncertainties exist regarding the specifics of the extent of the preoperative OSA evaluation.

Discernment of OSA status begins with a sleep-focused history and physical exam by the bariatric surgery team. The diagnostic features of OSA are discussed in Chapters 11 and 16. No cardinal symptom of OSA, such as snoring or excessive daytime sleepiness, is singularly sufficient to predict the presence of OSA or its severity in bariatric surgery candidates. Furthermore, no a single best metric of body habitus for predicting OSA has been identified.[3] Instead, a combination of symptoms and signs is more discriminatory, so many prediction formulas combining clinical parameters have been created to hone clinicians' detection of OSA. An example of a screening tool for OSA extensively studied in preoperative patients is the STOP-Bang instrument.[38] This questionnaire poses "yes-or-no" questions about **s**noring, **t**iredness, **o**bserved apneas, blood **p**ressure, **B**MI higher than 35 kg/m², **a**ge older than 50 years, **n**eck circumference greater than 40 cm, and male **g**ender, with likelihood of the presence of OSA increasing as the number of affirmative responses increases. Sensitivity (proportion of patients with OSA correctly identified by the STOP-Bang to have OSA) and specificity (proportion of patients without OSA correctly identified by the STOP-Bang to not have OSA) for moderate to severe OSA defined by AHI higher than 15 in patients with BMI of 35 kg/m² or greater preparing for nonbariatric operations depends on the cutpoints selected: score of 3 or higher: 97% (sensitivity) and 7% (specificity); score of 4 or higher: 86% and 28%; 5 or higher: 65% and 65%; and 6 or higher: 42% and 86%.[39] These figures highlight the tradeoff inherent in creating and implementing OSA prediction tools: As the threshold for the number of required OSA features is increased, those incorrectly labeled as having OSA (false positives) decreases, but detection of patients with OSA (true positives) also decreases. In general, most OSA prediction tools are more sensitive than specific, favoring detection of true positives (presence of OSA in patients identified as having the disorder) and thereby minimizing false negatives, at the expense of false positives (designating many patients as having OSA when in fact they do not). Severe OSA is unlikely to missed by OSA prediction tools, but reported sensitivities and specificities for a given screening tool have varied in the hands of different investigators, and the ideal preoperative OSA screening instrument has not been identified.[40]

Guidelines emerging from the anesthesiology literature[41-43] recommend incorporating an OSA prediction tool or checklist in the preoperative assessment of patients preparing for any surgery. The STOP-Bang is highlighted in several of these strategies[41,42]; the American Society of Anesthesiologists guideline for the perioperative management of patients with known or suspected OSA contains its own OSA prediction checklist.[43] Those patients judged to be at low risk for having OSA as determined by the screening instrument are cleared to proceed directly to surgery without further sleep testing, whereas those deemed to be at intermediate or high risk should proceed either to a formal sleep assessment or to surgery, with adjustment of their perioperative care for presumptive OSA, depending on the clinical status and the urgency of the surgical issue.

Attempts to create new OSA screening tools[37,44] or to validate existing[45,46] tools in bariatric surgery populations have not yielded powerfully discriminative sensitivity and specificity characteristics for the instruments tested. In the study by Gasa and colleagues,[44] the addition of sleep oximetry data did significantly enhance the sensitivity and specificity of their initial model based on anthropometric and clinical factors alone (age, waist circumference, systolic blood pressure, and witnessed apneas). The latest AACE-TOS-ASMBS bariatric surgery clinical practice guidelines[36] recommend "standardized screening" for OSA, with "confirmatory polysomnography to follow if screening tests are positive," but do not elaborate on the phrase, "screening tests." The guidelines label predictive modeling attempts "encouraging" but not definitive.[36] The current understanding of the role for OSA screening tools in the bariatric population will continue to evolve. At present, incorporation of an OSA screening tool into the preoperative evaluation of all bariatric surgery candidates by the surgical team should be considered as an initial minimum means to consistently ensure that OSA is deliberately contemplated in an organized manner and to enhance detection of the most severe OSA cases. Because the "best" OSA screening tool is not known, the decision about which tool to use must be made locally by the bariatric surgery team, ideally with guidance from their sleep medicine colleagues. The designation of OSA status by the screening tool output must be integrated with other pertinent information, such as collateral observations about the patient's breathing during sleep from the bed partner, history of airway difficulties with previous anesthetics, anticipated surgical approach (open versus laparoscopic), and comorbidity burden.

Laboratory-based, technologist-attended polysomnography remains the diagnostic "gold standard" modality for diagnosis of OSA.[47] A routine role for preoperative sleep testing (polysomnography or home sleep apnea testing) continues to be debated. Proponents for such a practice cite the high prevalence of OSA among severely obese patients, the potential for perioperative complications from unrecognized OSA, and the limited accuracy of clinical impression alone in OSA diagnosis. Opponents point to the lack of data demonstrating improved postoperative outcomes with preoperative initiation of CPAP in patients undergoing bariatric surgery, the uncertainty regarding the relative contribution of OSA to postoperative complications in this population, and potential clinical

overuse of such testings in patients deemed to be at low risk by clinical impression or OSA screening tool. The AACE-TOS-ASMBS bariatric surgery clinical practice guidelines[36] are vague: "routine preoperative screening with polysomnography should be considered." Performing sleep studies in all bariatric surgery candidates without exception, however, seems overly rigid. The reality is that if an OSA screening tool is systematically implemented, most patients will face the prospect of sleep testing before bariatric surgery because they will be judged to be at high risk by the OSA screening tool. For instance, in the study examining the performance of STOP-Bang in obese patients,[39] just 5% of preoperative patients with a BMI of 35 kg/m^2 or higher scored less than 2. Additionally, sleep testing may be needed to establish OSA as a weight-related comorbid condition in building justification for bariatric surgery, or if therapy for OSA is desired regardless of whether bariatric surgery is ultimately performed. In those patients without collateral sleep history or who are suspected of downplaying OSA symptoms, overnight oximetry monitoring may be an intermediate step between OSA screening by history and physical examination and a formal sleep study—that is, polysomnography. In bariatric surgery programs in which preoperative polysomnography or home sleep apnea testing is not routinely performed in every patient, preoperative consultation with a sleep specialist about the need for further sleep testing often is appropriate and is specifically recommended in situations of ambiguity about OSA status or its perioperative importance. Private insurers are increasingly mandating home sleep apnea testing in cases of suspected OSA, and the adult bariatric surgery candidate with a high pretest probability of having moderate to severe OSA and without significant comorbid cardiopulmonary disease may be an appropriate candidate for home sleep apnea testing followed by initiation of autoadjusting CPAP.[48] However, laboratory-based polysomnography is indicated and typically is covered by insurance carriers for the very obese suspects with OSA (BMI greater than 45 to 50 kg/m^2) or those with suspected OHS, because of the possible need for attended titration of modalities other than CPAP, such as bilevel (i.e., biphasic) positive airway pressure (BiPAP) and supplemental oxygen.

A high index of clinical suspicion should be maintained for the presence of OHS, because affected patients require more careful presurgical consideration. For several reasons, patients with OHS would be expected to be at higher risk than eucapnic obese patients with OSA during bariatric surgery. The diminished ventilatory responsiveness to hypoxia and hypercapnia in this patient group leads to increased sensitivity to sedatives and opioids, potentially greater problems with weaning from mechanical ventilation, and development of life-threatening obstructive apnea events, as well as acute worsening of hypercapnia with supplemental oxygen therapy unaccompanied by any ventilatory support such as BiPAP.[49] Rates of comorbid conditions such as systemic hypertension, pulmonary hypertension, cor pulmonale, and angina are higher in patients with OHS than in eucapnic obese patients.[50] OHS is a risk factor for development of venous thromboembolic (VTE) disease, which is a leading cause of postoperative death in bariatric surgery.[51]

OHS can be challenging to diagnose before bariatric surgery because patients may not always appear dramatically different than eucapnic obese patients with OSA. Patients with OHS more commonly have lower extremity edema, report moderate to severe dyspnea on exertion, exhibit higher AHIs and more profound minimum oxyhemoglobin saturations during sleep, spend greater time with an oxyhemoglobin saturation lower than 90% during sleep, have lower awake oxyhemoglobin saturations, are afflicted with higher BMIs, demonstrate greater restrictive changes on pulmonary function testing, and use more health care resources compared with eucapnic obese patients with OSA.[4,50] Serum bicarbonate of 27 mEq/L or more (reflecting metabolic compensation for chronic respiratory acidosis) is a sensitive but not specific marker for OHS in the obese patient with OSA.[52] If OHS is suspected on the basis of any or all of these factors, the following tests are recommended: arterial blood gas (hypoventilation manifests as hypercapnia, the severity of which should be determined), pulmonary function tests and chest radiograph (to search for other causes of chronic hypoventilation), echocardiogram (to assess the right heart pressures and function), complete blood count (to detect erythrocytosis), thyroid function tests (to rule out hypothyroidism, if not already done as part of routine testing of the obese patient), and polysomnography[4] (see Chapters 5, 11 and 16).

PAP therapy for moderate to severe OSA (AHI of 15 or higher) should be initiated preoperatively. Case-by-case decisions about CPAP are necessary in milder forms of OSA (e.g., position-dependent OSA); CPAP may be recommended preoperatively for a patient with AHI of 5 to 14 who also is hypersomnolent or in whom the degree of desaturation during obstructive apneas/hypopneas is of greater clinical concern, perhaps in the presence of comorbid conditions such as pulmonary hypertension. The elective nature of bariatric surgery should allow for follow-up assessment of titrated PAP therapy in the patient with newly diagnosed OSA or OHS before surgery. In many bariatric surgery centers, adherence to the preoperative PAP regimen for the candidate with OSA is a mandatory prerequisite; accordingly, failure to comply with this recommended therapy is a deal-breaker, because it points to the likelihood of poor adherence to other postoperative care requirements. The minimal preoperative PAP trial duration for achieving PAP acclimatization and garnering improvement in physical status is not known,[53] but because patterns of PAP use may be established within the first week of therapy,[54] close follow-up monitoring in the first few weeks to document adherence, address problems, and assess response is advised.[55] In the patient with OHS, a repeat measurement of arterial blood gases after 4 weeks of PAP therapy[4] may allow discontinuance of supplemental oxygen with confirmation of an adequate therapeutic response or may indicate the need for tracheostomy with or without ventilation when PAP fails to effect improvement.

Preoperative Assessment for Bariatric Surgery in the Patient with Established Obstructive Sleep Apnea

Patients with a known diagnosis of OSA and who are already on an established PAP regimen at the time they begin to explore the option of bariatric surgery should be asked preoperatively about suboptimal compliance, technical difficulties, persistent symptoms despite PAP, and increases in weight since their last sleep evaluation. Identification of any of these issues should prompt referral to a sleep specialist. Follow-up polysomnography is indicated for patients with substantial weight gain (i.e., 10% of baseline body weight or more) and

recurrent OSA symptoms despite PAP adherence.[47] Asymptomatic, PAP-adherent patients generally can proceed to surgery. They should be advised that PAP use will be required postoperatively and that they should bring their equipment to the hospital. Settings for PAP with or without supplemental oxygen usually are maintained postoperatively at preoperative levels, although acute adjustments may be necessary depending on the cumulative effects of factors such as opioid requirements and postoperative pulmonary disorders (e.g., VTE, pneumonia). Those patients with OSA treated previously with upper airway surgery who remain symptomatic, or in whom objective evidence of sleep-disordered breathing resolution is lacking, should be assumed to remain at risk for residual OSA and may benefit from a preoperative evaluation by a sleep specialist before bariatric surgery.[42,56] Such patients should be advised that temporary application of PAP may be necessary in the immediate postoperative period if upper airway obstruction occurs. The possibility of temporary outpatient use of PAP after surgery also should be discussed with bariatric surgery candidates who use an oral appliance for OSA management, because it may not be feasible to use their dental device immediately postoperatively.

Common Bariatric Surgical Procedures

Bariatric surgery procedures have been historically grouped into three categories based on anatomic components: predominately malabsorptive procedures, predominately restrictive procedures, and procedures with both malabsorptive and restrictive components. A majority of these operations are now performed by a less invasive, small-incision, laparoscopic approach. Ongoing research in animal models and human trials is aimed at further elucidation of the underlying mechanisms of action of bariatric surgery, which may ultimately allow a more sophisticated grouping of the surgical procedures based on their impacts on endocrine, neuronal, and behavioral physiologic variables.[57]

Roux-en-Y gastric bypass (RYGB) (Figure 22-2) combines creation of a small gastric pouch with modest intestinal or small bowel bypass. A traditional RYGB consists of transection of a small (15-mL) proximal gastric pouch along the lesser curvature of the stomach from the larger gastric segment, combined with a modest (encompassing 60 to 150 cm) intestinal bypass. The Roux-en-Y configuration allows biliopancreatic secretions and digestive juices to pass through the bile duct into the duodenum and then merge with the alimentary stream passing down from the stomach at the Y-type connection. The lengths of both the Roux and biliopancreatic limbs can be varied to produce more malabsorption. Most weight is lost in the first year, with long-term weight loss stabilizing at 2 to 3 years. Approximately 80% of patients typically experience weight stabilization, usually slightly above weight nadir, approximately 3 years after surgery. The remaining 20% of patients slowly regain excess weight over longer-term follow-up, and they risk becoming surgical failures.

The *laparoscopic adjustable gastric band* is an inflatable silicone prosthetic device that is placed around the top portion of the stomach, just below the esophagus (Figure 22-3), and restricts the upper stomach size to a small volume. The band is attached to a reservoir, with a port placed under the skin on the abdominal wall, and the inner lining of the band is a balloon that is adjustable by the addition or removal of saline

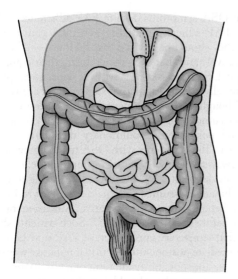

Figure 22-2 Roux-en-Y gastric bypass.

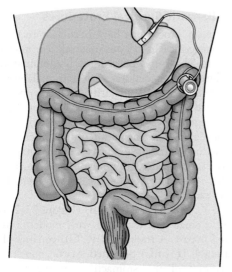

Figure 22-3 Gastric band procedure.

from the reservoir port. Inflation of the band increases the restriction of gastric outlet size and food flow. Postoperative management for patients who have undergone this procedure entails frequent follow-up visits for band adjustments/reservoir fills and strict adherence to dietary guidelines and lifestyle modification to achieve consistent weight loss. The weight loss trajectory after banding procedures is more gradual, with less weight lost than after RYGB. The favorable aspects of this procedure are that it is less invasive and requires less operating time, and that the band is both adjustable and removable. Use of the band procedure is declining with the increase in number of alternative surgical options being offered.[58]

The most recent major bariatric procedure to be introduced and growing in usage is the *vertical sleeve gastrectomy* (VSG).[59] This operation is a 70% vertical gastric resection, creating a long and narrow tubular gastric reservoir with no intestinal bypass. In many ways, VSG is intermediate between

bypass and banding in terms of complexity, risk, and weight loss results. Data on long-term results (beyond 1 to 2 years) with VSG are lacking.[60]

The less commonly used *biliopancreatic diversion* (BPD) and *BPD with duodenal switch* (BPDDS) procedures, which result in an extreme degree of malabsorption, are reserved for the treatment of "super-obese" patients. BPD combines a partial, subtotal gastrectomy and a very long Roux-en-Y anastomosis with a short common channel for nutrient absorption. With this procedure, patients can eat much larger quantities of food and still achieve and maintain weight loss. Disadvantages to the procedure include loose and foul-smelling stools, intestinal ulcers, anemia, vitamin and mineral deficiencies, and possible protein-calorie malnutrition. Because of these potential problems, patients who undergo BPD require lifelong dietary supplementation and close follow-up monitoring. With similar weight loss and complications, the BPDDS is a hybrid operation that combines a gastric sleeve resection with a long intestinal bypass in the Roux-en-Y configuration. In this procedure, ulcer rate is reduced, and dumping syndrome (the constellation of nausea, vomiting, abdominal pain or cramping, diarrhea, bloating, fatigue, palpitations, lightheadedness, sweating, and anxiety beginning within 15 to 30 minutes after eating) is eliminated by leaving intact the first portion of the intestine in the alimentary stream. BPD and BPDDS procedures are the most major and technically difficult procedures performed for weight loss and consequently should be offered only by experienced surgeons, and to patients who are able to undertake lifelong follow-up.

Debate continues regarding the selection of a specific procedure type for any given patient, and predictive data to meaningfully guide these decisions are lacking. Patients are provided with general guidelines about the different potential mechanisms of action, percent weight loss over time, and morbidity profile among procedures when making a final decision regarding surgery. The optimal choice of procedure depends in part on the expertise of the surgeon and the clinical facility, patient preference, and risk stratification.[36]

CLINICAL COURSE

Management of Obstructive Sleep Apnea Immediately after Bariatric Surgery

Many details regarding optimal care of the patient with OSA immediately after bariatric surgery remain unclear. The following general recommendations are based on experience, consensus expert opinion for generic surgical care,[41-43,56] and a limited peer-reviewed literature.

Airway extubation after bariatric surgery should be performed only when the patient is fully awake and alert and has demonstrated evidence of return of neuromuscular function (as evidenced by sustained head-lift for more than 5 seconds) and adequate vital capacity and peak inspiratory pressure.[43] Removal of the endotracheal tube should take place in the operating room, postanesthesia care unit (PACU), or special care unit so that airway control can be monitored closely and expertly addressed if lost.[43]

In the PACU, the patient should be maintained in the semiupright or lateral, not supine, position, if possible. Supplemental oxygen typically is provided under continuous pulse oximetry monitoring and titrated to the lowest level to maintain adequate oxygenation, especially in patients with OHS.

Ventilation also must be specifically monitored as supplemental oxygen may maintain adequate oxyhemoglobin saturation despite medication-exacerbated hypoventilation. Ventilation monitoring may include capnography, arterial blood gas testing, and scheduled assessments for respiratory events by PACU staff. In a study of a non–bariatric surgery perioperative patient population, recurrent respiratory events in the PACU powerfully predicted postoperative respiratory complications.[61] Respiratory events were scored during three consecutive 30-minute periods immediately after extubation and were defined as bradypnea (three or more episodes of fewer than 8 breaths/minute), apnea (one or more episodes of 10 seconds or longer of breathing cessation), desaturations (three or more episodes of oxyhemoglobin saturation below 90%), and pain-sedation mismatch (one or more episodes of high pain score and simultaneously high sedation score). Recurrent respiratory events meant that one or more of any of the PACU respiratory events occurred in at least two separate 30-minute time blocks and were associated with an odds ratio of 21 for postoperative respiratory complications.[61] In the PACU, PAP is instituted at the level prescribed before surgery in those patients who were using it preoperatively. In patients whose preoperative CPAP settings are not known or in whom initiation of CPAP is desired to address recurrent respiratory events emerging in the PACU, CPAP in autoadjusting mode can be applied or started at an empirically chosen level of 8 to10 cm H_2O and adjusted as needed, although acute initiation of such therapy in the PACU can be challenging in the PAP-naive patient. BiPAP, usually with oxygen, may be initiated to address acute hypoventilation. PACU staff must be capable of monitoring and managing PAP therapy, including addressing interface leaks and observing diligently for signs of breakthrough upper airway obstruction despite PAP, such as snoring, choking, witnessed apneas, cardiac dysrhythmias, or repetitive oxygen desaturation.

In the first 24 postoperative hours after bariatric surgery, patients are likely to be the most vulnerable to potential OSA-related complications,[62] although OSA propensity may be increased for at least several days after bariatric surgery because of the aggregate effects of ongoing sleep deprivation, rapid eye movement sleep rebound, and medication synergies.[56] Fortunately, the length of hospital stay usually is short (3.5 days and 1.6 days for gastric bypass and restrictive procedures, respectively).[63] Clinicians must consistently keep the possibility of OSA in mind in all patients as they consider postoperative analgesia, monitoring, oxygenation, and patient positioning[43] for the duration of the hospitalization. Systemic opioids should be used cautiously because of their ability to depress the respiratory drive and cause subsequent oxygen desaturation. The use of patient-controlled analgesia is controversial, although it may be an option if used without a basal rate and with restricted dosing. Nonsteroidal antiinflammatory agents may help decrease opioid dosing as recovery progresses but should be used cautiously in the postsurgical patient because of the enhanced potential for bleeding complications. Benzodiazepines should be avoided because of their negative effects on the respiratory control and upper airway musculature. Access to PAP should be available at all times during recovery—a seemingly obvious recommendation but one that may be overlooked by busy house staff, nurses unfamiliar with this ventilatory technique, and patients distracted or impaired by postoperative pain or pharmacologic obtundation. Properly

trained health care staff should be readily available to assist patients in PAP device placement, to troubleshoot interface problems, to observe for breakthrough upper airway obstruction, and to reassure patients struggling with a new PAP regimen.

Continuous pulse oximetry monitoring after discharge from the PACU is recommended for all post–bariatric surgery patients for as long as they are deemed to be at increased risk, which may be defined as the duration of intravenous opioid use or an oral opioid dose of greater than 60 mg of codeine every 4 hours.[42] Oximetry data should be continuously observed at the bedside in a critical care or stepdown unit, by telemetry on a hospital ward, or by a dedicated, trained observer in the patient's room. Choosing the optimal monitoring site will depend on the interplay of multiple factors. It is reasonable to consider intensive care unit (ICU) care for the first 24 to 48 hours after bariatric surgery in patients with one or more of the following features: age older than 50 years, BMI greater than 60 kg/m², significant comorbid cardiopulmonary disease, brittle diabetes mellitus, severe OSA/OHS with worrisome record of suboptimal PAP compliance, sluggish emergence from anesthesia, and intraoperative complications. In the University HealthSystem Consortium evaluation, a review of the bariatric programs at 29 academic medical centers in the United States, 7.7% of patients undergoing gastric bypass and 1.1% of patients undergoing a restrictive procedure required ICU support postoperatively.[5] Operative approach to bariatric surgery also must be considered. Case series from experienced surgery teams have reported that patients with established and treated OSA undergoing laparoscopic bariatric procedures do not require routine postoperative admission to the ICU.[64,65]

Incentive spirometry should be encouraged. If oxygen desaturations occur despite an appropriate PAP regimen, supplemental oxygen should be added while the provider searches for an explanation, such as transient worsening of upper airway obstruction requiring adjustment of PAP settings, VTE event, atelectasis, aspiration, pneumonia, or anastomotic leak. Caution with the use of supplemental oxygen without PAP during sleep is advised, because this strategy provides no protection against upper airway obstruction and will blunt detection of a disordered breathing event by oximetry monitoring. Postoperative supine positioning also should be avoided; instead, the head of the bed should be kept elevated in a semi-Fowler position (to at least 30 degrees) at all times. All post–bariatric surgery patients should be considered to be at moderate to high risk for VTE events; accordingly, thromboprophylaxis with low-molecular-weight heparin or low-dose unfractionated heparin, along with application of intermittent pneumatic compression stockings, is indicated in all patients.[36,66] The frequency of VTE after bariatric surgery with thromboprophylaxis is low at less than 1%.[66] Because most VTEs occur after hospital discharge, the AACE-TOS-ASMBS advises extended chemoprophylaxis (duration unspecified) for patients at higher risk for such events, such as those with a history of VTE or reduced activity level.[36] Prolonged respiratory failure after bariatric surgery is uncommon, occurring in less than 1% of cases, according to data from the American College of Surgeons' National Surgical Quality Improvement program encompassing approximately 32,000 patients who underwent bariatric surgery between 2006 and 2008; the impact of OSA on the rate of respiratory failure is not known, because OSA was not a risk factor assessed in the analysis.[67]

Laparoscopic bariatric surgery is performed in some patients in an ambulatory setting. A consensus statement from the Society for Ambulatory Anesthesia[41] warns against use of outpatient surgical procedures in patients with OSA if it is accompanied by a a nonoptimized comorbid condition; if an inability to control pain predominantly with nonopioid analgesic techniques can be anticipated; or if the patient displays unwillingness or inability to use PAP. Patients on PAP should be advised to bring their device to the ambulatory care facility for use during recovery. If the patient experiences recurrent respiratory events while in the PACU, hospital discharge should be delayed until the patient is observed to maintain adequate oxygenation (on PAP if necessary, if used preoperatively) in an unstimulated environment, preferably while sleeping.[43] Patients not on PAP should be advised to sleep exclusively nonsupine, and PAP users should wear their device during all sleep periods, including naps, for "several days" after surgery; all are advised to minimize use of opioids.

Benefits of Bariatric Surgery

Postoperative weight loss typically is reported as the mean percentage of excess weight loss, defined by the following formula:

$$(\text{Weight loss} \div \text{excess weight}) \times 100$$

where excess weight equals total preoperative weight minus ideal weight. In a review of 136 studies involving 22,000 bariatric surgery patients, Buchwald and colleagues[68] reported that the mean percentage of excess weight loss with bariatric surgery was 61.2%: 47.5% for gastric banding, 68.2% for gastric bypass (principally RYGB), and 70.1% for BPD and BPDDS. The mean decrease in BMI was 14.2 kg/m^2, whereas the mean decrease in absolute weight was 39.7 kg, similar to the 20- to 30-kg weight loss reported in the meta-analysis by Maggard and colleagues.[69] Comorbid conditions correspondingly decreased in severity with weight loss. Overall, diabetes mellitus completely resolved in 76.8%, hyperlipidemia decreased in degree in 70%, and arterial hypertension lessened in severity or resolved in 78.5%.[68] Weight loss, improvement with respect to comorbid conditions, and quality of life at 1 year, as well as rates of severe postoperative complications, are similar for RYGB and for VSG, both performed laparoscopically.[70] A retrospective cohort study comparing long-term mortality rates among 7925 patients who underwent gastric bypass and 7925 age-, sex-, and BMI-matched control subjects randomly selected from a state driver's license applicant registry demonstrated a 40% reduction in adjusted long-term mortality with bariatric surgery during a mean follow-up period of 7.1 years.[71]

No large randomized trials have compared bariatric surgery with medical management of obesity. The Swedish Obesity Study[72] was a large, prospective, nonrandomized, controlled trial that compared outcomes for 2010 obese subjects treated with bariatric surgery and for 2037 contemporaneously matched obese control subjects treated conventionally. At 2 years, weight had decreased by 23.4% in the surgery group but had increased by 0.1% in the control group, and after 10 years, weight had increased by 16.1% over presurgical weight in the surgery group but had increased by 1.6% in control subjects ($P < .001$ at both time points). Improvements in clinical

indices of diabetes, hypertriglyceridemia, and hypertension were more favorable in the surgery group, and the surgery group exhibited lower 2- and 10-year incident rates of diabetes than those for the control group. Maximal weight loss in the surgery group was assessed after 1 to 2 years, and at 10 years the maximal average losses were 32% for gastric bypass, 25% for vertical banded gastroplasty, and 20% for banding. Overall mortality was lower in the surgery group than in the control group.[73]

Long-term Impact of Bariatric Surgery on Obstructive Sleep Apnea

Weight loss induced by bariatric surgery is consistently associated with reductions in AHI.[74] Buchwald and coworkers' meta-analysis[68] of selected bariatric surgery outcomes reported that OSA resolved or decreased in severity in 83.6%. The weighted (i.e., weighting results by sample size) mean change in the AHI was 40 (events/hour), with a range of 16 to 52.8. Enthusiasm over these results must be tempered by several methodologic concerns. *Improvement* and *resolution* with respect to OSA were not explicitly defined. The studies included in the meta-analysis are not entirely specified, but a review of studies from the inclusion period (1990 to June 2003) revealed that reduction in OSA symptoms probably was sufficient in some studies to assess OSA response (i.e., postoperative polysomnography was not required in all subjects), the timing of polysomnography after surgery was nonuniform, and the results probably were variably reported (e.g., only preoperative and postoperative apnea indices were described, not AHIs).

Studies published since June 2003[75-78] corroborate earlier series reporting that surgically induced weight loss is associated with symptomatic improvement in OSA when reassessment occurs approximately 1 year or longer after surgery. However, many patients have residual OSA. Even though gastric banding resulted in a mean AHI reduction of 23.4 (events/hour), Lettieri and colleagues[79] found that 23 patients (96%) still met criteria for OSA (AHI higher than 5), 20 (83%) continued to experience transient nocturnal hypoxia (oxyhemoglobin saturation below 90%), and 13 (54%) had persistent sleepiness (Epworth Sleepiness Scale scores higher than 10) despite an average weight loss of 54 kg at a mean of 418 days postoperatively. In a metaanalysis of 12 studies involving 342 patients, Greenburg and colleagues[80] found that the pooled mean BMI decreased by 17.9 kg/m^2 and AHI decreased by 38.2, but the residual AHI averaged 15.8. Since that meta-analysis, a small randomized, controlled trial pitting bariatric surgery (laparoscopic adjustable gastric banding) ($n = 30$ patients) against a conventional weight loss program (individualized dietary, physical activity, and behavioral programs) ($n = 30$ patients) demonstrated that, although bariatric surgery produced significantly greater mean weight loss at 2 years than that achieved in the nonsurgical program (27.8 kg versus 5.1 kg), the reductions in AHI were statistically similar (25.5 versus 14; $P = .18$).[81] The mean residual AHI in the bariatric group was 39.5, and 73% of the bariatric group continued to have an AHI of 15 or higher. Accordingly, health care providers must remain vigilant for persistent OSA with a systematic postoperative follow-up program, because even dramatic changes in weight and symptoms do not guarantee objective cure of OSA. The optimal timing for postoperative polysomnography is not clear but depends in part on the patient's weight loss evolution. The CPAP requirement for residual OSA is likely to fall by at least 2 to 4 cm H_2O in the year after surgery.[82] Autotitrating CPAP after surgery may bridge the patient to polysomnography and obviate subjective pressure reductions or serial sleep studies.

The American Academy of Sleep Medicine concluded that bariatric surgery may be adjunctive in the treatment for OSA, but it rates this recommendation as an option, meaning that bariatric surgery is of uncertain clinical use in the management of OSA.[83] This designation is based on the lack of data at the Sackett level of evidence I to III and the potential for perioperative complications.

Risks and Complications of Bariatric Surgery

The Longitudinal Assessment of Bariatric Surgery (LABS) Consortium conducted a prospective, observation study of outcomes of bariatric surgical procedures at 10 clinical sites in the United States from 2005 to 2007. The rate of operative mortality, defined as death within the first 30 days, was 0.3% among 4610 consecutive patients who underwent RYGB or laparoscopic adjustable gastric banding: None of the 1198 patients who had a laparoscopic adjustable gastric band procedure died, 0.2% of the 2975 patients who underwent laparoscopic RYGB died, and 2.1% of the 437 patients who underwent open RYGB died.[84] A composite endpoint of death, deep vein thrombosis or venous thromboembolism, reintervention, and failure to be discharged by 30 days after surgery was reported in 4.1% of patients: 1% in the laparoscopic adjustable gastric banding group, 4.8% in the laparoscopic RYGB group, and 7.8% in the open RYGB group. Factors that were each independently associated with an increased risk of the composite endpoint were a history of venous thromboembolic disease, impaired functional status, and extreme values of BMI. Box 22-1 lists the postoperative adverse events from bariatric surgery, which can be grouped as early and late. A dreaded complication is anastomotic leak: In the University HealthSystem Consortium evaluation,[63] the anastomotic leak rate for gastric bypass procedures was 1.6%.

The extent to which OSA is linked to complications after bariatric surgery is not fully known. In a review of data for more than 3000 patients, OSA, older age, male sex, and revision gastric bypass were found to be independent predictors for anastomotic leak,[85] whereas OSA, hypertension, and less surgeon experience were identified by multivariate analysis as predictors of postoperative complications in a series of nearly 200 patients undergoing laparoscopic RYGB.[86] In the LABS analysis, OSA also was independently associated with increased risk for an adverse outcome, with a composite of such outcomes defined as the endpoint.[84] Accordingly, OSA has been linked to increased cost of postoperative care[87] and higher risk for prolonged postoperative hospital stay.[88] In other studies, however, the investigators have not identified OSA as an independent predictor of complications after bariatric surgery.[89-91] These reports are challenging to interpret and compare because of differences in procedures used and uncertainty over how aggressively OSA was pursued preoperatively and managed postoperatively, and many are single-center and possibly underpowered retrospective reviews, thus providing a lower grade of evidence. PAP initiated immediately after bariatric surgery does not appear to increase risk for anastomotic leaks.[92,93]

Box 22-1   COMPLICATIONS OF BARIATRIC SURGERY

Complications Common to All Bariatric Procedures

Early (up to 30 days after surgery)
Venous thromboembolic disease
Bleeding
Anastomotic leaks
Wound infections
Persistent nausea/vomiting, dehydration
Regional abdominal organ trauma
Incisional and internal hernias
Bowel obstruction
Atelectasis
Pneumonia
Cardiac dysrhythmias
Urinary tract infection
Death

Late (beyond 30 days after surgery)
Incisional and internal hernias
Bowel obstruction from adhesions
Nutritional deficiencies
Anastomotic strictures and marginal ulcers or erosions
Cholelithiasis
Anemia
Persistence or recurrence of obstructive sleep apnea
Need for body contouring
Weight regain

Procedure-Unique Complications/Adverse Effects
Roux-en-Y Gastric Bypass
Dumping syndrome

Laparoscopic Adjustable Gastric Banding
Band slippage or erosion
Port or device malfunction

Vertical Sleeve Gastrectomy
Refractory reflux

Biliopancreatic Diversion
Loose, foul-smelling stools
Protein-calorie malnutrition

PITFALLS AND CONTROVERSY

Controversy remains about the impact of OSA on bariatric surgery complications and thus to what extent must OSA be sought and treated preoperatively. Definitive data are not available. Bariatric surgery clinical practice guidelines[36] stipulate that OSA should be considered in all bariatric surgery candidates—but does that mean polysomnography is mandatory and that if it yields a positive result, PAP is required? The answer to both of these questions is likely to be "no." Instead, the history and physical findings pertinent to OSA, perhaps initially organized by a screening tool sensitive to OSA so that the search is consistent and systematized, must be combined with consideration of a host of other factors, both patient-related (comorbidity burden; OSA symptom severity; OHS likelihood) and procedure-related (open versus laparoscopic; inpatient versus ambulatory; anticipated postoperative opioid requirements), in deciding how to proceed. Those patients judged to be at low risk for having OSA as indicated by the collective clinical information (e.g., STOP-Bang score less than 3) can proceed directly to bariatric surgery without further sleep testing[42] *provided that* postoperative precautions are in place (e.g., careful monitoring in the PACU; minimization of opioid/sedative use; head of bed elevation; incentive spirometry) and the bariatric team is prepared to address OSA should it manifest during the immediate postoperative period. Patients deemed to be at intermediate or high risk for having OSA should proceed to a formal sleep assessment, with the sleep specialist guiding the ordering of sleep testing and the interpretation of findings.[42] PAP is started preoperatively for treatment of moderate to severe OSA (AHI of 15 or higher) and OHS. Preoperative PAP initiation allows the patient to begin accruing its neurobehavioral and cardiovascular benefits while working through other preparatory steps typically required for bariatric surgery. Furthermore, retrospective data suggest that it may decrease the risk of post–bariatric surgery complications[94] and is recommended by the AACE-TOS-ASMBS guidelines.[36]

CLINICAL PEARLS

- The sleep clinician should be mindful that bariatric surgery candidates are likely to have OSA, which requires careful consideration during the preoperative evaluation as well as in the postoperative period.
- Post–bariatric surgery patients should be expected to lose 20 to 50 kg by 1 to 2 years postoperatively, which current studies indicate should be accompanied by a 50% to 75% reduction in AHI and a drop in required PAP levels.
- Autotitrating CPAP may be a useful management modality as weight decreases after surgery.
- Despite dramatic weight loss, OSA may persist in many patients, so follow-up polysomnography is advised to reassess for this condition and to guide decisions about longer-term PAP use.

SUMMARY

The prevalence of obesity, a leading cause of preventable disease and death, is increasing. Nearly 70% percent of Americans currently are overweight or obese. Rates of overweight and obesity are higher among Mexican Americans and non-Hispanic black Americans than among non-Hispanic whites and Asian Americans. Excess weight is the strongest risk factor for OSA because of its adverse impact on upper airway neuromuscular function and anatomy. Bariatric surgery, comprising a variety of procedures that limit food absorption or restrict intake (or both), is indicated for severely obese patients in whom an adequate exercise and diet program has failed to achieve results and who have either a BMI of 40 kg/m^2 or greater or a BMI of 35 kg/m^2 or above in conjunction with one or more obesity-related severe comorbid conditions. The mean percentage of excess weight loss with bariatric surgery is approximately 60%, and in patients with major obesity-related conditions, such as diabetes mellitus and hypertension, consistent improvement in clinical indices is to be expected. Thirty-day mortality rate for bariatric surgery is less than 1%. OSA is almost universally present in bariatric surgery candi-

dates, sometimes in the context of OHS. The immediate post–bariatric surgery setting may exacerbate OSA, whereas OSA and its associated conditions may exacerbate challenges to the patient's immediate postoperative well-being. Systematic screening for OSA should therefore be a required component of preparation for bariatric surgery, with addition of a formal sleep evaluation for patients deemed to be at higher risk for OSA. Symptomatic improvement follows, but the OSA does not usually resolve with bariatric surgery–induced weight loss. The sleep clinician plays an important role in the bariatric surgery process, in preoperatively collaborating with the surgical team to identify OSA and by helping define its significance, determining which patients need OSA treatment, and initiating or optimizing OSA therapy to postoperatively determine the degree of residual OSA and the need for additional treatment.

Selected Readings

Abbas M, Cumella L, Zhang Y, et al. Outcomes of laparoscopic sleeve gastrectomy and roux-en-Y gastric bypass in patients older than 60. *Obes Surg* 2015;**25**(12):2251–6.

Arterbarn DE, Courcoulas AP. Bariatric surgery for obesity and metabolic conditions in adults. *BMJ* 2014;**349**:g3961.

Dudley KA, Tavakkoli A, Andrews RA, et al. Interest in bariatric surgery among obese patients with obstructive sleep apnea. *Surg Obes Rel Dis* 2015;**11**(5):1146–51.

Fouladpour N, Jesudoss R, Bolden N, et al. Perioperative Complications in Obstructive Sleep Apnea Patients Undergoing Surgery: A Review of the Legal Literature. *Anesth Analg* 2016;**122**(1):145–51.

Kushner RF, Ryan DH. Assessment and lifestyle management of patients with obesity. *JAMA* 2014;**312**:943–52.

Lettierri CJ, Eliasson AH, Greenburg DL. Persistence of obstructive sleep apnea after surgical weight loss. *J Clin Sleep Med* 2008;**4**:333–8.

The Longitudinal Assessment of Bariatric Surgery (LABS) Consortium. Perioperative safety in the longitudinal assessment of bariatric surgery. *N Engl J Med* 2009;**361**:445–54.

Mechanick JI, Youdim A, Jones DB, et al. Clinical practice guidelines for the perioperative nutritional, metabolic, and nonsurgical support of the bariatric surgery patient—2013 update: cosponsored by American Association of Clinical Endocrinologists, The Obesity Society, and American Society for Metabolic and Bariatric Surgery. *Obesity* 2013;**21**:S1–27.

Nguyen NT, Nguyen B, Gebhart A, Hohmann S. Changes in the makeup of bariatric surgery: a national increase in use of laparoscopic sleeve gastrectomy. *J Am Coll Surg* 2013;**216**:252–7.

North American Association for the Study of Obesity and the National Heart, Lung, and Blood Institute. *The practical guide: identification, evaluation, and treatment of overweight and obesity in adults.* NIH publication 00-4084. Bethesda (Md.): National Institutes of Health; 2000.

Ogden CL, Carroll MD, Kit BK, Flegal KM. Prevalence of childhood and adult obesity in the United States, 2011-12. *JAMA* 2014;**732**:806–14.

Piche ME, Auclair A, Harvey J, et al. How to choose and use bariatric surgery in 2015. *Can J Cardiol* 2015;**31**:153–66.

Schwartz AR, Patil SP, Laffan AM, et al. Obesity and obstructive sleep apnea: pathogenic mechanisms and therapeutic approaches. *Proc Am Thorac Soc* 2008;**5**:185–92.

Sjostrom L, Lindroos A-K, Peltonen M, et al. Lifestyle, diabetes, and cardiovascular risk factors 10 years after bariatric surgery. *N Engl J Med* 2004;**351**:2683–93.

Sjostrom L, Narbro K, Sjostrom CD, et al. Effects of bariatric surgery on mortality in Swedish obese subjects. *N Engl J Med* 2007;**357**:741–52.

Stefater MA, Wilson-Perez HE, Chambers AP, et al. All bariatric surgeries are not created equal: insights from mechanistic comparisons. *Endocr Rev* 2012;**33**:595–622.

Tsai A, Schumann R. Morbid obesity and perioperative complications. *Curr Opin Anaesthesiol* 2016;**29**(1):103–8.

A complete reference list can be found online at ExpertConsult.com.

Consequences

Obstructive Sleep Apnea and the Central Nervous System

Chapter

23

Ivana Rosenzweig; Terri E. Weaver; Mary J. Morrell

Chapter Highlights

- Patients with obstructive sleep apnea (OSA) demonstrate variable degrees of cognitive, emotional, and performance deficits.
- OSA is increasingly recognized as one of the potentially modifiable risk factors for dementia; its multiple effects on the central nervous system are acknowledged, albeit their nature and prognosis are yet to be fully understood.
- During nocturnal apnea-hypopnea episodes and sleep fragmentation, both maladaptive and adaptive pathways are likely initiated in the

brain of patients; the net result likely depends on the chronicity of process and idiosyncratic characteristics of each patient.
- Treatment of OSA with continuous positive airway pressure results in consistent improvement in cognition and performance, although the magnitude of improvement is variable.
- The role of continuous positive airway pressure and its long-term effectiveness with regard to cognitive and performance deficits need further study.

Obstructive sleep apnea (OSA) is one of the potentially modifiable risk factors for dementia,[1-4] and it is commonly associated with serious cardiovascular and metabolic comorbidities.[5-7] Nocturnal episodes of complete or partial pharyngeal obstruction in patients with OSA result in intermittent hypoxia, reoxygenation, hypercapnia, and sleep fragmentation.[8,9] An increase in respiratory effort, in association with hypoxemia or hypercapnia, triggers the frequent sleep arousals, which usually terminate the apneic episodes but also contribute to abnormal sleep architecture and lighter and less restorative sleep.[10] Progressive changes in sleep quality and structure, changes in cerebral blood flow, neurovascular and neurotransmitter changes, and the cellular redox status and neural regulation in OSA patients all may constitute contributing factors to cognitive decline.[8,11-13]

Increased road traffic accidents, reduced quality of life, excessive daytime sleepiness, labile interpersonal relationships, and decreased work and school efficiency have all been documented in OSA patients.[13] These impairments and deficits are not always reversed with treatment.[14] Beneficial effects of treatment on cognitive performance, sleepiness, and neural injury in OSA (Figure 23-1) are, however, documented in recent meta-analyses[15,16] and a meta review.[17] Two studies also suggest beneficial effects of continuous positive airway pressure (CPAP) therapy in minimally symptomatic, and older OSA patients, respectively.[18,19] In a recent study of a well-characterized longitudinal cohort (the Alzheimer's Disease Neuroimaging Initiative cohort), the self-reported presence of untreated sleep-disordered breathing, including "obstructive sleep apnea" and "sleep apnea," was associated with an earlier

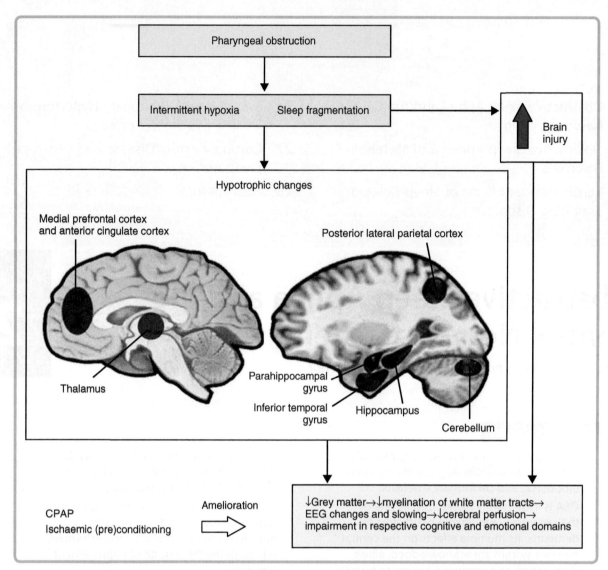

Figure 23-1 Brain regions and mechanisms involved in sleep apnea injury. The nocturnal episodes of complete or partial pharyngeal obstruction result in intermittent hypoxia and sleep fragmentation. Both intermittent hypoxia and sleep fragmentation can aggravate brain injury (*red arrow*) and cause hypotrophic changes in several brain regions shown.[128] Ensuing neurophysiologic and neurochemical changes can also manifest in cognitive and emotional deficits that can be ameliorated (*white arrow*) with continuous positive airway pressure therapy (CPAP) and/or ischemic preconditioning. EEG, Electroencephalography. (From Rosenzweig I, Glasser M, Polsek D, et al. Sleep apnoea and the brain: a complex relationship. *Lancet Respir Med* 2015;3:404–14.)

age at cognitive decline, up to a decade.[4] This association was found to be significant even when accounting for possible confounding factors such as sex, apolipoprotein ε4 status, diabetes, depression, body mass index, cardiovascular disease, hypertension, age at baseline, and education of participants. Moreover, this link appeared significantly attenuated in patients who used CPAP, suggesting that use of CPAP may delay progression, or onset, of cognitive impairment.[4] However, the effect of CPAP on delay in age at Alzheimer disease dementia onset was not demonstrated in this study.[4]

The current dearth of fully effective treatments for the central nervous system (CNS) sequelae of OSA is likely to be a reflection of an as yet poorly understood intricate interplay of both adaptive and maladaptive processes with the hypox-

emia, reoxygenation, hypercapnia or hypocapnia, and sleep fragmentation that occur in the CNS of OSA patients.[13] The overall net result of ongoing neuroinflammatory processes and ischemic preconditioning for each particular patient depends on the stage of this OSA-induced dynamic process, effects on other body systems, cognitive reserve, and idiosyncratic susceptibility.[11,13,20,21] Thus different therapeutic approaches might benefit different stages and conversely might aggravate damage in some patients.[11,13,20] This chapter addresses recent clinical and translational findings regarding the effects of intermittent hypoxia and sleep fragmentation on the CNS, describes the known cognitive and psychological deficits in patients with OSA, and proposes etiologic mechanisms behind the complex relationship between OSA and the CNS.

NEUROPATHOLOGY OF OBSTRUCTIVE SLEEP APNEA

Changes in cerebral blood flow that occur during obstructive apneas[22] and apnea-induced hypoxemia, combined with reduced cerebral perfusion, likely predispose patients to nocturnal cerebral ischemia.[23,24] In addition, an altered resting cerebral blood flow pattern in several CNS regions has been shown in OSA, along with hypoperfusion during the awake states.[25] Numerous clinical studies have demonstrated changes in the electroencephalogram of OSA patients compared with healthy individuals, including aberrant cortical excitability[26-28] and an associated array of neurocognitive deficits.[10] Taken collectively, such studies have also delineated a putative neurocircuitry "fingerprint" of OSA-induced brain injury and have suggested a disconnection of the frontal regions (Figure 23-2) and a disruption of the (cerebellar)-thalamocortical oscillator, with involvement of the hippocampal formation.[9,10] It has been previously suggested that the constellation of symptoms frequently encountered in OSA patients, such as depression, disturbances in attention, dysmetria of thought and affect, and executive and verbal memory deficits,[29-31] point to similarities with two other recognized neurologic clinical syndromes, frontal lobe syndrome and the cerebellar cognitive affective syndrome.[10,32]

The prefrontal model posits that the sleep disruption, intermittent hypoxemia, and hypercapnia experienced by OSA patients alter the normal restorative process that occurs during sleep, generating cellular and biochemical stresses that result in disruption of functional homeostasis and altered neuronal and glial viability within certain brain regions, primarily the prefrontal regions of the brain cortex.[33,34] This model has been proposed as a theoretical framework for the relationship between sleep fragmentation and nocturnal hypoxemia and predominantly frontal deficits (see Figure 23-2).[34] OSA-induced neuropathologic alterations can lead to destabilization of the executive system, causing behavioral disturbance in inhibition, maintenance of performance, self-regulation of affect and arousal, working memory, analysis and synthesis, and contextual memory.[33,34] Alterations in the executive system can adversely affect cognitive abilities, resulting in maladaptive types of behavior as depicted in Figure 23-2.[33,34] Nonetheless, unlike some other neurologic disorders, the impairments associated with OSA are more likely to produce inefficient performance rather than inability to perform.[34] For example, when memory- or divided attention–related neuronal circuitry is incapacitated, other CNS systems and circuitries likely get recruited in an effort to compensate.[33,34] However, if such systems are themselves affected by sleep fragmentation or hypoxemia, their compensatory contributions might be suboptimal. This may account for the increased activation of the prefrontal cortex under conditions of sleep deprivation documented by functional magnetic resonance imaging.[33,34] Impairments in performance of OSA patients can be further explained by deficits in elementary cognitive functions, specifically, sensory transduction, feature integration, and motor preparation and execution, which are required, even in simple response-time tasks.[34,35] Corresponding to the listed deficits in OSA patients, the neuroanatomic regions that have most commonly been reported in clinical and animal studies as affected in OSA suggest that both the cerebellar modulation of neural circuits and the normal state-dependent flow of information between thalamus (and basal ganglia) and frontoparietal cortex are likely to be affected in susceptible patients (see Figure 23-1).[10,36-41]

Some clinicians have argued against such a reductionist approach to OSA-induced brain injury and point out that emerging research indicates that the relationship between OSA disease severity and cognitive dysfunction is the product of a multitude of susceptibility and protective factors and that sleep fragmentation, hypoxemia, and cognitive reserve are only three such aspects.[9,10,16] Other commonly overlooked factors are duration of the disease, role of the blood-brain barrier, presence of hypertension, metabolic dysfunction, and systemic inflammation, levels of cerebral blood flow, and genetic vulnerability.[16] Further research is necessary to provide a clear understanding of the risk for neurocognitive dysfunction and the benefit and optimization of treatments.

Affected Neurocognitive Domains

Despite contradictory results and ongoing polemics in the field, most studies to date agree that patients with OSA can have significant deficits in attention and vigilance, long-term visual and verbal memory, visuospatial and constructional abilities, and executive function.[13,17,29] Several associations have been recognized, including the association between worsening global cognitive functioning and the severity of hypoxemia as well as the association between attention and vigilance dysfunction and the degree of sleep fragmentation.[13,17] Consensus is less strong on the effects of OSA on working memory and short-term memory.[17] In some studies,

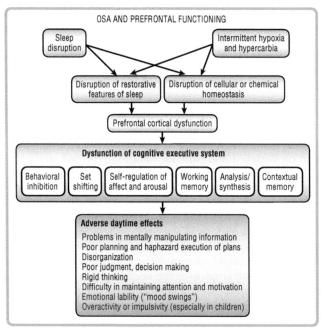

Figure 23-2 The proposed prefrontal model. In this model, obstructive sleep apnea–related sleep disruption and intermittent hypoxemia and hypercarbia alter the efficacy of restorative processes occurring during sleep and disrupt the functional homeostasis and neuronal and glial viability within particular brain regions, particularly the prefrontal regions of the brain cortex. (From Beebe DW, Gozal D. Obstructive sleep apnea and the prefrontal cortex: towards a comprehensive model linking nocturnal upper airway obstruction to daytime cognitive and behavioral deficits. *J Sleep Res* 2002;11:1–16.)

language ability and psychomotor functioning have been shown to be largely unaffected by OSA,[17] whereas others have pointed to psychomotor slowing as the most vulnerable cognitive domains and also the least responsive to treatment with CPAP.[42] Similarly, several studies showing impairments in language abilities in patients with severe OSA have not shown agreement on whether phonemic or semantic domains have the greatest effect.[43] Neurodevelopmental stages of adolescents and children with OSA appear to dictate a higher risk for this deficit.[44]

In children with OSA, the results of studies assessing cognitive performance and effects of treatment are similarly divergent.[45,46] In a recent study of children 7 to 12 years of age with sleep-disordered breathing (SDB), who were followed for 4 years, treatment of the SDB led to improvements in several aspects of neurocognition, collectively categorized as performance IQ.[45] Performance IQ represents fluid intelligence that is reflective of incidental learning, and it describes one's ability to adapt to new situations.[47] In this study, improvements were recorded in tasks associated with spatial visualization, visuomotor coordination, abstract thought, and nonverbal fluid reasoning.[45] However, overall improvements in academic ability or behavior were less clear. Furthermore, tendency to worsening of verbal IQ, which, unlike performance IQ, is more likely to be affected by formal education and learning experiences, was noted in a treated group.[45] A definitive explanation for this finding was not provided, and no statistically significant association between the reduction in verbal IQ performance and treatment was demonstrated.[45] Conversely, in another influential study, younger children with SDB followed for 12 months of treatment showed significant improvements in academic performance.[46] The different neurodevelopmental ages of children and different test parameters used provide for a complex clinical data set, against which no finite conclusions can be drawn. Nonetheless, particular patterns and associations seem to be emerging from this and earlier work, among which the association between performance IQ and slow wave activity (SWA) during non–rapid eye movement (NREM) sleep is perhaps the strongest one.[45,48] It has been argued that cognitive improvements in treated OSA patients may reflect increased stability of brain activity during sleep, allowing crucial synaptic repair and maintenance to occur and counteracting toxic effects of arousal and hypoxic effects of OSA.[45,49] This argument is concordant with findings showing that the neurochemical and gene environments of sleep and sleep activity patterns present crucial window periods during which the brain can restore cellular homeostasis, increase signal-to-noise ratio, and reinforce neuronal circuitry for subsequent cognitive processing demands.[12,50,51]

PROPOSED MECHANISTIC ROLE FOR PERTURBED SLEEP IN PATIENTS WITH OBSTRUCTIVE SLEEP APNEA

Sleep and sleep deprivation alter molecular signaling pathways that regulate synaptic strength, plasticity-related gene expression, and protein translation in a bidirectional manner.[51] Moreover, sleep deprivation can impair neuronal excitability, decrease myelination, and lead to cellular oxidative stress and misfolding of cellular proteins.[51,52] Frequent brief awakenings lead to fragmented sleep that negatively affects the next day's cognitive and emotional functioning, in a manner similar

to that of total sleep deprivation.[2] Several studies have attempted to assess whether OSA patients are more vulnerable to sleep-loss-induced performance deficits, with special emphasis on driving performance variables, with varied results.[53-56] From the practical point of view it is of major interest to develop reliable and practical bedside tests to help clinicians advise patients on their individual risk for traffic accidents.[13] Preclinical animal studies suggest that sleep fragmentation independently affects similar brain regions to those affected by intermittent hypoxia, as occurs in OSA.[8] Also, clinical studies of the effects of sleep deprivation on cognition in the general population suggest comparable cognitive impairments to those seen in OSA.[57] Frequent partial arousals during sleep in OSA patients contribute to abnormal sleep architecture and symptoms of excessive daytime somnolence (i.e., sleepiness).[8,9] An independent association between excessive daytime somnolence and cognitive impairment has been demonstrated, and several prospective studies have shown that excessive daytime somnolence is associated with an increased risk for cognitive decline and dementia.[1] Further, in a prospective cohort study of Japanese American men in the Honolulu-Asia Aging Study, lower nocturnal oxygenation and reduction in stage 3 (slow wave) NREM sleep were associated with the development of microinfarcts and brain atrophy.[58] Conversely, men with longer slow wave sleep time showed slower cognitive decline.[58]

The relationship between OSA and its effect on selected sleep stages merits particular attention, given that each of the sleep stages, with its attendant alterations in neurophysiology, is associated with facilitation of important functional learning and memory processes.[12] In OSA patients, the proportion of stage 2 NREM sleep (N2) has been shown to be increased, whereas proportions of stages 1 and 3 NREM sleep (N1, N3) and rapid eye movement (REM) sleep are decreased.[43] Limited experimental studies conducted to date have shown specific impairments of sleep-dependent consolidation of verbal declarative information in patients with OSA.[59] Furthermore, several recent clinical studies suggest disturbed spatiotemporal evolution of sleep spindles in patients with OSA during the night.[60,61]

However, dynamic analysis of sleep architecture is required to fully gauge the neurophysiologic effect of sleep fragmentation on sleep in OSA patients.[13] For example, in one study of mild OSA the exponential decay function of SWA was demonstrated to be significantly slower in OSA patients compared with controls.[62] This was due to the more even distribution of SWA throughout the night, without significant decrease in total slow wave and REM sleep time. These results show that mild sleep fragmentation can alter the dynamics of SWA, without significantly decreasing the amounts of slow wave and REM sleep, and emphasize the need to perform SWA decay analysis in sleep fragmentation disorders.[62] In the same study, a decrease in spindle activity was observed in N2 and N3 sleep that was not attributed to an increase of SWA.[60,62] Such a reduction in total spindle density has also been reported in sleep maintenance insomnia and is likely to be related to sleep fragmentation.[60-62]

The model proposed by Landmann and colleagues[63] suggests an integrative framework for the qualitative reorganization of memory during sleep.[63] It further builds on studies that have shown that sleep facilitates the abstraction of rules and the integration of knowledge into existing schemas during slow wave sleep.[50,51,63] REM sleep, on the other hand, has been shown to benefit creativity that requires the disintegration of existing patterns.[63] Both respective sleep stages have been commonly reported as reduced or fragmented in patients with OSA, and their dysregulation could underlie some of the frequently reported cognitive and performance deficits in OSA patients.[27,43] In line with this argument, one study that investigated the neurocognitive deficits in OSA found that the number of microarousals during the night was the best predictor of episodic memory deficit.[64] Traditionally, obstructive events during NREM sleep have been viewed as associated with greater cognitive deficits or impaired quality of life, whereas REM sleep events have been shown to be associated with greater sympathetic activity, arterial hypertension, and cardiovascular instability in patients with OSA.[65,66] Recently, the role for fragmented REM sleep in spatial navigational memory in OSA patients has been addressed with a physiologically relevant stimulus.[67] During this study, patients spent two different nights in the laboratory, during which they performed timed trials, before and after sleep, on one of two unique three-dimensional spatial mazes.[67] Normal consolidation of sleep was achieved with use of therapeutic CPAP throughout the first night, whereas during the second night CPAP was reduced only during the REM stages. Patients showed improvements in maze performance after a night of normal sleep, but those improvements were significantly reduced following a night of isolated REM disruption, without changes in psychomotor vigilance. Noted cognitive improvements were positively correlated with the mean REM run duration across both sleep conditions.[67]

It has been argued that the sense of excessive daytime sleepiness and of feeling unrefreshed in the morning in some OSA patients could be due to the inability to augment NREM SWA or REM sleep. Moreover, in some OSA patients, reduction of REM sleep can lead to dissociation of REM traits with other sleep stages, further affecting critical sleep windows for memory formation and consolidation.[12] Equally, it has been shown that when high homeostatic demands are not fully met during sleep, in the subsequent wake period microsleeps can occur in highly active regions of the brain[68] and can lead to concomitant disability for the function subserved by that region.[50,68] To what degree this takes place in OSA patients and whether this also contributes to attention-vigilance dysfunction and the higher frequency of traffic accidents noted for this patient group are yet to be fully defined.[13] Previously reported retarded SWA decay throughout the night, even in patients with mild OSA, further supports the notion of nonrestorative sleep in OSA.[62]

Several recent studies have aimed to discern the role of sleep in cognition and cognitive decline, with potential effect on the way we consider sleep in patients with OSA. For example, as depicted in Figure 23-3, *A*, it has been suggested that the amount of atrophy in the medial prefrontal cortex (mPFC), predicts the extent of disrupted slow wave (N3) sleep in older people, and consequent impaired overnight episodic hippocampal memory consolidation.[51,69] The mPFC area has been shown to be independently affected by OSA (see Figure 23-1) and has been known to be involved in the generation of slow waves.[13,69] It has been proposed that improving slow wave sleep in older adults (irrespective of their OSA status) may represent a novel treatment for minimizing cognitive decline in later life.[69]

The importance of sleep spindles in cognition has also gained interest over the past several years.[13,70] It has been shown that, during the night, OSA patients, unlike healthy controls, display a significant proportion of slow spindles in the frontal, central, and parietal regions.[60] One recent study has shown that older adults who express fewer prefrontal fast sleep spindles also exhibit a proportional impairment in hippocampal functioning during the subsequent wake periods and, with that impairment, a deficit in the ability to form new episodic memories.[71] Fast sleep spindles represent part of a coordinated NREM sleep–dependent memory mechanism, and it is thought that hippocampal sharp-wave ripples provide feedback excitation, which initiates neuroplasticity in spindle-activated cortical neurons.[51] Relative to slow sleep spindles, fast sleep spindle activity is associated with greater hippocampal activation and greater hippocampal-cortical functional connectivity.[2,71] The sleep architecture of even mild OSA patients shows a high degree of sleep fragmentation, which results in a different time course of SWA and a decreased sleep spindle index compared with controls.[62] Whether this deregulated spindle formation and activity present another contributory facet to cognitive complaints in patients in OSA, however, remains a conjecture at this point. Nonetheless, taken together, these studies suggest a possible role for OSA-induced brain injury in the acceleration, or even initiation, of cognitive decline in older adults (see Figure 23-3, *A*).[1-3,31,69] The exact pathophysiology of such an association remains elusive.[13]

Mental Health and Sleep Associations in Obstructive Sleep Apnea Patients

A bidirectional relationship between sleep and the function of the brain circuitry involved in emotions is increasingly supported by studies that further build on long-standing clinical observations of co-occurring mood and sleep disorders.[13,72] Unsurprisingly, then, a variety of mental health issues, such as affective disorders, emotional lability, and depression, have been reported as highly prevalent in individuals with OSA, with some studies reporting that up to 63% of OSA individuals are so affected[73] despite considerable heterogeneity and a high risk for bias in these studies.[13] Evidence from various studies is particularly suggestive of a role for REM sleep in selective emotional memory processing and sleep-dependent emotional memory depotentiation (see Figure 23-3, *B*).[72] Moreover, REM sleep is suggested to play a role in recalibrating the sensitivity and specificity of the brain's response to emotional events, both positive and negative.[72] This recalibration effect likely occurs, at least in part, as a result of modulation of noradrenergic brainstem activity and the responsive profiles of the amygdala and mPFC, two regions critically involved in detecting emotional salience.[13,72]

Of the psychiatric disorders, the evidence for increased prevalence of OSA is particularly strong in major depressive disorder and posttraumatic stress disorder (PTSD),[74,75] both independently associated with REM sleep disturbance.[13] Even though the causal relationship between these affective disorders and OSA is unclear and is likely to be multifactorial, the potential sleep mechanics of their interaction is worthy of further consideration.[13] PTSD is independently associated with decreases in the total time spent in REM sleep. It is also associated with marked fragmentation of REM sleep, indicative of arousal-related awakenings from REM sleep linked to

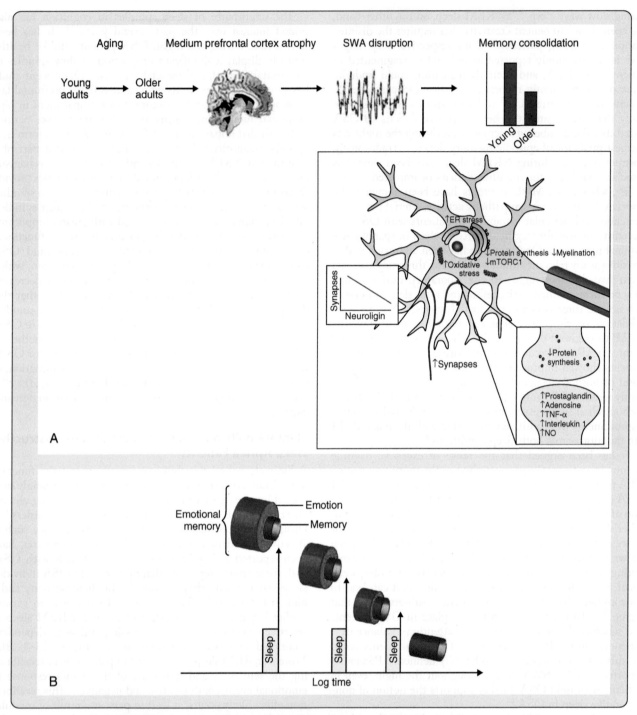

Figure 23-3 The proposed role for sleep in cognition and emotions. A, *Cognitive sleep:* Sleep apnea and aging can independently cause gray matter atrophy in the prefrontal cortex. Atrophy can mediate the degree of slow wave activity (SWA) disruption, whereas SWA in turn can mediate the degree of impaired memory retention.[69] SWA activity disruption likely also leads to cellular stress.[52] **B,** *Emotional sleep:* Conceptual schematics of "the sleep to forget and sleep to remember" model are shown, as described by Goldstein and Walker.[72] Over one or several nights and numerous repetitions of this REM mechanism, sleep transforms an emotional memory into a memory of an emotional event that is no longer emotional.[72] ER, Endoplasmic reticulum; IL-1, interleukin-1; mTORC1, mammalian target of rapamycin contact 1; NO, nitric oxide; TNF-α, tumor necrosis factor-α. (From Rosenzweig I, Glasser M, Polsek D, et al. Sleep apnoea and the brain: a complex relationship. *Lancet Respir Med* 2015;3:404–14.)

adrenergic surges.[72] CPAP adherence has been shown to be reduced in veterans with PTSD and comorbid OSA.[74] Based on the current knowledge of OSA-induced sleep deficits, it can be argued that in PTSD patients with comorbid OSA, the additive effect of sleep disturbances associated with the

OSA can further impair the quantity and quality of REM sleep. This would likely also affect the REM noradrenergic "housekeeping" function because it has been shown that REM sleep reduces, and thus likely restores, concentrations of CNS noradrenaline to baseline, allowing for optimal awake state functioning.[13,72] More specifically, several studies suggest that quiescence of locus coeruleus activity, a brainstem structure that is a source of noradrenergic input, during REM sleep throughout the night restores the appropriate next-day tonic-phasic response specificity within the emotional salience network (e.g., locus coeruleus, amygdala, mPFC).[72] It is hence feasible that OSA-induced REM fragmentation could further aggravate the hyperadrenergic state of some PTSD patients and lead to decreased connectivity between the PFC and amygdala and thus exaggerated amygdala reactivity.[72] The functional outcome may be an aggravated disease course and worse prognosis.[13,72] Of note, in the prospective Honolulu-Asia Aging Study, in which men (n = 3801) ages 71 to 93 years at baseline (1991) were followed until their death, higher nocturnal oxygenation during REM sleep was associated with less gliosis and neuronal loss in the locus coeruleus.[58]

Major depression, on the other hand, is associated with exaggerated REM sleep qualities and deficiency in monoamine activity.[72] The bidirectional-dual relationship between major depression and OSA has been suggested by findings of several studies.[31] In some OSA patients, fragmented REM sleep can precipitate a vicious cycle of impaired REM regulation and rebound REM augmentation.[13] This, along with concomitant changes in neurotransmitter systems caused by hypoxemia, could further lead to reduced monoamine activity, with associated increased negative rumination and ensuing depression, in genetically predisposed individuals.[13] Through its effects on REM sleep, comorbid OSA might also lead to dysfunctional consolidation and depotentiation of emotional memory from prior affective experiences.[13,72] It has been proposed that this may result in a condition of chronic anxiety within autobiographic memory networks (see Figure 23-3, B).[72] In support of this recent meta-analysis of randomized controlled trials of treatment of OSA, a significant improvement in depressive symptoms was reported.[76]

Even though the previously argued theoretical constructs of a bidirectional relationship between fragmented or disturbed sleep in OSA and psychiatric disorders are indirectly supported by animal and neuroimaging studies of sleep,[72] the underlying mechanics are likely to be more complex and, as such, require further well-designed studies.[13]

NEUROINFLAMMATION AND ISCHEMIC PRECONDITIONING

Cognitive and emotional complaints of OSA patients may also be explained by oxidative and neuroinflammatory effects of OSA on the CNS emotional salience network.[10,13,31] In OSA, repetitive occlusions of the upper airway lead to intermittent hypoxia and recurrent hypoxemia, typically characterized by short cycles of hypoxemia and reoxygenation.[20] However, the patterns vary greatly among patients, and, depending on the idiosyncratic characteristics of each individual, the end results might be either adaptive or maladaptive.[20] The outcome will likely depend on the dynamic interplay between the specific type and amount of reactive oxygen-nitrogen species produced, duration and frequency of such production, the intracellular localization, and microenvironmental antioxidant activity.[11] Additional interplay depends on factors such as genetic makeup, nutrition, and other lifestyle-related variables, all of which affect the redox status.[11,20] A variety of studies to date suggest that the severity of hypoxia,

its duration, and its cycle frequency are fundamental determinants of outcomes (Figure 23-4, A).[77,78] For example, it has been generally acknowledged that short, mild, and lower cycle frequencies of intermittent hypoxia may generate beneficial and adaptive responses in the brain, such as ischemic preconditioning.[20] Conversely, chronic, moderate to severe, and high-frequency intermittent hypoxia can induce maladaptive disruption of homeostatic mechanisms, leading to dysfunction and sterile neuroinflammation.[11,20]

Ischemic preconditioning represents a generalized adaptation to ischemia by a variety of cells.[21,79] In OSA, induction of ischemic preconditioning is thought to be due to the activation of several gene programs, including the hypoxia inducible factor-1, vascular endothelial growth factor, erythropoietin, atrial natriuretic peptide, and brain-derived neurotrophic factor.[80,81] Various end mechanisms and pathways have been shown to play a role in preconditioning, including those of long-term facilitation of phrenic motor output, chemoreflex activation, vascular remodeling, neo-angiogenesis, productive autophagy, reactive gliosis, various synaptic alterations, and modulation of adult hippocampal neurogenesis.[11,82,83] CPAP treatment of OSA has been shown to partially reverse structural imaging changes in gray matter of hippocampal regions and to ameliorate some of the associated cognitive deficits, possibly also by modulating adult neurogenesis.[84] In a recent neuroimaging study, coexistence of hypotrophic and hypertrophic changes in the brain of OSA patients was taken to reflect the evolving nature of OSA-associated brain injury.[36] It has been proposed that at any given time ongoing maladaptive neuroinflammatory processes likely exist alongside adaptive mechanisms of increased brain plasticity and ischemic preconditioning.[13] As a corollary to these findings, in a recent study that compared the cognitive performance of patients with high and low levels of OSA-related hypoxemia, controlling for demographic factors and other aspects of OSA severity, an unexpected advantage of higher levels of hypoxemia on memory was demonstrated in a carefully matched clinical cohort.[85]

Several studies also suggest that, under certain conditions, intermittent hypoxia can increase immune defenses without exacerbating inflammation.[11,20] Moreover, in animals, short-lasting hypoxic exposures mimicking OSA have been associated with recruitment of bone marrow–derived pluripotent stem cells, which exhibited upregulation of stem cell differentiation pathways, particularly involving CNS development and angiogenesis.[20]

Another powerful central neuroprotective adaptive mechanism for ischemic events has been demonstrated following the activation of the intrinsic neurons of the cerebellar fastigial nucleus.[86] Neurostimulation of these nuclei appears to provide "protective" reduced excitability of cortical neurons during subsequent ischemic episodes and to lead to reduced immunoreactivity of cerebral microvessels.[10] Also, a "compensatory" entraining of cerebellum by hypertrophic hippocampi has been proposed to occur in some younger patients with mild OSA.[36] Although there are no direct monosynaptic anatomic connections between hippocampi and cerebellum, their connectivity is thought to be important for the control of movement under states of heightened emotion and novel conditions and for associative learning.[10,13] Failed adaptation of cerebellar networks to injury, of any etiology, has been shown to lead to cognitive deficits and hyperactivity, distractibility, ruminative behaviors, dysphoria, and depression in some patients.[10,32]

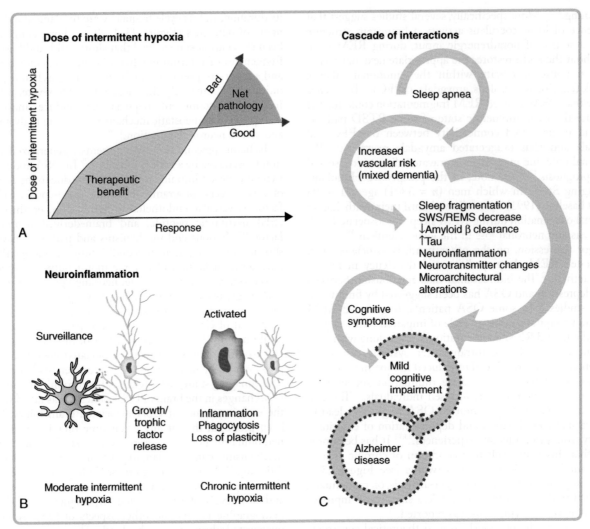

Figure 23-4 Adaptive and maladaptive processes induced by intermittent hypoxia. **A,** Conceptual presentation of the net effect of cycles of intermittent hypoxia, of varied length and frequency, over a period of time (minutes to days to weeks), as described by Dale and colleagues.[78] High doses still elicit neuroadaptive mechanisms, but the balance is shifted and maladaptive processes such as neuroinflammation **(B)** are likely to be instigated. Finding an optimal dose is key to developing effective treatment.[78] **C,** Possible cascade of interactions between sleep apnea and Alzheimer disease. (From Rosenzweig I, Glasser M, Polsek D, et al. Sleep apnoea and the brain: a complex relationship. *Lancet Respir Med* 2015;3:404–14.)

Neuroinflammation in Obstructive Sleep Apnea

There are, however, relevant maladaptive effects of intermittent hypoxia.[13] These include neuroinflammation, and, although the exact neurocellular sources for associated processes are still incompletely defined, activation of astroglia is likely to be important.[11,13,78] In addition, oligodendrocytes, myelin-producing cells of the CNS, have been shown to be selectively sensitive to hypoxia and sleep fragmentation.[87,88] The subsequent loss of buffering functions can ultimately contribute to pathologic processes, such as increased glial proliferation and microglial activation (see Figure 23-4, *B*).[13,78] Astroglial and microglial cells play critical roles in regional blood flow regulation and inflammatory processes in the brain, as well as critical coordination of bioenergetics through lactate transport.[78] Under normal conditions, microglia in the healthy CNS exhibit a surveillance phenotype that synthe-

sizes and releases neuroprotective growth and trophic factors.[78] However, severe and prolonged hypoxia can activate microglia toward a toxic, proinflammatory phenotype that triggers pathology, including hippocampal apoptosis, impaired synaptic plasticity, and cognitive impairment.[78] Neuroinflammation has been shown to independently increase the brain's sensitivity to stress, resulting in stress-related neuropsychiatric disorders, such as anxiety and depression.[13,89] Dynamic changes in transcription of inflammatory genes have been demonstrated following exposure to intermittent hypoxia.[13,78] Increased prostaglandin E_2 neural tissue concentrations have also been demonstrated in hippocampal and cortical regions accompanied by lipid peroxidation of polyunsaturated fatty acids.[78] Similarly, it has been shown that increased carbonylation- and nitrosylation-induced oxidative injury emerges in susceptible brain regions following exposure to intermittent hypoxia and promotes excessive daytime somnolence.[11,78] Recently, toll-like receptor 4 (TLR4) expression and activity have been demonstrated to be increased on monocytes of patients with OSA.[90] Similarly, ligands for TLR4 have been shown to be increased in the serum of children with OSA.[13,90] The microglia of the cortex and brainstem exhibit TLR4 expression after chronic intermittent hypoxia, when it is postulated to play a region-specific and differential (adaptive or maladaptive) role.[13,90] This finding is of particular interest because TLR4 has also been strongly implicated in several inflammatory and neurodegenerative disorders, including vascular dementia and Alzheimer disease.[90] In cognitively healthy adults, intermittent hypoxia has been correlated with increases in phosphorylated and total tau and amyloid β^{42} concentrations in cerebral spinal fluid, key components of Alzheimer pathology.[1,13] Similarly, cerebral amyloidogenesis and tau phosphorylation, along with neuronal degeneration and axonal dysfunction, have been demonstrated in the cortex and brainstem of animals exposed to intermittent hypoxia.[2] Taken together, these findings support the role for neuroinflammatory processes in cognitive and emotional deficits of OSA patients. They further suggest a close association between hypoxemia-induced maladaptive processes and dementia (see Figure 23-4, *C*).[13]

NEUROLOGIC DISORDERS AND COGNITIVE AND PERFORMANCE DEFICITS ASSOCIATED WITH OBSTRUCTIVE SLEEP APNEA

Several neurologic disorders have been associated with OSA.[10] For example, adults with epilepsy appear at increased risk for OSA.[91] Conversely, OSA is a recognized independent risk factor for stroke.[10] OSA has been associated with seizure exacerbations in older adults with epilepsy, and treatment with CPAP may represent an important avenue for improving seizure control in this population.[10,92,93] OSA-induced brain injury is believed to exacerbate neural damage during incident stroke as well as to increase the risk for a subsequent stroke.[94,95]

Additionally, an increasing body of evidence from animal studies suggests that cerebral amyloidogenesis and tau phosphorylation, two cardinal features of Alzheimer disease, can be triggered by intermittent hypoxia.[2] Intermittent hypoxia and associated generation of reactive oxygen species, known to occur during nocturnal apneic episodes, have been shown to initiate neuronal degeneration and axonal dysfunction in the cortex and brainstem of animals.[2,10] Also, oligodendrocytes, myelin-producing cells of the CNS, are selectively sensitive to hypoxia and sleep fragmentation.[10,88] However, it is not clear to what extent this particular vulnerability contributes to the widely reported hypotrophic white matter changes in the brains of some OSA patients, including the fornices and corpus callosum.[10,96,97] Impaired learning capabilities have been documented in children with OSA, along with increased hyperactivity and incidence of attention deficit disorders.[8] On the other end of the age spectrum, as noted earlier, several clinical studies have suggested that older patients with OSA might suffer accelerated brain atrophy, cognitive decline, and the onset and severity of dementia.[77,98,99]

It has been estimated that approximately 80% of OSA patients complain of both excessive daytime sleepiness and cognitive impairment, and half also report personality changes.[34] However, the exact prevalence of neurocognitive

deficits in patients with OSA remains unknown. One in four patients with newly diagnosed OSA has appreciable neuropsychological impairments.[34,100] Various studies suggest that memory impairments can be found in up to 9% of OSA subjects; 2% to 25% have problems with sustained attention, and 15% to 42% demonstrate difficulties with executive functioning.[34,101] Moreover, the increased frequency of work-related and traffic accidents in OSA patients may be taken as a surrogate indicator of neurobehavioral performance deficits.[34,102,103] Patients with OSA are 37 times more likely to complain of sleepiness compared with nonsnoring healthy controls. Work limitation in terms of difficulties with time management, mental tasks, interpersonal relationships, and work output have all been associated with excessive daytime sleepiness.[34] OSA patients are 7.5 times more likely to have difficulties with concentration at work, have a ninefold increase in difficulty learning new tasks, and are 20 times more likely to have problems performing monotonous tasks.[34,104] In addition, occupational accidents have been reported to occur in 50% of male OSA patients, whereas the risk for occupational accidents in women with OSA has been reported as six times greater than in controls.[34,102,105]

Of particular note is the finding that motor vehicle drivers, regardless of OSA status, do not always perceive their impairment and continue to drive while sleepy.[34,106] Overall, compared with normal controls, OSA patients are 2 to 13 times more likely to experience a driving-related traffic accident.[107] Such accidents are more likely to occur in those who manifest greater daytime sleepiness.[34,107] However, OSA has also been associated with motor vehicle crashes independent of daytime sleepiness.[108] Sleepiness due to work schedules and sleepiness due to OSA are independent risk factors for accidents.[34] For example, in commercial vehicle drivers, in whom both of these sleepiness-promoting conditions coexist, those with the highest level of sleepiness have a twofold increase in multiple accidents.[109] The data for OSA and automobile crashes are numerous and consistent: as a group, OSA patients' risk for motor vehicle collisions is increased twofold to fourfold (Videos 23-1 and 23-2).[34] On driving simulators, OSA patients hit more obstacles, have increased error in tracking and visual search, have increased response time to secondary stimuli, and drive out of bounds more times compared with non-OSA control subjects (Figure 23-5).[110] Still, not all OSA patients who drive have accidents, and as many as two thirds never have a collision.[106,110] A means to identify OSA patients at greatest risk for motor vehicle collisions is still not clear

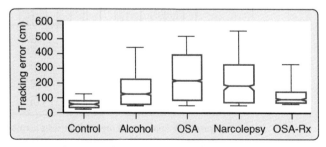

Figure 23-5 Summary of tracking errors in different groups on the Divided Attention Driving Task. *OSA,* Obstructive sleep apnea. (From George CF. Vigilance impairment: assessment by driving simulators. *Sleep* 2000; 23[Suppl. 4]:S115–18.)

based on available literature, and this complicates decision making from a medical and legal perspective.[34]

ASSESSMENT OF COGNITIVE AND NEUROBEHAVIORAL PERFORMANCE DEFICITS IN OBSTRUCTIVE SLEEP APNEA

To understand the cognitive and neurobehavioral performance deficits that affect patients with OSA, it is helpful to consider these from a categorical perspective.[34] The effects of sleep loss on performance include changes in cognitive performance, difficulty with working memory, slowing of response or inability to sustain attention across the duration of the task, declines in best effort or fastest response, lapses, and false responses.[34,111] As noted earlier, in OSA, hypoxemia-reoxygenation cycles with attendant biochemical and cellular alterations cause dysfunction of the prefrontal cortex, among other CNS regions.[34] This results in impaired executive function manifesting as false responses, problems with working memory and contextual memory, problems with cognitive processing in addition to deficits in the pattern of responses, and self-regulation of affect and arousal.[33,34] A description of the performance deficits and commonly used assessment techniques in OSA patients is given in Box 23-1.[34] Tests that can readily be performed in the clinical setting include the Digit Symbol Substitution Task (90-second test) to assess cognitive processing and the Psychomotor Vigilance Task (10-minute task) to evaluate the ability to sustain attention.[34] Summary information regarding the neurobehavioral tests may be found elsewhere.[112] The effects of OSA on cognitive processing, memory, sustained attention, and executive and

motor functioning are further shown in Figure 23-6, which reports the effects of OSA in patients relative to healthy adults.[34]

An additional issue to consider when assessing patients with OSA is their subjective cognitive and emotional complaints.[13] A detailed analysis of important studies in the field has suggested only a weak correlation between (subjective) cognitive complaints in patients with OSA and their objective cognitive functioning.[13,113] Divergent results of subjective versus objective complaints have been recognized in other medical populations, and several possible explanations for this in OSA patients have been suggested.[13] For example, an insufficient specificity of current tests for deficits documented in OSA is evident and largely acknowledged. Currently used and validated objective tests for cognition are frequently designed to assess deficits found in patients with traumatic brain injury and as such do not specifically assess impairments in OSA-induced brain injury.[13,113] Cognitive domains are not unitary constructs, and only the carefully deconstructed analysis of their different subcapacities and their vulnerabilities to a range of risks and protective factors specific to OSA can provide a more realistic assessment of an individual's disability.[13,16] Similarly, a number of impairments may be secondary to other symptoms of OSA, such as sleepiness itself, or they can be a sign of psychological distress.[113,114]

To date, subjective cognitive complaints have been largely ignored in randomized controlled trials of treatments for OSA patients. However, given that subjective cognitive complaints are linked to the quality of life, work productivity, and health care utilization of patients, it is important that future studies account for these.[113]

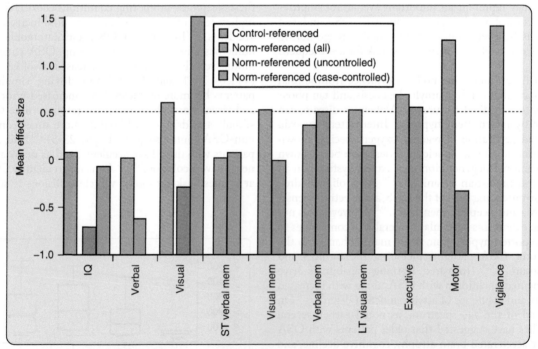

Figure 23-6 Summary of mean effect sizes across domains and data sets. Positive values indicate deficits relative to healthy adults, and negative values indicate strengths relative to healthy adults. The data set for moderate intelligence and visual functioning is split into case-controlled and uncontrolled samples for domains where study design (case-controlled versus uncontrolled) moderated the data. ST Mem, Short-term memory; LT Mem, long-term memory. (Modified from Beebe DW, Groesz L, Wells C, et al. The neuropsychological effects of obstructive sleep apnea: a meta-analysis of norm-referenced and case-controlled data. *Sleep* 2003;26:298–307, p. 302.)

Box 23-1 DEFINITION AND ASSESSMENT OF COGNITIVE AND NEUROBEHAVIORAL DEFICITS ASSOCIATED WITH OBSTRUCTIVE SLEEP APNEA

Cognitive Processing

Behavior

Decreased ability to digest information
- Slowing on task
- Increased errors
- Decline in total number correct and/or completed per unit of time

Measures Commonly Used to Assess Deficit

Self-paced tasks of short duration (1 to 5 minutes), including arithmetic calculations, communication, or concept attainment
- Paced Auditory Serial Addition Task (PASAT)
- Trail Making Test Parts A and B: sequencing numbers (A) or letters and numbers (B)
- Category Test: six sets of items organized around different principles with a seventh set comprising previously shown items
- Digit Symbol Substitution Test: supplying matching symbol given the corresponding number
- Digit Backward: stating verbally provided numbers in reverse order
- Letter Cancellation: cancellation of target alphabets from presentation of randomized alphabets

Memory

Behavior

Decreased ability to register, store, retain, and retrieve information

Measures Commonly Used to Assess Deficit

Short-term memory: timed tasks of up to 10 minutes that require free recall of words, numbers, paragraphs, or figures
- Probed, Recall Memory Task (words)
- Digit Span Forward (numbers)
- Wechsler Memory Scale Story Task (paragraph)
- Rey Auditory-Verbal Learning Test (figure)
Long-term memory: presenting the subject with lists of items that are longer than the seven-item memory capacity
- California Verbal Learning Test
Procedural memory: gradual acquisition and maintenance of motor skills and procedures
- Mirror Tracing Task
- Rotary Pursuit Task

Sustained Attention or Vigilance

Behavior

Inability to maintain attention over time.
- Slowing of response time (time on task)
- Increased errors

- Reduction in the fastest optimal response times
- Periods of delayed or no response (lapses)
- Response to stimuli when none presented (false responses)

Measures Commonly Used to Assess Deficit

Short-duration tasks (30 minutes)
- Psychomotor Vigilance Task (PVT)
- Four Choice Reaction Time Test
- Steer Clear
- Continuous performance tests

Divided Attention

Behavior

Inability to respond to more than one task or stimuli, such as with driving

Measures Commonly Used to Assess Deficit

Divided Attention Driving Test (DADT): mimics vigilant-related behavior essential to driving
- Tracking (the ability to stay within the driving lane)
- Visual search (looking for and avoiding obstacles, traffic lights, etc.)

Executive Functioning

Behavior

Problems with manipulating and processing information
Inadequate planning and execution of plans
Disorganization: poor judgment, decision making
Inflexible: emotional liability
Impulsivity
Difficulty maintaining motivation

Measures Commonly Used to Assess Deficit

Volition component or intentional behavior
- Assessed by asking the patients' preferences, what they like to do, or what makes them angry
Planning component
- Porteus Maze Test
- Tower Tests: Tower of London, Tower of Toronto, Tower of Hanoi
- Wisconsin Card Sorting Test
Purposive action
- Tinkertoy Test
Effective performance
- Random Generation Task

Modified from Dinges D. Probing the limits of functional capability: the effects of sleep loss on short-duration tasks. In: Broughton R, Ogilvie R, editors. *Sleep, arousal, and performance.* Boston: Birkhauser; 1992. p. 177–188.

EFFECT OF OBSTRUCTIVE SLEEP APNEA TREATMENT ON ASSOCIATED NEUROCOGNITIVE DEFICITS AND DISORDERS

Nonpharmacologic and pharmacologic treatments for OSA have been shown to improve cognitive outcomes in OSA patient subpopulations, as described in Chapter 16. The results of several meta-analyses suggest that CPAP treatment reduces sleepiness complaints and mood problems and that it improves objective cognitive functioning in OSA patients.[14,15,113,115,116] However, many questions regarding treatment with CPAP, the most pivotal of which are to whom, when, and for how long should CPAP treatment be administered, remain to be clarified.[13] The optimal treatment protocols, likely in combination with other lifestyle or pharmacologic approaches, may only be achieved once the full spectrum of the neuropathology of OSA and its dynamic fingerprinting are understood.[9,10,13] For example, it has been shown that in some treatment-compliant patients, the beneficial effect of CPAP on symptoms of sleepiness and sleep quality can be obtained after only few days of treatment. On the other hand, the effects on other subjective and objective cognitive symptoms are less well defined, and in to provide similar therapeutic effects, much longer duration of treatment may be required.[110,117] Two recent studies suggest that prolonged treatment might in fact be required in patients with severe OSA.[118,119] In one of these, an almost complete recovery of white matter tract pathology in patients with severe OSA was demonstrated in association with significant improvement in memory, attention, and executive functioning, only when 1 year of CPAP adherence was achieved.[118] The functional neuroanatomy of OSA has been highlighted in a study that documented that 3 months of treatment with CPAP improved cognitive function in several domains that corresponded to gray matter volume increases in frontal and hippocampal regions.[84] Most studies investigating treatments for OSA, however, fail to account for incomplete reversal of tissue damage or deficits in cognition, suggesting that early initiation of a prolonged treatment regimen might be necessary to optimize improvements in the neurocognitive disease process associated with OSA.[120-122]

The need for a longer duration of treatment with CPAP in elderly patients compared with younger patients has been suggested by the findings of a small pilot study that found that treatment of severe OSA in Alzheimer disease patients of mild to moderate severity was associated with significantly slower cognitive decline over 3 years.[119] Further, 1 year of CPAP treatment has been shown to improve sleepiness and quality of life in older people with OSA.[19]

Although less striking, limited evidence with drugs such as donepezil, physostigmine, and fluticasone also points to better cognitive outcomes in treated patients, likely necessitating longer treatments.[123,124] Pharmacologic treatment may also be required in patients with OSA who, despite adequate CPAP use, continue to complain of residual sleepiness.[125] It has been suggested that, among the most common explanations for persistent sleepiness in OSA patients, low CPAP compliance, inadequate CPAP titration leading to residual respiratory events and sleep fragmentation, mask or mouth leaks, treatment emergent central sleep apnea, behaviorally induced insufficient sleep syndrome, comorbid psychiatric disorders, sedative medication use, and undiagnosed coexisting sleep disorders predominate.[126] However, it has been recognized that some compliant CPAP users can still experience excessive daytime somnolence even after sleep hygiene improvement, optimization of CPAP treatment, and comorbid disorders management, and those patients are then considered as suffering from true residual sleepiness.[126] Although its pathophysiologic mechanisms remain unclear based on retrospective studies, the prevalence of such residual sleepiness can be estimated at approximately 10%.[126]

In clinical cases in which sleepiness is deemed severe enough to require treatment with an alerting drug, an objective evaluation at baseline should be done. This will allow for proper assessment of vigilance on treatment.[126] Of alerting drugs commonly used in other sleep disorders, modafinil and armodafinil have been shown to have some effects on CPAP-resistant sleepiness.[126] A recent meta-analysis of the effect of modafinil and armodafinil in patients with residual sleepiness suggested improved objective and subjective measures of sleepiness, wakefulness, and patients' perception of disease severity, with overall good tolerance and minimal side effects.[125] Moreover, a trend toward decreased CPAP after treatment with these agents was also observed.[125] Methylphenidate,[126] dexamphetamine, venlafaxine, and atomoxetine are yet to be tested specifically for this indication. Clinical trials of residual sleepiness treatment with histamine-3 receptor agonists are underway and may provide a useful alternative in countries where modafinil and armodafinil are not approved for the treatment of residual sleepiness.[127] Future large prospective studies are required to better define predictive baseline characteristics and possible causal mechanisms for residual sleepiness as well as to inform and guide clinicians in choosing the most appropriate pharmacologic treatments.

CLINICAL PEARLS

OSA is increasingly recognized as one of the potentially modifiable risk factors for cognitive and performance deficits and dementia in adults. During untreated apnea-hypopnea episodes, intermittent hypoxemia, reoxygenation, and hypercapnia or hypocapnia occur, along with sleep fragmentation and changes in cerebral blood flow. These may, independently and in combination, result in cognitive deficits and reduced daytime performance, with functional consequences for work and school efficiency. Clinician awareness of these impairments and their prompt treatment will reduce the burden of illness on the individual patient with OSA as well as the public health risk.

SUMMARY

Patients with OSA demonstrate variable degrees of cognitive and performance deficits. Such deficits are more easily identified in those with more severe OSA.[34] The long-term effectiveness of CPAP with regard to reducing cognitive and performance deficits in patients with mild OSA remains undetermined and needs further exploration.[34] The disruption of normal sleep physiology by OSA has been increasingly recognized as an underappreciated factor regarding such deficits, which, together with hypoxemia and other already recognized factors, may further aggravate age-related memory deficits in patients with OSA.[2,3,69,71] Clinically, this dynamic interplay underscores numerous subjective and objective cognitive and emotional complaints in some patients.[13,31,72] An understanding of the proportional effect of these factors in each individual OSA patient is a major challenge because they typically occur simultaneously and, in all likelihood, target similar neurocircuitry.[13] Persistent deficits, even after prolonged treatment with CPAP in some patients, suggest that early detection of the CNS sequelae in OSA is vital so that appropriate treatment can be administered before irreversible atrophic and metabolic changes occur. However, the optimal timing and duration of treatment and the optimal treatment population are still unclear and must be addressed in future prospective randomized controlled trials.[13] Studies discussed in this chapter strongly suggest that tapping into the therapeutic potential of ischemic preconditioning, while working on ameliorating the acute and chronic effects of neuroinflammation, may offer legitimate therapeutic targets in OSA.[2,11,78] Similarly, although they are in their infancy, studies of clinical approaches that target the sleep disturbance factors of this intricate equation advocate a significant future treatment intervention potential.[13]

Despite the need for more evidence regarding cognitive and performance deficits in community-acquired samples in sham CPAP–controlled studies, there is significant documentation that untreated and CPAP nonadherent OSA patients are at risk for traffic and occupational accidents.[34] Recent findings also raise valid questions about the mechanics of associations between OSA and dementia and further highlight the public health importance of detecting and targeting patients with OSA at highest risk for cognitive decline.

ACKNOWLEDGMENTS

Supported by the Wellcome Trust [103952/Z/14/Z] and the NIHR Respiratory Biomedical Research Unit at the Royal Brompton and Harefield NHS Foundation Trust, Imperial College, London.

Selected Readings

Dalmases M, Solé-Padullés C, Torres M, et al. Effect of CPAP on cognition, brain function and structure among elderly patients with obstructive sleep apnea: a randomized pilot study. *Chest* 2015;**148**(5):1214–23.

Ferini-Strambi L, Marelli S, Galbiati A, et al. Effects of continuous positive airway pressure on cognition and neuroimaging data in sleep apnea. *Int J Psychophysiol* 2013;**89**(2):203–12.

Gagnon K, Baril AA, Gagnon JF, et al. Cognitive impairment in obstructive sleep apnea. *Pathol Biol (Paris)* 2014;**62**(5):233–40.

Harper RM, Kumar R, Ogren JA, et al. Sleep-disordered breathing: effects on brain structure and function. *Respir Physiol Neurobiol* 2013;**188**(3):383–91.

Kheirandish-Gozal L, Yoder K, Kulkarni R, et al. Preliminary functional MRI neural correlates of executive functioning and empathy in children with obstructive sleep apnea. *Sleep* 2014;**37**(3):587–92.

Kilpinen R, Saunamäki T, Jehkonen M. Information processing speed in obstructive sleep apnea syndrome: a review. *Acta Neurol Scand* 2014;**129**(4):209–18.

Kim H, Joo E, Suh S, et al. Effects of long-term treatment on brain volume in patients with obstructive sleep apnea syndrome. *Hum Brain Mapp* 2016;**37**(1):395–409.

Lal C, Siddiqi N, Kumbhare S, Strange C. Impact of medications on cognitive function in obstructive sleep apnea syndrome. *Sleep Breath* 2015;**19**(3):939–45.

Lim DC, Pack AI. Obstructive sleep apnea and cognitive impairment: addressing the blood-brain barrier. *Sleep Med Rev* 2014;**18**(1):35–48.

Olaithe M, Bucks RS. Executive dysfunction in OSA before and after treatment: a meta-analysis. *Sleep* 2013;**36**(9):1297–305.

Stranks EK, Crowe SF. The Cognitive Effects of Obstructive Sleep Apnea: An Updated Meta-analysis. *Arch Clin Neuropsychol* 2016;pii: acv087.

Zhu Y, Fenik P, Zhan G, et al. Degeneration in arousal neurons in chronic sleep disruption modeling sleep apnea. *Front Neurol* 2015;**6**:109.

A complete reference list can be found online at ExpertConsult.com.

Obstructive Sleep Apnea and Metabolic Disorders

Mary Sau-Man Ip

Chapter Highlights

- With the common risk factor of obesity, obstructive sleep apnea (OSA) and metabolic disorders often coexist. Obesity itself is considered a metabolic disease. With global escalation of obesity trends, the current and future health care burdens of these conditions are of immense concern.

- OSA produces intermittent hypoxia and sleep disruption, with evidence for downstream cascades of sympathetic activation, oxidative stress, and inflammation—pathways that align with the pathogenetic mechanisms in metabolic disorders.

- Growing epidemiologic and clinical evidence suggests that OSA may modulate metabolic outcomes. The confounding effects of obesity on metabolic disorders have, however, been difficult to dissect. Of greater clinical relevance may be potential synergistic effects between OSA and obesity, mediated partly

through exacerbation of adipose tissue dysfunction.

- Animal and cell-based studies, mostly using intermittent hypoxia regimens as a surrogate model of OSA in humans, have provided evidence for deleterious effects on various tissues and cells in the pathogenesis of metabolic dysfunction and have elucidated relevant molecular pathways.

- Despite suggestive data from human observational studies, no definitive evidence has yet emerged to indicate that controlling OSA would result in improvement in metabolic function of significant clinical impact. Future studies need to address the challenges of small heterogeneous samples, diverse methodology for metabolic evaluation, and issues regarding withholding treatment for symptomatic OSA for substantial periods in longitudinal cohort follow-up or in randomized controlled studies.

Sleep modulates body metabolism, and sleep restriction or disturbance can have negative metabolic effects. Although each metabolic disorder has specific pathogenetic pathways, all share common grounds of engagement of hormones, oxidative stress, and inflammation, with obesity as a prevalent phenotypic feature.[1,2] Recurrent obstructed breathing events in obstructive sleep apnea (OSA) characteristically result in repeated cycles of hypoxia-reoxygenation with consequent disruption of sleep architecture, which may trigger downstream cascades that align with the mediating mechanisms for cardiometabolic dysfunction.[3,4] Hence, beyond the common link of obesity in the close partnership between OSA and metabolic disorders, great interest has focused on the potential role of OSA in the causation or aggravation of metabolic dysfunction per se, or in concert with other factors.

The metabolic network is one of intricate cross-talk among various organs, tissues, and cells and their respective signaling pathways. Thus the relationship between OSA and metabolic disorders is unlikely to comprise a set of discrete, one-to-one unidirectional connections but rather can be depicted as a complex network with interplay of various organs and tissues, along with multiple positive or negative feedback mechanisms.[1,2,5] Furthermore, metabolic function is subject to genetic as well as behavioral influences such as dietary intake and physical exercise, and these factors contribute to individual metabolic outcomes in persons with and without OSA.

OBSTRUCTIVE SLEEP APNEA AND METABOLIC DYSREGULATION: PATHOGENESIS AND MECHANISMS

Obesity and Adiposity

With advances in the understanding of adipose tissue biology, fat tissue, which traditionally has been viewed as a storage depot of energy, is now known as an active system with autocrine, paracrine, and endocrine functions, propagating signals to entrain metabolic cooperation of other organs and tissues.[2,5] Under conditions of positive energy balance, fat accumulates, and its distribution is crucial to health outcomes. Visceral fat in particular becomes dysfunctional, with altered nonesterified free fatty acid metabolism which may contribute to hepatic insulin resistance, dyslipidemia, and altered release of adipocytokines which are mediators of dysmetabolism.[2,6] The expansion of adipose tissue with hypertrophied adipocytes may cause cellular hypoxia, and oxidative stress and inflammation, initiating adipose tissue dysfunction.[6] Obesity is thus characterized by a state of chronic low-grade systemic and adipose tissue inflammation, fueling cardiometabolic dysfunction.[5,6,7]

Adiposity holds a unique role in the consideration of links between OSA and metabolic disorders. It is well established that obesity is a major risk factor for various metabolic disorders and a key component of the metabolic syndrome.[2,7]

Furthermore, obesity is now considered a metabolic disease in itself, with many systemic manifestations.[8] Obesity carries major public health impact, and its prevalence is escalating globally.[9] Obesity is the most common risk factor for OSA, although BMI accounts for only a small part of the variability of OSA severity as reflected in the apnea-hypopnea index (AHI), implying a multifactorial nature of OSA pathogenesis.[10] OSA and its severity have been reported to be associated with central obesity (involving the neck, trunk, and abdomen) and abdominal visceral fat, more so than with BMI, particularly in men.[10-12] Apart from affecting breathing mechanics predisposing to upper airway collapse, abdominal fat is a source of the adipokine leptin, which may modulate ventilatory control and upper airway function (see Chapter 30). In parallel, obesity also is the predominant risk factor for metabolic dysfunction. In clinical practice, abdominal obesity, as measured by waist circumference, is recommended as a useful screening tool for metabolic disorders.[13] The accumulation of visceral fat may result in lipid overflow, with further ectopic fat deposition in sites such as skeletal muscle and liver, and promote insulin resistance, whereas in the pancreas, lipid excess may impair insulin secretion.[2]

In OSA, neck fat deposition is considered to be of importance in upper airway dimensions and function, promoting structural narrowing and functional collapse.[10] Neck circumference, an established predictor of OSA, also has been shown to be a novel measure of cardiometabolic risk in the Framingham data.[14] Open to speculation, however, is whether neck circumference was a surrogate marker for OSA in those data in terms of cardiometabolic risk.

Inasmuch as obesity is a common and strong risk factor for both OSA and metabolic disorders, it is not surprising that patients with OSA not uncommonly have metabolic comorbid diseases. The ongoing enigma is whether and to what extent OSA per se is involved in the causation and/or aggravation of various metabolic disorders, including obesity. It is hypothesized that OSA exerts systemic effects on different end organs and tissues, with adipose tissue as one of the targets. With its strategic position in the metabolic network, dysfunctional adipose tissue is likely to play an important role in further metabolic dysfunction in OSA.[15] Additional evidence points to a more adverse metabolic profile even in lean subjects with OSA, compared with those without OSA.[16-18] It is not known, however, if OSA may act as a factor to convert presumably metabolically healthy adipose tissue in nonobese subjects to metabolically unhealthy tissue—a mechanism that has been proposed in metabolic dysgenesis.

It has been speculated that patients with OSA are inherently predisposed to weight gain and may experience difficulty in losing weight compared with subjects without OSA,[19] possibly relating to selective differences in body metabolism regulated by hormones such as insulin, leptin, or ghrelin. Repeated apneic spells and arousals during sleep are associated with excessive daytime sleepiness, which may reduce motivation to engage in physical activity and thereby predispose affected persons to weight gain over time. Furthermore, OSA may promote abdominal obesity through increasing insulin resistance, and/or disturbing sleep quality and quantity. The presence of sleep apnea in men with central obesity was found to attenuate metabolic improvement in response to a lifestyle intervention program, compared with men without OSA.[20]

Insulin Resistance and Glucose Metabolism

The body maintains glucose homeostasis mainly through the action of insulin on various tissues. In type 1 diabetes mellitus (DM), pancreatic beta cell failure of insulin secretion is the key defect, whereas in type 2 DM, which accounts for more than 90% of cases of DM globally, insulin resistance in muscle and liver is the primary pathophysiologic defect. Insulin is secreted in response to an increase in glucose concentration and reduces glucose levels by suppressing hepatic gluconeogenesis and promoting glucose uptake in skeletal muscle and fat. With increasing insulin resistance, pancreatic beta cells respond with a compensatory increase in insulin secretion such that glucose homeostasis and a constant blood glucose level can be maintained. When this compensatory mechanism is deficient or overwhelmed, impaired glucose tolerance and overt DM ensue.[21] Although the origins of insulin resistance can be traced to genetic background, the epidemic of DM is related to the parallel epidemic of obesity and physical inactivity. Insulin resistance is closely but not exclusively linked to visceral obesity, and worsening insulin resistance may further stimulate fat accumulation and encourage ectopic fat deposition.[2]

Insulin also regulates glycogenesis, lipogenesis, and protein synthesis, and insulin resistance may occur in many cells and tissues, within which there may be selective hormone resistance for different pathways.[22] In concert with other mechanisms, insulin resistance predisposes affected patients to endothelial dysfunction, which underlies many cardiometabolic diseases.[23]

In keeping with the common factor of obesity, it is not surprising that OSA is strongly associated with the spectrum of insulin-glucose dysmetabolism. OSA may contribute independently to insulin resistance and glucose dysmetabolism through its pathophysiologic profile of intermittent hypoxia, sympathetic activation, oxidative stress, and inflammation.[3] Such data are, however, subject to accuracy and variability of research methodology. A variety of methods for the evaluation of glucose metabolism have been deployed in sleep research[24,25] (Table 24-1). To accurately measure insulin sensitivity, it is necessary to use a method that observes in some fashion the metabolic effect of insulin given intravenously. Other methods are simpler to perform, but the results are affected by any degree of beta cell failure.[26,27] Furthermore, findings from epidemiologic or clinical studies are subject to the adequate control of the confounding factors. that are not easy to accurately identify or quantify.

Lipid Metabolism and Dyslipidemia

Lipids, including cholesterol, triglycerides, and others, are transported in the body as lipoprotein complexes in body fluids (plasma, interstitial fluid, and lymph) passing into and out of tissues, and metabolized through exogenous and endogenous pathways. The exogenous pathway operates for dietary lipids absorbed through the gastrointestinal tract, transporting them to the liver and other peripheral tissues, especially fat and muscles. The endogenous pathway refers to hepatic secretion and metabolism of lipoproteins, and their transport to peripheral tissues. As noted earlier, under conditions of positive energy balance, excess fat accumulates in adipose tissue and other organs as ectopic fat.[2,15] Lipid metabolism is regulated by both genetic and nongenetic factors. Secondary changes in plasma levels of lipids occur in a variety of diseases

Table 24-1   Assessment Tools for Glucose Metabolism in Clinical Practice and Research

Test	Brief Methodology	Parameter(s) Measured	Comments
Blood glucose	Fasting venous blood sample for plasma glucose level	Fasting glucose level	Conventional test for diagnosis of DM/impaired fasting glucose
Hemoglobin A_{1c} (HbA$_{1c}$)	Spot venous blood sample for glycated hemoglobin level	Glycemic status over past 2–3 months	Used in clinical practice to assess glycemic control in past 2–3 months in DM HbA$_{1c}$ ≥6.5% is used for diagnosis of DM (ADA/WHO); HbA$_{1c}$ of 5.7%–6.4% is used for diagnosis of prediabetes (ADA) Higher levels predict worse diabetic complications
Oral glucose tolerance test (OGTT)	Oral glucose loading (75 g) followed by evaluation of 2-hour post–blood glucose loading	Impaired glucose tolerance (IGT)	2-hour glucose ≥11.1 mmol/L for diagnosis of DM 7.8–11 mmol/L for diagnosis of IGT
	Oral glucose loading followed by evaluation of glucose every 30 minutes; simultaneous insulin levels measured	Insulin sensitivity	May be reflecting insulin secretion in response to glucose loading rather than insulin sensitivity Poor test reproducibility due to variability of gastrointestinal absorption and other factors
Hyperinsulinemic euglycemic clamp	A dose-response curve for data on exogenous insulin is generated by measuring the variable infusion rate of glucose required to maintain euglycemia	Insulin sensitivity	Gold standard for assessing insulin sensitivity The steady-state rate of peripheral glucose utilization (M value) is measured as milligrams of glucose used per kilogram of body weight per minute Labor-intensive investigation
Homeostasis model assessment (HOMA)	Fasting venous blood sample with glucose and insulin measurements HOMA-IR: insulin (μU/mL) × glucose (mmol/L)/22.5	Insulin resistance: HOMA-IR	First derived from epidemiologic studies Measures basal insulin resistance and insulin secretion
	HOMA-β: [20 × insulin (μU/mL)]/ [glucose (mmol/L) − 3.5]	Insulin secretion: HOMA-β	Reflects mainly hepatic insulin resistance
Frequently sampled intravenous glucose tolerance test (FSIGT, FSIVGTT)	Fasting baseline blood glucose (and insulin), followed by frequent sampling after glucose injection (for insulin sensitivity, insulin is injected 20 minutes later) for 3 hours. A computer model describing plasma dynamics (minimal model) is applied for deriving metabolic parameters	Assesses both pancreatic beta cell secretory capacity and peripheral glucose uptake in response to the bolus IV glucose Additional information on insulin sensitivity is gained by administration of insulin 20 minutes after the glucose load	Validated for insulin sensitivity against hyperglycemic euglycemic clamp No need for on-line measurements or external control of infusion Reflects whole-body insulin sensitivity
Short insulin tolerance test (SITT)	Administration of exogenous insulin followed by monitoring of fall in blood glucose over the next 30 minutes, to derive the glucose disappearance rate	Insulin sensitivity	Validated for insulin sensitivity against hyperglycemic euglycemic clamp No need for on-line measurements or external control of infusion

ADA/WHO, American Diabetes Association/World Health Organization; DM, diabetes mellitus; IV, intravenous.
From Lam DC, Lam KS, Ip MS. Obstructive sleep apnoea, insulin resistance and adipocytokines. *Clinic Endocrinol (Oxf)* 2015;82(2):165–77.

and clinical conditions, including obesity, smoking, insulin resistance, DM, and liver disorders. Obesity is frequently, although not invariably, accompanied by hyperlipidemia. An increase in fat mass is associated with increased release of free fatty acids to the liver, where they are reesterified in hepatocytes to form triglycerides, which are then packaged for secretion back into the circulation.[2] Obesity is a predisposing factor for development of fatty liver, in which disruption of hepatic biosynthesis of lipids occurs.[15]

Dyslipidemia is a major risk factor for atherosclerosis. In the clinical setting, lipids usually are classified as total cholesterol, high-density lipoprotein cholesterol (HDL cholesterol) and low-density lipoprotein cholesterol (LDL cholesterol), and triglycerides. The levels of these parameters have different implications regarding vasculopathy and cardiovascular disease (CVD). Multiple epidemiologic studies have demonstrated a strong relationship between serum cholesterol levels and coronary heart disease, and randomized controlled trials (RCTs) have unequivocally demonstrated that lowering cholesterol reduces clinical events due to atherosclerosis. LDL cholesterol is considered deleterious, whereas HDL cholesterol is believed to be protective, although in fact little evidence exists regarding the benefit of raising HDL cholesterol.[28] Elevated fasting triglyceride levels have not been correlated with significant CVD risk, but it has been suggested that postprandial hypertriglyceridemia may be a bigger CVD risk factor than fasting triglyceride levels.[29]

In the context of these biologic pathways and clinical outcomes, it is clear that the pathophysiology of OSA holds biologic plausibility regarding causation and/or promotion of dyslipidemia through modulation of fat or liver metabolism.

Liver Injury and Related Metabolic Dysregulation

As discussed previously, the liver plays a pivotal role in the regulation of both lipid and glucose metabolism. Obesity is known to result in liver injury as nonalcoholic fatty liver disease (NAFLD), which is another recently proposed addition to the list of disorders for inclusion in the metabolic syndrome.[30] Obesity causes intracellular accumulation of lipids in the liver, designated *hepatic steatosis* in light of the associated histopathologic changes observed. NAFLD ranges in severity from hepatic steatosis (presence of fat in more than 5% of hepatocytes), to steatohepatitis (i.e., nonalcoholic steatohepatitis [NASH]), to liver fibrosis and cirrhosis, and it may be a risk factor for hepatocellular cancer.

Obesity and insulin resistance are major risk factors for NAFLD; conversely, fat accumulation in the liver may cause hepatic insulin resistance with enhanced hepatic glucose production.[30] The reported prevalence of NAFLD varies, ranging between 30% and 100% in obesity and between 10% and 75% in type 2 DM.[31]

Obesity alone, however, does not appear to account for all cases of NAFLD. Although weight loss can significantly improve NASH histologic activity scores, the potential triggers for progression of NAFLD are not fully understood. OSA, possibly through the pathomechanism of intermittent hypoxia may promote the progression of simple steatosis to the more severe forms of NAFLD.[31]

Neurohumoral Activation

The hypothalamic-pituitary-adrenal (HPA) axis and the sympathetic nervous system play important roles in energy balance,

body metabolism, and the pathogenesis of obesity.[32] Other than exerting a prominent regulatory function on blood pressure, cortisol is an anabolic hormone that promotes insulin resistance and dyslipidemia, whereas catecholamines upregulate hormone-sensitive lipase and increase circulating free fatty acid levels, induce beta cell apoptosis, and adversely affect adipokine profile.

Recurrent asphyxia from obstructed breathing, as occurs in OSA, poses a potent stress to the body, resulting in the so-called "fight or flight" phenomenon. Stress-related neurohumoral activation is a potential mechanistic pathway for metabolic dysregulation in OSA. Animal models of chronic intermittent hypoxia (CIH) demonstrate sympathetic activation contributing to CIH-induced hypertension.[33] Experimental studies in healthy subjects subjected to short-term sleep deprivation, sleep fragmentation, or intermittent hypoxia have demonstrated alterations in hormonal profiles in association with altered glucose metabolism.[34] Sleep fragmentation induced by acoustic stimuli without hypoxia in healthy volunteers resulted in alterations in insulin-glucose metabolism, which were accompanied by alterations in daytime heart rate variability as a marker of sympathetic activation.[35,36] CIH may potentially sensitize the carotid body, contributing to increase in sympathetic nerve activity and increase in blood pressure.[37]

Studies of patients with OSA consistently demonstrate increased muscle sympathetic nerve activity even in the awake state, as well as increased output of urinary catecholamines, although the extent to which obesity itself contributes to such sympathetic activation remains unclear.[38,39] Robust data show that CPAP treatment of OSA can rapidly reduce sympathetic activity, indicating that OSA itself induces sympathetic activation.[40] In a study of subjects undergoing sleep study to investigate suspected OSA, the independent determinants of serum adiponectin levels included insulin resistance and urinary catecholamine levels but not the presence or severity of OSA, suggesting a complex relationship among these pathophysiologic parameters.[41]

The associations between OSA and other hormones from the HPA axis, such as cortisol, are not clear. In a study of obese subjects, despite a lack of difference in baseline cortisol levels between those with and those without OSA, the subjects in the OSA group showed a reduction in heart rate and greater cortisol suppression with dexamethasone after 3 months of CPAP treatment, suggesting that untreated OSA may lead to abnormally high activation of the sympathetic nervous system and HPA axis.[42] Overall, the literature on cortisol status and associated dysmetabolism in OSA has not been abundant or consistent.[43]

Intermittent Hypoxia

Recurrent apneas and hypopneas in OSA generate intermittent hypoxia, which appears to hold a pivotal position in the pathogenesis of metabolic dysfunction in OSA. The chronic if intermittent oxygenation deficit in OSA results in systemic tissue and cellular hypoxia, with a plethora of downstream effects. Mounting evidence suggests that intermittent hypoxia simulates ischemia-reperfusion and can activate oxidative stress and inflammation, which are key pathogenetic pathways in cardiometabolic dysfunction.[1,4]

Intermittent hypoxic exposure in animals in vivo or in cell cultures in vitro allows the controlled interrogation of cellular and molecular mechanisms that may occur in various tissues, organs, and cells under different conditions. Exposure to intermittent hypoxia for 6 to 8 hours in the 24-hour time clock over days or weeks, termed *chronic intermittent hypoxia* (CIH), as noted earlier in association with OSA in humans, often is used in experimental settings. A wide array of intermittent hypoxia regimens is used in different laboratories, which may partly explain the sometimes discrepant results. Different tissues and organs in murine models demonstrate individualized oxygenation profiles[44] and oxidative stress responses[45,46] to intermittent hypoxia challenge. For example, intermittent hypoxic exposure has been shown to cause oxygen partial pressure swings in the liver, whereas such fluctuations were found to be attenuated in muscle and markedly so in fat, which instead showed steady hypoxia.[44] Compared with lean mice, obese mice had lower baseline liver oxygen tension but similar fat and muscle tissue oxygen tensions, whereas both obese and lean mice exhibited similar tissue partial pressure changes with intermittent hypoxic exposure.[44] Another caveat regarding this mechanism as a pathogenetic trigger is the likely presence of adaptive mechanisms, and the balance or imbalance of these various otherwise poorly delineated factors probably determines eventual health outcomes.[47,48]

Intermittent hypoxia–induced upregulation of nuclear factor kappa B (NF-κB), the master transcriptional switch of inflammation, has been demonstrated in a variety of cells and tissues—leukocytes, vascular cells, fat cells, cardiovascular tissue, and liver tissue, with increased production of inflammatory gene products downstream of activation of NF-κB, such as tumor necrosis factor alpha (TNF-α), interleukin 6 (IL-6), and C-reactive protein (CRP).[44,45,49-53] Data have been controversial regarding intermittent hypoxia induction of hypoxia-inducible factor-1 (HIF-1), a transcription factor critical to physiologic responses to hypoxia, including erythropoiesis, angiogeneis, and glucose metabolism.[48] Severe, but not moderate, intermittent hypoxia has been found to elicit HIF-1 activation in PC12 pheochromocytoma cells,[54] whereas moderate intermittent hypoxia has been found to elicit preferential activation of NF-κB, but not HIF-1, in HeLa cells.[49]

In a lean mouse model of CIH (at 12 weeks), liver histologic examination showed marked accumulation of glycogen in hepatocytes, with evidence of increased hepatic levels of oxidative stress biomarkers and activation of NF-κB, and these changes were followed by sensitization to acetaminophen-induced liver toxicity.[52] Exposure to CIH in a mouse model of high-fat, high-cholesterol diet–induced obesity, compared with similar dietary manipulation alone, caused liver oxidative stress and hepatic inflammation in addition to hepatic steatosis.[53]

Taken collectively, animal and cell data indicate that CIH may act independently, or in concert with obesity, alcohol, or drugs, to promote oxidative stress, inflammation, and dysmetabolism. In rigorously controlled experimental settings, human volunteers have been exposed to intermittent hypoxic regimens to investigate specific metabolic responses. In some studies involving patients with OSA, dysmetabolism arising from OSA has been inferred to be due specifically to sleep hypoxemia, when the metabolic parameter studied showed significant correlations with deoxygenation parameters such as oxygen nadir, oxygen desaturation index, or duration of oxygen desaturation.

In a mouse model of intermittent hypoxia, insulin resistance increased in lean and genetically obese mice, as well as those with dietary obesity, and was dependent on the disruption of the leptin pathways.[55,56] With exposure to intermittent hypoxic regimens of increasing severity, progressively elevated insulin resistance and leptin levels were found in lean mice, whereas increase in leptin levels plateaued in obese mice, suggesting that adiposity may have overwhelmed the effect of the hypoxia on adipokine production.[44] Insulin resistance persisted in intermittent hypoxia–exposed mice that were subjected to pharmacologic denervation of the sympathetic and parasympathetic nervous systems,[56] which did not support the hypothesized mechanistic role of sympathetic activation on glucose dysmetabolism in OSA. Lean rats exposed to different regimens of CIH demonstrated "dose-related" increases in serum insulin, probably reflecting augmented beta cell secretion in response to increased insulin resistance, alongside a commensurate circulating adipocytokine profile with increases in leptin, IL-6, and TNF-α and a decrease in adiponectin.[50] Lean or obese mice exposed to CIH demonstrated evidence of oxidative stress in liver tissue, with upregulation of inflammatory markers; this line of evidence has given rise to the speculation that intermittent hypoxia may contribute to hepatic insulin resistance through the pathophysiologic changes of NASH.[52,53] However, one study of CIH exposure for 4 weeks demonstrated exacerbation of insulin resistance and induction of steatohepatitis in mice with diet-induced obesity, but not in lean mice.[57]

Intermittent hypoxia–induced alterations in adipose tissue and cell metabolism pave the way for adverse downstream effects on insulin resistance and glucose metabolism. In vitro studies of 3T3-L1 adipocytes have demonstrated hypoxic exposure dose–dependent upregulation of proinflammatory activities, represented by the profile of NF-κB, HIF-1, glucose transport factor-1, TNF, IL-6, leptin, and adiponectin.[50] Synthetic sympathomimetics also could suppress adiponectin gene expression in preadipocyte cell lines independently of the intermittent hypoxia mechanism.[58]

Intermittent hypoxia may modulate pancreatic beta cell function. Lean mice exposed to CIH and glucose infusion demonstrated pancreatic beta cell replication with increased insulin secretion,[59] whereas another study of CIH reported associated beta cell proliferation and enhanced cell death, which was mediated by oxidative stress.[60] Other than induction of insulin resistance and hepatocyte glucose output, intermittent hypoxic exposure for 14 days in lean mice increased oxidative stress in the pancreas and impaired beta cell function, and cessation of hypoxic exposure could not fully reverse observed changes in glucose metabolism.[61]

Intermittent hypoxia also has been shown to be a key factor in the upregulation of genes responsible for hepatic lipid biosynthesis, promotion of oxidation of serum lipids, and modulation of the neurohormonal axes that influence signaling pathways in lipid transport and synthesis.[62] Exposure to CIH has led to increase in circulating levels of triglycerides, total cholesterol, and LDL and VLDL cholesterol in a hypoxic dose-dependent manner in both lean and obese murine models.[63] CIH exposure in a mouse model of dietary obesity exacerbated diet-induced dyslipidemia, with evidence of atherosclerosis in the aorta.[64] At a molecular level, insulin's effects on lipogenesis were mediated predominantly by the transcription factor sterol regulatory element–binding protein (SREBP)-1c, which controls the expression of genes required for cholesterol, fatty acid, triglyceride, and phospholipid synthesis.[65] Mechanistic studies focusing on the liver have further demonstrated that intermittent hypoxia induces increased lipolysis with free fatty acid flux into the liver, with sequential upregulation of the master transcriptional factors HIF-1 and NF-κB, SREBP-1, and stearoyl coenzyme A desaturase-1 (SDC-1).[64,65] The outcomes are hepatic steatosis, aggravation of hepatic insulin resistance, and disruption of hepatic lipoprotein biosynthesis and secretion. A murine model of severe CIH was shown to result in poor clearance of triglyceride-rich lipoproteins, attributed to reduced lipoprotein lipase activity, which was decreased by 80% in adipose tissue.[66] These results resonate with the finding of postprandial hyperlipemia in subjects with OSA, which could be decreased with CPAP treatment.[67]

In human studies, intermittent hypoxia simulating that seen in OSA has been induced by altering inspired oxygen concentrations. Young healthy men exposed to 8 hours of intermittent hypoxia (through inhalation of "air" with 5% oxygen alternating with 21% oxygen) demonstrated impairment of insulin sensitivity, glucose disposal, and pancreatic islet cell function.[68]

Derangement of Sleep Quality and Quantity

The impact of sleep quality and sleep derangement on metabolism is significant. Recurrent obstructed breathing gives rise to cerebral arousals and disturbs sleep architecture, posing another trigger for metabolic dysregulation in OSA. Several epidemiologic studies have found a curvilinear relationship between sleep duration and obesity or glucose dysmetabolism, and subjects who reported shorter sleep durations, compared with those averaging more than 7 to 8 hours of sleep per night, exhibited greater degrees of obesity and glucose dysmetabolism.[69] Alterations in energy-regulating hormones including leptin and grhelin have been implicated.[70] Healthy subjects who were subjected to experimental sleep restriction demonstrated abnormal glucose metabolism[71] and impairment of insulin signaling in their subcutaneous adipocytes,[72] compared with after normal sleep. Studies using acoustic stimuli to induce sleep fragmentation,[36] with reduction of slow wave and REM sleep and preserved total sleep time,[35] showed that sleep disruption without hypoxia could lead to a decrease in insulin sensitivity, as well as impaired non–insulin-dependent glucose disposal and inadequate compensatory increase in insulin secretion.

In a study of 226 children, both obesity and OSA, and to a greater extent the combination of the two, were associated with reduced circulating levels of G protein–coupled receptor 120 (GPR120), a long-chain free fatty acid receptor protective against insulin resistance and systemic inflammation.[73] GPR120 levels correlated with insulin resistance, but not with dyslipidemia or CRP levels. Among the sleep parameters, GPR120 levels showed the strongest independent association with respiratory arousal index, which provoked the query of whether sleep curtailment or disruption, rather than the other pathophysiologic disturbance of OSA, was the etiologic mechanism.

Oxidative Stress

Oxidative stress is a state caused by imbalance between the production of reactive oxygen species (ROS) highly damaging to cells and the antioxidant activity that counteracts ROS. Oxidative stress activates redox-sensitive transcription factors

that regulate inflammatory processes and downregulate nitric oxide synthase, with consequent reduced nitric oxide in endothelial cells, leading to microvascular and macrovascular endothelial dysfunction. These cellular mechanisms also may be operative in other tissues and organs and may underlie the development of insulin resistance, dyslipidemia, arterial hypertension, and other cardiometabolic derangements.[6,74] The recurrent hypoxia-reoxygenation cycles in OSA (i.e., intermittent hypoxia and particularly CIH, as described previously) are thought to be analogous to ischemia-reperfusion injury known to produce ROS in the reperfusion phase. Evidence for occurrence of increased oxidative stress in OSA is not consistent, however. A majority of studies have found that subjects with OSA have increased biomarkers of oxidative stress compared with control subjects without OSA, which decreased after CPAP treatment of OSA, whereas a few studies reported reduced antioxidant activity.[4,75,76] For example, subjects with OSA were found to have an increase in lipid peroxidation, glycated end products of oxidation, serum or urinary reactive oxygen metabolites, ROS production from leukocytes or monocytes, and reduction of circulating nitric oxide, although there have also been negative studies.[4] Discrepant findings for the presence of oxidative stress in OSA may be related to the difficulty of assessing oxidative status accurately.[77] Furthermore, obesity itself has been associated with enhanced oxidative stress systemically and locally in adipose tissues, constituting a confounding factor in the study of oxidative stress potentially due to OSA.[6,15,75]

Inflammation and Alteration of the Adipocytokine Profile

Obesity and metabolic syndrome are known as proinflammatory states, with elevated circulating levels of proinflammatory mediators, often referred to as *adipocytokines* (see earlier text under Obesity and Adiposity).[7] Adiopokines are produced predominantly from adipose tissues, whereas cytokines are released by a variety of cells and tissues. Collectively, adipocytokines function as key mediators linking obesity and metabolic disorders.[7] It is hypothesized that OSA may modulate the expression and release of adipokines to favor adverse metabolism.[11] Intermittent hypoxia, oxidative stress, and sympathetic activity are capable of modulating release of proinflammatory adipocytokines from a variety of cells and tissues, including adipose tissues.[15,44,49-54] Investigation of alterations of adipocytokine regulation in subjects with OSA, however, have yielded highly variable results, which may be attributed to the presence of confounding factors, in particular obesity.[24]

OBSTRUCTIVE SLEEP APNEA AND METABOLIC DYSREGULATION: CLINICAL ASSOCIATIONS AND TREATMENT

Obesity

It has been estimated that a range of 15% to 90% of obese subjects have OSA, depending on age, gender, and BMI.[78] Generally, OSA prevalence is higher among persons with morbid obesity, and OSA severity is greater in obese than in leaner subjects.[10,78] Longitudinal data of the Wisconsin cohort indicated that a 10% gain in body weight increased the chance of developing moderate to severe OSA by a factor of 6, and that every 1% increase in body weight was associated with a 3% increase in AHI.[79] Conversely, weight loss reduced OSA severity but to a less substantial degree than that seen with exacerbation with weight gain. If OSA alters energy balance to promote obesity, it follows that treatment of OSA should mitigate obesity. However, studies on the impact of treatment of OSA on body weight or adiposity have not been supportive of a beneficial effect on body composition. In an RCT of CPAP treatment for OSA, therapeutic CPAP decreased daytime sleepiness and promoted physical activity over a 3-month period, but no change in body weight was seen.[80] Studies on the impact of CPAP treatment on abdominal fat have yielded conflicting data,[15] with randomized, sham-controlled trials for 8 and 12 weeks, respectively, showing no change in abdominal fat quantified by imaging.[81,82] In fact, a recent meta-analysis of data from randomized trials suggests that CPAP treatment of OSA may promote increase in BMI and body weight.[83] On the other hand, interventions including lifestyle modifications, antiobesity medications, and bariatric surgery (also termed *metabolic surgery*) can produce weight loss and have undoubted metabolic benefits as well as resulting in symptomatic improvement in obese subjects with OSA, although the relative impact of various weight reduction regimens in this regard remains underinvestigated.[84] In a controlled trial of surgical versus conventional therapy in severely obese subjects with OSA, greater weight loss in the surgical group did not translate to significantly greater reduction in AHI than that achieved with conventional weight loss approaches.[85] A daunting challenge is to find the optimal weight control measure that not only is effective in improving anthropometric aspects and various health outcomes but also is acceptable to the individual patient and sustainable in real-life situations.

Insulin and Glucose Metabolism

The clinical relationship between OSA and a range of glucose dysmetabolism disorders ranging from insulin resistance to overt diabetes has been extensively investigated and regularly reviewed.[3,86,87] Several population-based studies from the United States, Hong Kong, Korea, Brazil, and Europe consistently found that OSA was associated with increased insulin resistance or evidence of impaired glycemic status including DM, despite adjustment for obesity and other confounders.[17,88-93] The Sleep Heart Health Study (SHHS) cohort of 5874 subjects in the United States did not show an independent relationship between OSA and DM,[94] although in a subgroup of overweight, middle-aged men in the SHHS, an independent association was found between OSA and insulin resistance/glucose intolerance.[89] In 2014, the European Sleep Apnea Database (ESADA) reported its cross-sectional analysis of data on 6616 participants and found that increasing OSA severity was associated with increased likelihood of type 2 DM and worse glycemic control in the diabetic subjects despite adjustment for confounding variables.[93] The Wisconsin Sleep Cohort, which found an independent association between severity of untreated OSA and prevalence of DM at baseline, did not find any increase in incident DM at a 4-year follow-up evaluation.[88] Other longitudinal follow-up cohort studies from the United States[95] and Japan[96] have found associations between baseline OSA and incident diabetes over 3 to 4 years, as did another study from Australia, although the incidence of DM was very low in that cohort.[97] A historical cohort of 8678 patients undergoing diagnostic study for OSA in a single clinical center in Toronto showed that DM

developed in 1017 subjects with OSA (11.7%) over a median follow-up period of approximately 67 months.[98] With full adjustment for confounders, subjects with AHI greater than 30 had a 30% higher hazard of developing DM than those with AHI below 5. Adjusted odds ratios for the incidence of DM in moderate to severe OSA compared with those without OSA in different studies have ranged from 1.31[98] to 13.45.[87]

Conversely, a high prevalence of OSA has been reported among diabetic populations[94,99-104] (Figure 24-1). Several studies in diabetic subjects suggest that severity of OSA is associated with worse glycemic control,[93,102] although this correlation is not universally seen.[103]

A majority of studies analyzing nondiabetic subjects have reported independent associations between OSA and insulin resistance or sensitivity and/or other measures of glycemic health, with dose-dependent effect of OSA on such measures of metabolic impairment.[86] However, some studies found that such a relationship was confounded by obesity, such that the association was abolished after adjustments for BMI and/or other measures of adiposity.[86] The ESADA cohort study found that OSA severity independently predicted glycemic health assessed by HbA_{1c} in nondiabetic subjects.[92] Nonobese subjects with OSA, compared with BMI-matched or BMI-adjusted counterparts without OSA, also had more insulin resistance or glucose dysmetabolism.[16-18,105,106]

It has been proposed that excessive daytime sleepiness may be a phenotypic marker for insulin resistance in OSA. Associated abdominal or visceral obesity in OSA could contribute to sleepiness in OSA through hypercytokinemia.[107] Waist circumference and visceral fat have demonstrated high correlations with insulin resistance[13] and also with OSA prevalence[10,15] or severity.[12,15] Excessive daytime sleepiness was reported to be a useful indicator of moderate or severe OSA in white diabetic subjects,[108] but this was not the case in a Chinese diabetic population.[103] In a case-control study of nondiabetic subjects with similar BMI and AHI, those with excessive daytime sleepiness (as defined by a mean Epworth Sleepiness Scale [ESS] score of 16) had higher scores on homeostasis model assessment for insulin resistance (HOMA-IR) than those without sleepiness (mean ESS score of 4), and indices of insulin resistance were improved with CPAP treatment only in the group with baseline excessive sleepiness.[109]

Despite abundant positive data supporting an independent association of OSA and disturbance of glucose homeostasis, cross-sectional studies cannot be considered definitive for a causal link. Reported data on the effect of treatment of OSA, usually with CPAP, on insulin-glucose metabolism remain highly controversial.[86,87,110] A number of observational studies in either diabetics or non-diabetics with OSA suggested improvements in insulin resistance or glycemic status with CPAP treatment, but such results are by no means consistent, and most of the RCTs did not provide definitive evidence for an improvement in insulin-glucose metabolism in response to CPAP.[40] Several RCTs of CPAP treatment for OSA without DM ranging from 1 to 12 weeks in duration did not find consistent improvement in insulin resistance measured by HOMA-IR, or insulin sensitivity using OGTT or a hyperinsulinemic clamp.[111-113] Data from subset analysis or open continuation phase of these RCTS, and from observational studies, suggest that severity of OSA,[112] BMI,[111,114] CPAP adherence,[115] sample size, and/or treatment duration[113] may contribute to the determination of metabolic effects. Reported

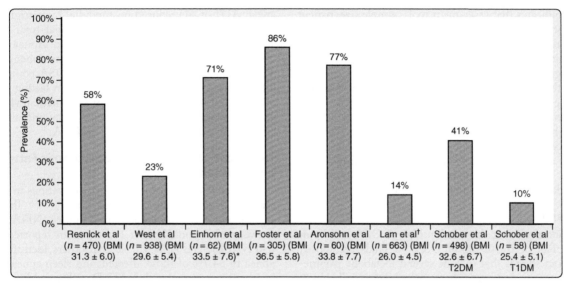

Figure 24-1 Prevalence of obstructive sleep apnea (OSA) in subjects with diabetes mellitus.*BMI available only in a bigger cohort of n = 279. †Chinese (Asian criteria for obesity: BMI greater than 25 kg/m²). T1DM, Type 1 diabetes mellitus; T2DM, type 2 diabetes mellitus. (Data from referenced studies: Resnick et al., 2003[94]; West et al., 2006[99]; Einhorn et al., 2007[100]; Foster et al., 2009[101]; Aronsohn et al., 2010[102]; Lam et al., 2010[103]; Schober et al., 2011—both cohorts.[104])

data on the confounding influence of obesity are controversial, with conflicting evidence that either obese (Chinese)[111] or nonobese (non-Asian white) subjects[114] can show more improvement in insulin sensitivity in response to CPAP. A rigorously conducted RCT that investigated the effects of CPAP alone versus weight reduction alone versus both interventions in a cohort of obese subjects with severe OSA showed that weight reduction but not CPAP alone over 24 weeks improved insulin sensitivity.[116] The beneficial effect was not further enhanced in the group receiving both interventions, suggesting that obesity has a more dominant impact than OSA on insulin resistance in persons with OSA. Because weight loss also may lead to changes in OSA, however, the absence of information on sleep-disordered breathing after the treatment period in those data disallows definitive analysis of the complicit interactions of multiple risk factors and conditions that occur in this patient population.[117]

In diabetic subjects with OSA, data from observational studies on treatment of OSA tend to be favorable regarding improvement in indicators of glycemic status.[86] In the only randomized sham-CPAP controlled study reported to date, neither HbA_{1c} nor insulin sensitivity measured with the hyperinsulinemic euglycemic clamp showed any improvement with CPAP over a 3-month period,[118] but the low average CPAP use of 2.5 hours per night in the "therapeutic" CPAP group is considered inadequate to produce any change in OSA-related sequelae. Rapid eye movement (REM)-related event frequency, as indicated by REM-AHI, but not NREM-related event frequency, was found to be associated with worse glycemic control in type 2 DM, suggesting potential treatment implications regarding the need for adequate inclusion of REM sleep periods in overnight CPAP usage.[119]

Recently, an RCT of CPAP in 39 subjects with prediabetes and OSA found that 8 hours of CPAP use every night for 2 weeks, documented by nightly in-laboratory sleep monitoring, could reduce glucose response to oral glucose tolerance testing and improve insulin sensitivity.[120] As with a previous 1-week

RCT in nondiabetic men,[111] these findings can be regarded as proof-of-concept for an adverse effect of untreated OSA on glucose metabolism, which is reversible with control of OSA, but the relevant clinical impact remains elusive.

In the face of increased insulin resistance, compensatory increase in insulin secretion occurs, but this homeostatic mechanism of beta cell function may be lost with chronic insult, ageing or pre-diabetic state. In clinical subjects or experimental human models of OSA, studies have shown conflicting data: pancreatic insulin secretion may be enhanced or impaired. In a study of 118 nondiabetic subjects with OSA evaluated with an intravenous glucose tolerance test (FSIVGGT), despite "OSA dose–dependent" impairment of insulin sensitivity, no increase in pancreatic beta cell insulin output was seen.[121] By contrast, in a study of 26 lean young men free of cardiometabolic disease, the presence of mild to moderate OSA was associated with insulin resistance and an increase in insulin secretion,[106] and a study of 45 severely obese adults also found that OSA was associated with increased beta cell function in those with normal glucose metabolism.[122]

Additional data indicate that coexistence of obesity, pregnancy, and OSA may well pose a conglomerate predisposition to gestational DM. Despite adjustment for pre-pregnancy BMI, a diagnosis of gestational DM has been strongly associated with a diagnosis of OSA.[123]

The diverse results regarding the effect of OSA or its treatment on glucose metabolism as illustrated above may be due to the use of different investigative tools that are not directly comparable, and to different sample characteristics. Host factors, intrinsic or extrinsic, play important roles in the determination of insulin-glucose metabolism in OSA, including age, BMI and adiposity, duration of OSA, prevailing glycemic status, genetic susceptibility, and variable exposures to external factors such as diet and exercise. Adherence to and duration of treatment for OSA also must be considered in the appraisal of any potential metabolic response. An overview of the literature indicates that assessment tools, sample size, patient characteristics, and treatment duration and adherence are factors that need to be carefully addressed in the design of future clinical studies.

Although current investigative data are dominated by studies of the action of OSA towards glucose homeostasis and DM, the possibility of diabetic autonomic neuropathy as a predisposing factor toward sleep-related pharyngeal collapse and OSA has been raised.[124] In subjects with type 1 DM in particular, who usually are not overweight or obese, a higher prevalence of OSA than in the general population raises the possibility of contribution by autonomic neuropathy,[104] although data are very limited in this regard.[124]

Dyslipidemia

Clinical data regarding the relationships of OSA and lipids and the effect of treatment of OSA on lipids are mostly gleaned from studies that include several metabolic parameters as end-points, and relatively few which specifically investigated dyslipidemia as the primary measure of interest. Epidemiologic studies comprising relatively large numbers of subjects have identified an association between OSA and dyslipidemia independent of confounding variables. In the American SHHS cohort with mean age of 62 years, stepwise regression models identified that the respiratory disturbance index was independently determined by higher total cholesterol levels in men, and lower HDL cholesterol levels in women.[125] The European SYNAPSE study of 846 participants with mean age of 68 years showed that severe OSA was independently associated with low HDL cholesterol.[126] Oxygen desaturation index and AHI were independent predictors of HDL cholesterol levels, and the relationships were more pronounced in those not receiving lipid-lowering agents.[126] The Brazilian San Paola sleep cohort found that an AHI of 15 or less and a longer duration of oxygen saturation below 90% were independently associated with elevated fasting glucose and triglyceride levels and HOMA-IR.[91] By contrast, no independent association was identified between OSA (defined by AHI of 5 or less) and cholesterol or triglyceride levels in community-dwelling middle-aged Chinese residents of Hong Kong.[90]

Clinical studies of patients with OSA have reported various adverse lipid profiles, including elevations of total cholesterol, triglycerides, LDL cholesterol or lower HDL cholesterol levels.[62] Apart from promoting a dyslipidemic profile of cholesterol or triglycerides, subjects with OSA have been shown to have higher levels of oxidized or dysfunctional lipids which are more atherogenic, ascribed to increased oxidative stress.[127,128]

Observational intervention studies and RCTs regarding the effect of OSA treatment on dyslipidemia profiles have demonstrated variable changes in lipid parameters,[15,40] although some studies with short treatment durations may not have allowed adequate time for changes in circulating lipid levels. In a single-center longitudinal follow-up study of 127 patients with OSA, positive airway pressure treatment for 6 months significantly increased HDL cholesterol levels.[129] Pooled data from two RCTs on metabolic profile in OSA suggested that CPAP treatment of OSA results in a lowering of serum total cholesterol.[130] In a randomized controlled cross-over trial with dyslipidemia as the primary end point, therapeutic CPAP treatment for 2 months compared with placebo CPAP in 30 subjects with severe OSA (defined as mean AHI of 41) reduced postprandial hypertriglyceridemia and also lowered fasting and postprandial total cholesterol levels.[67] However, in the Icelandic Sleep Apnea Cohort, a 2-years follow-up assessment of CPAP treatment outcomes in 199 subjects with newly diagnosed OSA compared with 118 nonusers did not show any change in fasting lipid levels with CPAP treatment.[131] A recent systematic review of randomized controlled studies did not show any alteration in lipid levels with CPAP treatment of OSA.[40]

Hepatic Dysfunction and Nonalcoholic Fatty Liver Disease

A number of reports of liver enzyme elevations in adults and children with OSA have been published.[31,132,133] The National Health and Nutrition Examination Survey (NHANES) data between 2005 and 2010 for 10,541 adults reported that 15% had NAFLD and 7.2% had sleep disorders, identified as sleep apnea in 64.7% of those affected, and sleep apnea was independently associated with NAFLD with an odds ratio of 1.39 (95% confidence interval, 0.98 to 1.97).[134] Definitive evidence of liver injury in OSA was mostly derived from findings in morbidly obese subjects who underwent liver biopsy during bariatric surgery.[15] As with other metabolic dysfunction, the association of fatty liver with OSA is substantially confounded by obesity, and an independent relationship has not been firmly established.[31]

In studies of obese subjects, those with moderate or severe OSA and severe sleep-related hypoxemia exhibited more significant changes in indices of hepatic inflammation than those with mild OSA,[135,136] and in a series of subjects undergoing bariatric surgery, the absence of OSA was found to be an independent predictor of normal findings on liver histologic analysis.[137] Patients with severe OSA (AHI greater than 50) were found to have more insulin resistance and to have higher percentage of steatosis, as well as higher prevalence of necrosis and fibrosis, than patients with milder OSA with similar BMI.[138] In a study of 65 consecutive children with biopsy-proven NAFLD, 60% were shown to have OSA on polysomnography, and the presence and severity of OSA were associated with features of NASH and fibrosis, independently of BMI, abdominal adiposity, metabolic syndrome, and insulin resistance.[139] This relationship held in the nonobese children with NAFLD. Of note, the duration of oxyhemoglobin saturation below 90% correlated with increased hepatocyte apoptosis and fibrogenesis.

Despite the concern that OSA may worsen NAFLD, the major causes of premature death in subjects with NAFLD have been identified as type 2 DM and CVD, rather than the liver disease itself.[140] This correlation serves, however, as a reminder of the potential role of additional liver injury from OSA as a pathway to greater cardiometabolic burden.

Inflammation and Alteration of Adipocytokines

Multiple studies have addressed the profile of proinflammatory mediators in OSA, and results have been diverse and confounded by obesity.[24] A meta-analysis of 51 studies found higher levels of CRP, TNF-α, IL-6, and other molecules in patients with OSA than in control group subjects.[141] The Icelandic cohort study of 454 subjects with untreated OSA showed that OSA severity, as reflected by the degree of nocturnal oxygen desaturation, but not AHI, correlated significantly with levels of IL-6 and CRP.[142] An association of

BMI with IL-6 was found only in obese participants, and an independent association of OSA severity and CRP levels was found for minimum oxygen saturation only. Although a meta-analysis found that treatment of OSA with CPAP improved levels of CRP, TNF-α, and IL-6, the studies pooled for this analysis generally were small, nonrandomized trials,[143] and well-designed studies have failed to demonstrate that CPAP alters inflammation markers in OSA.[24,40]

Leptin regulates appetite and energy intake, and hyperleptinemia in obesity reflects leptin resistance. Hyperleptinemia is associated with increased insulin resistance and cardiometabolic morbidities. Subjects with OSA have consistently been found to have elevated plasma leptin levels compared with healthy subjects, although whether the increase is related independently to OSA or is simply due to the concomitant adiposity remains controversial.[24] Some studies have suggested that nocturnal hypoxemia, rather than AHI itself, is a better indicator of the effect of OSA on leptin levels. The Icelandic Sleep Apnea Cohort study of 452 patients with untreated OSA (mean BMI, 32.7 kg/m^2) showed that the dominant determinants of leptin levels were still obesity and gender, although OSA severity as measured by AHI explained a significant variance (3.2%) in leptin levels in the nonhypertensive group, with the relationship strongest in nonobese, nonhypertensive subjects.[144] Adiponectin has insulin-sensitizing, antiinflammatory, and antiatherogenic properties, and hypoadiponectinemia is associated with reduced insulin sensitivity, type 2 DM, and the metabolic syndrome. A majority of relevant studies in OSA have found that hypoadiponectinemia strongly correlates with obesity and insulin resistance as in general populations, but the relationship of adiponectin levels and OSA is heavily confounded by obesity.[24] One study suggested that the degree of sympathetic activation, rather than sleep-disordered breathing indices, contributed to the determination of adiponectin levels.[41] Another study found that nonobese men with severe OSA, compared with nonobese control subjects who did not have OSA, demonstrated more impaired insulin resistance (higher HOMA-IR) and a profile of higher 24-hour levels of leptin, CRP, IL-6, and TNF-α but similar levels of adiponectin.[18]

Obstructive Sleep Apnea and Metabolic Syndrome

Although the considerable disagreement in the medical community over terminology and diagnostic criteria has yet to be resolved, *metabolic syndrome* is conceptually accepted as a clustering of multiple metabolic risk factors for CVD and DM.[13] The key features of metabolic syndrome are abdominal obesity, insulin resistance, atherogenic dyslipidemia, a prothrombotic state, and an inflammatory profile. This constellation of metabolic aberrations often is accompanied by arterial hypertension and/or type 2 DM, in keeping with the relevant genetic or exogenous predispositions.[2] Different sets of clinical criteria for definition of metabolic syndrome have been reached by various expert panels,[13] and one widely used set of criteria from the National Cholesterol Education Program Adult Treatment Panel III is presented in Table 24-2[145,146] for reference. Besides the core components, an increasing number of conditions are proposed to be included in the metabolic syndrome "family," and OSA is one such condition because of its strong associations with other core factors and its potential role in causing CVD and glucose dysmetabolism.[146,147]

Table 24-2 Definition of Metabolic Syndrome of the National Cholesterol Education Program Adult Treatment Panel III (NECP-ATIII)

Risk Factor	Defining Level
Abdominal obesity (waist circumference)	
Men	>102 cm
Women	>88 cm
Triglycerides	≥150 mg/dL
High-density lipoprotein cholesterol (HDL cholesterol)	
Men	<40 mg/dL
Women	<50 mg/dL
Blood pressure	≥130/≥85 mm Hg
Fasting glucose	≥110 mg/dL
Asian criteria for abdominal obesity*	
Men	≥90 cm
Women	≥80 cm

*Asian abdominal obesity criteria: data from *The IDF consensus worldwide definition of the metabolic syndrome*. Brussels: International Diabetes Federation; 2006. <http://www.idf.org/webdata/docs/IDF_Meta_def_final.pdf>.
Data from National Cholesterol Education Program (NCEP) expert panel on detection, evaluation, and treatment of high blood cholesterol in Adults (Adult Treatment Panel III). Third report of the National Cholesterol Education Program (NCEP) Expert Panel on Detection, Evaluation, and Treatment of High Blood Cholesterol in Adults (Adult Treatment Panel III) final report. *Circulation* 2002; 106:3113–421.

As illustrated in previous sections of this chapter, strong and probably independent associations of OSA with various individual clinical components of the metabolic syndrome are likely. Studies have demonstrated a 5- to 7-fold increase in the association of OSA with this phenotypic entity, compared with those without OSA, and the association was independent of BMI and age; a similar association has been found in subjects with versus those without metabolic syndrome.[3,11] Of a total of 228 patients referred for OSA evaluation, 146 patients proved to have OSA, of whom 60% had metabolic syndrome, whereas of those without significant OSA, only 40% had metabolic syndrome.[148] The presence of OSA in subjects with classical metabolic syndrome as defined by current international guidelines may add to the associated inflammatory and cardiometabolic burden.[149] To date, definitive evidence that treating OSA reduces the occurrence of conventionally defined metabolic syndrome is lacking. With respect to clinical impact, this may be just a matter of threshold—if indeed treatment of OSA can produce adequate improvement in individual components of the metabolic syndrome, it is reasonable to anticipate improvement in the adverse cardiometabolic outcomes predicted by metabolic syndrome. However, despite increasing research focus in this area, treatment of OSA has not yet been associated with consistent and clinically important improvement in the metabolic components of obesity, insulin-glucose dysmetabolism, dyslipidemia, or systemic inflammation.[40,150]

CONCLUSIONS AND PERSPECTIVES

The strong association between OSA and metabolic disorders has received intense interest, against the background of a

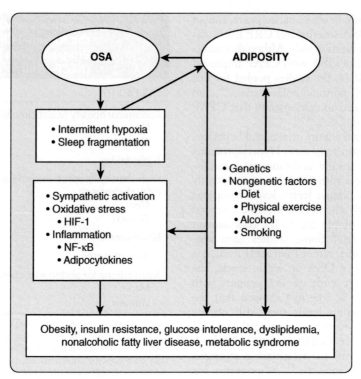

Figure 24-2 Proposed mechanistic links of obstructive sleep apnea (OSA) and metabolic disorders. HIF-1, Hypoxia-inducible factor-1; NK-κB, nuclear factor kappa B.

global epidemic of obesity and obesity-related diseases, and the modern lifestyle of sleep curtailment. In human disease, despite growing evidence for an independent or additive adverse effect of OSA on metabolic function, the relationship remains controversial owing to the strong potential confounding effect of obesity and the unaccounted influence of numerous intrinsic or exogenous factors that may affect body metabolism. Furthermore, the influence of OSA and metabolic dysfunction may be bidirectional, and the putative alterations of metabolic function by OSA, such as increased insulin resistance with promotion of visceral adiposity, may in turn aggravate OSA, allowing a vicious circle to be established (see Figure 24-2). The demonstration of a beneficial metabolic effect of treatment of OSA, moreover, has been elusive. Overall, many studies are of limited sample size and/or heterogeneous sample characteristics, and because of the need for symptomatic treatment in this condition, conducting RCTs or longitudinal follow-up studies of untreated disease with adequate duration is inherently difficult. Treatment results for children, young adults, and a range of middle-aged to elderly adults can hardly be directly compared; obese subjects may behave differently from lean subjects metabolically, and the difference may not be adequately resolved with adjustment for BMI. Furthermore, factors such as the duration of OSA before sleep study diagnosis are not possible to define accurately, owing to the nonspecific and insidious onset of symptoms in most cases, and the prevailing metabolic status in the individual patient influence whether "reversibility" could still be attained with treatment of OSA even if it is the culprit for dysmetabolism. Finally, any metabolic benefits that are demonstrated in the study setting, especially in short-term studies, need to be reproducible in real life, where lifestyle factors and treatment adherence interpose.

Animal and cellular studies using intermittent hypoxia or other surrogate models for OSA allow manipulation of experimental conditions to provide insights into the physiologic or molecular mechanisms that may be at play in the human disease. Accordingly, such studies can be expected to pave the way for extension into translational work in humans.

SUMMARY

In view of the many factors that may influence metabolic health and disease, it is unrealistic to expect that one unifying path applies to all. Although any demonstrated adverse impact of OSA on metabolic function may be of limited clinical effect, the economy of scale would translate such effect into an enormous health care burden when coupled with the sweeping epidemic of obesity and anticipated escalation of rates of related morbidity in the coming decades. Meanwhile, holistic care mandates a multidimensional approach, in both clinical practice and research, to the management of patients presenting with either OSA or a metabolic disorder. Strong evidence suggests that controlling body weight is of pivotal importance in improving metabolic health, including in subjects with OSA. OSA is gaining professional recognition as a serious comorbid condition to be accorded appropriate attention in the management of cardiometabolic disorders.[151,152] Recent clinical practice guidelines note that OSA should be identified and appropriately treated in the comprehensive care of patients with DM.[152] It is of pivotal importance that both the medical profession and the public be aware of the clustering of OSA and metabolic disorders, with the consequent need for determination of optimal methods of prevention, early recognition, and relevant clinical management.

CLINICAL PEARL

Strong associations are recognized between OSA and various metabolic disorders, notably obesity, type 2 DM, dyslipidemia, and NAFLD. Despite abundant suggestive evidence for independent associations between OSA and metabolic dysfunction, a causal or aggravating role for OSA in dysmetabolism is not yet delineated, and treatment of OSA has not been definitively shown to prevent or improve metabolic dysfunction. A reasonable holistic clinical approach mandates high vigilance regarding the clustering of these conditions, with relevant screening and specific management considered accordingly. The need for appropriate body weight control measures is particularly relevant in this regard.

Selected Readings

Alberti KG, Eckel RH, Grundy SM, et al. Harmonizing the metabolic syndrome: a joint interim statement of the International Diabetes Federation Task Force on epidemiology and prevention; National Heart, Lung, and Blood Institute; American Heart Association; World Heart Federation; International Atherosclerosis Society; and International Association for the Study of Obesity. *Circulation* 2009;**120**(16):1640–5.

Arnardottir ES, Lim DC, Keenan BT, et al. Effects of obesity on the association between long-term sleep apnea treatment and changes in interleukin-6 levels: the Icelandic Sleep Apnea Cohort. *J Sleep Res* 2015;**24**(2):148–59.

Bonsignore MR, McNicholas WT, Montserrat JM, et al. Adipose tissue in obesity and obstructive sleep apnoea. *Eur Respir J* 2012;**39**(3):746–67.

Chirinos JA, Gurubhagavatula I, Teff K, et al. CPAP, weight loss, or both for obstructive sleep apnea. *N Engl J Med* 2014;**370**(24):2265–75.

Kent BD, Grote L, Bonsignore M, et al. Sleep apnoea severity independently predicts glycaemic health in nondiabetic subjects: the ESADA study. *Eur Respir J* 2014;**44**(1):130–9.

Lam JC, Mak JC, Ip MS. Obesity, obstructive sleep apnoea and metabolic syndrome. *Respirology* 2012;**17**(2):223–36.

Lavie L. Oxidative stress—a unifying paradigm in obstructive sleep apnea and comorbidities. *Prog Cardiovasc Dis* 2009;**51**(4):303–12.

Martínez-Ceron E, Fernández-Navarro I, Garcia-Rio F. Effects of continuous positive airway pressure treatment on glucose metabolism in patients with obstructive sleep apnea. *Sleep Med Rev* 2016;**25**:121–30.

Pamidi S, Wroblewski K, Stepien M, et al. Eight hours of nightly CPAP treatment of obstructive sleep apnea improves glucose metabolism in prediabetes: a randomized controlled trial. *Am J Respir Crit Care Med* 2015;**192**(1):96–105.

Preis SR, Massaro JM, Hoffmann U, et al. Neck circumference as a novel measure of cardiometabolic risk: the Framingham Heart study. *J Clin Endocrinol Metab* 2010;**95**:3701–10.

Salord N, Fortuna AM, Monasterio C, et al. A Randomized Controlled Trial of Continuous Positive Airway Pressure on Glucose Tolerance in Obese Patients with Obstructive Sleep Apnea. *Sleep* 2016;**39**(1):35–41.

Strand LB, Carnethon M, Biggs ML, et al. Sleep disturbances and glucose metabolism in older adults: the cardiovascular health study. *Diabetes Care* 2015;**38**(11):2050–8.

A complete reference list can be found online at ExpertConsult.com.

Cardiovascular Effects of Sleep-Related Breathing Disorders

Virend K. Somers; Shahrokh Javaheri

Chapter Highlights

- The cycle of apnea and recovery causes hypoxemia and reoxygenation, hypercapnia and hypocapnia, changes in intrathoracic pressure, and arousals. These consequences of sleep apnea, both obstructive and central apnea, adversely affect cardiovascular function. The cardiovascular effects of sleep apnea may be mediated by redox-sensitive gene activation, altered autonomic nervous system activity, oxidative stress, and release of inflammatory mediators. Pathophysiologic consequences of sleep apnea elicit acute and chronic cardiovascular changes.

- Hypoxemia has direct (decreased myocardial oxygen delivery) and indirect (activation of sympathetic nervous system, promotion of endothelial cell dysfunction, and pulmonary arteriolar vasoconstriction) cardiac and vascular effects. Reoxygenation may cause additional damage through further production of free radical species. Hypoxemia-reoxygenation, with intermittent and profound alterations in the partial pressure of oxygen (PO_2), may occur hundreds of times during sleep.

- Because of potentiated chemoreflex responses to hypoxemia-hypercapnia, the sympathetic and consequent presser responses to hypoxemia-hypercapnia, particularly in the absence of inhibitory effects of breathing, are marked. Nighttime sympathetic activation carries over into daytime wakefulness.

- Large negative intrathoracic pressures are generated during episodes of obstructive apnea. Negative intrathoracic pressure increases the transmural pressure (pressure inside minus pressure outside) of the intrathoracic vascular structures, including aorta, pulmonary vascular bed, and ventricles.

- Bradycardias may be especially severe and are elicited because of activation of the diving reflex by the combination of hypoxemia and apnea. Episodes of up to 10 seconds or more of sinus arrest may occur because of chemoreflex-mediated vagal activation.

- Sleep apnea has been implicated in systolic and diastolic heart failure, ventricular arrhythmias, and atrial fibrillation. However, whether treating sleep apnea prevents heart failure and arrhythmias or improves survival remains to be determined from randomized controlled trials.

Hemodynamic changes have been most studied in patients with obstructive sleep apnea (OSA), and in these studies, acute apnea-induced hemodynamic changes have been documented. Chronic exposure may also result in left ventricular systolic and diastolic dysfunction and in increased atrial volume. A limited number of studies have shown that treatment of OSA with nasal continuous positive airway pressure (CPAP) devices or tracheostomy can result in reversal of left ventricular dysfunction and arrhythmias. Whether treatment of sleep apnea reduces cardiovascular events or cardiovascular mortality remains to be demonstrated in randomized control trials. However, several observational studies have reported that treatment of sleep apnea improves survival primarily because cardiovascular events are reduced.

Periodic breathing is characterized by cyclic changes in tidal breathing with intervening episodes of obstructive or central apnea or hypopnea. These disordered breathing events result in three basic pathophysiologic consequences: (1) intermittent arterial blood gas abnormalities characterized by hypoxemia-reoxygenation and hypercapnia-hypocapnia, (2) arousals and a shift to light sleep stages, and (3) large negative swings in intrathoracic pressure (Figure 25-1).[1-3] These pathophysiologic consequences of apnea and hypopnea, both obstructive and central, adversely affect cardiovascular function, acutely and chronically.

ARTERIAL BLOOD GAS ABNORMALITIES AND THEIR CONSEQUENCES

Periodic breathing consists of cyclic changes in breathing pattern that include episodes of apnea and hypopnea, resulting in hypoxemia and hypercapnia. After apnea and hypopnea,

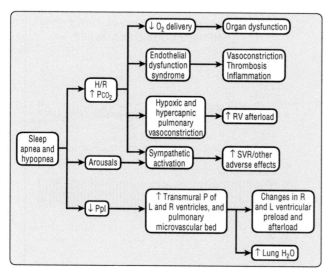

Figure 25-1 Pathophysiologic consequences of sleep apnea and hypopnea. Pleural pressure (Ppl) is a surrogate of the pressure surrounding the heart and other vascular structures. H/R, Hypoxia-reoxygenation; L, left; P, pressure; R, right; RV, right ventricular; SVR, systemic vascular resistance; ↑, increased; ↓, decreased. (Modified from Javaheri S. Sleep-related breathing disorders in heart failure. In: Mann DL, editor. *Heart failure: a companion to Braunwald's heart disease.* Philadelphia: Saunders; 2003. p. 478.)

hyperpnea ensues, resulting in reoxygenation and hypocapnia. These alterations in blood gases affect the cardiovascular system in different ways.

Hypoxemia and Reoxygenation

Hypoxemia has direct (decreased myocardial oxygen delivery) and indirect (activation of sympathetic nervous system, promotion of endothelial cell dysfunction, and pulmonary arteriolar vasoconstriction) cardiac and vascular effects. Hypoxemia with reoxygenation may be analogous to ischemia with reperfusion, and reoxygenation may cause additional damage through further production of free radical species. Biochemical injury due to hypoxemia-reoxygenation has considerable relevance to sleep apnea-hypopnea, where intermittent and profound alterations in the partial pressure of oxygen (Po_2) may occur hundreds of times during sleep.

Direct Effects of Hypoxia on Myocardium

Decreased myocardial oxygen delivery may result in an imbalance between myocardial oxygen consumption and demand, resulting in myocardial hypoxia, particularly if there is already coronary artery disease. At the same time, myocardial oxygen demand may be elevated because of concomitant tachycardia. Potential clinical consequences of myocardial hypoxia include nocturnal angina, nocturnal myocardial infarction,[4] arrhythmias, and even nocturnal sudden death.[5] Hypoxia may also impair myocardial contractility and cause diastolic dysfunction.[6]

Hypoxemia-Reoxygenation and Coronary Endothelial Dysfunction

Coronary vessel endothelial cells play a central role in vasoregulation, coagulation, and inflammation.[7] Blood flow and coagulation are modulated by production and release of vasoactive substances that include vasodilators and platelet deaggregators (e.g., nitric oxide, prostacyclin) and vasoconstrictors

and platelet aggregators (e.g., endothelin and thromboxane). The balance between vasoregulatory agents is important in modulating coronary blood flow and coagulation status in both health and disease.

Through activation of certain transcription factors such as hypoxia-inducible factor-1 and nuclear factor-κB,[8,9] hypoxia increases the expression of a number of genes such as those encoding endothelin-1, a potent vasoconstrictor with proinflammatory properties, vascular endothelial growth factor, and platelet-derived growth factor. In contrast, it suppresses the transcriptional rate of endothelial nitric oxide synthase,[10] resulting in decreased production of nitric oxide, which is vasodilatory and has antimitogenic properties. Hypoxia also enhances expression of adhesion molecules and promotes leukocyte rolling and endothelial adherence,[11] and it is involved in induction of endothelial and myocyte apoptosis.[12]

Some of the aforementioned adverse effects of sustained hypoxia have also been observed with intermittent hypoxia (i.e., hypoxia-reoxygenation).[13-23] In this context, intermittent hypoxia has been proposed to be more deleterious than sustained hypoxia.[18,19] Reoxygenation through delivery of oxygen molecules provides a substrate for additional production of oxygen radicals and may contribute to oxidative stress.

The pathophysiologic consequences of hypoxemia-reoxygenation could lead to vascular inflammation and remodeling, similar to atherosclerosis.[7,23] Endothelial dysfunction has been demonstrated in a number of cardiovascular disorders, including hypertension, myocardial infarction, and stroke. Interestingly, these disorders have been also associated with OSA. It is therefore conceivable that endothelial dysfunction caused by sleep-related breathing disorders may contribute to worsening of atherosclerosis, atherothrombosis, and left ventricular dysfunction.[1,24]

The inflammatory and neurohormonal (see Obstructive Sleep Apnea and Systolic Heart Failure, later) consequences of altered blood gas chemistry have been best studied in patients with OSA, which is associated with increased sympathetic activity, high concentrations of endothelin, adhesion molecules, inflammatory cytokines, activation of white blood cells, oxidative stress, endothelial dysfunction, and hypercoagulopathy.[1,22,24-39] These autonomic, biochemical, and functional alterations may be reversed with use of nasal CPAP to treat OSA. However, such systematic studies are lacking for central sleep apnea, with the exception of studies showing increased overnight and morning sympathetic activity and increased concentration of endothelin and brain natriuretic peptide in patients with heart failure with central sleep apnea compared with those without central sleep apnea (for details, see Chapter 28).[40]

Hypoxemia-Hypercapnia and the Autonomic Nervous System

Sleep apneas and hypopneas, both obstructive and central (Figures 25-2 and 25-3), increase sympathetic activity through complex mechanisms. Hypoxemia stimulates the peripheral arterial chemoreceptors in the carotid bodies, triggering reflex increases in sympathetic activity.[41,42] Hypercapnia stimulates the peripheral and the central chemoreceptors located in the region of the brainstem, also increasing sympathetic activity.

Both hypoxemia and hypercapnia increase ventilation, which, acting through thoracic afferents, buffers the increases

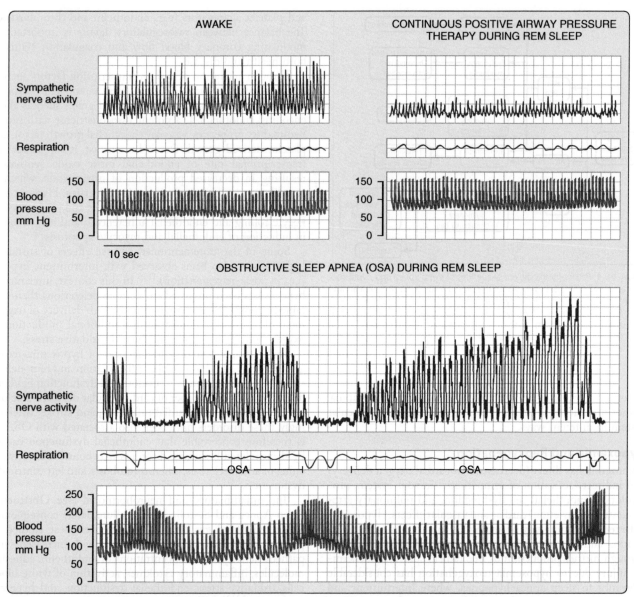

Figure 25-2 Recordings of sympathetic nerve activity, intraarterial blood pressure, and breathing in a normotensive patient with obstructive sleep apnea (OSA) during resting normoxic wakefulness (*top left*). The patient was free of any other overt cardiovascular disease and on no medications. Note the high levels of sympathetic nerve traffic even in the absence of apneic events. During REM sleep (*bottom*), the repetitive hypoxemia and hypercapnia elicit chemoreflex-mediated sympathetic activation and vasoconstriction. At the end of apneas, with increases in cardiac output and severe vasoconstriction, intraarterial blood pressure can reach levels from 130/60 mm Hg during wakefulness to a peak of 220/130 mm Hg during apneas. At the end of apneas, there also is abrupt inhibition of sympathetic traffic because of the increase in blood pressure acting through the baroreflexes and the sympathetic inhibitory effects of the thoracic afferents. After treatment of OSA with continuous positive airway pressure (*top right*), there is a marked reduction in sympathetic traffic and in blood pressure. (From Somers VK, Dyken ME, Clary MP, et al. Sympathetic neural mechanisms in obstructive sleep apnea. *J Clin Invest* 1995;96:1897–904.)

in sympathetic drive during hypoxemia and to a lesser extent during hypercapnia.[41,42] Thus when hypoxemia or hypercapnia occurs during apnea, the absence of ventilatory inhibition results in a potentiation of sympathetic activation and consequent vasoconstriction and blood pressure surges. In this context, and especially when there are potentiated chemoreflex responses to hypoxemia-hypercapnia,[43,44] the sympathetic and consequent pressor responses to hypoxemia-hypercapnia,

particularly in the absence of inhibitory effects of breathing, are marked.

Nighttime sympathetic activation carries over into daytime wakefulness. Repetitive hypoxemia may be implicated because after 2 weeks of chronic intermittent hypoxia, healthy normal subjects manifested an increase in sympathetic outflow, together with increased chemoreflex gain and blunted baroreflex function.[45]

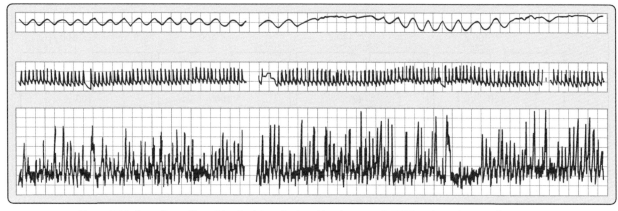

Figure 25-3 Recordings of breathing (*top*), beat-by-beat blood pressure (*middle*), and muscle sympathetic nerve activity (MSNA) (*bottom*) in a patient with severe congestive heart failure, during normal breathing on the *left* and during Cheyne-Stokes breathing on the *right*. Oxygen saturation was 94% during normal breathing and oscillated between 97% and 90% during Cheyne-Stokes breathing. MSNA total burst amplitude increased from 1533 arbitrary units per minute during normal breathing to 1759 arbitrary units per minute during Cheyne-Stokes breathing. Mean blood pressure was 70 mm Hg during normal breathing and peaked at 82 mm Hg during the hyperventilation that followed central apnea. Patients with heart failure have high levels of sympathetic drive even during normal breathing. During central apneas, there is a modest but significant further increase in sympathetic activity. (From Van de Borne P, Oren R, Abouassaly C, et al. Effect of Cheyne-Stokes respiration on muscle sympathetic nerve activity in severe congestive heart failure secondary to ischemic or idiopathic dilated cardiomyopathy. *Am J Cardiol* 1998;81:432–6.)

Alveolar Hypoxia-Hypercapnia and Pulmonary Arteriolar Vasoconstriction

Alveolar hypoxia, in part through release of endothelin, and hypercapnia cause pulmonary arteriolar vasoconstriction and hypertension, which could adversely affect right ventricular function (see Chapter 26).

Hypocapnia

Episodes of hyperpnea after apneas and hypopneas result in hypocapnia. Hypocapnia may impair myocardial oxygen delivery and uptake by coronary artery vasoconstriction[45] and shifting of the oxygen-hemoglobin dissociation curve to the left. Hypocapnia may also contribute to arrhythmogenesis.

Arousals, Shift to Light Sleep Stages, and the Autonomic Nervous System

Compared with wakefulness, the balance of activity of sympathetic and parasympathetic nervous system reverses in normal sleep.[46,47] Normally, there is a progressive reduction in sympathetic nerve traffic, heart rate, and blood pressure during the deepening stages of non–rapid eye movement (NREM) sleep, such that sympathetic activity, heart rate, and blood pressure in stage 4 sleep are substantially lower than during supine resting wakefulness.[46,47] During phasic rapid eye movement (REM) sleep, there is an abrupt increase in sympathetic activity, resulting in intermittent and brief surges in blood pressure and heart rate. On average, blood pressure and heart rate during REM sleep are similar to levels recorded during wakefulness. Thus during normal sleep, there is a well-regulated pattern of alteration in autonomic and hemodynamic measures, modulated by changes in sleep stage. These organized responses to normal sleep are disrupted in patients with sleep-related breathing disorders, both obstructive and central sleep apnea. Sleep architecture is dramatically altered in patients with OSA-hypopnea and also in patients with

heart failure and central sleep apnea. There is a shift to light sleep stages. Most important, however, apneas and hypopneas commonly result in arousals that are also associated with an increase in sympathetic activity and a decrease in parasympathetic activity,[47,48] and increasing blood pressure and heart rate. In OSA, arousals occur at the end of the apnea and with resumption of breathing. In patients with central sleep apnea and Hunter-Cheyne-Stokes breathing pattern, arousals occur at the peak of hyperventilation.

In addition to arousals, sleep-related breathing disorders may increase sympathetic activity by hypoxemia, hypercapnia, and changes in ventilation, as noted previously.

There are multiple adverse cardiac consequences of sympathetic activation. These include increased systemic vascular resistance and left ventricular afterload, venoconstriction with increased right ventricular preload, increased myocardial contractility, hypertrophy, tachycardia, and arrhythmias. Furthermore, increased myocardial norepinephrine may cause myocyte toxicity and apoptosis.[49,50]

Central sleep apnea and OSA increase sympathetic activity as measured by either microneurography or blood and urinary norepinephrine levels.[51-56] Treatment of obstructive[54-56] and central sleep apnea[52,57] decreases sympathetic activity, with important implications. First, with regard to central sleep apnea in heart failure, increased sympathetic activity is associated with poor survival; therefore a reduction in sympathetic activity should have favorable prognostic implications. OSA causes nocturnal increases in sympathetic activity and blood pressure, which carry over into the daytime. OSA is a known cause of hypertension, and in some patients blood pressure decreases relatively quickly with effective treatment of OSA with CPAP (see Chapter 26).

In summary, pathophysiologic consequences of sleep-related breathing disorders, such as increased periods of wakefulness (interruption insomnia), arousals, hypoxemia, and hypercapnia, collectively contribute to increased sympathetic activity.

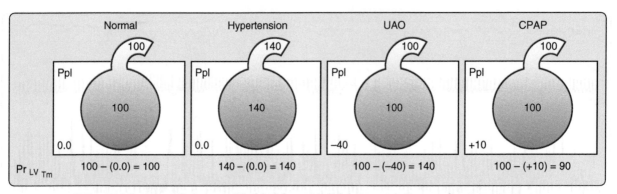

Figure 25-4 Transmural (Tm) pressure (Pr) of the left ventricle (LV) during systole. Because of an obstructive apnea (upper airway occlusion [UAO]), a negative pleural pressure (Ppl) of −40 mm Hg is generated. This increases left ventricular transmural pressure from 100 to 140 mm Hg, which is equivalent to an increase in systolic aortic blood pressure from 100 to 140 mm Hg. Note the reduction in left ventricular transmural pressure with application of nasal continuous positive airway pressure (CPAP). (Modified from Javaheri S. Sleep-related breathing disorders in heart failure. In: Mann DL, editor. *Heart failure: a companion to Braunwald's heart disease.* Philadelphia: Saunders; 2003. p. 480.)

Exaggerated Negative Intrathoracic Pressure and Its Consequences

Large negative intrathoracic pressures are generated during episodes of obstructive apnea. In central sleep apnea, relatively large negative pressure deflections occur during hyperpnea, particularly in the face of less compliant (stiff) lungs (due to heart failure). However, pleural pressure changes are usually more pronounced in obstructive than in central sleep apnea.

A number of studies have addressed the cardiovascular consequences of both negative and positive pressure deflections affecting right and left ventricular function.[58,59] Negative intrathoracic pressure increases the transmural pressure (pressure inside minus pressure outside) (Figure 25-4) of the intrathoracic vascular structures, including aorta, pulmonary vascular bed, atria, and ventricles.

According to Laplace's law, increased transmural myocardial pressure increases wall tension and myocardial oxygen consumption. Furthermore, negative intrathoracic perivascular pressure could increase extravascular lung water by favoring fluid transudation across the pulmonary microvascular bed and by diminishing lymph outflow from the lung.[60] This may account in part for cases of flash pulmonary edema reported in OSA, and sleep apnea may contribute to excess lung water and pulmonary edema in congestive heart failure. In addition, decreased intrathoracic pressure increases venous inflow, resulting in increased right ventricular diastolic filling, which in turn may decrease left ventricular compliance and volume, a phenomenon called *ventricular interdependence.* Application of nasal CPAP to treat sleep apnea, both obstructive and central, reduces transmural pressure by two mechanisms. First, and most important, it decreases or eliminates apneas, desaturation, and arousals, which as noted previously collectively increase sympathetic activity and result in cyclic surges in arterial blood pressure. Second, nasal CPAP not only attenuates steep surges in intrathoracic pressure but also actually increases the pleural pressure, thus decreasing transmural pressures across intrathoracic structures (see Figure 25-4).

ACUTE HEMODYNAMIC EFFECTS OF SLEEP APNEA

The circulatory responses to individual apneas and hypopneas are governed by the interaction of stresses and physiologic consequences described previously.[61,62] Hemodynamic changes are related to development of hypoxemia, hypercapnia, presence or absence of breathing, changes in intrathoracic pressure, and the consequent mechanical effects.

Hemodynamic changes have been best studied in human OSA.[61,63,64] The evolution of a cycle of apnea and recovery is complex and represents an unsteady hemodynamic state. For these reasons, hemodynamic changes occur during the course of an apnea, and these changes are different from those occurring during the immediate or late postapneic periods. During recovery, arousals and ventilation further affect hemodynamics. Cyclic changes in heart rate and systemic and pulmonary arterial blood pressure paralleling periodic breathing occur commonly.[61,63-66] In some patients, there is a very clear and progressive bradycardia toward the end of apnea, with abrupt development of tachycardia with resumption of breathing, because of the vagolytic effects of lung inflation and arousals. This manifests as a pattern of repetitive bradycardias or tachycardias during sleep, which may be evident on Holter monitoring and may signify the presence of OSA. In experimental sleep apnea, decreases in heart rate are more severe during central than obstructive apnea, reflecting lack of activation of thoracic afferents.[62]

The bradycardias may be especially severe,[65,66] and they are elicited because of activation of the diving reflex by the combination of hypoxemia and apnea. Episodes of up to 10 seconds or more of sinus arrest may occur because of the chemoreflex-mediated vagal activation. The consequent absence of perfusion, because of asystole, may have implications for patients with preexisting severe cerebral or cardiac ischemia.

At the termination of obstructive apneas, there are surges in blood pressure. This cyclic change in blood pressure is one of the most consistent hemodynamic findings in patients with OSA. Multiple mechanisms are involved. During apnea, the increased hypoxemia and hypercapnia, acting through the chemoreflexes, progressively elicit sympathetic activation and vasoconstriction.[53] With resumption of breathing, because of the inspiratory increase in right ventricular filling, stroke volume may increase. Vagolytic effects of inspiration result in tachycardia. The increased stroke volume and heart rate result in an increased cardiac output entering a vasoconstricted peripheral circulation, with consequent acute increases in blood pressure.[53] However, just after termination of an obstructive apnea, there is abrupt inhibition of sympathetic activity to the peripheral blood vessels, in part because the deep breathing inhibits sympathetic activity through thoracic afferents and in part because of baroreflex inhibition of sympathetic activity secondary to the postapneic blood pressure surge. Nevertheless, despite the interruption in sympathetic nerve traffic, vasoconstriction persists for several seconds after termination of the sympathetic nerve discharge because of the kinetics of norepinephrine uptake, release, and washout at the neurovascular junction.

Another consistent finding is a mild reduction in stroke volume during obstructive apnea, which has been documented using noninvasive techniques for measuring beat-to-beat cardiac output.[61] This probably results from a decrease in left ventricular preload and an increase in afterload. Changes in stroke volume after termination of the apnea depend on where in the recovery cycle it is being measured.[61]

Obstructive Sleep Apnea, Left Ventricular Dysfunction, and Heart Failure

The relationship between central sleep apnea and heart failure is discussed in Chapter 28. In this section, we review OSA as a cause of heart failure.

Obstructive Sleep Apnea and Systolic Heart Failure

In a canine model mimicking severe OSA,[67] within a 1- to 3-month period of exposure to apneas during sleep, left ventricular systolic dysfunction developed. Left ventricular ejection fraction, measured during the daytime, decreased significantly because of an increase in left ventricular systolic volume.

In humans, there are two kinds of studies relating left ventricular systolic dysfunction and OSA—first, studies in which patients with OSA have been assessed for the presence of left ventricular dysfunction,[68-71] and second, studies in patients with established left ventricular systolic dysfunction who have been assessed to determine the prevalence of OSA.[72,73] In some studies,[74-75] changes in left ventricular ejection fraction in response to treatment for OSA have also been described.

Results of studies assessing left ventricular systolic function in OSA patients are conflicting.[68-70] However, in the two studies[69,70] in which technetium-99m was used to assess left ventricular systolic function, OSA was associated with left ventricular systolic dysfunction. Use of radionuclide ventriculography to assess left ventricular function is important because in obese subjects, echocardiography, which has been used in some studies, may be associated with technical difficulties.

Alchanatis and colleagues[69] studied 29 patients with severe OSA (apnea-hypopnea index [AHI] greater than 15/hour; mean AHI, 54/hour; lowest arterial oxygen saturation, 62%) and 12 control subjects (AHI, 9/hour; lowest saturation, 92%).

The subjects were without known cardiovascular disease. The mean left ventricular ejection fraction was significantly lower in patients with OSA compared with the control group (53% vs. 61%; $P < .003$). Six months after treatment with CPAP, left ventricular ejection fraction increased significantly to 56% ($P < .001$). Left ventricular diastolic dysfunction also improved significantly (see later).

In a large study[70] of 169 patients with OSA (AHI greater than 10/hour; mean AHI, 47/hour), 13 subjects (8%) had left ventricular systolic dysfunction (range, 32% to 50%). Left ventricular systolic dysfunction was not the result of ischemic disease as evidenced by echocardiography and dipyridamole stress testing. In seven patients who were treated for OSA (six with CPAP and one with upper airway surgery), 1 year after therapy, mean left ventricular ejection increased significantly from 44% to 63%.[70]

In the cross-sectional analysis of more than 6000 patients enrolled in the Sleep Health Heart Study,[71] the presence of OSA increased the likelihood of having a history of heart failure by an odds ratio of 2.5. Furthermore, there was a significant dose-dependent correlation between AHI and the prevalence of heart failure.

In studies of patients with established left ventricular systolic dysfunction undergoing polysomnography (reviewed in Chapter 28), the prevalence of OSA, defined as an AHI of at least 15/hour, ranged from 12% to 32%.[76] This wide range is not particularly surprising. The prevalence depends on a number of factors, including the number of obese patients with heart failure enrolled in each study and the different polysomnographic criteria used by various investigators for diagnosis of OSA. Another important issue is the difficulty in accurately classifying hypopneas into central versus obstructive, which is a determinant of prevalence of the phenotype of sleep-disordered breathing.

In a prospective study[72] of 81 patients with known systolic dysfunction and in whom no question was asked regarding snoring or other symptoms associated with OSA, 11% had OSA, with a mean AHI of 36/hour and a lowest arterial oxygen saturation of 72%. In a retrospective study[73] of 450 patients with systolic dysfunction who were referred for a sleep study because of snoring and other symptoms of sleep apnea, 32% had OSA. From the aforementioned studies, however, it cannot be determined whether OSA preceded heart failure. Yet, as is discussed later, treatment of OSA with nasal CPAP increases left ventricular ejection fraction,[74,75] indicating that OSA contributes to worsening of left ventricular systolic dysfunction.

The mechanisms by which OSA may impair left ventricular systolic function are multiple. Hypoxemia plays a critical role, both by impairing myocardial contractility and through a host of neurohormonal mechanisms. In addition, increases in left ventricular wall stress and transmural pressure occur because of additive effects of the excess negative juxtacardiac pressure (during obstructive apneas) and development of hypertension.

The effects of positive airway pressure therapy on left ventricular ejection fraction in patients with OSA and systolic heart failure have been reported in five randomized clinical trials, two of which were double blind (Table 25-1). In three of the studies in which CPAP was used, including the only two double-blind randomized clinical trials, the rise in left ventricular fraction was minimal or not at all. It should be

Table 25-1   Effects of Positive Airway Pressure Therapy on Left Ventricular Ejection Fraction in Patients with Obstructive Sleep Apnea and Systolic Heart Failure

Variable	Kaneko Open	Mansfield Open	Egea DB	Smith DB	Khayat Open	Khayat Open
n	12	19	20	23	11	13
AHI (n/hr)	40	25	44	36	30	34
LVEF (%)	25	35	29	30	29	26
Increase in LVEF (%)	9*	5*	2.2*	0.0	0.5	8.5*
Duration	4 wk	3 mo	3 mo	6 wk	3 mo	3 mo
PAP titration	CPAP yes	CPAP yes	CPAP yes	Auto CPAP	CPAP yes	Bilevel yes
Compliance (hr)	6.2	5.6	NR	3.5	3.6	4.5

*Indicates a statistically significant change.
AHI, Apnea-hypopnea index; CPAP, continuous positive airway pressure; DB, double blind; NR, not reported; PAP, positive airway pressure.
Data from Kaneko Y, Flores JS, Usui K, et al. Cardiovascular effects of continuous positive airway pressure in patients with heart failure and obstructive sleep apnea. *N Engl J Med* 2003;348:1233–41; Mansfield DR, Gollogly, NC, Kaye DM, et al. Controlled trial of continuous positive airway pressure in obstructive sleep apnea in heart failure. *Am J Respir Crit Care Med* 2004;169:361–6; Egea CJ, Aizpuru F, Pinto JA, et al. Cardiac function after CPAP therapy in patients with chronic heart failure and sleep apnea: a multicenter study. *Sleep Med* 2008;9:660–6; Schmidt LA, Vennelle M, Gardner RS, et al. Autotitrating continuous positive airway pressure therapy in patients with chronic heart failure and obstructive sleep apnea: a randomized placebo controlled trial. *Eur Heart J* 2007;28:1221–7; Khayat RN, Abraham WT, Patt B, et al. Cardiac effects of continuous and bilevel crowded airway pressure for patients with heart failure and obstructive sleep apnea: a pilot study. *Chest* 2008;134:1162–8.

noted, however, that in at least two of these studies compliance with CPAP was also limited. In the two open studies in which compliance hours with CPAP were more than those in the double-blind studies, ejection fraction increased between 5% and 9%. In one open randomized clinical trial of CPAP versus a bilevel device, the ejection fraction increased significantly only with bilevel therapy.

Obstructive Sleep Apnea and Diastolic Heart Failure

Isolated left ventricular diastolic heart failure with relative preservation of left ventricular systolic function is the most common form of heart failure in elderly subjects. The pathophysiologic consequences of this form of heart failure relate to a hypertrophied, noncompliant left ventricle, shifting the pressure-volume curve upward and to the left. Therefore, for a given left ventricular volume, left ventricular end-diastolic pressure increases, resulting in elevated left atrial and pulmonary capillary pressure and in pulmonary congestion and edema.

As noted previously, hemodynamic studies[63,64] of patients with OSA have documented that pulmonary capillary pressure increases during the course of an obstructive apnea, indicating development of diastolic dysfunction. During obstructive apnea, left ventricular transmural wall tension increases because of an increase in aortic blood pressure and a simultaneous decrease in juxtacardiac pressure. Furthermore, hypoxemia may impair left ventricular relaxation, further impairing diastolic function.[77] Repeated exposure to nocturnal hypertension and hypoxemia and consequent development of OSA-induced systemic hypertension and increased left ventricular mass may also contribute to left ventricular diastolic dysfunction.

Most studies show that OSA is associated with an increase in left ventricular mass,[78-81] and suggest that the OSA-related cardiac structural changes may resolve with CPAP treatment.[80] An early study[78] reported that OSA may cause left ventricular hypertrophy even in the absence of daytime systemic hypertension. This finding was later supported by

another study[79] comparing patients with OSA (AHI >20/hour) and those without OSA (AHI <20/hour).

In the largest study,[81] consisting of 2058 Sleep Heart Health Study participants, left ventricular mass was associated with both apnea-hypopnea and hypoxemia indexes after adjustment for age, sex, ethnicity, study site, body mass index, smoking, systolic blood pressure, antihypertensive medication use, diabetes mellitus, myocardial infarction, and alcohol consumption. Although there are considerable data[72,73,82] regarding the prevalence of sleep apnea in patients with systolic heart failure (reviewed by Javaheri[76]), the prevalence of OSA in diastolic heart failure has been studied only in one large systematic study.[83] Bitter and colleagues evaluated 244 consecutive patients (87 women) with heart failure with a preserved ejection fraction (HFpEF). All underwent polygraphy, right heart catheterization, and echocardiography. The two major causes of HFpEF were systemic hypertension (44%) and coronary artery disease (33%). Forty-eight percent had an AHI of 15 or more per hour, a prevalence similar to that seen in patients with heart failure with a reduced ejection fraction (HFrEF). Among patients with an AHI of 15/hour or more, 23% had central sleep apnea. Consistent with the observation in HFrEF, patients with HFpEF and central sleep apnea had lower Pco_2 and higher left ventricular end-diastolic and pulmonary capillary wedge pressure than OSA patients.

As noted earlier, isolated diastolic heart failure is highly prevalent in elderly subjects. Furthermore, elderly subjects have a high prevalence of OSA. It is speculated that OSA could be the cause of diastolic heart failure, or the presence of OSA could contribute to the worsening of left ventricular diastolic dysfunction. In this regard, a preliminary study reported that treatment of OSA improves left ventricular diastolic dysfunction,[69] an observation confirmed by the only randomized, placebo (sham CPAP)-controlled trial[80] showing that after 12 weeks on effective CPAP therapy, there was a significant increase in E/A ratio (the ratio of early to late diastolic filling) and a significant decrease in isovolumic relaxation and mitral deceleration. These observations are similar to the improvement seen in systolic function when patients with heart failure and OSA are treated with CPAP (see Table 25-1).[74-76]

Arrhythmias in Obstructive Sleep Apnea

Obstructive Sleep Apnea Predisposing to an Arrhythmogenic Substrate

Repetitive nocturnal apneas elicit severe derangements in cardiovascular homeostasis. Hypoxemia, hypercapnia, acidosis, adrenergic activation, increased afterload, and rapid fluctuations in cardiac wall stress would reasonably be expected to be conducive to tachycardia-brachycardia oscillations and atrial and ventricular arrhythmias (Figures 25-5 and 25-6). A variety of atrioventricular arrhythmias, including complete heart block and ventricular asystole during sleep, have been observed in patients with OSA[84-86] and have been eliminated by either tracheostomy or use of nasal CPAP.[84,85] Profound OSA-induced arrhythmias can occur in the absence of any major structural abnormalities in the conduction system.[87]

Although the normal heart would be less likely to manifest malignant arrhythmias in the setting of severe obstructive apnea, the ischemic, hypertrophied, or failing heart may be more susceptible.[88] Nevertheless, activation of the diving reflex[66,89] during apneas can often elicit severe bradyarrhythmias, even in the setting of a normal myocardium and normal cardiac electrophysiologic function.

Tachycardia-Bradycardia Oscillations

Patients undergoing Holter monitoring may be noted to have repetitive cyclic episodes of tachycardias and bradycardias during the night.[90,91] These cyclic fluctuations may be attributable to obstructive apneas, although this cannot be confirmed because standard Holter monitoring does not incorporate simultaneous measurements of either breathing pattern or oxygen saturation.

These oscillations in cardiac rate are for the most part explained by changes in cardiac autonomic drive related to breathing pattern. During the course of apnea, incremental hypoxemia elicits the diving reflex so that bradycardia becomes progressively more marked. With termination of apnea, hyperpnea occurs with consequent activation of thoracic afferents, which is vagolytic.[92] Thus with resumption of breathing, abrupt lung inflation interrupts vagal drive to the heart, resulting in rapid-onset tachycardia. Furthermore, increased cardiac-bound sympathetic drive and withdrawal of parasympathetic activity because of arousals should also contribute to the tachycardia seen with termination of obstructive apnea. It is interesting that tachycardia persists even though blood pressure increases strikingly with termination of apnea. The vagolytic effects of inspiration and the arousal-associated changes in the autonomic nervous system not only interrupt the chemoreflex-mediated cardiac vagal drive but also blunt the expected cardiac vagal drive that would occur secondary to baroreflex activation by the postapneic surge in blood pressure.

Because of the repetitive nature of nocturnal apneas, Holter or other electrocardiographic monitoring at night manifests as a tachycardia-bradycardia pattern. This cardiac rate oscillation is less apparent in patients with autonomic dysfunction, such as patients with long-standing diabetes or cardiac transplant recipients with denervated hearts. Although the changes in cardiac rate are predominantly reflex mediated, breathing-related changes in cardiac filling, as well as rapid changes in cardiac transmural pressures resulting from the Müller maneuver, also modulate heart rate by variations in stretch of cardiac conduction tissue.

Bradyarrhythmias

The primary response to hypoxia is bradycardia.[89] When hypoxia is accompanied by the action of breathing, the bradycardic response is masked because of inhibition of cardiac vagal drive by ventilation.[66] The sympathetic response to hypoxemia, although evident to some extent during breathing, is also attenuated by ventilation and is therefore potentiated during apnea.[93,94] Patients with OSA may be particularly susceptible to hypoxia-induced bradyarrhythmias because their peripheral chemoreflex is heightened, so that even during

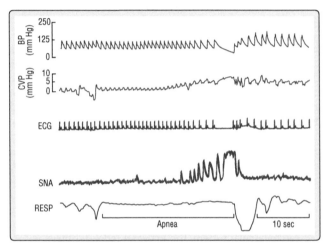

Figure 25-5 Recordings of intraarterial blood pressure (BP), central venous pressure (CVP), electrocardiogram (ECG), sympathetic nerve activity (SNA), and respiratory patterns (RESP) in a healthy subject during voluntary end-expiratory apnea. During apnea, there is a progressive increase in the RR interval on the ECG with eventual sinus pause and atrioventricular block. Accompanying this is increased sympathetic activity. The simultaneous sympathetic activation to peripheral blood vessels and vagal activation of the heart is characteristic of the diving reflex. Note the rapid increase in heart rate and sympathetic inhibition during resumption of breathing. This occurs in part because thoracic afferents activated by inspiration inhibit both sympathetic traffic and vagal cardiac drive. (From Somers VK, Dyken ME, Mark AL, Abboud FM. Parasympathetic hyperresponsiveness and bradyarrhythmias during apnea in hypertension. *Clin Auton Res* 1992;2:171–6.)

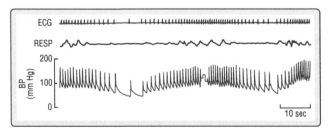

Figure 25-6 A patient with sleep apnea manifesting prolonged and profound bradyarrhythmias with absence of either atrial or ventricular contraction. The beat-by-beat blood pressure (BP) recording confirms the absence of any perfusion during the bradycardia. ECG, electrocardiogram; RESP, respiratory pattern. (From Somers VK, Dyken ME, Mark AL, Abboud FM. Parasympathetic hyperresponsiveness and bradyarrhythmias during apnea in hypertension. *Clin Auton Res* 1992;2:171–6.)

voluntary apneas, hypoxemia elicits greater bradycardia than is seen in closely matched control subjects.[95] The arterial baroreflexes serve as an important buffer to diminish chemoreflex gain.[96] Impaired baroreflex sensitivity, such as is seen in hypertension[97] and heart failure,[98] may be associated with further increased chemoreflex drive. Thus patients with hypertension or heart failure who have OSA may manifest even greater sympathetic, and perhaps bradycardic, responses to obstructive apneas.

Profound bradyarrhythmias may have important consequences, particularly in patients with underlying cardiovascular disease. As an example, in the absence of recognition of OSA as a potential cause of the bradyarrhythmia, patients may receive pacemaker implantation, even though their cardiac conduction system may be completely normal and the bradyarrhythmias could be abolished by effective treatment with CPAP.[83,84,99] Second, prolonged episodes of asystole result in absence of perfusion (see Figure 25-6). Absence of perfusion in the setting of apnea-induced hypoxemia, occurring repetitively through the night, may have important implications for ischemic damage to end organs in which there may already be preexisting circulatory compromise.

Ventricular Arrhythmias

There is an extensive literature on sleep apnea inducing nocturnal angina and cardiac ischemia evidenced by ST-segment depression.[100,101] Thus there is a potential contribution of OSA to ventricular arrhythmias through ventricular ectopy during profound bradycardia as well as polymorphic ventricular tachycardia due to cardiac hypoxia-ischemia. These episodes occur primarily with severe desaturation,[83,84] are more common in patients with coronary heart disease,[86] and are virtually eliminated with treatment.[83,84,99] The prevalence of these arrhythmias is low in patients without premorbid cardiorespiratory disease or severe desaturation.[102]

Atrial Fibrillation

In patients cardioverted for atrial fibrillation, those with polysomnographically proven OSA who were not receiving effective CPAP treatment had a 12-month recurrence rate of 82% compared with a 42% recurrence rate in patients with OSA receiving effective CPAP.[103] In patients cardioverted for atrial fibrillation in whom no sleep study had been done, the recurrence rate was 53%. This risk for recurrence in the patients with atrial fibrillation without a previous sleep study suggests that undiagnosed OSA may be present in a large proportion of patients with atrial fibrillation. In addition, among the untreated patients with OSA, those experiencing a recurrence of atrial fibrillation had more severe nocturnal hypoxemia than those without a recurrence. Furthermore, the increased recurrence in patients with untreated OSA could not be explained by factors such as antiarrhythmic medication, body mass index, hypertension, cardiac function, or atrial size.

Mooe and colleagues[104] observed that after coronary artery bypass surgery, patients with OSA were more likely to experience postoperative atrial fibrillation. However, it is not clear whether this was explained by other variables in the patients with OSA.

In a recent longitudinal study of several thousand patients, those with OSA had an increased risk for developing new-onset atrial fibrillation compared with those who did not have OSA. This risk was evident in patients age 65 or younger, and it was especially marked in those with more severe nocturnal hypoxemia.[105]

There are many reasons that OSA may be conducive to atrial fibrillation. Hypoxemia, presser surges, and sympathetic activation are all potential mechanisms leading to atrial fibrillation. High levels of C-reactive protein may also independently predict the development of atrial fibrillation.[106] Patients with OSA may have increased levels of C-reactive protein.[107-110] Furthermore, abrupt and dramatic changes in intrathoracic negative pressures may especially affect the atria because of their relatively thin walls compared with the ventricles. Increased pressure gradients with consequent increased atrial wall stretch, occurring repetitively through the night, may be expected to induce mechanical and electrical changes that are also conducive to atrial fibrillation.[111-113] Autonomic mechanisms may be pivotal. Animal models suggest that ganglionated plexus ablation may profoundly inhibit the development of atrial fibrillation in response to hypoxemia and apnea.[114]

About 50% of patients presenting for cardioversion have a high risk for sleep apnea compared with 30% of patients from a general cardiology clinic.[115] Even in patients with comorbid OSA undergoing pulmonary vein isolation, recurrence of atrial fibrillation is more than twofold greater in those not treated with CPAP compared with those receiving CPAP therapy.[116]

CLINICAL PEARLS

- Apnea and recovery cycles result in three basic abnormalities: alterations in blood gases, arousals, and changes in intrathoracic pressure.
- Hypoxemia-reoxygenation has deleterious effects on the cardiovascular system. This activates redox-sensitive genes, resulting in synthesis of vasoconstrictor and inflammatory mediators; increases sympathetic activity; and causes oxidative stress. These alterations have been best studied in patients with OSA.
- Untreated OSA may increase the risk for recurrence of atrial fibrillation after cardioversion.
- Sleep apnea can induce severe bradyarrhythmias, including prolonged periods of asystole and heart block, even in the setting of a normal myocardium and cardiac electrophysiologic function.
- OSA should be considered in patients who have ST-segment depression or angina occurring primarily at night.
- Heart failure may be significantly linked to the presence of either central sleep apnea or OSA.

SUMMARY

Sleep-related breathing disorders affect cardiovascular function in a variety of ways. OSA and central sleep apnea act through multiple mechanisms to elicit acute circulatory responses, which have implications for the development of chronic vascular and cardiac dysfunction. The acute responses to apnea are mediated in large part by the effects of apnea on blood gas chemistry, which exerts important cardiovascular effects directly on the myocardium and blood vessels and also acts through reflex mechanisms. Acute neural, circulatory, endothelial, inflammatory, and other responses to repetitive nocturnal hypoxemia and hypercapnia may act to induce long-term damage to the myocardium and to the coronary and other vascular beds. With the development of functional and structural cardiovascular disease, the consequences of acute apneas are magnified. For example, severe hypoxemia in the setting of sleep apnea is more easily tolerated by an overtly healthy cardiovascular system compared with one in which myocardial ischemia or left ventricular dysfunction is present, with consequent diminished cardiovascular reserve. Small, short-term studies have suggested that effective prevention of recurrent apneas may favorably affect surrogates of cardiovascular disease outcome, such as sympathetic activity, blood pressure, and left ventricular ejection fraction. The importance of large randomized controlled trials in establishing the benefits, if any, of treating sleep apnea in patients with heart failure are highlighted by the results of the recently completed SERVE-HF Study.[117] In patients with stable systolic heart failure (LVEF ≤ 45%) and predominantly central sleep apnea, treatment with adaptive servo-ventilation (ASV) versus usual care was not accompanied by any reduction in the primary endpoint of hospitalization for worsening heart failure or mortality. This was despite a significant improvement in central sleep apnea with ASV. In fact, there was an increase in all cause mortality and in cardiovascular mortality in the treated group. It is important to note that these findings cannot be extended to similar patients with unstable heart failure, to patients with heart failure with preserved ejection fraction, or to heart failure patients with OSA.

Selected Readings

Cowie MR, Woehrle H, Wegscheider K, et al. Adaptive Servo-Ventilation for Central Sleep Apnea in Systolic Heart Failure. *N Engl J Med* 2015;**373**(12):1095–105.

de Burgh Daly M, Angell-James J, Elsner R. Role of carotid-body chemoreceptors and their reflex interactions in bradycardia and cardiac arrest. *Lancet* 1997;**1**:764–7.

Gami AS, Howard DE, Olson EJ, et al. Day-night pattern of sudden cardiac death in obstructive sleep apnea. *N Engl J Med* 2005;**352**:1206–14.

Ghias M, Scherlag BG, Lu Z, et al. The role of ganglionated plexi in apnea-related atrial fibrillation. *J Am Coll Cardiol* 2009;**54**:2075–83.

Hoyos CM, Melehan KL, Liu PY, et al. Does obstructive sleep apnea cause endothelial dysfunction? A critical review of the literature. *Sleep Med Rev* 2015;**20**:15–26.

Javaheri S. A mechanism of central sleep apnea in patients with heart failure. *N Engl J Med* 1999;**341**:949–54.

Javaheri S. Heart failure. In: Kushida CA, editor. *The encyclopedia of sleep*, vol. 3. Waltham, MA: Academic Press; 2013. p. 374–86.

Javaheri S, Parker TJ, Liming JD, et al. Sleep apnea in 81 ambulatory male patients with stable heart failure: types and their prevalences, consequences and presentations. *Circulation* 1998;**97**:2154–9.

Jelic S, Padeletti M, Canfield S, et al. Inflammation, oxidative stress and repair capacity of the vascular endothelium in obstructive sleep apnea. *Circulation* 2008;**117**:2270–8.

Kaneko Y, Floras JS, Usui K, et al. Cardiovascular effects of continuous positive airway pressure in patients with heart failure and obstructive sleep apnea. *N Engl J Med* 2003;**348**:1233–41.

Kim Y, Koo YS, Lee HY, Lee SY. Can Continuous Positive Airway Pressure Reduce the Risk of Stroke in Obstructive Sleep Apnea Patients? A Systematic Review and Meta-Analysis. *PLoS ONE* 2016;**11**(1):e0146317.

Mansukhani MP, Wang S, Somers VK. Sleep, death, and the heart. *Am J Physiol Heart Circ Physiol* 2015;**309**(5):H739–49.

Punjabi NM, Beamer BA. C-reactive protein is associated with sleep disordered breathing independent of adiposity. *Sleep* 2007;**30**:29–34.

Somers VK, Dyken ME, Clary MP, et al. Sympathetic neural mechanisms in obstructive sleep apnea. *J Clin Invest* 1995;**96**:1897–904.

Somers VK, Dyken ME, Mark AL, et al. Sympathetic-nerve activity during sleep in normal subjects. *N Engl J Med* 1993;**328**:303–7.

Somers VK, White DP, Amin R, et al. Sleep apnea and cardiovascular disease: an American Heart Association/American College of Cardiology Foundation scientific statement from the American Heart Association Council for High Blood Pressure Research Professional Education Committee, Council on Clinical Cardiology, Stroke Council, and Council On Cardiovascular Nursing. In collaboration with the National Heart, Lung, and Blood Institute National Center on Sleep Disorders Research (National Institutes of Health). *Circulation* 2008;**118**:1080–111. and *J Am Coll Cardiol* 2008;**19**;(52):686–717.

A complete reference list can be found online at ExpertConsult.com.

Systemic and Pulmonary Hypertension in Obstructive Sleep Apnea

F. Javier Nieto; Terry Young; Paul E. Peppard; Shahrokh Javaheri

Chapter Highlights

- Cross-sectional and prospective cohort studies in both population and clinical settings show an association between obstructive sleep apnea (OSA) and risk for systemic hypertension that appears to be independent of obesity, age, and other potential confounding factors.

- The strength, consistency, and dose-response relationship shown across studies suggest that the association is causal.

- In support of a causal relationship, recent meta-analysis of randomized trials shows that treatment with positive airway pressure results in a reduction of blood pressure among hypertensive patients with OSA that is likely to be of clinical and therapeutic significance. This effect is most pronounced in patient with

- baseline elevated blood pressure, those who have severe OSA, and those who are adherent to therapy.

- Using the current definition of pulmonary hypertension, about 10% of patients with OSA have mean pulmonary artery pressure of 25 mm Hg or greater. Mild pulmonary arterial hypertension may occur in patients with OSA without daytime hypoxemia or chronic obstructive pulmonary disease, although pulmonary hypertension could be more severe in the presence of chronic lung disease, heart failure, and obesity hypoventilation.

- Studies, mostly observational, suggest that treatment of OSA improves pulmonary hypertension.

Although the clinical association between obstructive sleep apnea (OSA) and hypertension has long been reported[1-3] in sleep medicine, the potential importance of OSA in patients with elevated blood pressure and cardiovascular disease is gaining recognition beyond the field of sleep research. As early as 1998, a committee of experts gathered by the World Health Organization (WHO) recognized OSA as a likely cause of secondary pulmonary arterial hypertension.[4] A few years later, the increasing evidence that OSA has a causal role in the development of hypertension was discussed in two influential taskforce statements.[5,6] Furthermore, the 2013 guidelines for the management of hypertension by the European Society of Hypertension and the European Society of Cardiology include OSA as one of the "special conditions" that need to be evaluated and treated in hypertensive patients.[7] In the United States, even though OSA was recognized as an identifiable cause of hypertension in the seventh report of the Joint National Committee for the Prevention, Detection, Evaluation, and Treatment of High Blood Pressure,[8] surprisingly, the recently updated eighth report does not include reference to OSA—or any sleep-related disorder—in relation to hypertension management.[9]

An accurate estimate of the fraction of systemic hypertension that can be causally attributed to OSA is lacking, and data on OSA and pulmonary hypertension (PH) are sparse; however, clinical recognition of both the high prevalence of hypertension in people with OSA[10,11] and the high occurrence of OSA in hypertensive patients[12-14] is imperative. The aim of this chapter is to present the epidemiologic and clinical evidence in support of a role of OSA in systemic and PH and

to describe the clinical issues in identification and treatment of patients with OSA and hypertension.

SYSTEMIC HYPERTENSION

Epidemiologic Evidence for a Role of Obstructive Sleep Apnea in Systemic Hypertension

The early observations of hypertension in patients with sleep apnea stimulated several cross-sectional clinic- and community-based studies that attempted to determine whether there was an association between OSA and hypertension that was not explained by excess body weight or other factors common to both OSA and hypertension.[11] Results were mixed, but many of the studies had methodologic shortcomings, such as inadequate sample size, flawed comparison groups, substantial measurement error, or limited statistical analysis.[15,16] Since then, findings from both population and clinical studies have shed important new light on this association.

Reports from several well-designed epidemiology studies, summarized in Table 26-1, generally show associations of polysomnography (PSG)-determined OSA and hypertension that remain significant after adjustment for potential confounding factors.[17-19] The strongest epidemiologic evidence for a causal association comes from longitudinal analyses of data from the Wisconsin Sleep Cohort Study of middle-aged state employees.[20,21] The incidence of new hypertension, defined as systolic blood pressure of at least 140 mm Hg, diastolic blood pressure of at least 90 mm Hg, or use of antihypertensive medication at follow-up, was significantly dependent on

Table 26-1   Associations of Polysomnographically Determined Sleep-Disordered Breathing and Hypertension in Four Population Studies

Study Design	Participants (n)	Odds Ratio* for Hypertension[†] (95% CI)				
		AHI Category				
		<1.0[‡]	1 to 4.9	5 to 14.9	15 to 30	≥30
Wisconsin Sleep Cohort Study,[20] state employees, ages 30 to 65 years, prospective, 4–8 years' follow-up	709	1.0	1.2 (1.1–1.8)	2.0 (1.3–3.2)	2.9 (1.5–5.6)	
Sleep Heart Health Study,[19,25] multicenter, ages 40–97 years						
a. Cross-sectional[25]	6132	1.0	1.1 (0.9–1.3)	1.2 (1.0–1.4)	1.3 (1.9–1.6)	1.4 (1.0–1.8)
b. Prospective, 2- and 5-year follow-up[19]	2470	1.0		0.9 (0.7–1.2)	1.1 (0.8–1.5)	1.5 (0.9–2.5)
Southern Pennsylvania,[23] population sample through random-digit dialing, ages 20–100 years, cross-sectional	1741	1.0		2.3[§] (1.4–3.6)	6.9[§] (2.0–26.4)	
Vitoria-Gasteiz, Spain,[24] random census sample, ages 30–70 years, cross-sectional						
a. Cross-sectional[24]	552	1.0	2.5 (1.1–5.8)	1.3 (0.5–4.1)	2.3 (0.9–5.7)	
b. Prospective, 7.5-year follow-up[22]	1180	(RDI <3) 1.0	(3 ≤ RDI <7) 1.1 (0.8–1.5)	(7 ≤ RDI <14) 0.9 (0.6–1.3)	(RDI ≥14) 1.0 (0.6–1.6)	

*Odds ratios are all adjusted for age, sex, body mass index (BMI), neck circumference, alcohol intake, and cigarette smoking. Additional adjustments are made for baseline hypertension and waist circumference in the Wisconsin study; for ethnicity and waist-to-hip ratio in the Sleep Heart Health Study; for ethnicity, menopause, and hormone replacement therapy in the Southern Pennsylvania study; and for coffee consumption and fitness level in the prospective Spanish study.
[†]Defined by systolic blood pressure ≥140 mm Hg, diastolic blood pressure ≥90 mm Hg, or use of antihypertensive medication.
[‡]Reference category for odds ratio.
[§]Estimated at the mean age and BMI of the sample.
AHI, Apnea-hypopnea index; CI, confidence interval; RDI, respiratory disturbance index.

baseline level of OSA. After considering confounding factors, the odds of developing new hypertension over 4 years was twofold greater for those with an apnea-hypopnea index (AHI) of 5 to 15 events/hour and threefold greater for those with an AHI of greater than 15 at baseline, compared with participants without OSA at baseline (i.e., AHI <1). Longitudinal analyses of OSA as a predictor of 5-year incidence of hypertension in the Sleep Heart Health Study (SHHS)[19] and 7.5-year incidence of hypertension in the Vitoria-Gasteiz (Spain) Cohort[22] did not find the same strong association as was found in the Wisconsin cohort; however, the SHHS findings were consistent with about a 50% increased risk for incident hypertension in persons with severe OSA.

Cross-sectional analyses of baseline data from three population cohorts (Southern Pennsylvania,[23] Spain,[24] and the SHHS[25]) using measurements, definitions, and statistical adjustment models similar to those used in the Wisconsin Sleep Cohort have also shown OSA to be a statistically significant risk factor for hypertension (Figure 26-1; see Table 26-1). Collectively, the relationship between OSA and hypertension has been assessed with state-of-the-art measurements in more than 10,000 men and women from the general population, and results have been generally consistent. Confidence in the validity of the findings is increased as a result of the care taken by investigators to evaluate the effects of methodologic limitations.[20,26] If the epidemiology findings do reflect a

causal relationship, as is suggested by most of the population-based data, a harder look must be taken at the importance of preventing OSA or at treating even mild OSA, discussed more fully below.

The largest population study, the cross-sectional examination of OSA and prevalent hypertension of Nieto and colleagues,[22] had sufficient power to describe the strength of the association across a wide spectrum of moderate to severe OSA. The findings suggest a dose-response association between OSA and hypertension up to a moderate level of OSA severity, with the association "flattening" across the severe range (AHI >30). It is possible that a flattening threshold exists, but methodologic limitations may account for it as well. This feature may reflect a survival bias against persons with high-severity OSA and cardiovascular disease, thus potentially missing subjects with the strongest associations from the analysis, as well as greater measurement error of OSA severity at higher AHI levels. Alternatively, a flattening threshold may be due to the presence of pathophysiologic consequences of severe OSA, such as heart failure, that could reduce blood pressure. In regard to heart failure, severe OSA has been associated with left ventricular systolic dysfunction[27]; in the SHHS, there was a dose-dependent relation between AHI and prevalence of heart failure.[28] If left ventricular systolic dysfunction occurs as OSA becomes more severe, adequate left ventricular stroke volume may not be maintained to

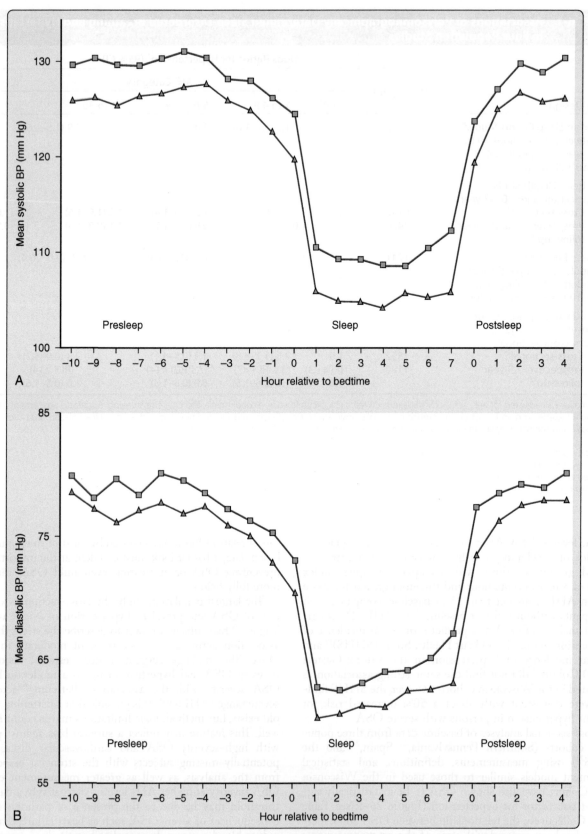

Figure 26-1 Ambulatory blood pressure (BP) during presleep, sleep, and postsleep by apnea-hypopnea index (AHI) category (Wisconsin Sleep Cohort Study). *Triangles:* AHI ≤5 events/hour; number of participants, 537. *Squares:* AHI ≥5, number of participants, 231. **A,** Systolic blood pressure. **B,** Diastolic blood pressure. Mean blood pressure values are adjusted for age, sex, and body mass index.

sustain a high blood pressure. Additionally, mechanisms mediating hypertension in OSA may be become saturated at greater OSA severity levels. In a two-arm study[29] of therapeutic and subtherapeutic positive airway pressure (PAP) in OSA, there were no changes in systemic arterial blood pressure from baseline in the subtherapeutic PAP trial arm despite a decrease in average AHI from 65 to 33. These results are consistent with a flattening of the OSA-hypertension association at greater OSA severity levels.

Obstructive Sleep Apnea and Hypertension in Population Subgroups

Determining the association of OSA with hypertension by subgroups (e.g., sex, age, ethnicity, body habitus) will increase understanding of physiologic mechanisms and may help target health care to appropriate subgroups. Most population cohort studies have reported a lack of sex differences in the association of OSA and hypertension. This message is particularly important because of past underdiagnosis and undertreatment of OSA in women; less-aggressive evaluation and treatment of OSA in women may lead to a relative survival disadvantage for them.[30]

Few studies have included sufficient population diversity to determine whether the association of OSA and hypertension varies by ethnicity. Recent population studies of OSA and hypertension in older adults have expanded the focus beyond OSA in middle age. Cross-sectional regression analyses of two large cohort studies with age ranges that include sufficient older people have suggested a negative interaction between age and AHI with respect to hypertension. Bixler and coworkers found that odds ratios (ORs) for hypertension decreased as age increased when patients with an AHI of 30 or greater were compared with those with an AHI of zero, and there was essentially no risk for hypertension associated with OSA for those 70 years and older.[23] Similar findings were reported by the SHHS: after stratifying their sample with a cutoff age of 65 years, the OR for hypertension with an AHI of greater than 30 versus an AHI of less than 1.5 was lower and not statistically significant for ages 65 years and older (OR = 1.23), compared with ages 40 to 65 years (OR = 1.64).[25] Further analysis of the SHHS data revealed that OSA was not associated with isolated systolic hypertension, the most common form of hypertension in older people.[31]

In contrast, cross-sectional analysis of the Bay Area Sleep Cohort of 129 older adults found a significant association between frequent (10 or more) apnea and hypopnea events during rapid eye movement sleep and diastolic blood pressure greater than 90 mm Hg.[32] This study of adults with a mean age of 72 years also linked occult sleep-disordered breathing to markers of cardiovascular disease. The authors concluded that a role of OSA in cardiovascular disease in older adults should not be ruled out.

Although it is possible that OSA outcomes differ in older versus younger people, methodologic difficulties arising from high comorbidity and survival bias are inherent in studying health effects of OSA in older populations and could cause a spurious age effect. Clinical practice should not be influenced by the notion that health risks of OSA in older people are lower until there are conclusive data—especially considering that even if relative risks relating OSA and hypertension are attenuated in older adults, corresponding absolute risk differences may well not be.

The prevalence of being overweight, a strong risk factor for both OSA and hypertension, is increasing worldwide. Most studies, using multiple regression analysis, have demonstrated that even after consideration of the strong associations of OSA and obesity, they both persist as independent factors in the development of hypertension.[5] However, understanding of specific mechanisms as well as precise effect sizes are limited by many analytic issues, including identification of relevant measures of body habitus, how the variables should be modeled in analyses, and the time course for OSA to have an effect on blood pressure. Adjusting for a marker of obesity (e.g., body mass index [BMI]) in multiple regression analysis of the relationship between OSA and hypertension is justified under the assumption that obesity is a confounder (i.e., obesity is a risk factor for both OSA and hypertension); however, if the relationship between OSA and obesity is bidirectional (e.g., if metabolic changes associated with OSA lead to an increase in body weight), adjustment for obesity in regression models of OSA and hypertension may lead to bias.

Furthermore, the interaction of obesity and OSA with respect to the development of hypertension is not clear. That is, does the strength of the OSA-hypertension association vary by body habitus? Findings from two of the large cohort studies have indicated that OSA is more strongly predictive of hypertension in leaner than in obese individuals: BMI was a significant modifier of the OSA-hypertension association in studies by Young and coworkers[33] and Bixler and coworkers.[23] The OR for hypertension and OSA increased in magnitude with decreasing BMI, indicating that in leaner people, those with OSA compared with those without may be at particularly high risk for hypertension. This finding has clinical implications, particularly in primary care, where sleep apnea is not likely to be suspected in nonobese patients, even in the presence of symptoms.

Obstructive Sleep Apnea and Diurnal Blood Pressure

Hypertension defined by chronic elevated daytime blood pressure is generally considered to be the outcome of interest; however, OSA-related nocturnal perturbations also include repeated spiking of pressures that exceed hypertension cutoff points (blood pressure load) and elevated average nighttime blood pressure as well as a carryover effect resulting in elevated daytime blood pressure.[5] Early studies of hemodynamics in patients with OSA involved invasive blood pressure monitoring; more recent studies of circadian patterns of blood pressure rely on ambulatory monitors that sample blood pressure at 15- to 30-minute intervals with arm cuff inflation–based methods.

Most studies with ambulatory blood pressure monitoring have been conducted on patients with sleep apnea. A Marburg study of 93 OSA patients[34] showed that the number of oxygen desaturation events per hour of presumed sleep was linearly related to both daytime and nighttime systolic and diastolic blood pressures, and it was related more strongly to nighttime pressures. In Great Britain, Davies and colleagues[35] performed ambulatory blood pressure studies on 45 pairs of sleep apnea patients and community controls matched to the patients on age, BMI, and treated hypertension. Sleep apnea patients had significantly higher diastolic pressures during the day and night, higher systolic pressures during the night, and a notably smaller nocturnal dip.

Data from population studies with PSG and nocturnal blood pressure measures are sparse. In a preliminary study of 147 Wisconsin Sleep Cohort Study subjects,[36] OSA was consistently associated with elevated blood pressure measured by 24-hour ambulatory monitoring. Average systolic and diastolic blood pressures during wake and sleep, and systolic blood pressure load during wake and sleep, were all statistically significantly higher in the participants with mild to more severe OSA. Findings from an update with a much larger cohort sample ($n = 768$) are shown in Figure 26-1. Blood pressures, adjusted for confounding factors, were higher at every hour before, during, and after sleep for those with an AHI of greater than 5 versus an AHI of less than 5.

Nocturnal blood pressure relative to daytime pressure has been of special interest because studies have shown that the lack of the normal nighttime decline (nondipping) in blood pressure, usually considered to be a nighttime drop of at least 10% of the daytime pressure, is related to adverse cardiovascular outcomes independent of hypertension.[37] Findings from relatively small clinic-based samples do suggest that patients with OSA have a smaller nocturnal decline in blood pressure.[34,35,37-42] Prospective data from the Wisconsin Sleep Cohort study strengthen the evidence that acute effects of apnea and hypopnea episodes lead to a less favorable nighttime pattern of blood pressures.[43] Baseline and 7-year follow-up data from PSG and ambulatory blood pressure on a subsample of 328 participants in the Wisconsin cohort, free of nondipping at baseline, were analyzed. There was a dose-response increase in the odds of developing a pattern of nondipping in systolic blood pressure: Compared with subjects with an AHI of less than 5 at baseline, ORs, adjusted for confounding factors, were 3.1 (95% confidence interval [CI], 1.3 to 7.7) and 4.4 (95% CI, 1.2 to 16) for an AHI of 5 to 14 and for an AHI of 15 or greater, respectively.

Collectively, the ambulatory blood pressure studies do support an association between OSA and elevated blood pressure during both the nighttime and the daytime, and some studies suggest that the effect is greater during nighttime. These findings are particularly important because elevated ambulatory blood pressure has been shown to predict cardiovascular events independently of office-measured blood pressure and other cardiovascular risk factors.[44]

Blood Pressure Changes in Patients with Obstructive Sleep Apnea after Positive Airway Pressure Treatment

Studies of the effect of PAP on blood pressure have evolved from clinical observations of treated patients to sophisticated, randomized, double-blind trials, with sham PAP as the control condition and objectively measured compliance. Results from these studies are important, even though they do not necessarily directly address the basic question of whether OSA caused the initiation (incidence) of hypertension. This is because the effect of OSA on vasculature hemodynamics might be different at different stages in the natural history of OSA and hypertension, both chronic conditions evolving over a lifetime. However, even with this important caveat, clinical trial results generally show that successful treatment of OSA in patients who are also hypertensive tends to result in lower blood pressure levels.

The results of these studies are not uniformly consistent, likely because of differences in study design, sample size, patient populations, treatment regimens, and compliance from study to study. However, as reviewed in the following paragraphs, the pattern emerging from the overall body of literature on the subject, and especially when the most recent and highly powered studies are considered, strongly suggests that treatment of OSA does have a measurable effect in lowering blood pressure.

With respect to observational evidence, a prospective study that followed 55 patients (35 of whom were men) with both OSA and hypertension for 2 years,[45] a significant decrease was shown only for diastolic blood pressure (−2.2 mm Hg [95% CI, −4.2 to −0.1]), but not in systolic or 24-hour mean arterial blood pressure. Subgroup analyses, however, showed that 24-hour mean blood pressure did decrease significantly in patients with incompletely controlled hypertension at entry (−4.4 mm Hg, $P = .01$) as well as in those with high PAP compliance (−5.3 mm Hg, $P = .01$).

The predictors of change in blood pressure associated with PAP treatment in patients with OSA were examined in another observational prospective cohort study that recruited 86 patients treated for daytime sleepiness with PAP.[46] After 6 months, the average fall in 24-hour mean blood pressure was 4.9 mm Hg (95% CI, −7.1 to −2.1); the main predictors of blood pressure fall were the change in level of self-reported sleepiness and baseline BMI. These results are consistent with another observational study addressing a slightly different question: whether PAP treatment prevents new-onset hypertension. In this study, the hypertension incidence was assessed among 1889 patients who were referred for a PSG study and were free of hypertension at baseline and followed for up to 17 years (median, 12.2 years).[47] Compared with controls in this study, the adjusted hazard ratio of hypertension was 1.33 in patients with OSA who were not eligible for PAP treatment, 1.96 among OSA patients who declined PAP treatment, and 1.78 among patients not adherent to PAP (all $P < .05$). In contrast, patients with OSA who received PAP treatment had a statistically significant lower risk for hypertension incidence than controls (hazard ratio, 0.71; 95% CI, 0.53 to 0.94).

Evidence from randomized controlled trials has been growing in recent years, and even though not all of the studies are consistent, the evidence supports the notion that PAP treatment results in a moderate but clinically significant lowering of blood pressure. Some of the early studies showed a significant lowering of blood pressure in patients with OSA, even though most of these studies did not select according to hypertension status.[29,48-50] In some of these studies, the effects were stronger or exclusively observed among the PAP-compliant patients.[29,49]

Other randomized trials, however, have shown minimal or nonsignificant effects of PAP in blood pressure.[51-56] Aside from the small sample size and limited statistical power, a potentially important limitation of some of these studies is that many of the patients included in the trial were not hypertensive, and thus there might be limited room for a lowering of blood pressuring effect as well as limited compliance with the treatment.

To address the latter, Hla and coworkers[57] investigated the effect of 3 weeks of PAP on blood pressure in hypertensive subjects with and without OSA to control for effects that PAP might have on blood pressure independent of an effect from elimination of apnea and hypopnea events. Newly diagnosed, unmedicated hypertensive men from primary care settings were assessed for OSA by laboratory PSG to identify 14 men with an AHI of greater than 5 (mean AHI, 25) and 10 men with an AHI of less than 5 (mean AHI, 1). The OSA group received therapeutic PAP, and the non-OSA group received PAP at a pressure of 5 cm H_2O for 3 weeks. Ambulatory blood pressure monitoring indicated that nocturnal blood pressure in the OSA group dropped significantly with PAP (−10.3 mm Hg systolic, −4.5 mm Hg diastolic) but was essentially unchanged with PAP in the non-OSA group. There was a greater but statistically nonsignificant difference in blood pressure drop in the OSA versus non-OSA group in daytime blood pressure (−2.4 mm Hg systolic, −0.6 mm Hg diastolic).

In a meta-analysis of 16 trials conducted between 1996 and 2006 and including a total of 818 patients,[58] a small but statistically significant mean net change in systolic (−2.5 mm Hg; 95% CI, −4.3 to −0.6) and diastolic (−1.8 mm Hg; 95% CI, −3.0 to −0.6) blood pressures was observed. Net reductions in blood pressure were not statistically different between daytime and nighttime. This meta-analysis had some limitations that might reduce its generalizability (e.g., most studies included predominantly or exclusively obese middle-aged men, some studies were not blinded, and compliance was often limited). Furthermore, the duration of PAP treatment in all of these studies was relatively short, ranging from 2 to 24 weeks[58]; longer treatment may be associated with different effects on systemic blood pressure.

These limitations notwithstanding, it is remarkable that a more recent meta-analysis including 28 studies published between 1980 and 2012 (representing 1948 patients) obtained results that were highly consistent with those of the previous study[59]: The weighted mean difference in diurnal systolic blood pressure (−2.58 mm Hg; 95% CI, −3.57 to −1.59 mm Hg) and diastolic blood pressure (−2.01 mm Hg; 95% CI, −2.84 to −1.18 mm Hg) both significantly favored PAP treatment over control arms. The effects were stronger in studies that included patients who were younger, were sleepier, had more severe OSA, and exhibited a higher degree of adherence to PAP.[59] The estimated effects were even stronger (3- to 5-mm Hg decrease in 24-hour blood pressure values) in another meta-analysis focusing on studies of resistant hypertension[60] and in another recent multicenter study in Spain.[61]

In one of the largest and more carefully conducted randomized controlled trials to date, Gottlieb and colleagues recruited 318 patients with cardiovascular disease or multiple cardiovascular risk factors from cardiology practices, that is, patients who were presumably subject to proper blood pressure control.[62] Among the 281 patients who had 24-hour blood pressure data at baseline and 12-week follow-up in this study, mean 24-hour arterial blood pressure was significantly lower in the group receiving PAP than in the control group (−2.4 mm Hg; 95% CI, −4.7 to −0.1; $P = .04$). Remarkably, the estimated reduction in blood pressure achieved by PAP is almost identical to that estimated in the two meta-analyses described previously.[58,59]

The focus of most of the previous studies and meta-analyses was primarily on changes in blood pressure associated with different types and length of PAP treatment in a variety of patient populations (e.g., some with OSA, some with hypertension, combinations of both). The results of one of the few randomized studies looking at the effect of PAP treatment on the *incidence* of hypertension were inconclusive.[63] In this Spanish multicenter study, 725 patients with OSA but without baseline hypertension and symptoms of daytime sleepiness were randomized to PAP treatment or no active treatment and followed up for a median of 4 years; even though a slight reduction (17%) in the combined incidence of hypertension and cardiovascular events was observed in the study, the result was not statistically significant, probably owing to the small number of events and limited statistical power.

A possible mechanism that might explain the putative improvement in blood pressure associated with PAP treatment is an improvement in vascular function. OSA may increase sympathetic activity, which is reversed by therapy with PAP. Other mechanisms are likely to be involved. In a randomized controlled trial including 29 patients with OSA associated with desaturation, compared with placebo, 6 weeks of PAP was associated with an improved forearm blood flow in response to both endothelial and non–endothelium-dependent stimuli.[64] Previous non–placebo-controlled studies have also demonstrated an association between PAP and either biochemical markers of vascular function[65] or forearm flow-mediated dilation measures.[55] Overall, the results of both observational and experimental studies on the effect of PAP therapy are consistent with evidence from both animal and human epidemiologic (particularly longitudinal) studies showing OSA as a possible cause of hypertension (see above). All this evidence, coupled with biologic plausibility studies defining mechanisms linking OSA to hypertension and the reversal of such mechanisms with PAP, support the hypothesis of a contribution of OSA to elevated blood pressure.

Clinical Relevance of the Role of Obstructive Sleep Apnea in Hypertension

In contrast to the state of evidence two decades ago, findings in support of a role for OSA in the development of hypertension are now difficult to dismiss as spurious.[66-68] Translating these findings to clinical settings, however, poses challenges. These findings, as well as new guidelines on hypertension detection and treatment, support case-finding for OSA in patients with hypertension in primary care settings, but what is the next step? Although diagnosis and treatment of a patient with hypertension and symptomatic OSA are priorities, a critical and much-debated question is the course of action that should be taken if a hypertensive patient has mild OSA without daytime symptoms of sleepiness. Is treatment of mild, asymptomatic OSA without complaints of sleepiness warranted on the basis of potential cardiovascular consequences? Arguments against treatment point to the lack of conclusive data. Based on the average effect of PAP on change in blood pressure, the predicted effect on an individual is likely to be small and of uncertain clinical significance and thus would not warrant replacing antihypertensive drugs for controlling blood pressure.[69]

On the other hand, there are arguments for considering PAP treatment in nonsleepy patients with mild, asymptomatic OSA and coexisting hypertension.[70,71] Worsening of mild sleep apnea over time is likely, and cardiovascular consequences that might be attributable to severe OSA could be prevented.[71] Some data suggest that PAP treatment for patients with OSA and drug-resistant hypertension may be of benefit in lowering blood pressure.[60,72] Also, as noted by Gottlieb and colleagues,[62] even an average reduction of 2 mm Hg in systolic blood pressure—the approximate mean effect of PAP treatment from meta-analyses of OSA treatment trials described previously—might be expected to substantially lower stroke rates (by ~10%) and heart disease mortality rates (by ~7%) in treated populations.[73]

Primary health care providers increasingly recognize markers for OSA, such as snoring, and are becoming more aware of the OSA-hypertension association. Consequently, referrals of patients with mild, asymptomatic OSA for sleep evaluations will very likely increase, heightening the dilemma of whom to treat in the face of limited medical resources. Further understanding of the costs and benefits of OSA treatment in preventing the incidence and progression of hypertension and other cardiovascular diseases is needed before this problem can be satisfactorily addressed.

Meanwhile, clinicians providing care for OSA patients using PAP should underscore the importance of full compliance as well as adequate control of disordered breathing events with PAP, as evidenced by studies showing the importance of treatment adherence in lowering blood pressure.[29,48] As indicated earlier, long-term small changes in blood pressure have major preventive effects. In prospective studies of 420,000 persons, a decrease of 5 mm Hg in diastolic blood pressure lessened the incidence of stroke and coronary heart disease by approximately 34% and 21%, respectively, and there was a dose-dependent reduction in blood pressure and incident cardiovascular diseases.[74] Therefore, in patients with OSA, long-term compliance with PAP may be effective in preventing adverse cerebrovascular and cardiovascular diseases.

PULMONARY HYPERTENSION

Obstructive Sleep Apnea as a Cause of Pulmonary Hypertension

In 1998, the second WHO conference on pulmonary arterial hypertension[4] recognized sleep-disordered breathing as a secondary cause of PH. The classification of PH has been revised by a more recent WHO conference.[75,76] There are five groups, each with a number of subgroups consisting of various causes of PH. The first group, pulmonary arterial hypertension, includes idiopathic pulmonary arterial hypertension. The second class is pulmonary venous hypertension, which is most commonly due to elevated left heart filling pressures such as left ventricular diastolic dysfunction. PH secondary to OSA falls into the third category, which also includes chronic obstructive pulmonary disease (COPD), interstitial lung diseases, and PH chronic exposure to high altitude. The basic pathophysiologic mechanism underlying PH in this group of disorders is hypoxemia. However, as will be emphasized later, OSA can cause PH through left ventricular diastolic dysfunction, as it occurs in group 2. Group 4 is PH due to thromboembolic pathologic disorders, and group 5 consists of miscellaneous disorders that cannot be easily classified in the other four groups.

The gold standard for diagnosis of PH is right heart catheterization. As noted earlier, the WHO defines the presence of PH as resting mean pulmonary artery pressure of 25 mm Hg or greater. Investigators in the field of sleep apnea have mostly used a mean pulmonary artery pressure of 20 mm Hg or greater, a threshold that is lower than that defined by WHO. However, a resting mean pulmonary artery pressure of 20 mm Hg or greater is generally considered abnormal. In this chapter, we defined PH according to the WHO criteria, which have become the rule independent of the cause of the PH. We also emphasized that right heart catheterization is essential for phenotyping PH, assessing its severity and the targeted therapy.

In patients with OSA, the prevalence of abnormal mean pulmonary artery pressure varies considerably, from 15% to 70%.[77-84] This variation in part depends on inclusion in some studies of patients with COPD, hypercapnic OSA (obesity hypoventilation syndrome), and obesity, which contribute to increased frequency, prevalence, and severity of PH in OSA. Meanwhile, in patients with OSA without comorbid disorders, PH is usually mild, although it could also be severe in advanced OSA, resulting in cor pulmonale, a feature of pickwickian syndrome (hypercapnic OSA syndrome).

An early study[1] of 12 patients with OSA who had undergone right heart catheterization showed cyclic changes in pulmonary artery pressure coinciding with episodes of OSA. A marked degree of hypoxemia and hypercapnia was associated with these hemodynamic abnormalities. In some of these patients, systolic pulmonary artery pressure exceeded 60 mm Hg. During wakefulness, four patients had abnormal mean pulmonary artery pressure ranging from 20 to 22 mm Hg. One of these four patients had an elevated pulmonary capillary wedge pressure of 16 mm Hg. With exercise, most of the patients had mean pulmonary artery pressure of about 30 mm Hg. In some of these patients, the wedge pressure increased with exercise, unmasking left ventricular diastolic dysfunction. This study indicated that OSA impaired the physiologic processes that normally operate to enable pulmonary circulation and left ventricular function to maintain pulmonary artery pressure close to normal in the face of increases in cardiac output.

Since the study of Tilkian and colleagues,[1] many studies have demonstrated presence of PH in patients with OSA. Box 26-1 summarizes the four largest studies in which full-night PSG and right heart catheterization, the gold standard for diagnosis of OSA and PH, were performed. In a French study[78] involving 220 consecutive patients with an AHI of greater than 20, 37 patients (17%) had a resting mean pulmonary artery pressure of at least 20 mm Hg (range, 20 to 44 mm Hg), and in 17 patients (8%) the mean pressure was 25 mm Hg or greater. Patients with a resting mean pulmonary artery pressure of at least 20 mm Hg had more severe OSA, a higher $Paco_2$, a higher BMI, and a lower Pao_2 than patients without PH. Furthermore, these patients had higher prevalence of both obstructive and restrictive pulmonary defects. $Paco_2$ and forced expiratory volume in 1 second (FEV_1) were the two major predictors of high resting mean pulmonary artery pressure. When PH was defined as a mean pressure of 30 mm Hg with exercise, virtually all patients met this criterion; in 23 patients (62%) the mean pressure exceeded 40 mm Hg.

In an Australian study[79] of 100 consecutive patients with an AHI of 20 or more, 42% had elevated pulmonary artery pressure, with the mean pressure ranging from about 20 to 52 mm Hg. Some patients had overlap syndrome. In 24% of the patients, the mean pressure was more than 25 mm Hg. In this study, $Paco_2$, Pao_2, and FEV_1 accounted for about 33% of vital capacity (FVC) of less than 60% predicted. The study involved 44 patients, 12 of whom (27%) had mean pulmonary artery pressure greater than 20 mm Hg, all with pulmonary capillary wedge pressure of less than 15 mm Hg. Importantly, 8 patients (18% of all patients) had PH with mean pulmonary artery pressure of 25 mm Hg or greater. The authors reported that mean pulmonary artery pressure was positively correlated with BMI and negatively correlated with Pao_2. Patients with elevated mean pulmonary artery pressure had significantly lower values for FVC and FEV_1. The mechanisms by which BMI positively correlated with PH could have been multifactorial and related to restrictive lung defect and hypoxemia.

Combining the results of the aforementioned four studies using PSG to determine the presence of OSA, and right heart catheterization to define PH, 51 of the 456 patients (11%) satisfy the current WHO criteria for PH.

In conclusion, mild PH is common in patients with OSA and may occur in the absence of COPD and daytime hypoxemia. However, severe OSA, severe hypoxemia, hypercapnia (obesity hypoventilation syndrome), obstructive or restrictive lung defects, and left heart disease are more commonly associated with PH and contribute to its severity. In addition, as noted, increased pulmonary artery pressure either becomes manifest or is augmented by exercise and can cause dyspnea and exercise intolerance.[82]

Mechanisms of Pulmonary Hypertension in Patients with Obstructive Sleep Apnea

Intermittent nocturnal rises in the pulmonary artery pressure in association with upper airway collapse have been well documented. Multiple mechanisms mediate nocturnal rises in pulmonary artery pressure.[85] These include alterations in blood gases (i.e., intermittent hypoxemia and hypercapnia), cardiac output, lung volume, intrathoracic pressure, compliance of pulmonary circulation, and left ventricular diastolic dysfunction. With time and in the long run, nocturnal PH spills over to diurnal hypertension.

Diurnal PH in patients with OSA could be precapillary, capillary, or postcapillary, depending in part on comorbid disorders that may contribute to the development of PH (Box 26-2). Postcapillary PH (pulmonary venous hypertension) is common and results primarily from elevated left heart filling pressures, specifically owing to their left ventricular hypertrophy and diastolic dysfunction caused by diurnal systemic hypertension and nocturnal consequences of OSA noted

variability in pulmonary artery pressure. Six patients with abnormal pulmonary artery pressure had normal Pao_2.

In a German study[80] of 92 consecutive patients with an AHI of greater than 10 and with COPD as an exclusion criterion, 20% had a mean pulmonary artery pressure of 20 to 25 mm Hg. Only one patient met the current criterion of PH with a mean of 25 mm Hg. Eight patients had increased pulmonary capillary wedge pressure, and all of these patients had systemic hypertension that was presumably causing left ventricular diastolic dysfunction. Pulmonary capillary wedge pressure and time spent with a saturation of below 90% were the independent variables predicting PH.

The presence of PH in patients with OSA but without COPD was also confirmed in another French study (see Box 26-1).[81] In this study, however, COPD was defined by an FEV_1 of less than 70% predicted and a ratio of FEV_1 to forced previously. In regard to the latter, left ventricular hypertrophy could be present in patients with OSA even in the absence of daytime systemic hypertension,[86] presumably because of cyclic changes in systemic artery blood pressure and hypoxemia[84] during sleep. In the presence of a hypertrophied or noncompliant left ventricle, end-diastolic pressure increases, resulting in backward passive increase in pulmonary venous, capillary, and pulmonary artery systolic and diastolic pressures. This acute postcapillary PH is reversible, if the etiologic factor (e.g., OSA) is effectively treated. Otherwise, with persistent PH, remodeling of pulmonary vascular bed occurs and vascular resistance increases, which in time may become reversible even if the etiology of left heart disease is effectively treated.

As noted earlier, as a cause of PH, OSA is categorized in group 3 along with COPD and other lung diseases. Here, the underlying pathophysiology is hypoxemia. However, because of intermittent partial or complete pharyngeal collapse during sleep, repeated episodes of hypoxemia and hypercapnia occur, both of which have been shown to acutely induce pulmonary arteriolar vasoconstriction, increasing pulmonary vascular resistance. With time, however, distinct pathophysiologic sequelae ensue that may be irreversible. In any case this is the precapillary PH, which is another potential mechanism of OSA-induced PH. Therefore the combination of hypoxic-hypercapnic pulmonary arteriolar vasoconstriction and pulmonary venous hypertension could result in severe PH in patients with OSA. Similarly, when OSA is comorbid with COPD, which is in the same group with OSA as a potential cause for PH, the combination could result in severe PH.

Detailed molecular mechanisms underlying PH in OSA are beyond the scope of this chapter. However, production of mediators eventually results in endothelial cell damage, vascular cell proliferation, and aberrant vascular remodeling. In addition, with endothelial cell dysfunction, there is reduced nitric oxide production and increased endothelin,[86,87] both of which contribute to further PH. As noted earlier, the initial cascade of events is potentially reversible, emphasizing the importance of early recognition and treatment of OSA.

Loss of vascular surface area, as may occur in patients with COPD, is an important cause of capillary PH, and it may significantly contribute to PH in patients with OSA. Several studies[77-79] have shown that COPD and a low FEV_1 are predictors of PH in patients with OSA. COPD could also contribute to PH by way of arteriolar vasoconstriction due to hypoxemia and hypercapnia as noted previously.

An important mechanism mediating PH in patients with OSA is the presence of factors that cause constriction of pulmonary arterioles, leading to precapillary PH. The best-known stimulus is alveolar hypoxia, and it is not surprising that hypoxemia is an independent predictor of PH in OSA (see Box 26-1). However, hypercapnia could also increase pulmonary arterial blood pressure. The molecular mechanisms of PH in general are complex and multifactorial. Both acquired and genetic factors are involved. Disordered endothelial cell function, in part caused by hypoxia (and reoxygenation) and manifested biochemically by an imbalance between concentrations of local vasodilators (e.g., nitric oxide and prostacyclins) and vasoconstrictors (e.g., endothelin-1, thromboxane, serotonin), as occurs in endothelial dysfunction syndrome, appears to mediate the development of PH.[87,88] It is also conceivable that if OSA is long-standing, pulmonary vascular remodeling similar to that in COPD could occur because a

number of mediators such as vascular endothelial growth factor are proliferative and angiogenic.

In summary, the consequence of OSA on pulmonary circulation may vary from those of cyclic nocturnal PH, which occurs in virtually all patients, to daytime PH, right ventricular dysfunction, and eventually cor pulmonale, a feature of pickwickian syndrome. However, even in the absence of cor pulmonale, which is the manifestation of long-standing severe PH, presence of PH increases right ventricular afterload and myocardial oxygen consumption. If PH develops as a result of increases in cardiac output (e.g., with exercise), it may cause dyspnea and exercise intolerance.

Changes in Pulmonary Artery Pressure after Positive Airway Pressure Treatment of Obstructive Sleep Apnea

Because mechanisms of PH in OSA are multifactorial (see Box 26-2), the behavioral response of pulmonary circulation to therapy for OSA probably depends on several factors. For example, if loss of vascular surface area due to the presence of COPD or other comorbid pulmonary disorders is contributing to PH in OSA, this component is irreversible.[89] Similarly, if remodeling of the pulmonary vascular bed has occurred, long-standing effective therapy is necessary to effect any reversal component (reverse remodeling). Therefore, if PAP is used to treat OSA, long-term compliance with therapy is critical and needs to be confirmed by covert monitoring. Large, long-term systematic studies considering these important factors are necessary to determine the effects of treatment of OSA on pulmonary circulation. Lack of such considerations may lead to serious underestimation of effects.

Effective treatment of OSA could improve PH. Here we review the studies that have implemented right heart catheterization both at baseline as well as long term. In an early study when tracheotomy was the best therapeutic option, Fletcher and colleagues[89] studied three groups of OSA patients. Nine patients with hypercapnic OSA and mostly with COPD underwent the operation, and repeat right heart catheterization was performed about 6 months later. Six of nine patients had baseline right heart catheterization, and five of them met the current criteria for PH. The resting mean pulmonary artery pressure was 39 mm Hg in these six patients. About 12 months later, the mean resting pulmonary artery pressure was 25 mm Hg. Mean pulmonary artery pressure decreased in five of the six patients. It did not change significantly in the single patient who had mean pulmonary artery pressure of about 24 mm Hg. Meanwhile there was a significant rise in right ventricular ejection fraction in association with a reduction in the pulmonary artery pressure and vascular resistance. Motta and coworkers[90] also performed tracheostomy on six patients with OSA. However, the mean pulmonary artery pressure did not change significantly in these patients. Importantly, only one patient met the current criterion of PH with a mean pressure of 28 mm Hg.

Another negative study was reported by Sforza and colleagues.[91] The authors treated 54 patients with OSA with CPAP. The mean pulmonary artery pressure did not change significantly. However, similar to the study of Motta and colleagues, none of the patients met the current criterion for PH.

Alchanatis and colleagues[92] studied 29 patients with OSA and without COPD. Three of the 29 patients met the current criterion for PH with baseline values of 30, 30, and 28 mm Hg.

Six months after therapy with CPAP, the mean pulmonary artery pressure had dropped below 25 mm Hg in these 3 patients. Respective values were about 23, 22, and 20 mm Hg.

In another French study of OSA patients who were treated with long-term CPAP, Chouat and associates[92] reported no significant changes in mean pulmonary artery pressure in 44 patients who had undergone right heart catheterization. The mean pulmonary artery pressure at baseline, however, was normal at 16 mm Hg. After an average of 64 months of CPAP use, the mean pressure was 17 mm Hg. The authors reported that in 11 patients whose average value of the mean pulmonary artery pressure was 24 mm Hg at baseline (authors considered a value of 20 mm Hg or greater as PH), the pressure decreased to 20 mm Hg, although this value was not statistically significant. It is not clear how many of the 11 patients met the current criterion for PH. However, if the mean pressure is within normal range it may not be expected to decrease significantly with intervention.

The last a study using right heart catheterization was reported by Sajkov's group[93] who studied 20 patients with OSA (average AHI, 49 or greater) before and 4 months after treatment with PAP. In this study, PAP compliance was objectively monitored, and the average was 5 hours per night. Patients had normal lung function. Five patients who had abnormal pulmonary artery pressure (range, 20 to 32 mm Hg) showed the most dramatic decrease to less than 20 mm Hg after 4 months of effective treatment with PAP. Two of the 5 patients met the current criterion for PH with mean pulmonary artery pressures of 31 and 27 mm Hg. Four months after therapy with CPAP, respective pressures were 18 and 13 mm Hg. Interestingly, the authors showed a time-dependent progressive decrease in mean pulmonary artery pressure with right heart catheterization, which was performed at 1 and 4 months of intervention. In a subject who was not compliant with CPAP, there was no change in pulmonary artery pressure. Although this was a single observation, this finding and those reported for systemic hypertension strongly indicate that effective use of PAP is necessary to lower systemic and pulmonary artery pressures.

We now review relevant randomized clinical trials. Arias and colleagues[94] randomized 23 middle-aged patients with severe OSA (AHI, 44 or greater) to either sham PAP or PAP therapy. In this crossover trial, after 12 weeks of PAP therapy, pulmonary artery systolic pressure decreased significantly from a mean of about 30 to 24 mm Hg. The reduction was greatest (8.5 mm Hg) in patients with PH defined as pulmonary artery systolic pressure of 30 or more determined by echocardiography. In the second randomized study[95] sham CPAP was used as placebo. Arias and colleagues[95] performed a crossover study of 12 weeks' duration in 27 consecutive newly diagnosed men with OSA and abnormal echocardiographic left ventricular filling pattern. Twelve weeks of effective CPAP therapy resulted in significant increases in E/A ratio and reduction in mitral deceleration isovolume relaxation times. We must emphasize that based on the design of this important study, the main and perhaps the only pathologic reason causing left ventricular diastolic dysfunction was OSA; among the exclusion criteria were presence of known hypertension, ischemic or valvular heart disease, diabetes, morbid obesity, and daytime hypoxemia. Therefore the results of this study demonstrate that OSA could be a cause of the reversible diastolic dysfunction. As noted earlier, impaired left ventricular filling could be an important cause of PH in patients with OSA.

The American College of Cardiology and American Heart Association expert consensus document recommends PSG to rule out OSA for all patients with PH. The recommendation is based on the idea that targeted therapy of OSA could either improve or prevent further deterioration in central hemodynamics.

CLINICAL PEARLS

- Epidemiologic studies support a causal role of OSA in systemic hypertension independent of BMI, measures of fat distribution, age, sex, and other possible confounding factors.
- Randomized double-blind placebo (sham PAP)–controlled trials of patients with hypertension demonstrate that effective treatment of OSA with PAP lowers blood pressure. A decrease in blood pressure is most pronounced in those with the most severe OSA and those who are the most compliant.
- Even small decrements in blood pressure, maintained for the long term, have been shown to significantly lessen the incidence of cerebrovascular and cardiovascular diseases. Thus the potential lowering of blood pressure from PAP treatment holds promise for decreasing cerebrovascular or cardiovascular disease. However, adequate control of OSA and compliance with PAP, particularly in patients with severe OSA, are critical.
- Several observational studies show that OSA, particularly when severe, is a cause of mortality. Treatment with PAP decreases mortality risk.
- OSA is a cause of secondary PH, and this has been recognized by international health organizations. PH as defined by a mean pulmonary artery pressure of 25 mm Hg or greater is usually mild, although it could be severe, particularly in the presence of severe OSA or OSA with hypercapnia, obesity, and comorbid disorders such as COPD. Treatment of OSA with PAP may improve or prevent further deterioration in pulmonary pressures. All patients with PH, independent of the cause, should undergo PSG and targeted therapy when indicated. This may halt deterioration in central hemodynamics.

SUMMARY

Findings from investigations based on diverse populations and different study designs support a role for OSA in systemic hypertension and PH. Population-based epidemiology studies have shown that persons with moderate to severe OSA (15 or more apnea or hypopnea events per hour) have greater probability of having or developing hypertension than persons who do not have OSA. These associations are only partly explained by confounding factors such as age or increased BMI. In epidemiologic studies that use 24-hour ambulatory blood pressure monitoring, OSA–blood pressure associations are seen with both sleep and wake blood pressures. PH, too, is prevalent in patients with OSA. Mild pulmonary arterial hypertension may occur in patients with OSA without daytime hypoxemia or COPD, but these comorbidities are more common in patients with severe OSA.

OSA treatment trials also support a causal association between OSA and hypertension, with most studies of systemic or pulmonary blood pressures before and after PAP therapy demonstrating blood pressure reductions. Intervention trials generally show modest reductions in systemic blood pressure (2 to 10 mm Hg reductions), with the largest effects seen in effectively treated patients with severe OSA. Importantly, small changes in blood pressure, if maintained, have the potential to significantly decrease the population incidence of cerebrovascular and cardiovascular disease.

Selected Readings

Barbé F, Durán-Cantolla J, Sanchez de la Torre M, et al. Effect of continuous positive airway pressure on the incidence of hypertension and cardiovascular events in nonsleepy patients with obstructive sleep apnea: a randomized controlled trial. *JAMA* 2012;**307**:2161–8.

Campos-Rodriguez F, Perez-Ronchel J, Grilo-Reina A, et al. Long-term effect of continuous positive airway pressure on BP in patients with hypertension and sleep apnea. *Chest* 2007;**132**:1847–52.

Cano-Pumarega I, Durán-Cantolla J, Aizpuru F, et al. Obstructive sleep apnea and systemic hypertension: longitudinal study in the general population: the Vitoria Sleep Cohort. *Am J Respir Crit Care Med* 2011;**184**:1299–304.

Damiani MF, Zito A, Carratù P, et al. Obstructive Sleep Apnea, Hypertension, and Their Additive Effects on Atherosclerosis. *Biochem Res Int* 2015;**2015**:984193.

Floras JS. Hypertension and sleep apnea. *Can J Cardiol* 2015;**31**:889–97.

Gottlieb DJ, Punjabi NM, Mehra R, et al. CPAP versus oxygen in obstructive sleep apnea. *N Engl J Med* 2014;**370**:2276–85.

Ismail K, Roberts K, Manning P, et al. OSA and pulmonary hypertension: time for a new look. *Chest* 2015;**147**(3):847–61.

Javaheri S, Javaheri S, Javaheri A. Sleep apnea, heart failure and pulmonary hypertension. *Curr Heart Fail Rep* 2013;**10**:315–20.

Marin JM, Agusti A, Villar I, et al. Association between treated and untreated obstructive sleep apnea and risk of hypertension. *JAMA* 2012;**307**:2169–76.

Martinez-Garcia MA, Capote F, Campos-Rodriguez F, et al. Effect of CPAP on blood pressure in patients with obstructive sleep apnea and resistant hypertension: the HIPARCO randomized clinical trial. *JAMA* 2013;**310**:2407–15.

Montesi SB, Edwards BA, Malhotra A, Bakker JP. The effect of continuous positive airway pressure treatment on blood pressure: a systematic review and meta-analysis of randomized controlled trials. *J Clin Sleep Med* 2012;**8**:587–96.

Motta J, Guilleminault C, Schroeder JS, et al. Tracheostomy and hemodynamic changes in sleep-induced apnea. *Ann Intern Med* 1978;**89**:454–8.

O'Conner GT, Caffo B, Newman AB, et al. Prospective study of sleep-disordered breathing and hypertension; the Sleep Heart Health Study. *Am J Respir Crit Care Med* 2009;**179**:1159–64.

A complete reference list can be found online at ExpertConsult.com.

Coronary Artery Disease and Obstructive Sleep Apnea

Yüksel Peker; Karl A. Franklin; Jan Hedner

Chapter Highlights

- Obstructive sleep apnea is overrepresented in patients with coronary artery disease and occurs in about 50% (36% to 66%) of such patients, most of them without complaints of excessive daytime sleepiness.
- Sleep apnea is even more prevalent during the presentation of myocardial infarction and may explain a peak incidence of sudden cardiac death during midnight and early morning hours.
- Increased oxygen demand and reduced oxygen supply after obstructive apneas may trigger nocturnal angina in patients with low oxygen reserve because of lack of ventilation.
- Patients with sleep apnea and coronary artery disease have an increased risk for developing stroke, but it is still unclear whether they have an increased risk for early death independent of other comorbidities.

- Obstructive sleep apnea is suggested as an independent risk factor for atherosclerosis because of repeated apnea-induced hypoxemia and reoxygenation-induced oxidative stress with immediate and sustained sympathetic activation, endothelial dysfunction, and inflammation.
- Prospective studies report a reduction of nocturnal ischemia during elimination of obstructive events with continuous positive airway pressure treatment and lowering of the risk for recurrent myocardial infarction, without any reports of adverse events.
- Randomized controlled trials examining the effect of continuous positive airway pressure treatment on long-term cardiovascular outcomes are underway.

Epidemiologic data suggest that obstructive sleep apnea (OSA) is overrepresented in patients with coronary artery disease (CAD). Other studies suggest that the clinical course of CAD is initiated or accelerated by the presence of sleep-related breathing disorders. A rapidly evolving field of experimental data demonstrates that OSA, by phenomena such as hypoxemia and reoxygenation, may trigger a sequence of events involved in the development of atherosclerotic disease.

Development of vascular disease and CAD is influenced by several risk factors that also have been associated with OSA. Sleep apneic events induce a state of increased cardiac oxygen demand but are also often associated with low oxygen reserve because of lack of ventilation. Nocturnal angina can therefore be triggered by sleep apneas in patients with CAD. There is growing evidence that elimination of the sleep disorder can benefit patients with OSA at risk for CAD. Other data suggest that treatment of OSA improves prognosis in patients undergoing coronary revascularization. This chapter reviews the evidence of an association between these two conditions.

EPIDEMIOLOGY

The risk for experiencing angina pectoris or an acute coronary syndrome such as unstable angina, acute myocardial infarc-

tion (MI), or sudden cardiac death (SCD) has long been known to be increased during the late hours of sleep or in the hours soon after awakening.[1] This association may be explained in part by occurrence of OSA. A retrospective analysis showed an overrepresentation of peak time in sudden death from the cardiac causes during the sleeping hours in patients with OSA, which contrasted with a nadir in sudden death from cardiac causes in subjects without OSA and in the general population.[2] The same group addressed whether OSA independently increases the risk for SCD in a longitudinal follow-up of 10,701 consecutive adults.[3] During an average follow-up of 5.3 years, 142 patients had resuscitated or suffered from SCD (annual rate, 0.27%). In a multivariate analysis, SCD was associated with an apnea-hypopnea index (AHI) of at least 20 events/hour (hazard ratio [HR] = 1.60), mean nocturnal oxygen saturation of less than 93% (HR = 2.93), and oxygen nadir saturation of less than 78% (HR = 2.60; all $P < .001$). The authors concluded that OSA predicted incident SCD. Another small prospective study addressing the time of onset of MI showed a higher likelihood of having OSA in those with an onset of MI during midnight hours.[4] Moreover, a recent study also demonstrated that the incidence of MI onset between 6:00 AM and 12:00 PM was higher in OSA patients (AHI ≥5) than in control patients (38% vs. 25%; $P = .039$). Moderate to severe OSA (AHI ≥15) significantly enhanced this circadian variation (odds ratio [OR] = 2.0) after adjustment for age, body mass index (BMI), and comorbidities.[5]

In general, there is a stronger relationship between OSA and CAD in clinical cohorts than in the general population because clinical cohort studies are particularly influenced by comorbidity and confounding factors, including obesity, diabetes mellitus, hypertension, smoking, and hyperlipidemia. This circumstance also suggests that OSA constitutes an additive or synergistic risk factor for development of CAD.

Prevalence of Obstructive Sleep Apnea and Coronary Artery Disease in the General Population

The largest study to date addressing OSA and CAD in the general population is the Sleep Heart Health Study.[6] The investigators performed a cross-sectional analysis of 6132 subjects undergoing unattended full-night home polysomnography. There was a modest risk increase (peaking at an OR of 1.27) for self-reported CAD when the highest and lowest AHI quartiles were compared. The weak association in this general population study may be explained by a proportionally high age and a low median AHI.

Prevalence of Coronary Artery Disease in Patients with Obstructive Sleep Apnea

Clinical studies of CAD in sleep clinic cohorts generally involve patients with OSA and with daytime symptoms. Consequently, compared with studies in the general population, these studies deal with symptomatic patients, those likely to suffer from more severe sleep apnea, and potentially patients with excess comorbidities such as diabetes, obesity, and cardiovascular disorders. Available data are to a large extent based on uncontrolled studies. For example, in a sleep clinic cohort of 386 subjects,[7] CAD was present in almost one fourth of subjects with OSA, and the percentage of patients with CAD was high among those with moderate to severe OSA.

In another study,[8] simultaneous polysomnography and electrocardiographic recordings demonstrated that episodes of nocturnal ischemia were more common in patients with OSA who also had CAD, and mainly so during rapid eye movement (REM) sleep, during periods of high apnea activity, and during sustained hypoxemia. Moreover, ST-segment depression on electrocardiography was not uncommon during sleep in patients with OSA but without a history of CAD, and these changes were eliminated by continuous positive airway pressure (CPAP).[9] Studies using invasive measures, including angiography, verified CAD in more than 20% of investigated subjects with OSA,[10] and an even higher prevalence (68%) was reported in a slightly larger study of unselected patients with OSA.[11] Collectively these data suggest a proportionally high prevalence of CAD in sleep clinic cohorts.

Prevalence of Obstructive Sleep Apnea in Patients with Coronary Artery Disease

Sleep-disordered breathing appears to be common in patients with CAD. An early small study demonstrated OSA or central sleep apnea with Cheyne-Stokes breathing in 13 of 17 male patients with angiographically verified CAD.[12] A subsequent Australian case-control study that investigated middle-aged male survivors of acute MI and age-matched controls provided the first clinic-based epidemiologic evidence of an increased prevalence of OSA in patients with CAD.[13] OSA (apnea index [AI] ≥5 events/hour) was found in

approximately one third of the patients, compared with only 4% of age-matched healthy controls, and constituted an independent predictor of MI after adjustment for traditional risk factors.

A larger case-control study provided a similar OSA prevalence (31%), whereas the prevalence in the control group was 20%.[14] In this population, an AHI of 20 was associated with a history of MI (OR = 2.0; 95% confidence interval [CI], 1.0 to 3.8). In a tightly age-, sex-, and BMI-matched Swedish case-control study of 62 patients, OSA, based on an AHI of greater than 10, provided an independent OR of 3.1 (95% CI, 1.2 to 8.3) for CAD adjusted for several cardiovascular risk factors.[15] A recent matched Spanish case-control study found OSA (based on AHI ≥15) in 35% of patients with acute MI compared with 15% in the control group ($P < .001$).[16] The adjusted OR for acute MI was 12.2 (95% CI, 2.0 to 72.6), applying the AHI cutoff value of 15 for OSA diagnosis.

There are also data suggesting that the OSA and CAD association may be influenced by sex and age. In patients with angiographically verified CAD, an AI of greater than 10 was almost twice as common in men,[17] but three times more common in women[18] younger than 70 years, compared with age-matched controls. An uncontrolled study of 50 randomly selected CAD patients demonstrated OSA in 50% based on an AI of greater than 10.[19] Another uncontrolled German study reported an OSA prevalence of 35% applying AHI of 10 or more events/hour as the diagnostic criterion in 74 men with significant stenosis of one or more coronary arteries but failed to establish a significant relationship between AHI and number of coronary vessels involved.[20] A subsequent uncontrolled follow-up study found OSA (AHI ≥10) in 57% of 89 subjects with acute coronary syndrome undergoing percutaneous coronary intervention (PCI).[21] A similar high prevalence of OSA (66%) was reported in another investigation based on AHI of 10 or greater.[22] Two other uncontrolled studies performed in CAD patients undergoing PCI demonstrated OSA (AHI ≥15) in 43% and 66%, respectively.[23,24] One study based on a retrospective chart review of 798 consecutive patients with acute MI demonstrated that OSA was initially suspected only in 12% of the patient records, whereas after overnight polysomnography, 41% of patients presented an AHI of 15 or greater, suggesting that OSA was common but unrecognized in patients with CAD.[25] Moreover, baseline data of a randomized controlled trial (RCT) among 662 revascularized CAD patients in Sweden (the Randomized Intervention with CPAP in Coronary Artery Disease and Sleep Apnoea [RIC-CADSA] trial) revealed that 64% had an AHI of 15 or greater (Figure 27-1), but most did not report daytime hypersomnolence.[26] Of note, the occurrence of OSA in this cohort was more common than the prevalence of hypertension, diabetes, obesity, and current smoking. Finally, a similar prevalence (64%) of sleep-disordered breathing, defined as an oxygen desaturation index (ODI) of greater than 5 based on a WatchPAT-100 sleep study, was reported recently in prospective evaluation of 180 patients with acute MI.[27] However, no distinction was made between OSA and central sleep apnea or CSR in that cohort.

The possibility that OSA may trigger episodes of nocturnal angina in patients with disabling CAD was addressed in an interventional study.[28] OSA was found in 9 of 10 investigated patients with CAD who had nocturnal angina, and episodes of ischemia were reversed after elimination of the apneic

Results of the Home Sleep Studies in 662
Patients with Coronary Artery Disease

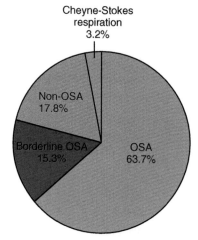

Figure 27-1 Classification of the groups based on the results of the unat-tended cardiorespiratory sleep recordings in patients with revascularized coronary artery disease. Obstructive sleep apnea (OSA) refers to apnea-hypopnea-index (AHI) of 15 or more events/hr; borderline OSA, AHI 5 to 14.9 events/hr; Non-OSA, AHI <5 event/hr. (Modified from Glantz H, Thun-ström E, Herlitz J, et al. Occurrence and predictors of obstructive sleep apnea in a revascularized coronary artery disease cohort. *Ann Am Thorac Soc* 2013;4:350–6.)

events with CPAP treatment. A subsequent larger cross-sectional study found signs of silent nocturnal myocardial ischemia in 31% of 226 patients with CAD but failed to demonstrate a general and immediate temporal relationship between OSA and episodes of myocardial ischemia.[29] However, a direct association could be documented in a small subgroup of patients, and, in general, episodes of silent ischemia appeared to be more frequent in those with more severe OSA. A retrospective evaluation of more than 200 patients undergoing electron-beam computed tomography within 3 years of an overnight sleep recording addressed the occurrence of subclinical coronary artery calcification.[30] With multivari-ate adjustment, the OR for coronary artery calcification was 3.3 in the most severe AHI quartile (mean, 63.4 events/hour).

The effect of OSA on the prognosis of CAD has been addressed in several studies. In a study of patients with CAD who were undergoing elective PCI, concomitant OSA was significantly related to increased late lumen loss and restenosis after an average follow-up time of 7 months.[31] In another study, the incidence of adverse cardiac events (cardiac death, reinfarction, and target vessel revascularization) was reported to be almost 24% among patients with OSA, compared with 5% among those without OSA, during a 6-month follow-up.[21] Moreover, patients with CAD who had concomitant OSA were found to have an increased risk for cardiovascular mor-tality over a 5-year period.[32,33] Conversely, another study dem-onstrated no effect of OSA on readmission rate of PCI-treated patients with CAD who had concomitant OSA during a 6-month follow-up period[22] and no significant difference regarding the 10-year survival rate for patients with CAD and with OSA compared with those without OSA at baseline.[34] Moreover, a recent clinical report (mentioned previously)[27] found no association between sleep apnea in the setting of acute MI and adverse clinical outcomes, including death, heart failure, and new MI, during a median follow-up of 68 months. On the other hand, the incidence of stroke was reported to

be increased in patients with CAD who had concomitant OSA.[35] Stroke occurred in 18% of patients with CAD and sleep apnea, compared with 5% of those without sleep apnea, during 10 years of follow-up after a coronary angiography was performed. After adjustments for confounders, including hypertension and atrial fibrillation, the patients with sleep apnea had an adjusted HR of 2.9 (95% CI, 1.4 to 6.1) for a stroke.[35]

Hence OSA is common in patients with MI, but their mean AHI is relatively low in most published reports (Table 27-1).[13-15,17-22,27,36] Moreover, the prevalence of OSA is higher in patients with MI than in those with angina pectoris. This finding may be explained by the occurrence of Cheyne-Stokes breathing as a result of reduced ejection fraction.[19] Indeed the definition of the ideal timing for OSA screening after an acute MI remains unresolved. One study reported that 50% of CAD patients had an AHI of 15 or greater at the time of acute presentation in the coronary care unit, whereas 28% had remaining OSA based on the same AHI cutoff at least 6 weeks after hospital discharge.[37] A later study demonstrated occurrence of OSA (AHI ≥10) within the first 2 days after hospital admission in 54% of patients with acute coronary syndromes and preserved left ventricular ejection fraction, whereas 22 of 28 patients (79%) had residual OSA 1 month after the acute event, and only 6 of the 28 patients (21%) were diagnosed as having OSA at 6-month follow-up.[36] Thus OSA may be transient and, to some degree, related to the acute phase of the CAD, to more supine position of patients in the coronary care units, or to medications (sedatives and analge-sics). Available studies accumulating some 2324 patients with CAD demonstrated an OSA prevalence of about 47% (see Table 27-1). Despite the differences in the diagnostic proce-dures (full polysomnography or cardiorespiratory sleep record-ings) as well as varying cutoff values of AI, AHI, or ODI for definition of the sleep-disordered breathing, there seems to be enough evidence to advocate for overnight sleep recordings in individuals with MI given that concomitant OSA may worsen long-term outcomes in patients with CAD.

Incidence of Coronary Artery Disease in Longitudinal Studies

The first report on incident CAD data in a sleep clinic cohort was a smaller observational study demonstrating CAD devel-opment in almost one fourth of untreated patients with OSA during a 7-year follow-up period.[38] The corresponding numbers in treated sleep apnea patients and nonapneic snorers were 4% and 6%, respectively. Moreover, more than 50% of a normotensive cohort not treated for OSA developed at least one cardiovascular disease during the 7-year follow-up (Figure 27-2).[39] In that cohort, new CAD cases were also found among normotensive patients, suggesting that development of CAD in part may be independent of diurnal systemic hyper-tension induced by OSA. A larger observational study of a sleep clinic cohort, containing close to 1300 subjects with OSA, with a mean follow-up of 10 years, found a three to four times higher incidence of fatal and nonfatal cardiovascu-lar events in patients with severe OSA compared with simple snorers.[40] Multivariate analysis showed that the risk for fatal cardiovascular events was significantly increased in severe untreated patients with OSA (OR = 3.2; 95% CI, 1.1 to 7.5) compared with healthy controls. Another prospective observational study of a sleep clinic cohort including 1436

Table 27-1   Prevalence of Obstructive Sleep Apnea in Patients with Coronary Artery Disease

Study	Patients (no.)	Sex	Prevalence (%)	Diagnostic Criteria (events/hr)	Controlled?
Hung et al., 1990[13]	101	Male	36	AI >5	Yes
Andreas et al., 1996[19]	50	Male, female	50	AI >10	No
Mooe et al., 1996[17]	142	Male	37	AHI ≥10	Yes
Mooe et al., 1996[18]	102	Female	30	AHI ≥10	Yes
Koehler & Schafer, 1996[20]	74	Male	35	AHI ≥10	No
Peker et al., 1999[15]	62	Male, female	31	AHI ≥10	Yes
Schafer et al., 1999[14]	223	Male	31	AHI ≥10	Yes
Skinner et al., 2005[37]	26	Male, female	50	AHI ≥15	No
Mehra et al., 2006[22]	104	Male, female	66	AHI ≥10	No
Nakashima et al., 2006[23]	86	Male, female	43	AHI ≥15	No
Yumino et al., 2007[21]	89	Male, female	57	AHI ≥10	No
Lee et al., 2009[24]	105	Male, female	66	AHI ≥15	No
Konecny et al., 2010[25]	74	Male, female	41	AHI ≥15	No
Schiza et al., 2012[36]	52	Male, female	54	AHI ≥10	No
Garcia-Rio et al., 2013[16]	192	Male, female	35	AHI ≥15	Yes
Glantz et al., 2013[26]	662	Male, female	64	AHI ≥15	No
Aronson et al., 2014[27]	180	Male, female	64	ODI >5	No
Total or mean	2324	—	47	—	—

AHI, Apnea-hypopnea index; AI, apnea index; ODI, oxygen desaturation index.

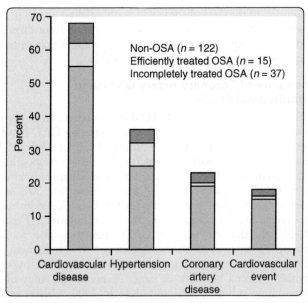

Figure 27-2 Incidence of cardiovascular disease during a 7-year follow-up in middle-aged men otherwise healthy at baseline. The fraction of individuals with incidence of cardiovascular disease, hypertension, coronary artery disease, and cardiovascular event (stroke, myocardial infarction, or cardiovascular death) is shown. Depicted are data from patients without OSA (Non-OSA) as well as from those incompletely or efficiently treated for their sleep and breathing disorder. (Modified from Peker Y, Hedner J, Norum J, et al. Increased incidence of cardiovascular disease in middle-aged men with obstructive sleep apnea: a seven-year follow-up. *Am J Respir Crit Care* 2002; 166:159–65).

consecutive subjects demonstrated that OSA (AHI ≥5) was associated with an increased risk for CAD events or death from cardiovascular causes (adjusted HR = 2.1; 95% CI, 1.1 to 3.9) during a follow-up period of almost 3 years.[41] Moreover, there was a dose-response relationship between AHI and composite outcome of CAD events or cardiovascular death (adjusted HR = 2.8; 95% CI, 1.5 to 5.5) in patients with severe OSA (AHI ≥30) compared with those without OSA (AHI <5).[41] Similarly, the 18-year follow-up study of the population-based Wisconsin Sleep Cohort sample reported an adjusted HR of 5.2 (95% CI, 1.4 to 19.2) for cardiovascular mortality in patients with severe OSA (AHI ≥30) and not using CPAP compared with those without OSA.[42] The longitudinal analysis of the Sleep Heart Health Study, including 1927 men and 2495 women free of CAD and heart failure at baseline, demonstrated a significant but weak association between severe OSA and incident CAD (adjusted HR of 1.7 for those with AHI ≥30 compared with those with AHI <5) in middle-aged men, but not in women.[43] In contrast to this population-based report, a recent observational follow-up study of 1116 women from two Spanish sleep clinic cohorts reported that untreated severe OSA was linked to increased cardiovascular mortality with an adjusted HR of 3.5 for those with AHI of 30 or greater compared to those with AHI of less than 10.[44] Another recent report from the same clinical cohorts demonstrated an adjusted HR of 2.8 (95% CI, 1.4 to 5.6) for the incidence of CAD or stroke in women with untreated OSA (AHI ≥10) compared with the control group without OSA.[45]

Effect of Obstructive Sleep Apnea Treatment on Coronary Artery Disease

The first-line treatment of OSA is CPAP, which is known to reduce daytime sleepiness and to improve quality of life.[46] A retrospective analysis of 55 subjects and comorbid OSA over an average follow-up time of 7.3 years showed a significantly lower occurrence of the composite end point of cardiovascular death, acute coronary syndrome, hospitalization for cardiac failure, or need for revascularization in those compliant with prescribed CPAP therapy.[47] In another follow-up study over 7.5 years, deaths from cardiovascular disease were less frequent in patients with OSA treated with CPAP compared with those without treatment.[48] Moreover, a review of 371 revascularized patients with OSA with concomitant CAD suggested a significantly lower cardiac death rate (3%) among 175 patients treated with CPAP compared with 10% among 196 untreated patients during a follow-up period of 5 years.[49] In the investigation of the sleep clinic cohort (mentioned earlier),[40] treatment with CPAP significantly reduced cardiovascular risk in men with severe OSA. Similar to that report, adequate CPAP treatment seemed to reduce the risk for composite end point of incident CAD or stroke in women with OSA.[45]

Plenty of evidence suggests that CPAP treatment reduces the number of ischemic events in patients with nocturnal angina and concomitant OSA in the short term.[28] A recent observational study addressed the effect of CPAP on recurrent episodes in patients with acute MI and concomitant OSA.[16] After adjustment for confounding factors, treated OSA patients who were compliant with CPAP had a lower risk for recurrent MI and revascularization (adjusted HRs = 0.16 and 0.15, respectively) than untreated patients and a similar risk to non-OSA patients (Figure 27-3). Of note, some patients with CAD and OSA may not experience daytime sleepiness (i.e., they are asymptomatic), and less is known regarding the adherence to CPAP therapy in these patients. However, a study of a sleep clinic cohort with concomitant CAD suggested a comparable compliance between sleepy and nonsleepy patients.[50] Observational studies might be criticized for potential bias because patients adhering to CPAP may have specific baseline characteristics, may be adhering to other medical therapy, or may otherwise have a healthier lifestyle. Observed benefits of CPAP in an observational study therefore provides a lower scientific evidence value compared with an RCT. Several RCTs examining the effect of CPAP on cardiovascular outcomes are underway.[51-54]

PATHOGENESIS

Obstructive sleep apnea is associated with considerable immediate hemodynamic change (see Chapter 25). During the cycle of the apneic event, there is increased work of breathing, considerable negative intrathoracic pressure swings, recurrent hypoxia and reoxygenation, and fluctuating autonomic activity (see Chapter 25). Heart rate and blood pressure also fluctuate through the cycle, but the relative contribution of each of these changes to development of cardiovascular disease is unknown. Increased oxygen demand and reduced oxygen supply (i.e., hypoxemia) after sleep-disordered breathing may trigger an attack of angina pectoris in patients with CAD, who already have reduced coronary flow reserve.[31] Nocturnal oxygen desaturations have been related to the severity of coronary atherosclerosis in patients with CAD[55] and may be an important contributor to coronary restenosis in patients with CAD who are treated with PCI.[56] Another study reported signs of apnea-induced ischemia predominantly during REM sleep,[8] a finding that may be explained by the often more prolonged and severe apneic events that commonly occur in this sleep stage. OSA is also associated with long-term alteration of cardiac structure, hemodynamic reflex function, and vascular structure or function. A recent report from the baseline echocardiographic investigations of the CAD patients

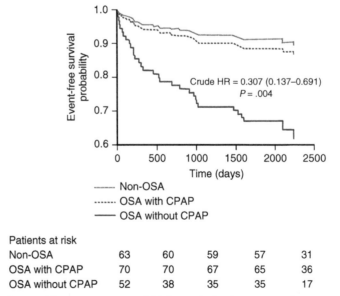

Patients at risk						
Non-OSA	63	60	59	57	31	12
OSA with CPAP	70	70	67	65	36	19
OSA without CPAP	52	38	35	35	17	9

Figure 27-3 Time until first recurrent myocardial infarction in the three groups of patients with coronary artery disease. Crude hazard ratio (HR) of treated versus untreated OSA is presented. CPAP, Continuous positive airway pressure; OSA, obstructive sleep apnea. (From Garcia-Rio F, Alonso-Fernandez A, Armada E, et al. CPAP effect on recurrent episodes in patients with sleep apnea and myocardial infarction. *Int J Cardiol* 2013;168:1328–35.)

with preserved left ventricular ejection fraction in the RIC-CADSA cohort demonstrated a poorer diastolic function (OR = 1.9; 95% CI, 1.1 to 3.2) in patients with OSA (AHI ≥15) after adjustment for traditionally recognized risk factors.[57] The OSA is associated with immediate and sustained sympathetic activation.[58] Baroreceptor and chemoreceptor responsiveness is altered,[59] and vascular reactivity in terms of responsiveness to hypoxemia or vasoconstrictors appears to be elevated.[60] A series of studies demonstrated that vascular endothelial function, expressed in terms of nitric oxide vascular dilating capacity, appears to be reduced in OSA.[61] Changes are specific to OSA in the sense that they are reversed by CPAP (see Chapter 25).[62-66]

The mechanisms responsible for endothelial cell damage and dysfunction are not entirely understood. However, investigations have shown that oxidative stress, potentially as a result of periodic hypoxia and reperfusion, is enhanced.[67] Oxidative stress results in compromised nitric oxide bioavailability and leads to an activation of redox-sensitive gene expression. Ensuing steps in this chain of events include increased expression of adhesion molecules by an activated endothelium and leukocytes, which finally leads to acceleration of a vascular inflammatory cascade that promotes atherosclerosis and vascular dysfunction.

This hypothesis (see Chapter 25)[67] is supported by data from patients with OSA demonstrating increased free radical production,[63] increased plasma-lipid peroxidation, increased adenosine and uric acid levels,[67] and increased levels of redox-sensitive gene expression products, including vascular endothelial growth factor[68] and inflammatory cytokines.[69] Interestingly, there was an improvement of endothelial function in patients with OSA following inhibition of xanthine oxidase by allopurinol[70] or supplemental vitamin C.[71] Circulating levels of adhesion molecules[72] as well as adhesion molecule–dependent monocyte to endothelial cell avidity appear to be increased in OSA.[73] Finally, sleep apnea appears to provide an additive stimulus for adhesion molecule expression in patients with CAD.[74] Increased levels of circulating markers of inflammation, including tumor necrosis factor-α,[75] C-reactive protein (CRP),[69,76] and interleukin-6 (IL-6),[69] have been inconsistently found to be increased in OSA. A recent report from the Icelandic Sleep Apnea Cohort containing 454 untreated OSA patients (AHI ≥15) demonstrated that OSA severity was an independent predictor of levels of CRP and IL-6, but this association was found only in obese patients.[77] Another recent report from the RICCADSA cohort demonstrated an association between OSA and elevated CRP and IL-6 also in nonobese patients.[78] This suggests that established CAD may be associated with vascular inflammation in OSA patients irrespective of comorbid obesity and that determinants of these markers are, besides OSA, also influenced by multiple comorbid risk factors for cardiovascular disease.

However, given the knowledge about ischemic preconditioning as a cardioprotective maneuver for reducing experimental myocardial infarct size,[79] it has been proposed that intermittent nocturnal hypoxia in OSA may provide future protection against myocardial ischemic insults by the regulation of critical mechanisms in the coronary endothelium.[80] Indeed, a recent study in patients with acute MI demonstrated a greater mobilization of endothelial progenitor cells and increased endothelial growth factor expression in patients

with mild to moderate sleep apnea.[81] Moreover, an observational study of 136 patients with an acute nonfatal MI found lower high-sensitivity troponin-T (hs-TnT) levels in patients with more severe OSA, suggesting a possible cardioprotective role by ischemic preconditioning in OSA.[82] On the other hand, there are data suggesting an independent association between increasing AHI and increasing hs-TnT levels in 1665 individuals without cardiovascular disease.[83] Over a median of 12.4 years' follow-up, hs-TnT was related to risk for death or incident heart failure in all OSA categories, suggesting that subclinical myocardial injury caused by OSA may play a role in the subsequent risk for cardiac disease.[83] Thus the short-term benefits of a possible ischemic preconditioning due to intermittent hypoxemia may be counteracted by other adverse outcomes in the long run.

The tentative association between OSA and CAD is supported by experimental data suggesting oxidative stress, endothelial dysfunction, and acceleration of vascular inflammation as a result of OSA. All of these mechanisms facilitate the onset and progression of atherosclerosis. One study found signs of atherosclerosis in large arteries of OSA patients without other risk factors for CAD, and the severity of the signs of atherosclerosis was correlated to the severity of OSA.[84] In another study by the same researcher group, these signs of early atherosclerosis in OSA patients were responsive to CPAP.[85] Finally, a higher atherosclerotic plaque volume in the coronary vessels of the stable CAD patients with OSA was demonstrated using a three-dimensional intravascular ultrasound technique.[86] A more recent study found that the frequency of noncalcified or mixed plaques was much higher in patients with OSA than in non-OSA patients who were investigated by noninvasive coronary computed tomography angiography.[87] Thus atherosclerotic plaque formation may jeopardize coronary flow reserve and generate symptoms of nocturnal angina during periods of increased flow demand. Such episodes occur repeatedly in sleep apnea, and they are associated with hypoxemia that further enhances the vulnerability for ischemia. On the other hand, most heart attacks (i.e., acute MI, sudden cardiac death) stem from sudden rupture of less-obtrusive plaques, which triggers thrombus formation in coronary vessels.[88] As mentioned earlier, it is suggested that sleep-disordered breathing influences the circadian acute coronary event distribution. OSA may lead to a disproportionate number of events that occur during or soon after the sleeping period.

CLINICAL COURSE AND PREVENTION

Early recognition and treatment of OSA may be beneficial in terms of CAD prevention. A retrospective analysis of a sleep laboratory cohort followed over 7 years found a reduction (relative risk, 0.29; 95% CI, 0.10 to 0.82) of incident CAD in patients with effectively treated OSA compared with ineffectively treated or untreated patients.[38] On the other hand, in a group of patients with CAD followed for 5 years, mortality was higher in those with comorbid OSA (38%) than in those with no OSA (9%).[32] Although the higher mortality was in part explained by the presence of other traditional risk factors, there was an independent influence of the breathing disorder. Another study followed 408 patients with stable angina and angiographically verified CAD for 5 years after sleep apnea recordings. The risk for a cerebrovascular event, including stroke and transient ischemic attack, was tripled in patients with CAD and concomitant OSA.[33,35]

Patients with CAD and nocturnal angina should be considered for sleep recording because nasal CPAP reduces angina attacks and nocturnal myocardial ischemia.[28] In the study of 10 severely disabled patients with a history of frequent nocturnal angina, 9 had sleep apnea.[28] Treatment with CPAP reduced episodes of nocturnal ischemia. There is no evidence to suggest that medication used for treatment of CAD affects the severity of the breathing disorder. A double-blind crossover study of nitrates in patients with OSA with or without CAD found lower oxygen saturation during apnea-associated ischemic episodes than during ischemia not associated with apnea (77.3% vs. 93.1%), and nitrate administration did not reduce the number of ischemic episodes associated with apnea.[89]

Although there is scientific support for a considerable effect of OSA on vascular structure and function, it is likely that development of CAD and other forms of vascular disease is determined by multiple genotypic and phenotypic factors. The absolute role of OSA in this concerted influence should evidently be better clarified. However, with the increasing recognition of OSA as an independent, additive, or even synergistic risk factor for CAD, we are facing a need for early identification of high-risk persons and a consensus on well-defined treatment strategies in such patients. Although more evidence is needed to address CPAP treatment as a useful therapy in patients with CAD and nonsymptomatic OSA, research in this field is growing rapidly, and the results from these ongoing RCTs[51-53] may soon add further insights.

CLINICAL PEARLS

- Recurrent apneas during sleep lead to a sequence of events that independently or in concert with other recognized risk factors are likely to have adverse effects on vascular structure and function.
- Not only may phenomena such as hypoxemia, reoxygenation, and recurrent vascular wall stress induce CAD, but also the events themselves may aggravate already-existing compromised coronary artery flow reserve.
- The adverse health effects of OSA in terms of CAD development, progression, and proneness to complications are likely to depend on genotypic and phenotypic factors. Markers or predictors for identification of high-risk persons in this context are still lacking.
- Almost 50% of patients with CAD have OSA defined according to conventional criteria. A large fraction of these patients do not exhibit daytime sleepiness. Additional data on different phenotypes of OSA as well as compliance with CPAP treatment, especially for nonsleepy patients with OSA and CAD, are needed.
- OSA identifies patients at risk for CAD and may represent a highly prevalent and modifiable risk factor.
- Recognition of the adverse effect of OSA on vascular disease will open a perspective of new primary and secondary prevention models for CAD that involve identifying and eliminating the sleep-disordered breathing.

SUMMARY

Recurrent apneas during sleep lead to a sequence of events that, independently or in concert with other recognized risk factors, are likely to have harmful effects on vascular structure and function. OSA-related phenomena, including hypoxemia, reoxygenation, and recurrent vascular wall stress, may induce CAD, and the events may aggravate already existing compromised coronary artery flow reserve. The epidemiologic support for a causal relationship between OSA and CAD is increasing but is not fully confirmed. This relationship is stronger in clinical cohorts than in the general population, which suggests that comorbid OSA in obese, hypertensive, smoking, and hyperlipidemic patients may provide an additive or synergistic risk factor for development of CAD.

Patients with CAD, including nocturnal angina, should therefore be considered for diagnostic sleep recording because elimination of apneas by nasal CPAP during sleep has been shown to reduce angina attacks and nocturnal myocardial ischemia. Moreover, prospective cohort data point to a reduction of recurrent myocardial infarction and revascularization in CAD patients treated with CPAP. The long-term tentative causal association between OSA and CAD is supported by experimental data suggesting endothelial dysfunction, acceleration of vascular inflammation, and development of atherosclerotic disease as a result of the breathing disorder. Increased recognition of the adverse effect of OSA on vascular disease may open a perspective of new primary and secondary prevention models for CAD that involve identification and elimination of the OSA.

Selected Readings

Arzt M, Hetzenecker A, Steiner S, Buchner S. Sleep-disordered breathing and coronary artery disease. *Can J Cardiol* 2015;**31**(7):909–17.

Damiani MF, Zito A, Carratù P, et al. Obstructive Sleep Apnea, Hypertension, and Their Additive Effects on Atherosclerosis. *Biochem Res Int* 2015;**2015**:984193.

Franklin KA, Nilsson JB, Sahlin C, et al. Sleep apnea and nocturnal angina. *Lancet* 1995;**345**:1085–7.

Gami AS, Olson EJ, Shen WK, et al. Obstructive sleep apnea and the risk of sudden cardiac death. *J Am Coll Cardiol* 2013;**62**:610–16.

Garcia-Rio F, Alonso-Fernandez A, Armada E, et al. CPAP effect on recurrent episodes in patients with sleep apnea and myocardial infarction. *Int J Cardiol* 2013;**168**:1328–35.

Lutsey PL, McClelland RL, Duprez D, et al. Objectively measured sleep characteristics and prevalence of coronary artery calcification: the Multi-Ethnic Study of theroslcerosis Sleep study. *Thorax* 2015;**70**(9):880–7.

Maeder MT, Schoch OD, Rickli H. A clinical approach to obstructive sleep apnea as a risk factor for cardiovascular disease. *Vasc Health Risk Manag* 2016;**12**:85–103.

Peker Y, Carlson J, Hedner J. Increased incidence of coronary artery disease in sleep apnoea: a long-term follow-up. *Eur Respir J* 2006;**28**:596–602.

Querejeta Roca G, Redline S, Punjabi N, et al. Sleep apnea is associated with subclinical myocardial injury in the community: the ARIC-SHHS study. *Am J Respir Crit Care Med* 2013;**188**:1460–5.

Thunström E, Glantz H, Fu M, et al. Increased inflammatory activity in nonobese patients with coronary artery disease and obstructive sleep apnea. *Sleep* 2015;**38**(3):463–71.

Valo M, Wons A, Moeller A, Teupe C. Markers of myocardial ischemia in patients with coronary artery disease and obstructive sleep apnea: effect of continuous positive airway pressure therapy. *Clin Cardiol* 2015;**38**(8):462–8.

A complete reference list can be found online at ExpertConsult.com.

Heart Failure

Shahrokh Javaheri

Chapter Highlights

- Multiple studies from across the globe showing that about 50% of patients with heart failure, both heart failure with reduced ejection fraction and preserved ejection fraction, have moderate to severe sleep apnea with an apnea hypopnea index ≥15/hour.

- Both obstructive and central sleep apneas may occur concomitantly in the same patient. Therapy will depend, in part, on predominant apnea type, which is determined by polysomnography.

- Multiple studies also indicate that both obstructive and central sleep apneas are independently associated with readmission to the hospital and excess mortality. Furthermore, effective treatment has been shown to decrease the number of readmissions and premature mortality.

- For treatment of obstructive sleep apnea, continuous positive airway pressure therapy is the treatment of choice. Importantly, survival benefits are encountered in only those who are compliant with the device.

- For patients whose sleep apnea is not suppressed by continuous positive airway pressure, including almost 50% of patients with central sleep apnea, we recommend the use of adaptive servo-ventilation if LVEF is greater than 45%. Most of the studies using adaptive servo-ventilation have shown improvement in cardiac biomarkers, and readmission, but the impact on survival may be negative if LVEF is low.

Heart failure has been known for more than 2 centuries to be associated with abnormal breathing patterns, and John Cheyne and William Stokes have been credited for its description—hence the eponym *Cheyne-Stokes breathing*.[1,2] However, 37 years earlier, John Hunter,[3,4] a British physician, was the first to describe this breathing pattern, which is characterized by gradual crescendo–decrescendo changes in tidal volume, commonly with an intervening central apnea (Figure 28-1).[5-9] We therefore refer to this pattern as *Hunter-Cheyne-Stokes breathing* (HCSB). Periodic breathing is a pattern of breathing characterized by cyclic fluctuations in the amplitude of airflow and tidal volume.[10] It consists of recurring cycles of apnea or hypopnea, or both, followed by hyperpnea. The apneas and hypopneas may be obstructive (i.e., the result of upper airway occlusion) or central.[10] Obstructive sleep apnea (OSA)–hypopnea is the most common form of periodic breathing in persons without heart failure. However, in patients *with* heart failure, both obstructive and central periodic breathing are common and frequently occur together, although one phenotype is predominant.

HCSB is a form of periodic breathing with central sleep apnea (CSA) and hypopnea that occurs in patients with heart failure and has a long cycle time.[11] The latter is an important feature of HCSB breathing and reflects the prolonged circulation time that is a pathologic feature of heart failure. HCSB is a subjective description and is not readily quantifiable. For these reasons, the term *central sleep apnea* is preferable, and it also avoids misrepresentation, because credit for the discovery of breathing pattern has not been given to the original discoverer.

CSA observed in awake patients with heart failure has been considered an indicator of a terminal prognosis. However, like obstructive apnea, central apnea occurs primarily during sleep, and polysomnographic studies have reported a high prevalence of this disorder in ambulatory patients with stable heart failure.[8,9,12-14]

EPIDEMIOLOGY OF HEART FAILURE AND SLEEP-RELATED BREATHING DISORDERS

Heart failure has become a major public health problem.[15] In the United States, approximately 5.1 million adults 20 years and older have heart failure, and 0.8 million individuals are newly diagnosed each year.[15] Furthermore, it is projected that the prevalence of heart failure will increase 46% from 2012 to 2030, resulting in more than 8 to 9.5 million people ≥18 years of age with heart failure. It is estimated that heart failure may contribute directly or indirectly to about 280,000 deaths each year.[15] The death rate increases progressively with advanced symptomatology, with a 5-year survival rate approaching 50%.

Heart failure is the largest single Medicare expenditure because it is the leading cause of hospitalization for patients older than age 65 years. Annually, more than 1 million patients with heart failure need hospitalization. Currently more than $30 billion is spent annually on heart failure.[15]

Left ventricular (LV) myocardial failure is the most common cause of heart failure in adults, and it could be predominantly diastolic, referred to as *heart failure with preserved ejection fraction* (HFpEF), or manifested by combined systolic and diastolic dysfunction, referred to as *heart failure with*

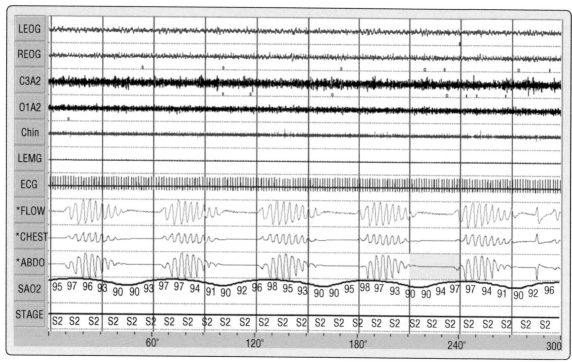

Figure 28-1 A 10-minute epoch of a patient with systolic heart failure and Hunter-Cheyne-Stokes breathing. Note recurrent hypoxia/reoxygenation as a result of central sleep apnea. (From Kryger MH. *Atlas of clinical sleep medicine.* 2nd ed. Philadelphia: Saunders; 2014.)

reduced ejection fraction (HFrEF). The principal hallmark of HFrEF is a depressed left ventricular ejection fraction (LVEF), which is commonly associated with an increase in end-diastolic and systolic volumes. The symptoms, which result from both diminished cardiac output and the concomitant diastolic dysfunction, include shortness of breath, orthopnea, nocturnal dyspnea, nocturia, fatigue, and exercise intolerance. Many of these symptoms overlap with those of sleep apnea, making it difficult to suspect sleep apnea when comorbid with heart failure.

Meanwhile, it is estimated that 20 million people may have asymptomatic LV systolic dysfunction, and, with time, these persons are likely to develop HFrEF. As will be discussed later, overall, about 50% of individuals with LV systolic dysfunction both asymptomatic or symptomatic suffer from moderate to severe sleep apnea.

The other phenotype, HFpEF, is the most common form of heart failure in elderly patients. The pathophysiologic consequence of LV diastolic dysfunction relates to a hypertrophied or a noncompliant left ventricle shifting the pressure volume curve upward and to the left. Therefore, for a given LV volume, LV end-diastolic pressure increases, resulting in elevated left atrial and pulmonary capillary pressures, pulmonary congestion, and edema. Similar to asymptomatic LV systolic dysfunction, which, with time, leads to HFrEF, asymptomatic LV diastolic dysfunction is also independently associated with incident overt heart failure and is predictive of all-cause death.[16]

Sleep Apnea in Heart Failure with Reduced Ejection Fraction

The prevalence of sleep-related breathing disorders has been systematically studied in patients with HFrEF.[5] Poly-somnographic studies[6-14,17-25] and studies using respiratory channels[26-29] show a high prevalence of sleep apnea in this population. Most recent large studies of consecutive patients with HFrEF are depicted in Table 28-1.

High prevalence rates have been reported in patients who have HFrEF, HFrEF patients awaiting transplantation,[18] patients with valve heart disease,[19] and those with an implanted cardiac defibrillator.[20]

The most systematic prospective study of HFrEF[17] involved 100 ambulatory male patients with stable, treated heart failure. Using an apnea-hypopnea index (AHI) of 15 events per hour or greater as the threshold, 49 patients (49% of all patients) had moderate to severe sleep apnea–hypopnea, with an average AHI of 44. In comparison, a population study of subjects without heart failure[30] showed that 13% of working men and 6% women ages 30 to 70 years had an AHI of greater than 15. An AHI of 5 or greater has been used to define the presence of a significant number of disordered-breathing events in OSA–hypopnea syndrome.[23] Therefore, with a much higher prevalence of sleep apnea observed in patients with heart failure than in the general population, HFrEF should be the leading risk factor for sleep apnea in the general population. In our studies,[9,17] about 10% of the patients were on beta blockers; however, recent studies continue to show a high prevalence of sleep apnea, both central and obstructive, despite the widespread use of beta blockers. Table 28-1 shows the prevalence of central and OSA in the largest recent studies.[17,23-29] Combining the results of these recent series, which reported an AHI of 15 per hour of sleep as the threshold, 53% of 1607 patients with HFrEF had moderate to severe sleep apnea, 34% had CSA, and 19% had OSA (Figure 28-2). However, there has been considerable variation in the reported prevalence of these two forms of sleep apnea

Table 28-1   Prevalence of Sleep Apnea in Recent Studies of Systolic Heart Failure

COUNTRY (year)	N	%AHI ≥15/h	%CSA	%OSA	%β Blockers
USA (06)* Javaheri	100	49	37	12	10
USA (08) McDonald	108	61	31	30	82
Canada (07)* Wang	218	46	21	26	80
UK (07)* Vazir	55	53	38	15	78
Germany (07) Oldenberg	700	651	32	19	85
Germany (09)* Hagenda	50	64	44	20	100
Germany (10)* Jilek	273	64	50	14	88
Portugal (10)* Ferreira	103	45	nr	nr	90
Total	1607	53	34	20	81

*In these studies, brain waves were not recorded.
AHI, Apnea–hypopnea index (the threshold used to define the presence of the disorder in each study); CSA, central sleep apnea; nr, not reported; OSA, obstructive sleep apnea.
Modified from Kryger MH. *Atlas of clinical sleep medicine.* 2nd ed. Philadelphia: Saunders; 2014.

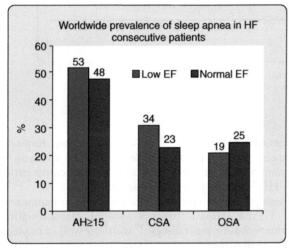

Figure 28-2 Prevalence of sleep apnea in heart failure with reduced ejection fraction (HFrEF) or preserved ejection HFpEF). The data presented combine a series of world sleep studies (see Table 28-1) in consecutive patients with HFrEF, and 244 consecutive patients with HFpEF.[31] AHI, Apnea–hypopnea index; CSA, central sleep apnea; OSA, obstructive sleep apnea. (From Kryger MH. *Atlas of clinical sleep medicine.* Philadelphia: Elsevier; 2014.)

in patients with HFrEF (see Table 28-1), which depends on a number of issues. The major reasons are the criteria used to define hypopnea, the accuracy of classification of disordered-breathing events (obstructive versus central, particularly in regard to hypopneas), the criteria used to define predominant obstructive versus CSA, the number of obese patients with heart failure enrolled, the level of arterial Pco_2, and the severity of LV systolic dysfunction.

Sleep Apnea in Heart Failure with Preserved Ejection Fraction

There is also a high prevalence of sleep apnea in HFpEF.[31,32] The largest prospective study[31] to date evaluated 244 consecutive patients (87 women). All underwent polygraphy, right heart catheterization, and echocardiography. The two major causes of HFpEF were systemic hypertension (44%) and coronary artery disease (33%). Forty-eight percent had an AHI of 15 or more per hour, of whom 23% had CSA. Patients

with CSA had lower Pco_2 but higher LV end-diastolic and pulmonary capillary wedge pressure. The latter finding is critical to the development of periodic breathing and CSA because increased wedge pressure and pulmonary congestion decrease the Pco_2 reserve, the major mechanism underlying CSA.[33] We must emphasize that there is a vicious cycle between HFpEF and sleep apnea. Hemodynamic studies show that pulmonary capillary pressure increases during the course of obstructive apnea, indicating the development of LV diastolic dysfunction (see Chapter 25). Chronic repetitive exposure to negative swings in intrathoracic pressure, cyclic nocturnal hypertension and hypoxemia, and diurnal systemic hypertension could eventually result in worsening the LV hypertrophy, dysfunction, and heart failure. In this regard, studies[34,35] suggest that OSA is associated with an increase in LV mass and dysfunction. In the largest study,[36] consisting of 2058 Sleep Heart Health Study participants, LV mass was associated with both apnea–hypopnea and hypoxemia indices after adjustment for age, sex, ethnicity, body mass index, smoking, systolic blood pressure, antihypertensive medication use, diabetes mellitus, prevalent myocardial infarction, and alcohol consumption. Furthermore, in an observational study,[34] treatment of OSA patients with CPAP resulted in a reversal of diastolic dysfunction. In another observational study,[35] an adaptive servo-ventilation (ASV) device was used to treat patients with HFpEF and HCSB and severe CSA. ASV treatment led to a significant decrease in left atrial diameter and early-to-atrial (E/A) filling velocity ratio, whereas the early filling to early diastolic mitral annular velocity ratio increased significantly. It therefore appears that treatment of both OSA and CSA results in remodeling of the left heart structures. These observational findings have been confirmed by a randomized placebo (sham CPAP)–controlled trial,[37] showing that, after 12 weeks on effective CPAP therapy, there was a significant increase in the E/A ratio, a significant decrease in isovolemic relaxation and mitral deceleration time. The results of these studies have important therapeutic implications for HFpEF because, to date, there are no approved therapies to reduce hospitalization or mortality for this disorder, which is on the rise, and the growing elderly population in whom HFpEF is the predominant phenotype of heart failure guarantees additional burden.[38] In addition, similar to asymptomatic LV systolic dysfunction, which, as noted earlier, will eventually lead to HFrEF, it has been shown that LV diastolic dysfunction is a precursor to HFpEF.[16]

In summary, the prevalence of moderate to severe sleep apnea is about 50% in both forms of heart failure, HFrEF and HFpEF (Figure 28-2), and introduction of beta blockers in the therapeutic armamentarium of heart failure has had no impact on the prevalence of sleep apnea. In contrast to OSA (which is the predominant form of the disorder in the general population with a rare episode of central apnea in the pattern, in heart failure), central and OSA commonly occur together. Sleep physicians reviewing the polysomnogram, therefore, have to determine the predominant form of the disorder for therapeutic options. The predominant phenotype, obstructive versus central, is quite variable and, in large part, depends on the categorization of hypopneas into central or obstructive.

Sex and Sleep-Related Breathing Disorders in Heart Failure

In the general population, the prevalence of OSA is much higher in men than in women. This also holds true for CSA in HFrEF. Combining the results of several studies of patients with HFrEF,[12-14,18,39] 40% of the male patients and 18% of the female patients have CSA (Figure 28-3). A similar trend was found for OSA.

The results of population studies of subjects without heart failure (reviewed by Young and colleagues[40]) suggest that menopause may be a risk factor for OSA, and that the risk is probably reduced by hormone replacement therapy. In women with congestive heart failure and systolic dysfunction, the risk of CSA was six times higher in those ages 60 years and older than in those younger than 60 years.[12] A similar difference was also reported for OSA–hypopnea before and after age 60 years.[12] Thus female hormonal status plays a role in the development of sleep-disordered breathing in women with and without heart failure.

Progesterone is a known respiratory stimulant, and its effects on the respiratory system may, in part, explain the lower prevalence of central and OSA in menstruating women. Progesterone increases ventilation[41] and the tone of the dilator muscles of the upper airway.[42] Furthermore, premenopausal women have a significantly lower apneic threshold than men.[43] This should decrease the probability of developing central apnea during sleep in female subjects (see the following section on mechanisms of CSA). In contrast to progesterone, administration of testosterone to premenopausal women results in diminution of the Pco_2 reserve,[44] which should increase the likelihood of developing apnea during sleep.[32] The results of these two studies suggest that the balance of progesterone/testosterone is critical in determining the Pco_2 reserve.

MECHANISMS OF SLEEP-RELATED BREATHING DISORDERS IN HEART FAILURE

Mechanisms of Central Sleep Apnea in Heart Failure

The mechanisms of periodic breathing and CSA in heart failure are complex and multifactorial (see Chapter 15).[5,33,45,46] In heart failure, alterations occur in various components of the negative feedback system controlling breathing that increase the likelihood of developing periodic breathing, during both sleep and wakefulness. In addition, there are specific sleep-related mechanisms that explain the genesis of CSA and the reason periodic breathing becomes so prevalent during sleep.

Mathematical models of the negative feedback system predict that increased arterial circulation time (which delays the transfer of information regarding changes in Po_2 and Pco_2 from pulmonary capillary blood to the chemoreceptors, referred to as *mixing gain*), enhanced gain of the chemoreceptors, and enhanced plant gain (e.g., decreased functional residual capacity), which are the three components of the loop gain, collectively increase the likelihood of periodic breathing.[10,11,33,45-48]

Loop gain is the engineering term that defines the tendency of the negative feedback loop toward instability in response to a ventilatory disturbance. As an example, normally, a short pause in breathing, an apnea, or hypopnea causes a compensatory increase in ventilation. If the magnitude of the increase in ventilation is greater than or equal to the magnitude of the preceding respiratory disturbance, that is, loop gain is ≥1, the system becomes unstable and will fluctuate between underventilation and overventilation.

Delay in transfer of information due to prolonged circulation time, that is, increased mixing gain, plays a fundamental role in destabilization of a negative feedback system.[11,33,47] It has the potential to convert a negative feedback system to a positive feedback system. In heart failure, arterial circulation time may be increased for a variety of reasons, including dilation of cardiac chambers, increased pulmonary blood volume, and decreased cardiac output. However, patients with heart failure invariably have increased circulation time. Therefore, although increased circulation time is necessary to develop periodic breathing, it does not explain why only some heart failure patients have periodic breathing. The second component of the loop gain that increases the likelihood of occurrence of periodic breathing (and also central apnea during sleep) is the gain of the chemoreceptors.[8] In persons with increased sensitivity to CO_2 (or hypoxia), the chemoreceptors elicit a large ventilatory response whenever the Pco_2 rises (or the Po_2 decreases). The consequent intense hyperventilation,

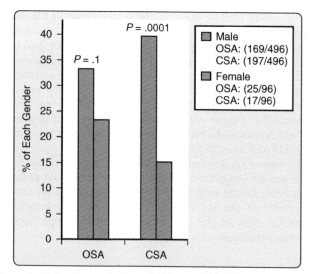

Figure 28-3 Prevalence of obstructive sleep apnea (OSA) and central sleep apnea (CSA) in men and women with systolic heart failure. The prevalence of CSA is much lower in women than in men. A similar trend is found in OSA, although it is not statistically significant. (From Javaheri S. Sleep related breathing disorders in heart failure. In: Mann DL, editor. *Heart failure: a companion to Braunwald's heart disease.* Philadelphia: Saunders; 2004. p. 471–87.)

by driving the P_{CO_2} below the apneic threshold, results in central apnea. As a result of central apnea, P_{CO_2} rises (and P_{O_2} falls), and the cycles of hyperventilation and hypoventilation (hypopnea) or central apnea are maintained.[7] Differences in the gain of the chemoreceptors among patients with heart failure may, in part, explain why only some patients with heart failure develop periodic breathing and CSA.

The third component of the loop gain that may contribute to the development of periodic breathing in heart failure is decreased functional residual capacity, which results in underdamping.[5,33,45] This means that, for a given change in ventilation (e.g., a pause in breathing), changes in the controlled variables—namely P_{O_2} and P_{CO_2}—will be augmented (referred to as *increased plant gain*). In turn, the augmented changes in P_{O_2} and P_{CO_2} result in a pronounced compensatory ventilatory response, and overcompensation tends to destabilize breathing. Patients with heart failure may have decreased functional residual capacity for a variety of reasons, including pleural effusion, cardiomegaly, and decreased compliance of the respiratory system. Functional residual capacity may decrease further in the supine position, facilitating the development of periodic breathing in this position.

The aforementioned mechanisms that collectively increase the loop gain and the likelihood of periodic breathing are present during both sleep and wakefulness. However, in the supine position and during sleep, further changes, such as a reduction in functional residual capacity, metabolic rate (another factor in the plant gain), and cardiac output, occur that will augment the likelihood of developing periodic breathing beyond that observed during wakefulness. Furthermore, loop gain, as described previously, differs from the dynamic loop gain during sleep when periodic breathing is present and steady state is absent.[33]

Meanwhile, like obstructive apnea, central apnea usually occurs during sleep or when a subject is awake but dozing. The genesis of CSA during sleep relates specifically to the removal of the nonchemical drive of wakefulness on breathing and to the unmasking of the apneic threshold—the level of P_{CO_2} below which rhythmic breathing ceases.[33] The difference between two P_{CO_2} set points—the prevailing P_{CO_2} minus the P_{CO_2} at the apneic threshold, referred to as *P_{CO_2} reserve*—is a critical factor for the occurrence of CSA. The smaller the difference, the greater the likelihood of occurrence of apnea.

Normally, with the onset of sleep, ventilation decreases and P_{CO_2} increases. As long as the prevailing P_{CO_2} is above the apneic threshold, rhythmic breathing continues. However, in some patients with heart failure, the awake prevailing P_{CO_2} does not significantly rise with onset of sleep.[49,50] Importantly, however, heart failure patients who develop central apnea have increased CO_2 chemosensitivity below eupnea[50] while asleep, as well as above eupnea while awake, as discussed previously.[48] Because of increased CO_2 chemosensitivity below eupnea,[50] the prevailing P_{CO_2} and the apneic threshold P_{CO_2} are close together, increasing the likelihood of developing central apnea during sleep. The increased chemosensitivity above eupnea becomes particularly pathophysiological during arousals occurring following apneas, when excessive ventilatory response lowers the prevailing P_{CO_2} toward or below the apneic threshold.[48]

The reason for the lack of the normally observed rise in P_{CO_2} in some patients with heart failure is not clear. It could result from the lack of the normally observed sleep-induced decrease in ventilation. Conceivably, because of increased venous return in the supine position, and in the presence of a stiff left ventricle, pulmonary capillary pressure could rise. This results in an increase in respiratory rate and ventilation, preventing the normally observed rise in P_{CO_2}. At the same time, the increase in pulmonary capillary pressure increases the chemosensitivity below eupnea and decreases the P_{CO_2} reserve, promoting the likelihood of developing central apnea. This was demonstrated in naturally sleeping dogs in whom pulmonary capillary pressure could be increased to different levels by inflating a balloon placed in the left atrium.[51] The mechanisms remain to be fully elucidated, although vagal afferents have been shown to have significant influences on the responsiveness of both carotid bodies as well as central chemoreceptors.[32] Several studies[52-54] have shown that patients with heart failure and low arterial P_{CO_2} have a high probability of developing central apnea during sleep. Predictive value of a low steady-state arterial P_{CO_2} (<35 mm Hg) is about 80%.[54] The reason for this association lies on the fact that a low arterial P_{CO_2} is caused by increased pulmonary wedge pressure, which, per se, sensitizes carotid bodies and the central chemoreceptors promoting CSA, as noted previously.[48] Meanwhile, although an awake low arterial P_{CO_2} is highly predictive of CSA, it is not a prerequisite. Many patients with heart failure and CSA have a normal awake arterial P_{CO_2}.[55] What is important is the proximity of the apneic threshold to the arterial P_{CO_2}, and an increased CO_2 chemosensitivity below eupnea.

Mechanisms of Obstructive Sleep Apnea in Heart Failure

As noted earlier, OSA and hypopnea are also common in heart failure. The mechanisms are multifactorial.[7,56-59] First, periodic breathing resulting from heart failure predisposes the susceptible subjects to develop upper airway occlusion during the nadir of the ventilatory cycles of periodic breathing.[7,56] For this reason, we observed multiple episodes of upper airway obstruction frequently following central apneas.[7]

Second, increased venous congestion and pressure resulting from right heart failure may diminish upper airway size[57] and facilitate upper airway occlusion. Venous congestion of the upper airway may be worse in the supine (than in the erect) position, and rostral fluid shift, particularly in the presence of edema in the lower extremities and redistribution of fluid into vascular space, may further compound upper airway patency.[58] Third, patients with heart failure and OSA are commonly obese, and obesity may compromise upper airway patency. While currently 35% of patients with HFrEF are obese, almost 53% of those with HFpEF suffer from this disorder[59] for which reason the prevalence of OSA is higher in patients with HFpEF than in HFrEF.[31,32]

In summary, decreased upper airway size resulting from both venous congestion and obesity may predispose patients with heart failure to develop upper airway occlusion during the nadir of the ventilatory cycles of periodic breathing, when the tone of the dilator muscles of the upper airway decreases the most.

PATHOLOGIC CONSEQUENCES AND PROGNOSTIC SIGNIFICANCE OF SLEEP-RELATED BREATHING DISORDERS

The cycles of apnea–hypopnea and hyperpnea, both obstructive and central, are associated with three adverse

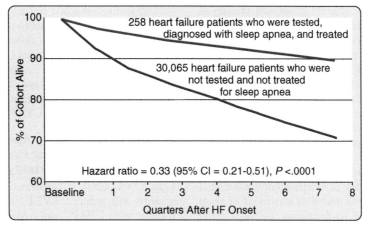

Figure 28-4 Data were from Medicare beneficiaries who were diagnosed with new heart failure. The 2-year survival of the 258 patients who were tested, diagnosed, and treated for sleep apnea was much better than the survival of the 30,065 patients who were not tested for sleep apnea. The survival was adjusted for age, gender, and Charlson Comorbidity Index. (Modified from Javaheri S, Caref B, Chen E, et al. Sleep apnea testing and outcomes in a large cohort of Medicare beneficiaries with newly diagnosed heart failure. *Am J Respir Crit Care Med* 2011;183:539–46.)

consequences. These include arterial blood gas abnormalities characterized by intermittent hypoxemia–reoxygenation and hypercapnia–hypocapnia, excessive arousals and shift to light sleep stages, and large negative swings in intrathoracic pressure (see Chapter 25). The pathophysiologic consequences of obstructive and CSAs and hypopneas are qualitatively similar (but worse in OSA than in CSA), adversely affect various cardiovascular functions, and are potentially most detrimental in the presence of established coronary artery disease and LV systolic and diastolic dysfunction. In the long run, these adverse consequences result in excess morbidity, hospital readmission, and mortality of patients with heart failure.

Effects of Obstructive Sleep Apnea on Sympathetic Activity, Cardiovascular Function, Hospital Readmission, and Mortality

In patients with heart failure, the presence of OSA is associated with increased sympathetic activity[60] and reduced LVEF, which are reversed if sleep apnea is effectively treated with nasal CPAP.[54-57] There are five randomized clinical trials[61-65] of CPAP therapy for OSA in patients with HFrEF. In three of these studies,[61-63] LVEF increased significantly (when compared with the control group) by about 10%, 5%, and 2%. In two[63,64] of these five studies, sham CPAP was used in the control group; in one,[63] LVEF increased significantly but slightly (2%), and, in the other one,[64] ejection fraction did not increase. In the latter study,[64] auto-CPAP was used, and the adherence hours to CPAP were less than in the two previous studies,[61,62] which had demonstrated 10% and 5% increases in ejection fraction. In the most recent study,[64] 45 patients with OSA (mean AHI = 27/hour of sleep) and HFrEF (mean LVEF = 36%) were randomized to CPAP ($n = 22$) or no CPAP ($n = 23$) for 6 to 8 weeks. Comparing the two groups, there were no significant changes in LVEF.

In patients with established coronary artery disease, OSA is an independent prognostic factor for recurrent cardiovascular disorders and survival.[66-67] Similarly, in heart failure, OSA is an independent predictor of mortality,[23] and two observational studies (Figure 28-4), one from Japan[68] and the other from the United States,[69] confirm this association and further

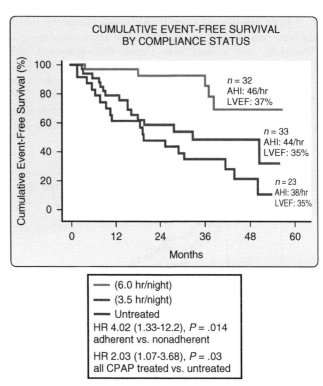

Figure 28-5 Probability for hospitalization and mortality of heart failure patients with obstructive sleep apnea decrease if they are treated with continuous positive airway pressure (CPAP) and adhere to therapy. AHI, Apnea–hypopnea index; HR, hazard ratio; LVEF, left ventricular ejection fraction. (From Kryger MH. *Atlas of clinical sleep medicine*. Philadelphia: Elsevier; 2010; modified from Kasai T, Narui K, Dohi P, et al. Prognosis of patients with heart failure and obstructive sleep apnea treated with continuous positive airway pressure. *Chest* 2008;133:690–6.)

suggest that therapy with CPAP improves survival, particularly in those who are most compliant with it (Figure 28-5).[68] This latter observation in patients with heart failure is similar to that in patients with hypertension, as studies indicate that the reduction in blood pressure is most prominent in those who are most adherent to CPAP therapy (see Chapter 26). In the U.S. study,[69] a random sample of Medicare beneficiaries newly diagnosed with heart failure was enrolled. Of the 30,719 subjects, only 1263 (4%) were clinically suspected to have sleep apnea. Of these, 553 (2% of the total cohort) underwent sleep study, and some were treated mostly with CPAP. After adjustment for age, sex, and comorbidities, subjects with heart failure who were tested, diagnosed, and treated had a better 2-year survival rate compared with subjects with heart failure who were not tested (hazard ratio, 0.33 [95% confidence interval, 0.21–0.51]; P = .0001; Figure 28-4).

One important issue not previously emphasized is that, in patients with heart failure, OSA is independently associated with excess hospital readmission and that treatment of sleep apnea could lower the rate of readmissions. In the United States, Medicare began financially penalizing hospitals with excess readmissions in 2012, and, starting in October 2013, readmission penalties doubled to 2% of reimbursement. In one study from a heart hospital, Khayat and colleagues[70] demonstrated that severe OSA was independently associated with 1.5 times higher readmission when compared to heart failure patients without OSA. Importantly, these authors accounted for a large number of relevant pathologic variables, which otherwise could have associated with excess readmission. Meanwhile, two studies have shown that treatment with CPAP decreases the rate of readmission. In a study of Medicare beneficiaries with congestive heart failure, readmission costs for those treated for sleep apnea (mostly with CPAP) were much lower than for those suspected of having sleep apnea but who were not referred for sleep studies and,

consequently, remained untreated.[69,71] Another retrospective study[72] of patients admitted to the hospital for a cardiac cause, including congestive heart failure who underwent polygraphy and found to have sleep apnea (AHI ≥ 5/hour, mostly OSA), hospital readmission or emergency department visit for a cardiac issue within 30 days of discharge was quite high in those who refused or were nonadherent to CPAP compared to those who adhered to CPAP therapy (P = .025).

Effects of Central Sleep Apnea on Sympathetic Activity, Cardiovascular Function, Hospital Readmission, and Mortality

Like OSA, CSA is associated with increased sympathetic activity and reduced LVEF, which is reversed by effective therapy with CPAP[73] and oxygen.

Several studies,[21,29,74-86] but not all,[84,85] have suggested that presence of CSA decreases survival among patients with HFrEF. In one[84] of the two studies[84,85] noted, there was a tendency for excess mortality in heart failure patients with CSA, although this was not significant, probably because of the small number of patients.

We followed 88 heart failure patients with (n = 56) or without (n = 32) CSA with a median follow-up of 51 months.[81] After controlling for 24 confounding variables, CSA was associated with excess mortality (hazard ratio, 2.14; P = .02; Figure 28-6). The average survival of heart failure patients without CSA was 90 months compared with 45 months for those with CSA. That CSA contributes to excess mortality in heart failure is supported by the observation that effective treatment of CSA with CPAP in HFrEF[80] and with ASV in HFpEF[87]

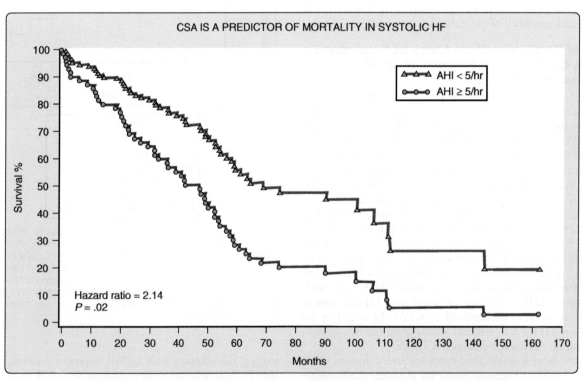

Figure 28-6 Probability of survival in patients with systolic heart failure (HF) according to the presence or absence of central sleep apnea (CSA). AHI, Apnea–hypopnea index. (From Kryger MH. *Atlas of clinical sleep medicine.* Philadelphia: Elsevier; 2010; modified from Javaheri S, Shukla R, Zeigler H, Wexler L. Central sleep apnea, right ventricular dysfunction, and low diastolic blood pressure are predictors of mortality in systolic heart failure. *J Am Coll Cardiol* 2007;49:2028–34.)

improves survival. The first study[80] was based on the post-hoc analysis of the Canadian randomized clinical trial, and the second one was a randomized trial involving the small number of patients with HFpEF.[87] The results of a relatively large observational study[29] of patients with predominantly CSA who agreed to use ASV are consistent with those of the aforementioned randomized trials.[81,87]

Similar to findings in OSA, CSA has been found to be an independent predictor of hospital readmission within 30 days after discharge. Khayat and colleagues[70] performed a prospective observational study of consecutive patients with HFrEF (LVEF = 22%), 165 with CSA and 139 without sleep apnea. In patients with CSA, the rate ratio for cardiac readmission within 1 or 6 months was 1.5 ($P = .03$) higher than patients without sleep apnea. The authors accounted for age, gender, body weight, blood pressure, coronary artery disease, hemoglobin, serum sodium and creatinine concentration, diabetes mellitus, and length of stay. Further, treatment of CSA has been shown to be associated with decreased hospital readmission.[88-91] Virtually all of these studies[88-91] are from Japan, are observational, the end points were a combination of premature mortality and readmission due to heart failure, and ASV devices were used to treat CSA, or when mixed with OSA.

CLINICAL PRESENTATION OF OBSTRUCTIVE AND CENTRAL SLEEP APNEAS IN PATIENTS WITH HEART FAILURE

Obesity is an important risk factor for development of OSA in patients with heart failure,[9,12,16] as it is for patients without heart failure.[29] Patients with HFrEF and OSA are significantly heavier and snore habitually (Figure 28-7). They may also have a higher systemic arterial blood pressure than subjects with CSA.[9,12] Aside from obesity and habitual snoring, it is often difficult to clinically suspect the presence of sleep apnea in patients with heart failure because (1) the prevalence of sleepiness is similar in heart failure patients with and in those without sleep apnea[9,16] (see Figure 28-7), and (2) the symptoms of heart failure and sleep apnea overlap. The overlapping symptoms of sleep apnea and heart failure include sleep-onset and maintenance insomnia, nocturia, waking up with shortness of breath (orthopnea, paroxysmal nocturnal dyspnea, hyperpnea due to periodic breathing), unrefreshed sleep, and daytime fatigue. The overlapping of the symptoms of heart failure and sleep apnea undoubtedly contributes to the underdiagnosis of sleep-related breathing disorders in patients with heart failure. CSA, in particular, is most difficult to diagnose,[8] because obesity and habitual snoring, which are the two hallmarks of OSA (see Figure 28-7), are commonly absent in heart failure patients with CSA.[8,9] However, there are some clues that, when present, should increase the probability of the presence of CSA. These include a high-numbered class in the New York Heart Association classification, low LVEF, and steady-state arterial Pco_2, atrial fibrillation, and nocturnal ventricular arrhythmias (Figure 28-8).[9]

Indications for Polysomnography in Heart Failure

As noted, patients with heart failure and sleep apnea do not generally present with symptoms that distinguish them from heart failure patients without sleep apnea. Furthermore, because heart failure is common, it is not possible to perform sleep studies on all patients with heart failure. However, there are a number of clinical and laboratory findings that, when present in patients with heart failure, should increase clinical suspicion for sleep apnea. These markers are different for obstructive and CSA.

Risk factors for OSA–hypopnea in patients with heart failure are similar to those in patients without heart failure. They include obesity, increased neck size, habitual snoring, and hypertension. These risk factors and others, such as

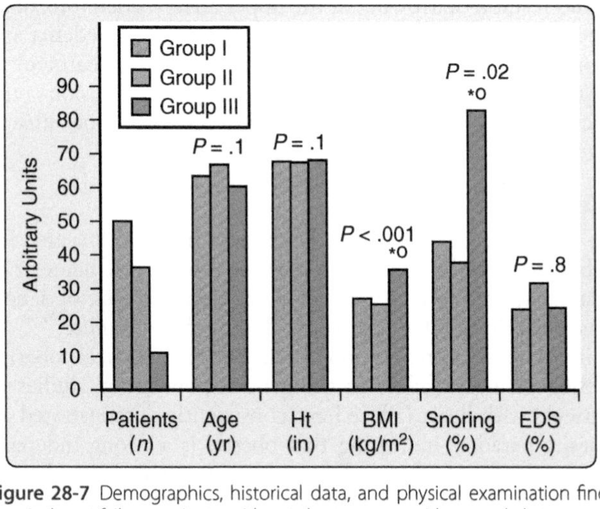

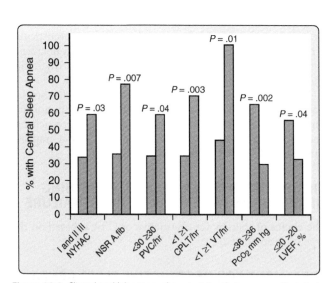

Figure 28-7 Demographics, historical data, and physical examination findings in heart failure patients without sleep apnea, with central sleep apnea (CSA), and with obstructive sleep apnea (OSA). Patients with OSA were more obese and had a higher prevalence of habitual snoring than patients with CSA. There was no difference in prevalence of excessive daytime sleepiness between the patients with heart failure and the patients without sleep apnea. BMI, Body mass index; EDS, excessive daytime sleepiness; Ht, height. (From Kryger MH. *Atlas of clinical sleep medicine*. Philadelphia: Elsevier; 2010; modified from Javaheri S. Sleep disorders in systolic heart failure: a prospective study of 100 male patients—the final report. *Int J Cardiol* 2006;106:21–8.)

Figure 28-8 Clinical and laboratory characteristics that are more likely to be associated with central sleep apnea. A. fib, Atrial fibrillation; CPLT, couplets; LVEF, left ventricular ejection fraction; NSR, normal sinus rhythm; NYHAC, New York Heart Association Class; PVC, premature ventricular contractions; VT, ventricular tachycardia. (From Javaheri S. Sleep disorders in systolic heart failure: a prospective study of 100 male patients—the final report. *Int J Cardiol* 2006;106:21–8.)

witnessed apnea, waking up unrested, and excessive daytime sleepiness, when present, should increase the level of suspicion for the presence of OSA. The following are symptoms that should alert the clinician to the possibility of apnea in heart failure patients:

Nocturnal angina—substernal chest pain that awakens the patient—should increase suspicion for sleep apnea in the general population and for patients with coronary heart disease and heart failure.

Paroxysmal nocturnal dyspnea characteristically awakens the patient with shortness of breath, which is relieved with resumption of an erect position. However, this symptom may be a perception of shortness of breath occurring during the hyperpneic phase of periodic breathing, suggesting presence of sleep apnea.

Restless sleep, maintenance insomnia, and *leg movements* may reflect periodic arousals and movements after apneas and hypopneas. Periodic limb movement, however, is also found in patients with systolic heart failure.[16,92,93]

Patients with heart failure and progressive ventricular systolic or diastolic dysfunction or patients who remain in New York Heart Association classes III or IV, despite intensive medical therapy, should have a diagnostic sleep study.

The prevalence of sleep apnea is high in patients with an implanted cardioverter or defibrillator,[20] and those awaiting cardiac transplantation.[17] The waiting period for transplantation is long, and a large number of patients succumb to the consequences of heart failure while waiting. It is conceivable that survival of these pretransplant patients may improve if their sleep apnea is diagnosed and appropriately treated. If so, the chance of receiving cardiac transplantation may increase.

As noted earlier, several studies[52-54] have shown that heart failure patients with low arterial Pco_2 have a high prevalence of CSA. The predictive value of low Pco_2 (<35 mm Hg) is about 80%.[54] However, many patients with heart failure have CSA apnea without daytime hypocapnia.[54,55]

Several studies have shown that heart failure patients with sleep apnea have a higher prevalence of atrioventricular arrhythmias, especially atrial fibrillation[9,12,16,94] and nocturnal ventricular arrhythmias.[9,16,95] Presence of these arrhythmias should increase suspicion for the presence of CSA.

In the presence of the aforementioned risk factors for obstructive and CSA, polysomnography should be performed for diagnosis and response to therapy. Such an approach has been shown to decrease hospital readmission and improve survival, as discussed previously.

TREATMENT OF SLEEP-RELATED BREATHING DISORDERS IN PATIENTS WITH HEART FAILURE

The choice of therapy for obstructive or CSA is based on the type of sleep apnea.[96]

TREATMENT FOR OBSTRUCTIVE SLEEP APNEA

In general, treatment of OSA–hypopnea is similar in patients with and without heart failure, although there are some differences (Box 28-1). In the presence of cardiovascular disease, every attempt should be made to treat OSA with positive airway pressure devices.

Box 28-1 TREATMENT OF OBSTRUCTIVE SLEEP APNEA IN PATIENTS WITH HEART FAILURE OPTIMIZATION OF CARDIOPULMONARY FUNCTION

- To eliminate or improve periodic breathing
- To decrease right atrial and central venous pressure upper airway congestion/edema, which may increase upper airway size
- To improve functional residual capacity, which may increase upper airway size as lung volume increases
- Avoidance of benzodiazepines, opioids, alcoholic beverages, sildenafil, tadalafil, and vardenafil
- Weight loss if applicable
- Nasal positive airway pressure devices (see Chapter 18):
  - Continuous positive airway pressure (CPAP)
  - Bilevel positive airway pressure
- Oral appliances (see Chapter 19):
  - Supplemental nocturnal nasal oxygen to minimize desaturation and to decrease periodic breathing
- Upper airway procedures (see Chapter 21):
  - Uvulopalatopharyngoplasty
  - Laser surgery
  - Radiofrequency volume reduction

Optimization of Cardiopulmonary Function

Optimal treatment of heart failure by improving both periodic breathing and lower extremity edema may decrease the likelihood of developing upper airway occlusion. Upper airway narrowing and occlusion may occur at the nadir of the ventilatory cycle of periodic breathing,[56] and, in some patients with heart failure, the first few breaths after central apneas are obstructed.[7] Furthermore, in biventricular heart failure, elevated right atrial and central venous pressure may result in pharyngeal congestion and edema, which along the fluid from lower extremities translocated cephalad in supine position could result in narrowing of the upper airway. Therefore, therapeutic measures to decrease the lower extremity edema and venous pressure[57,58] are advisable. Also, optimal treatment of heart failure to decrease lung water and pleural effusion could increase lung volumes, which should increase upper airway size, which is dependent on lung volume.

Weight Loss

In the general population, obesity is a major risk factor for OSA, and weight reduction improves OSA (see Chapter 22). Similarly, obesity is associated with increased risk of a new onset cardiovascular disease, including heart failure.[97,98] In spite of these aforementioned relationships between obesity, OSA, and heart failure in the general population, studies of patients with heart failure have consistently demonstrated an obesity paradox, indicating that obesity is a strong independent predictor of improved outcomes for patients with chronic heart failure. However, many patients with heart failure and OSA are obese,[9,12,16] and OSA per se has been shown to be a risk factor for the development of heart failure.[99] For this reason, we generally advise weight loss for obese patients with OSA, irrespective of heart failure. However, studies are needed to determine optimal body weight and whether purposeful weight loss in congestive heart failure comorbid with OSA improves cardiac function.

Avoidance of Alcoholic Beverages, Benzodiazepines, and Phosphodiesterase-5 Inhibitors at Bedtime, and Smoking

The use of alcoholic beverages and benzodiazepines may increase the likelihood of upper airway occlusion by promoting the relaxation of the muscles of the upper airway. We also advise patients that phosphodiesterase inhibitors used to treat erectile dysfunction (e.g., sildenafil [Viagra], vardenafil [Levitra], and tadalafil [Cialis]) may worsen OSA. In a randomized double-blind placebo-controlled study,[100] it was shown that 50 mg of sildenafil significantly increased the obstructive AHI and desaturation in a group of patients with OSA.

Smoking, via mechanisms mediated by nicotine, the active chemical in tobacco, increases efferent sympathetic activity (at least, in part, due to stimulating peripheral chemoreceptors in the carotid bodies, which contain excitatory nicotinic receptors) and plasma catecholamine resulting in increases in blood pressure, heart rate, and myocardial oxygen consumption.[101] In addition, nicotine decreases oxygen availability and causes coronary vasospasm, all promoting ventricular tachyarrhythmia. In a recent study[101] of 87 patients with HFrEF, smoking was associated with nocturnal ventricular tachycardia with an odds ratio of about 10. This is not surprising because excessive adrenergic overactivity is the underlying mechanism of arrhythmias and heart failure, in particular, when comorbid with sleep apnea is already a hyperadrenergic state.

Positive Airway Pressure Devices

Positive airway pressure devices are the treatment of choice and have been most successfully used to treat OSA in the general population and in patients with heart failure. First-night application of nasal CPAP results in a significant decrease in disordered breathing, arterial oxyhemoglobin desaturation, and arousals.[102] Short-term use of CPAP in patients with heart failure and OSA improves LVEF, blood pressure, and ventricular systolic volume,[61-63] but adherence to CPAP is a critical factor. For CPAP-noncompliant subjects who complain of a high expiratory pressure, bilevel pressure devices should be tried. As noted earlier, two recent observational studies[68,69] of patients with heart failure have shown that effective treatment of OSA with CPAP improves survival, particularly in those who are compliant with CPAP (see Figures 28-4 and 28-5).[68]

Supplemental Nasal Oxygen

For subjects with heart failure who cannot tolerate positive air pressure devices, oxygen is an alternative for treating OSA. The rationale for use of nocturnal supplemental nasal oxygen is to improve both hypoxemia and periodic breathing. Minimizing desaturation and hypoxemia–reoxygenation may have important therapeutic implications. Furthermore, as noted earlier, improvement in periodic breathing may decrease in obstructive disordered-breathing events that occur at the nadir of ventilation. We emphasize, however, that there are no systematic studies treating OSA of patients with heart failure with oxygen.

Upper Airway Surgical Procedures

Upper airway surgical procedures are performed for treatment of OSA in the general population, but there are no data in patients with heart failure.

Oral Appliances

Oral appliances are used to treat OSA, particularly in patients who cannot tolerate CPAP (see Chapter 19). Limited data are available in heart failure.[103] We speculate that efficacy of these devices in heart failure patients with OSA is similar to that in the general population. After application, a sleep study is recommended to ensure effectiveness.

TREATMENT FOR CENTRAL SLEEP APNEA

Figure 28-9 shows our approach to treatment of patients with CSA in heart failure.

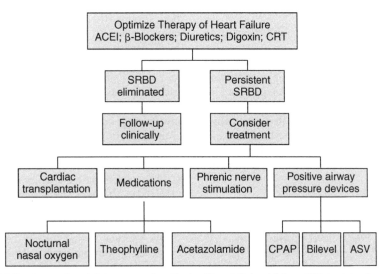

Figure 28-9 Treatment of central sleep apnea in patients with systolic heart failure. *ACEI,* Angiotensin-converting enzyme inhibitor; *APSSV,* adaptive pressure support servo-ventilation; *CRT,* cardiac resynchronization therapy; *nCPAP,* nasal continuous positive airway pressure; *PAP,* positive airway pressure; *SRBD,* sleep-related breathing disorder. (Modified from Javaheri S. Sleep-related breathing disorders in heart failure. In: Mann DL, editor. *Heart failure: a companion to Braunwald's heart disease.* Philadelphia: Saunders; 2004. p. 482.)

Optimization of Cardiopulmonary Function

Intensive therapy for heart failure with diuretics, angiotensin-converting enzyme inhibitors, beta blockers, and cardiac resynchronization therapy (CRT) can improve periodic breathing.[5] Because pulmonary congestion and edema are associated with narrowing of Pco_2 reserve,[51] reduction in wedge pressure should be associated with widening of Pco_2 reserve and improvement in CSA. Furthermore, with therapy, arterial circulation time decreases (as stroke volume increases and cardiopulmonary blood volume decreases), and functional residual capacity may increase (because of a decrease in cardiac size, pleural effusion, and intravascular and extravascular lung water). These changes contribute to the stabilization of breathing.

Beta blockers, by increasing stroke volume and decreasing pulmonary capillary pressure, should be particularly helpful in improving periodic breathing in systolic heart failure. An additional beneficial effect of beta blockers may relate to their counterbalancing of nocturnal cardiac sympathetic hyperactivity, resulting from repetitive arousals and desaturation. The reduction in cardiac sympathetic activity may have contributed to improved survival in trials of beta blockers in patients with heart failure. One particular side effect of beta blockers, however, is related to their effect on melatonin. Melatonin, a sleep-promoting chemical, is secreted via the cyclic adenosine monophosphate–mediated beta-adrenergic signal transduction system. Some beta blockers (exceptions include carvedilol), by inhibiting this process, decrease melatonin secretion[104,105] and could potentially contribute to worsening of sleep.

Regarding improvement in cardiac function and CSA, a few studies of CRT[106-110] showed some improvement in CSA, particularly noticeable in those with CRT-induced hemodynamic improvement. However, CRT devices are ineffective for OSA; although, in one study,[106] OSA improved, and improvement correlated with a decrease in circulation time.

If periodic breathing persists after cardiopulmonary function is optimized, several approaches are possible (see Figure 28-9).

Cardiac Transplantation

Preliminary studies, reviewed by Javaheri,[5] and a study of 45 patients with heart failure[111] have shown that, after cardiac transplantation, CSA is virtually eliminated. However, with time, a large number of cardiac transplant recipients develop OSA.[92] In this study, 36% had an AHI of 15 per hour or greater.[111] OSA developed in those who had gained the most weight after transplantation, and it was associated with habitual snoring, poor quality of life, and systemic hypertension. Cardiac transplantation was also associated with a high prevalence of restless legs syndrome and periodic limb movements (Figure 28-10).[111]

Positive Airway Pressure Devices

Continuous Positive Airway Pressure

Several devices, including CPAP, bilevel pressure, and ASV, have been used to treat CSA in patients with heart failure.

In contrast to treatment of OSA, where application of nasal CPAP invariably results in virtual elimination of obstructive disordered-breathing events, treatment of CSA in patients with heart failure is difficult, and response to therapy is not uniform.[112] In our study,[102] first-night CPAP titration was

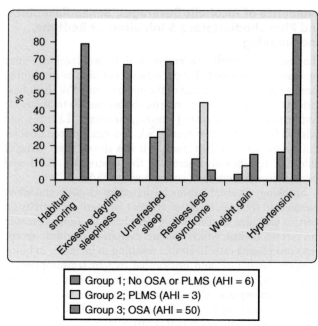

Figure 28-10 Phenotype of patients after heart transplantation. Group 1 did not have obstructive sleep apnea (OSA) or periodic limb movements during sleep (PLMS), Group 2 had PLMS, and Group 3 had OSA. AHI, Apnea–hypopnea index. Weight gain is in kilograms since the transplantation. (Modified from Javaheri S, Abraham W, Brown C, et al. Prevalence of obstructive sleep apnea and periodic limb movement in 45 subjects with heart transplantation. *Eur Heart J* 2004;25:260–6.)

effective in improving CSA in 43% of the patients (57% were considered CPAP nonresponsive). In the multicenter Canadian trial,[113] 47% of the patients were considered CPAP nonresponsive at 3 months. In this trial,[113] 132 patients were randomized to the control group and 128 to the CPAP arm. The baseline features were similar in the two randomized groups. The patients in the therapeutic arm were adapted to CPAP over 1 to 3 nights (without formal titration), and the maximum pressure was set at 10 cm H_2O or lower at whatever was tolerated.

A second polysomnography was performed at 3 months in both groups. There was no significant change in AHI in the control group. In the CPAP arm, the average AHI decreased by 50%, with considerable improvement in desaturation. Furthermore, the average plasma norepinephrine level decreased, and LVEF increased (all statistically significant). These measurements remained unchanged in the control group. However, after an interim analysis was performed, the safety-monitoring committee recommended termination of the study. This, in part, was related to worsened transplantation-free survival (primarily due to increased number of deaths from progressive heart failure and sudden death) of the CPAP-treated patients compared with the control group ($P = .02$). Although the survival curves diverged after about 3 years (favoring the CPAP arm), the difference was not statistically significant ($P = .06$).

We speculated that CPAP therapy could have resulted in excess early mortality for several reasons, including the following[114]: (1) Those who died were heart failure patients with CSA, whose periodic breathing was CPAP nonresponsive; and (2) those who died were heart failure patients whose ventricular function (according to the Frank-Starling curve) was preload dependent.

If right and LV function is preload-dependent, any reduction in venous return by the increased intrathoracic pressure, with application of CPAP, could decrease right ventricular stroke volume and return to the left ventricle, decreasing LV stroke volume and causing hypotension, diminished coronary blood flow, myocardial ischemia, and arrhythmias. Any such effect of CPAP on blood pressure is further augmented during sleep when blood pressure normally decreases.

The aforementioned assumptions that, in the Canadian trial, excess cardiovascular death due to CPAP occurred primarily in CPAP nonresponders were confirmed by a post-hoc analysis of mortality of patients with CSA (Figure 28-11).[80] In those whose CSA responded to CPAP, transplantation-free survival was significantly improved when compared with the untreated control group. In addition, the mortality of CPAP nonresponders appeared to be the worst, although the number of patients was small for statistical significance.

In the Canadian trial[113] at 3 months, 43% of heart failure patients with CSA were CPAP nonresponsive, compared with 57% in our study[102] of first-night use. Typically, CPAP-responsive patients had less severe CSA than CPAP-nonresponsive patients. In our study,[102] in CPAP-responsive patients, the average AHI decreased from 36 to 40 per hour, with elimination of desaturation. An important observation was that the number of premature ventricular contractions, couplets, and ventricular tachycardia decreased. This effect was presumed to result from decreased sympathetic activity, because arousals decreased and saturation improved. Heart failure patients with severe CSA (57% of the patients) did not respond to CPAP, and use of CPAP had no significant effect on ventricular irritability.

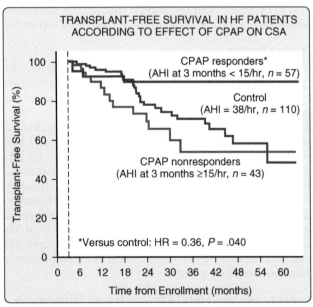

Figure 28-11 Probability of survival in patients with systolic heart failure (HF) comparing continuous positive airway pressure (CPAP) responders to a control group (patients with systolic heart failure and similar apnea–hypopnea index [AHI]) and to CPAP nonresponders. CPAP responders had a significantly increased probability of survival compared with the control group. CPAP nonresponders tended to have a poor survival when compared with the control group, although this was not significant. CSA, Central sleep apnea; HR, hazard ratio. (From Kryger MH. *Atlas of clinical sleep medicine.* Philadelphia: Elsevier; 2010; modified from Artz M, Floras JS, Logan AG, et al. Suppression of central sleep apnea by continuous positive airway pressure and transplant-free survival in heart failure. *Circulation* 2007;115:3173–80.)

The mechanisms of improvement in CSA in CPAP-responsive patients are multifactorial. One may relate to improvement in pulmonary congestion, which should widen Pco_2 reserve.[51] CPAP may improve stroke volume by decreasing LV afterload, which decreases arterial circulation time. CPAP should increase functional residual capacity, which decreases underdamping, and CPAP opens the upper airway, which is a benefit for those patients with CSA in whom upper airway closure occurs.

Adaptive Servoventilation

However, as noted earlier, 43% to 57% of heart failure patients with CSA are nonresponsive to CPAP. For these patients, and those who are intolerant to CPAP, until recently ASV devices were recommended (see end of this section).[72] These devices provide varying amounts of anticyclic inspiratory pressure support during different phases of periodic breathing, augmenting ventilation when the patient's minute ventilation decreases below a target and withdrawing support when the patient's ventilation is above the target.[112] In this way, periodic breathing is eliminated while on the device. In addition, the device initiates a breath on a timely basis, preventing development of a central apnea. Finally, the new generation of these devices is equipped with automatic end expiratory positive pressure algorithms[71,112,115] that operate to eliminate obstructive disordered breathing events. Having this virtue, these devices were expected to be advantageous for treatment of complex sleep-related breathing disorders when both CSA and OSA and hypopneas are present. Specifically in patients with heart failure, such complex breathing events are frequently observed during polysomnography. In addition, the phenotype of sleep apnea may vary during progression of heart failure and during acute decompensation when excess fluid from the lower extremities translocate to the neck area in supine position. Under such circumstances, upper airway obstruction could occur,[57,58] and a fixed end expiratory positive airway pressure with either a CPAP or bilevel device is inadequate to eliminate obstructive events.

ASV devices have been used to treat CSA in patients with congestive heart failure, generally with favorable results. In an acute (1-night) study[116] in 14 subjects with HFrEF and CSA, the ASV device decreased the AHI more than oxygen, CPAP, and bilevel devices. Indeed, in a meta-analysis of patients with congestive heart failure, in whom ASV therapy was compared to a control arm (the control arm could be medical therapy, oxygen, CPAP or bilevel), we concluded that ASV was much more effective in reducing AHI.[117] Specifically, in crossover studies, the mean AHI decreased from about 50/hour to 6/hour, compared to 20/hour. Multiple long-term studies with ASV have been reported, and these have been reviewed recently.[112,117] In general, most (but not all) of these studies show significant improvement in biomarkers of heart failure, LVEF, and reduction in primary end points, commonly a combination of mortality and readmission to the hospital, as noted previously.[83,88-91,118]

In a prospective parallel design, randomized controlled trial[119] from Norway, 51 patients with congestive heart failure and CSA, ages 57 to 81 years, were randomized to either an ASV or a control group; 30 patients completed the study (15 from each group). Three months treatment with ASV significantly improved LVEF from 32% to 36%, 6-minute walk, and a New York Heart Association classification. These variables did not change significantly in the control group. These results were somewhat different from a similarly designed German study,[120] in which significant but equal increments in LVEF occurred after 3 months, both in the ASV arm and the control group. However, consistent with the results of the previous study,[119] reduction in N-terminal pro-brain natriuretic peptide was significantly greater in the ASV arm. However, in our meta-analysis[119] discussed previously, ASV therapy significantly improved LVEF when compared to the control. Furthermore, in a recent well-designed trial,[120] in which 23 patients with persistent CSA (in spite of using CPAP for 3 months) were randomized to either continued CPAP (n = 11) or ASV (n = 12), LVEF increased significantly (32% to 38%) in the ASV group. Furthermore, reductions in plasma B-type natriuretic peptide and urinary norepinephrine and an increase in 6-minute walk distance and quality of life as measured by short form 36 were significantly greater with ASV than CPAP.

Meanwhile, as noted previously, with automatic variable end expiratory positive pressure algorithms, ASV devices are effective in treating both CSA and OSA. In the three trials[122-124] that compared CPAP versus ASV in patients with heart failure and coexistent OSA and CSA, ASV was significantly more effective in improving LVEF than CPAP. Because both obstructive and central sleep disorders commonly occur together, and the phenotype may change with time (e.g., obstructive events becoming prominent during acute decompensation of the heart failure), ASV devices with automatic end expiratory positive pressure rhythm can be quite effective under such circumstances.

A large multi site international clinical trial (SERVE-HF)[124a] that evaluated the effect of treating central sleep apnea with an ASV device in patients with heart failure and reduced ejection fraction (HFrEF) has raised serious concerns about the safety of ASV in these patients. Not only was ASV ineffective, but also post-hoc analysis found excess cardiovascular mortality in treated patients. The cause of the excess mortality is unknown; the authors hypothesized that CSA might be a compensatory mechanism with a protective effect in HFrEF.

However, there are several other (perhaps more) plausible explanations for the excess cardiovascular mortality in the trial. These include methodological issues, the use of the old generation ASV device, which is no longer manufactured by the sponsor of the trial, residual sleep-disordered breathing with significant oxygen desaturation, patient selection, data collection, and treatment adherence as well as group crossovers as potential confounding factors (Javaheri et al, unpublished). Below, only the device-related issues are briefly reviewed.

The data from the trial[124a] show that the device was ineffective in a number of patients (note the large range of AHI values downloaded from the ASV devices across the months of follow-up in Table S4 in the supplementary appendix of reference 124a). There could be multiple reasons for these residual events. Two important issues regarding the algorithm of the first generation ASV device used in SERVE-HF could have been contributory: First, it allows for only fixed expiratory positive airway pressure (EPAP), and second, there are flaws in the inspiratory pressure support algorithm that were addressed and improved considerably in the latest generation models.[122] Regarding fixed EPAP, it is known that the

phenotype of sleep-disordered breathing may change over time from predominantly central to predominantly obstructive events, and data from Table 2 in the study[124a] are confirmatory. In that case, in the face of obstructive apneas and the fixed expiratory pressure of the device, the ASV device used was equipped with only one strategy for suppressing these events: progressively increasing inspiratory pressure support in an attempt to open the closed airway. Once the airway opened, the prevailing high pressures may have resulted in an excessive rise in intrathoracic pressure with consequent adverse hemodynamic effects. In addition, excess ventilation due to excessive inspiratory pressure support could result in hyperventilation and alkalemia which is arrythmogenic, and at the same time the baseline Pco_2 could be lowered excessively promoting recurrence of apneas. The current generation of ASV devices can be set to increase EPAP automatically in response to obstructive apneas and would not have been subject to this failure.

Independent of the reasons why the trial failed, manufacturers of ASV devices have declared that ASV devices are contraindicated for heart failure patients with central sleep apnea when LVEF is 45% or less. Because we no longer use ASV, our current approach to such patients is to first make sure that heart failure is maximally treated, both pharmacologically and device-wise, when indicated. Then gentle CPAP titration is performed with maximum pressure not to exceed 10 to 12 cm H_2O. If the AHI decreases below 15/hour of sleep, long term CPAP therapy is recommended. Otherwise nocturnal O_2 titration is recommended with the least amount of supplemental O_2 needed to eliminate hypoxia and maintain arterial oxyhemoglobin saturation above 92%, avoiding hyperoxia.

Meanwhile we are anxiously waiting for the results of the ADVENT trial[124b] and the remede trial.[124c] The latter uses a transvenous phrenic nerve pacemaker (see also Chapter 15).

Cardiac Pacing

In 15 subjects with predominantly mild to moderate CSA, some of whom had mild LV systolic dysfunction, atrial overdrive pacing improved periodic breathing.[125] These subjects had permanent atrial-synchronized ventricular pacemakers placed for symptomatic sinus bradycardia. Atrial overdrive (an average of 72 beats per minute versus spontaneous 57 beats per minute) moderately (but significantly) decreased the AHI from 28 to 11, improved arterial oxyhemoglobin desaturation, and decreased arousals. The mechanism remains unclear, but it could have been the improved cardiac output. However, if cardiac pacing improves CSA, biventricular pacing[126] should be more effective than atrial pacing overdrive,[106-110] as discussed earlier. In one study,[108] CRT decreased central AHI from 31/hour to 17/hour. There was no effect on obstructive disordered breathing events.

Transvenous Unilateral Phrenic Nerve Stimulation

Most recently, transvenous unilateral phrenic nerve stimulation has been used to stimulate phrenic nerve and treat CSA. In this acute study,[127] 16 patients underwent two successive nights of polysomnography—one night with and one night without phrenic nerve stimulation from either the right brachiocephalic vein or the left pericardiophrenic vein. Stimulation resulted in significant improvement in the AHI Central Apnea Index, arousal index, and oxygen desaturation index 4%. No significant changes occurred in the Obstructive Apnea

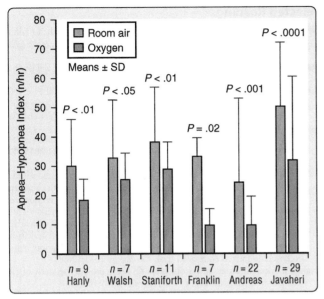

Figure 28-12 Effects of supplemental nasal oxygen on apnea–hypopnea index in patients with systolic heart failure.

Index or AHI. This approach may represent a novel therapy for CSA and warrants further study. Currently, a randomized clinical trial is in progress.

Medications

Nasal Nocturnal Oxygen. Systematic studies in patients with systolic heart failure[128-133] have shown that nocturnal therapy with supplemental nasal oxygen improves CSA (Figure 28-12). Oxygen therapy may also decrease arousals and improve the hypnogram by shifting sleep structure to deep sleep stages. In addition, randomized placebo-controlled double-blind studies have shown that short-term (1 to 4 weeks) administration of nocturnal supplemental nasal oxygen improves maximal exercise capacity[130] and decreases overnight urinary norepinephrine excretion.[131]

Three randomized clinical trials of nocturnal nasal oxygen therapy[133-136] for 9-, 12-, and 52-week periods, reported that, when compared with the control group, oxygen therapy improved CSA and desaturation and significantly increased LVEF and quality of life of patients with heart failure. In the oxygen-treated group, LVEF increased 5% (versus 1% in the control group) in the 12-week study,[136] and 5.5% (versus 1.3% in the control group) in the 52-week study.[135]

Supplemental administration of nasal oxygen may decrease periodic breathing by several mechanisms.[134] These include an increase in the difference between the prevailing Pco_2 and the Pco_2 at the apneic threshold; a reduction in the ventilatory response to CO_2 and perhaps to hypoxemia; and an increase in body stores (e.g., lung contents) of oxygen, which increases damping. Prospective placebo-controlled long-term studies, however, are necessary to determine whether nocturnal oxygen therapy has the potential to decrease mortality of patients with systolic heart failure.

Theophylline. Open[7,137] and blind studies[138] have shown the efficacy of theophylline in the treatment of CSA in heart failure. In a double-blind randomized placebo-controlled crossover study of 15 patients with treated, stable systolic heart failure, oral theophylline at therapeutic plasma concentration (11 μg/mL, range 7 to 15 μg/mL) decreased the AHI by about 50% and improved arterial oxyhemoglobin saturation.[137]

Mechanisms of action of theophylline in improving central apnea remain unclear.[123] At therapeutic serum concentrations, theophylline competes with adenosine at some of its receptor sites. In the central nervous system, adenosine is a respiratory depressant, and theophylline stimulates respiration by competing with adenosine. Conceivably, therefore, an increase in ventilation by theophylline decreasing the plant gain could decrease central apnea during sleep. Theophylline does not increase ventilatory response to CO_2.

Potential arrhythmogenic effects and phosphodiesterase inhibition are common concerns with long-term use of theophylline in patients with heart failure. Therefore, further controlled studies are necessary to ensure its safety. If theophylline is used to treat CSA, frequent and careful follow-ups are necessary.

Acetazolamide. In a double-blind placebo-controlled crossover study[139] of 12 patients with heart failure, acetazolamide, administered at about 3 mg/kg one-half hour before bedtime, decreased the central AHI significantly from about 57/hour (in the placebo arm) to 34/hour. Acetazolamide improved arterial oxyhemoglobin desaturation significantly. Furthermore, patients reported improved subjective perceptions of the following: overall sleep quality, feeling rested on awakening, falling asleep unintentionally during daytime, and fatigue. Acetazolamide, therefore, could have other advantageous effects when used in patients with heart failure and CSA, including acting as a mild diuretic and also normalizing the alkalemia (caused by loop diuretics) commonly present in patients with heart failure. In our patients, arterial blood pH decreased from 7.43 to 7.37.[139]

Acetazolamide improves CSA by decreasing the plant gain as shown in naturally sleeping canine experiments[140] and patients with heart failure with CSA.[141]

Benzodiazepines. Benzodiazepines, by decreasing arousals, may decrease CSA. However, a placebo-controlled double-blind study[142] showed a reduction in arousals but failed to show any improvement in CSA in patients with systolic heart failure. Although benzodiazepines do not increase the number of central apneas, their use may increase the likelihood of developing obstructive apneas in some heart failure patients.

Inhaled CO_2 and Addition of External Dead Space. Several studies have shown that low-level inhalation of CO_2 and addition of external dead space (by increasing Pco_2) improve CSA.[145-147] However, studies[146,147] show that CO_2 inhalation increases spontaneous arousals, which are associated with increased sympathetic and decreased parasympathetic activity. One study[145] also showed that addition of dead space was associated with increased arousals. Knowing the adverse cardiovascular effects of increased sympathetic overactivity in heart failure, use of CO_2 and external dead space to treat CSA in heart failure should be avoided. However, dynamic CO_2 inhalation,[148-150] when it can be inhaled intermittently within a part of breathing cycle, could eventually prove useful.

CLINICAL PEARLS

- Because of the increased average life span and improved therapy of ischemic coronary artery disease and hypertension, the prevalence of heart failure remains high.
- Periodic breathing is common in heart failure and is characterized by apnea, hypopnea, and hyperpnea, which cause sleep disruption, arousals, hypoxemia/reoxygenation, hypercapnia/hypocapnia, and changes in intrathoracic pressure. Periodic breathing includes both obstructive and central sleep-related breathing disorders. All of these adversely affect sleep and cardiovascular function.
- Periodic breathing may contribute to the remodeling of LV dysfunction and to the progressively declining course of heart failure.
- Several studies have demonstrated that both CSA and OSA are associated with increased mortality of patients with heart failure and systolic dysfunction.
- There are only a few long-term studies on treatment of sleep apnea in systolic heart failure. These show that effective treatment of both CSA and OSA with CPAP improves mortality of patients with heart failure.
- At this time ASV is not recommended in CHF when LVEF is less than 45%.

SUMMARY

Heart failure is a common disorder that has a significant economic impact and is associated with excess morbidity and mortality. Because of increased average life spans and improved therapy for hypertension and ischemic coronary artery disease, the incidence and prevalence of heart failure remain high.

One factor that may contribute to the progressively declining course of heart failure, hospital readmission, quality of life, and premature mortality is the occurrence of periodic breathing, with repetitive episodes of apnea, hypopnea, and hyperpnea. Episodes of apnea, hypopnea, and the following hyperpnea collectively cause hypoxemia and reoxygenation, hypercapnia and hypocapnia, changes in intrathoracic pressure, and sleep disruption and arousals. These pathophysiological consequences of sleep-related breathing disorders have deleterious effects on the cardiovascular system, and they may be most pronounced in the setting of established heart failure and coronary artery disease.

Multiple studies have demonstrated increased readmission and premature mortality independently associated with obstructive and CSA comorbid with heart failure. In addition, multiple studies have also demonstrated that effective treatment of both obstructive and CSA decreases hospital readmission and improves survival, particularly in those patients who are most adherent to therapy.

ASV devices with automatic inspiratory pressure support and automatic end expiratory positive pressure algorithms, along with a backup rate, are quite effective in the treatment of hybrid sleep-related breathing disorders consisting of both central and OSA but are not recommended when LVEF is less than 45%. The best approach for patients with low LVEF is not clear, and future research will be needed to guide the management of these patients.[151]

Selected Readings

Bitter T, Faber L, Hering D, et al. Sleep-disordered breathing in heart failure with normal left ventricular ejection fraction. *Eur J Heart Fail* 2009;**11**:602–8.

Bradley TD, Flores JS. ADVENT-HF investigators. The SERVE-HF trial. *Can Respir J* 2015;**22**(6):313.

Costanzo MR, Augostini R, Goldberg LR, et al. Design of the remedē System Pivotal Trial: a prospective, randomized study in the use of respiratory rhythm management to treat central sleep apnea. *J Card Fail* 2015;**21**(11):892–902.

Cowie MR, Woehrle H, Wegscheider K, et al. Adaptive servo-ventilation for central sleep apnea in systolic heart failure. *N Engl J Med* 2015;**373**:1095–105.

Galetke W, Ghassemi BM, Priegnitz C, et al. Anticyclic modulated ventilation versus continuous positive airway pressure in patients with coexisting obstructive sleep apnea and Cheyne–Stokes respiration: a randomized crossover trial. *Sleep Med* 2014;**15**:874–9.

Hetland A, Haugaa KH, Olseng M, et al. Three-month treatment with adaptive servo-ventilation improves cardiac function and physical activity in patients with chronic heart failure and Cheyne-Stokes respiration: a prospective randomized controlled trial. *Cardiology* 2013;**126**:81–96.

Javaheri S. Sleep disorders in systolic heart failure: a prospective study of 100 male patients. The final report. *Int J Cardiol* 2006;**106**:21–8.

Javaheri S, Brown L, Randerath W. Positive airway pressure therapy with adaptive servo ventilation (part 1: operational algorithms). *Chest* 2014;**146**:514–23.

Javaheri S, Brown L, Randerath W. Positive airway pressure therapy with adaptive servo-ventilation (part II: clinical applications). *Chest* 2014;**146**:855–68.

Javaheri S, Caref B, Chen E, et al. Sleep apnea testing and outcomes in a large cohort of Medicare beneficiaries with newly diagnosed heart failure. *Am J Respir Crit Care Med* 2011;**183**:539–46.

Javaheri S, Dempsey JA. Central sleep apnea. *Compr Physiol* 2013;**3**:141–63.

Jilek C, Krenn M, Sebah D, et al. Prognostic impact of sleep disordered breathing and its treatment in heart failure: an observational study. *Eur J Heart Fail* 2011;**13**:68–75.

Kasai T, Kasagi S, Maeno K-I, et al. Adaptive servo-ventilation in cardiac function and neurohormonal status in patients with heart failure and central sleep apnea nonresponsive to continuous positive airway pressure. *JACC Heart Fail* 2013;**1**:58–63.

Kasai T, Narui K, Dohi T, et al. Prognosis of patients with heart failure and obstructive sleep apnea treated with continuous positive airway pressure. *Chest* 2008;**133**:690–6.

Koyama T, Watanabe H, Igarashi G, et al. Effect of short-duration adaptive servo-ventilation therapy on cardiac function in patients with heart failure. *Circ J* 2012;**76**:2606–13.

Koyama T, Watanabe H, Igarashi G, et al. Short-term prognosis of adaptive servo-ventilation therapy in patients with heart failure. *Circ J* 2011;**75**:710–12.

Oldenburg O, Lamp B, Faber L, et al. Sleep disordered breathing in patients with symptomatic heart failure: a contemporary study of prevalence in and characteristics of 700 patients. *Eur J Heart Fail* 2007;**9**:251–7.

Priou P, d'Ortho MP, Damy T, et al. Adaptive servo-ventilation: How does it fit into the treatment of central sleep apnoea syndrome? Expert opinions. *Rev Mal Respir* 2015 Nov 20. pii: S0761-8425(15)00364-2.

Suzuki S, Yoshihisa A, Miyata M, et al. Adaptive servo-ventilation therapy improves long-term prognosis in heart failure patients with anemia and sleep-disordered breathing. *Int Heart J* 2014;**55**:342–9.

Yoshihisa A, Suzuki S, Yamaki T, et al. Impact of adaptive servo-ventilation on cardiovascular function and prognosis in heart failure patients with preserved left ventricular ejection fraction and sleep-disordered breathing. *Eur J Heart Fail* 2013;**15**:543–50.

Yumino D, Redolfi S, Ruttanaumpawan P, et al. Nocturnal rostral fluid shift: a unifying concept for the pathogenesis of obstructive and central sleep apnea in men with heart failure. *Circulation* 2010;**121**:1598–605.

Zhang J, et al. Exploring quality of life in patients with and without heart failure. *Int J Cardiol* 2016;**202**:676–84.

A complete reference list can be found online at ExpertConsult.com.

Overlap Syndromes of Sleep and Breathing Disorders

Chapter

29

Jose M. Marin; Santiago J. Carrizo

Chapter Highlights

- Sleep depresses the central control of breathing and muscle tone. These changes have no health effects in healthy subjects. However, in patients with pulmonary diseases such as chronic obstructive pulmonary disease (COPD), asthma, and interstitial lung diseases, these changes may aggravate gas exchange abnormalities and induce significant hypoxemia and hypercapnia, especially during rapid eye movement sleep.

- As COPD, asthma, and obstructive sleep apnea (OSA) are prevalent disorders in adults, overlap of OSA and either COPD or asthma is frequent in clinical practice. Such overlap, termed *overlap syndrome*, carries an excessive risk for worsened sleep- and awake-related outcomes than any one of these conditions alone, including

increased risk of COPD exacerbations and mortality.

- Practitioners should identify the coexistence and severity of OSA in patients with COPD or asthma and the presence and severity of the overlap syndrome, and they should establish a personalized treatment in each case. A sleep study should be considered in any patient with COPD or asthma with signs and symptoms of OSA, such as snoring and excessive daytime sleepiness, or with inappropriate awake hypoxemia.

- Noninvasive ventilation (continuous positive airway pressure, bilevel positive airway pressure), with supplemental oxygen if necessary, should be prescribed after an appropriate titration process.

OVERVIEW

Sleep is associated with adaptive changes of the airways, lungs, and chest wall mechanics. In patients with chronic pulmonary diseases, such physiologic changes as well as the pathophysiologic changes of sleep breathing disorders, such as obstructive sleep apnea (OSA), may result in acute and chronic adverse effects, including precipitation or worsening of hypoxemia, hypercapnia, and bronchoconstriction, which in the long term

can contribute to worsened outcomes in these chronic pulmonary disorders. This chapter reviews the clinically imperative concepts of overlap syndromes, defined as the coexistence in the same patient of OSA and one or more of the following chronic respiratory conditions: chronic obstructive pulmonary disease (COPD), asthma, and pulmonary hypertension (PH). The clinical relevance of identifying the coexistence of a primary sleep disorder such as OSA in patients with these chronic respiratory disorders lies not only in the diagnosis of an overlap syndrome; it also involves a worse prognosis for these coexistent respiratory diseases and the need for specific treatment of the concomitant sleep-disordered breathing (SDB). Physicians who care for patients with such respiratory disorders should recognize these associations.

CHRONIC OBSTRUCTIVE PULMONARY DISEASE

According to the latest version of the Global Initiative for Chronic Obstructive Lung Disease (GOLD) strategy document,[1] COPD is defined as a preventable and treatable disease, characterized by persistent airflow limitation that is usually progressive and associated with an enhanced chronic inflammatory response in the airways and the lung to noxious particles or gases. A clinical diagnosis of COPD should be considered in any patient with dyspnea, chronic cough, or sputum production and a history of exposure to risk factors for the disease. Spirometry is required to make the diagnosis in this clinical context; a postbronchodilator forced expiratory volume in the first second of expiration to forced vital capacity (FEV_1/FVC) ratio of less than 0.7 confirms the presence of persistent airflow limitation and thus of COPD.

Sleep disturbance is common in COPD without other coexistent primary sleep disorders. In a large survey conducted in North America and Europe, 40% of patients reported problems with their sleep.[2] In a European survey, 78.1% of patients with COPD reported some degree of nighttime symptoms, including one or more of the following: dyspnea, cough with increased sputum production, wheezing, and difficulty with maintenance of sleep. The prevalence of such nighttime symptoms was positively correlated with the severity of spirometrically measured airflow obstruction.[3] Polysomnography (PSG) studies show that these patients have problems initiating or maintaining sleep, reduced rapid eye movement (REM) sleep, and frequent microarousals. This poor sleep quality increases in parallel with the frequency of nocturnal respiratory symptoms, like cough and wheezing,[4] and COPD severity.[5]

In COPD patients, sleep is associated with reduced rib cage contribution to breathing, diaphragmatic inefficiency, and increased accessory muscle contribution to breathing.[6] The result is a reduction in functional residual capacity, which may augment ventilation-perfusion mismatching and hypoxemia. More than 50% of COPD patients with daytime arterial oxygen saturation of hemoglobin (Sao_2) above 90% on breathing room air, and without concomitant OSA, experience significant oxygen desaturation during sleep, defined as spending at least 30% of the night with Sao_2 below 90%.[7] Daytime gas exchange abnormalities are, however, somewhat predictive of sleep oxygen desaturation among COPD patients.[8] Given the shape of the oxyhemoglobin dissociation curve, patients on the steep portion of the curve (e.g., Pao_2 <60 mm Hg on breathing room air during the daytime) would be expected to have a greater fall in Sao_2 during sleep, particularly during REM sleep. Accentuated physiologic hypoventilation in COPD is also the consequence of decreased central respiratory drive response to chemical and mechanical inputs,[9] increased upper airway resistance due to a loss of tone in the upper pharyngeal muscles,[10] and reduced efficiency of diaphragmatic contraction due to lung hyperinflation.[11] The consequences of nocturnal hypoxemia and hypercapnia are well known and include arrhythmias and PH. In addition, recent data suggest that disturbed sleep is an independent risk factor of COPD exacerbations and mortality.[12]

Chronic Obstructive Lung Disease and Obstructive Sleep Apnea Overlap Syndrome

Definitions and Classifications

The GOLD definition of COPD also underlines that "exacerbations and comorbidities contribute to the overall severity in individual patients."[1] OSA is recognized as one of these comorbidities. OSA is characterized by sleep-related pathologically increased upper airway resistance, repetitive decrease or absence of inspiratory and expiratory airflow, sympathetic activation, and intermittent oxyhemoglobin desaturation and hypercapnia.[13] The diagnosis of OSA requires a PSG study, with five or more apneas or hypopneas per hour of sleep (i.e., the apnea-hypopnea index [AHI]) consistent with OSA.[14] The consensus definitions of severity in OSA, mild (AHI ≥5 and <15 episodes/hour), moderate (AHI ≥15 and <30 episodes/hour), and severe (≥30 episodes/hour), are in part based on published literature that has found an association between such severity definitions of OSA and risk of excess mortality in this sleep-related breathing disorder.[15-19]

The coexistence of COPD and OSA was first described as the overlap syndrome by David Flenley 30 years ago.[20] He pointed out that PSG should be considered in COPD patients with obesity, snoring, or morning headache associated with nocturnal oxygen therapy to assess for the presence of associated OSA. He believed that the clinical course and prognosis of such "overlap patients" were worse than for patients suffering from COPD or untreated OSA alone. These opinions remain valid today. Nevertheless, at present, the term *overlap syndrome* is not a formal diagnostic designation for patients suffering from OSA and COPD. In the individual patient, it is better to describe the underlying lung disease and the associated abnormality of the sleep disorder. A classification of severity for this entity is not available, and health outcomes appear to depend on the severity of OSA and COPD independently.

Epidemiology of COPD/OSA Overlap Syndrome

In pulmonary clinics, OSA and COPD are two of the most prevalent chronic respiratory disorders. It is estimated that 10% of the general population has moderate to severe COPD as defined by an FEV_1/FVC ratio of less than 0.7 plus an FEV_1 of less than 80% predicted.[21] The prevalence of COPD increases with age and is directly related to the prevalence of tobacco smoking, but outdoor and indoor air pollution are also major COPD risk factors. The prevalence and burden of COPD are projected to increase in the coming decades because of continued exposure to COPD risk factors and the aging of the world's population.

Among men and women between the ages of 30 and 60 years, 20% and 9%, respectively, had an AHI of at least 5 events/hour in the Wisconsin Sleep Cohort Study.[22] Since this report was published 20 years ago, data from the same ongoing cohort provide prevalence estimates of moderate to severe SDB of the sleep apnea type (AHI ≥ 15 events/hour), thus showing a substantial increase during the last 2 decades.[23] The sex disparity of OSA ends at around the age of 55 years, with a sharp rise among postmenopausal women.[23-25]

There are, however, no studies that directly assess the prevalence of the OSA/COPD overlap syndrome. Because COPD and OSA are each increasing throughout the world in association with an aging population, presumably the overlap syndrome is becoming more prevalent. In clinical series, it has been noted that approximately 11% of patients with at least moderate OSA, as defined by an AHI of more than 20 events/hour, have airflow limitation on spirometry.[26] In a European population study of patients with predominantly mild COPD, the coincidence of OSA syndrome (AHI >5 events/hour accompanied by excessive daytime sleepiness) occurred in 1% of the total population.[27] The Sleep Heart Health Study, a community-based cohort study that included 5954 participants who had PSG and spirometry at baseline, found that 19% had airway obstruction (defined as FEV_1/FVC <0.7) that was predominantly mild. The prevalence of OSA, defined as a respiratory disturbance index of more than 10 events/hour, was not higher in subjects with airway obstruction (defined as FEV_1/FVC <0.7) compared with the nonobstructed population.[28] There were 254 participants (4.3%) who had both characteristics: obstructive airways disease and sleep apnea. As expected, respiratory disturbance index increased with higher body mass index (BMI) in participants with and without airway obstruction. Age effect was not specifically addressed in this study. In short, the few available population studies of the association between COPD and OSA (i.e., overlap syndrome) show great variability in the prevalence of this association. It does appear that the world's adult population is affected in a range between 1% and 4%. This range likely reflects, at least to some extent, differences in the criteria used to define OSA and the age and weight of the subjects studied.

Sleep in Patients with COPD/OSA Overlap Syndrome

In the Sleep Heart Health Study, patients with OSA/COPD overlap syndrome had a lower total sleep time, lower sleep efficiency, and higher daytime sleepiness as assessed by the Epworth Sleepiness Scale[29] than did patients with COPD alone. They were also more likely to have greater sleep-related oxygen desaturation compared with participants with OSA or airway obstruction alone.[28] Most important, patients with overlap syndrome, compared with patients with either COPD or OSA alone, display more profound oxygen desaturation during sleep as well as worse daytime hypoxemia and hypercapnia.[26]

Risk Factors for COPD/OSA Overlap Syndrome

Patients with COPD can incur specific OSA risks, including obesity irrespective of airflow obstruction severity,[30] active smoking,[31,32] and both pharyngeal and lower extremity edema associated with episodic use of oral corticosteroids and impaired cardiac output.[33] There is also evidence that patients with advanced COPD who lose weight may show reduced diathesis for upper airway obstruction.

Sleep and Breathing Pathophysiology of COPD/OSA Overlap Syndrome

Because obesity also reduces functional residual capacity during sleep, overweight and obese patients with COPD/OSA overlap syndrome are particularly subject to a reduction of alveolar volume and greater gas exchange abnormalities during sleep apneas and hypopneas (Figure 29-1). Further, respiratory control center output is reduced during sleep, especially during REM sleep,[34] including blunted ventilatory responses and mouth occlusion pressure responses to CO_2.[35] During obstructive apneic episodes, to overcome the upper airway resistance and to maintain adequate airflow to the lung, increased diaphragmatic and abdominal muscle effort is required. This can be particularly difficult in COPD patients who already have increased intrathoracic airway resistance and lung hyperinflation at baseline. When COPD patients develop such obstructive apnea episodes, the compensatory response of the respiratory center is slower, apneas are longer, and changes in Pao_2 and Pco_2 are more intense compared with non-COPD subjects. Patients with COPD/OSA overlap syndrome who have awake hypoxemia are especially prone to nocturnal oxygen desaturation by being on the steep portion of the oxyhemoglobin dissociation curve.

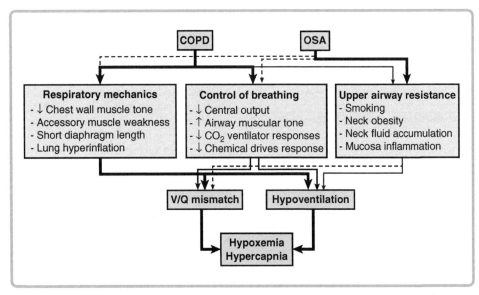

Figure 29-1 Pathways involved in producing sleep-related hypoxemia and hypercapnia in chronic obstructive pulmonary disease (COPD) and obstructive sleep apnea (OSA) overlap syndrome.

Clinical Features of COPD/OSA Overlap Syndrome

Compared with patients with COPD alone or OSA alone, overlap patients of similar ages tend to be more obese and to have more comorbid conditions.[36] They also report more daytime sleepiness[28] and poorer quality of life[37] than either COPD or OSA patients without overlap syndrome. Sleep recordings of patients with COPD/OSA overlap show a lower total sleep time, lower sleep efficiency, and greater sleep fragmentation than those with COPD or OSA alone. More severe nocturnal O_2 desaturation is also a characteristic feature in COPD/OSA overlap patients compared with either condition alone. Subjects with OSA alone return to a normal O_2 saturation (Sao_2) in sleep between obstructive events (i.e., intermittent hypoxemia), whereas in COPD alone, as a result of the diathesis to sleep-related hypoventilation and ventilation-perfusion mismatch as noted before, nocturnal O_2 saturation characteristically decreases more evenly throughout sleep and at the termination of an apnea or hypopnea episode tends not to return to the initial baseline level (Figure 29-2). A typical patient with COPD/OSA overlap syndrome has a reduced awake and asleep baseline Sao_2, a lower mean sleep-related Sao_2, and a longer time in hypoxemia than patients with OSA or COPD alone.

The majority of patients with OSA alone do not develop significant sleep-related hypercapnia because of interapnea hyperventilation. However, if the patient also has COPD, the abnormal mechanical and chemical ventilatory responses as noted before may result in postapnea CO_2 levels that do not return to baseline. Over time, a progressive desensitization of the respiratory center in response to OSA-related hypoxic-hypercapnic episodes develops, such that patients with COPD/OSA overlap syndrome can remain hypercapnic during sleep.[38] Of note, continuous positive airway pressure (CPAP) treatment for the OSA (see Diagnosis and Management of COPD/OSA Overlap Syndrome) can partially reverse this phenomenon.[39] Although daytime hypercapnia can develop in OSA without COPD, awake hypercapnia is much more frequent in the patient with overlap syndrome.[40] Both daytime hypoxemia and hypercapnia have been found to be predictors of right-sided heart failure in COPD

patients,[41] and therefore these should be considered potentially treatable markers of otherwise poorer prognosis in COPD/OSA overlap.

Excessive sleepiness in patients with OSA alone is associated with decrements in school and work performance.[42] Further, there is also a strong association between OSA severity, as measured by the AHI, and the risk of traffic accidents.[43] It is reasonable to expect that in patients with COPD/OSA overlap syndrome, such performance decrements and risks reflect the sum of the severity of the sleep disorders of both entities, but such consequences of the COPD/OSA overlap syndrome have not been evaluated specifically. Similarly, whereas OSA is considered an independent risk factor for insulin resistance, with OSA severity predicting risk for incident diabetes,[44] neither COPD alone nor COPD/OSA overlap has been specifically linked with risk of metabolic disorders.

Both OSA and COPD alone are associated with an increased risk of cardiovascular morbidity and mortality. For example, epidemiologic data show a strong association between OSA and incident arterial hypertension,[45] particularly refractory hypertension. In COPD alone, however, arterial hypertension prevalence is similar to that of the general population, and patients with COPD/OSA overlap appear to have the same prevalence rates as patients with OSA alone.[36] Untreated OSA patients are also particularly susceptible to development of atrial fibrillation,[46] as are patients with COPD alone, likely related to nocturnal O_2 desaturation.[47,48] A community-based retrospective cohort analysis, including data collected on 2873 patients older than 65 years, confirmed an increased risk of new-onset atrial fibrillation in COPD/OSA overlap syndrome compared with OSA or COPD alone.[49]

Epidemiologic data indicate that incidence of coronary artery disease, stroke, and heart failure is increased in OSA[15,16,50] and COPD[51]; no such incidence data are available for COPD/OSA overlap. However, Chaouat et al[26] demonstrated that patients with COPD/OSA overlap syndrome have increased daytime pulmonary vascular resistance compared with patients with OSA alone, whereas Sharma et al[52] recently documented a higher right ventricular mass and remodeling indices in overlap syndrome compared with patients with COPD alone. In addition, arterial stiffness, a surrogate marker of subclinical atherosclerosis, has also been found to be significantly higher in subjects with COPD/OSA overlap than in those with OSA alone.[53] Finally, whereas increased oxidative stress is associated with both COPD and OSA, with evidence of increased circulating proinflammatory cytokines and leukocytes in both disorders, no specific data exist regarding COPD/OSA overlap syndrome and risk and prevalence of such oxidative stress compared with COPD or OSA alone. Potential key risk factors for endothelial dysfunction, atherosclerosis, and ultimately cardiovascular diseases are depicted in Figure 29-3.

In both COPD alone and OSA alone, the risk of excess all-cause mortality increases in association with increasing severity of these disorders. The excess of mortality is most marked in younger individuals with OSA[54] and in more elderly patients with COPD.[55] Overall, evidence indicates that mortality is increased in COPD/OSA overlap patients. For example, in OSA patients studied at sleep clinics, the coexistence of COPD has been found to increase the risk of

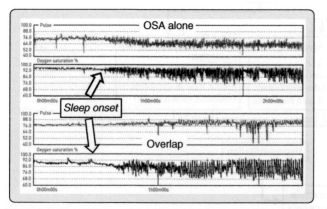

Figure 29-2 Typical pattern during sleep of a patient with obstructive sleep apnea (OSA) alone (*upper panel*) and chronic obstructive pulmonary disease (COPD)/OSA overlap syndrome (*lower panel*). Note the pattern of persistent O_2 desaturation in overlap patients; in contrast to the OSA patients, O_2 saturation does not return to baseline between apnea episodes.

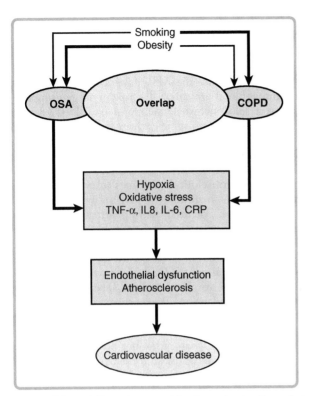

Figure 29-3 Schematic illustrating potential pathways involved in producing accelerated cardiovascular disease as a result of obstructive sleep apnea (OSA), chronic obstructive pulmonary disease (COPD), and COPD/OSA overlap syndrome. COPD, Chronic obstructive pulmonary disease; CRP, c-reactive protein; IL, interleukin; TNF-α, tumor necrosis factor-alpha.

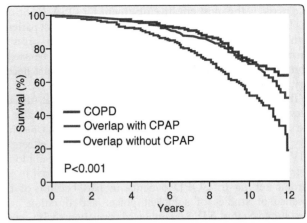

Figure 29-4 Kaplan-Meier survival curves of chronic obstructive pulmonary disease (COPD) patients without obstructive sleep apnea (OSA), patients with COPD and coexisting untreated OSA (overlap group), and patients with overlap syndrome treated with continuous positive airway pressure (CPAP). The differences in survival for COPD alone and COPD/OSA overlap syndrome treated with CPAP are statistically different compared with patients with untreated overlap syndrome ($P < .001$). (Reprinted with permission of the American Thoracic Society. Copyright © 2014 American Thoracic Society. Marin JM, Soriano JB, Carrizo SJ, et al. Outcomes in patients with chronic obstructive pulmonary disease and obstructive sleep apnea: the overlap syndrome. *Am J Respir Crit Care Med* 2010;182:325–31. Official Journal of the American Thoracic Society.)

death compared with patients with OSA alone.[56] We have recently confirmed this in a large cohort of patients with an average age of 57 years, referred with suspected SDB. In addition to PSG, all patients underwent spirometry as a routine procedure.[36] During a median follow-up period of more than 9 years, all-cause mortality was higher in the overlap group untreated for OSA (42.2%) than in the COPD-only group (24.2%) (Figure 29-4). In the COPD patients, comorbid untreated OSA remained a risk factor for death even after adjustment for FEV_1 percentage predicted as a surrogate of COPD severity. There was a significantly higher number of cardiovascular deaths in patients with COPD only and untreated overlap syndrome compared with overlap patients treated appropriately for their OSA with CPAP. Interestingly, the second most frequent cause of death was cancer in patients with both OSA and COPD alone.[57,58]

Nocturnal death risk appears to be increased in COPD compared with the general population, mainly during COPD exacerbations.[59] Nocturnal hypoxemia, an important pathophysiologic feature of OSA, is associated with sudden cardiac death (SCD). Gami et al[60] reported on 10,701 consecutive adults undergoing diagnostic PSG and sought to identify the risk of SCD associated with OSA. During an average follow-up of 5.3 years, 142 patients had resuscitated or fatal SCD. Independently of well-established risk factors, SCD was best predicted by age older than 60 years, AHI above 20, mean nocturnal Sao_2 below 93%, and nadir nocturnal Sao_2 below 78%. No data are available in this study regarding the risk of nocturnal death in patients with COPD/OSA overlap versus COPD or OSA alone. Nevertheless, the report by

McNicholas and FitzGerald[59] documented that nocturnal death was higher among patients admitted for acute exacerbation of chronic bronchitis or emphysema than in patients admitted for other causes. It is possible that an increased sympathetic activity along with a reduction in the perfusion of oxygen to the myocardium can increase the risk of arrhythmias and mortality during nighttime hours in COPD patients. Whether the coexistence of OSA (i.e., COPD/OSA overlap) increases this risk remains unknown.

Diagnosis and Management of COPD/OSA Overlap Syndrome

There are no specific guidelines for the diagnosis or treatment of COPD/OSA overlap syndrome. In the appropriate clinical context, PSG and spirometry should be performed to confirm the existence of the syndrome and to establish its severity. It has been appropriately stated that PSG should be considered in patients with COPD "when OSA is suspected because of either symptoms or the development of hypoxemic complications—cor pulmonale and polycythemia—with daytime Pao_2 greater than 60 mm Hg."[61]

The therapeutic management of identified COPD/OSA overlap syndrome patients should, in general, be based on optimizing treatment for both conditions (COPD and OSA) following corresponding clinical recommendations.[1,43] The goal of such therapy includes improvement in subjective outcomes, such as sleep fragmentation, sleep quality, and daytime sleepiness, as well as optimization of more objective data regarding daytime alertness and function and COPD- and OSA-specific cardiopulmonary outcomes, such as frequency of COPD exacerbation. Correction of hypoxemia and hypercapnia during sleep is considered especially important to reduce cardiovascular complications and to increase survival.

Noninvasive ventilation (NIV), currently typically applied as positive airway pressure (PAP) delivery thorough a nasal or face mask, is the most effective treatment for OSA. Continuous PAP (CPAP) is the optimal PAP therapy for most patients with OSA; bilevel PAP, which delivers a higher pressure during inspiration than during expiration, may also be used if a pressure gradient that increases alveolar ventilation is necessary, effective, and tolerated.

In COPD, NIV in a specifically ventilatory mode (usually bilevel PAP) is consistently shown to be highly effective in the setting of acute and acute-on-chronic hypercapnic respiratory insufficiency. In contrast, data regarding the effects of NIV on quality of life, lung function, gas exchange, and long-term survival have been contradictory when it is used in the chronic setting in COPD patients, in part because of the absence of studies of sufficient power and duration.[62] In the United States, NIV is reimbursed for patients with severe COPD and all of the following criteria: (1) OSA has been ruled out; (2) awake $Paco_2$ is 52 mm Hg or higher; and (3) sleep oximetry shows Sao_2 of 88% or less for 5 minutes or more while breathing supplemental O_2 at 2 liters/minute or at the patient's prescribed Fio_2.[63]

Data have now accrued specific to OSA/COPD overlap syndrome regarding nocturnal NIV, specifically CPAP. In a long-term cohort study, overlap syndrome patients not treated with CPAP demonstrated both an increased risk of death from any cause and an increased risk of hospitalization for COPD exacerbation compared with overlap patients who were treated with and adhered to CPAP.[36] In another observational study, the use of CPAP added to long-term oxygen therapy improved survival among overlap patients with chronic respiratory failure.[64] Finally, a retrospective analysis of 227 patients with COPD/OSA overlap syndrome treated with CPAP revealed that a greater time on CPAP was associated with a reduced risk of death after controlling for common risk factors.[65]

The choice between CPAP and bilevel PAP can be determined during the titration session, based on the pattern of SDB. In cases in which OSA predominates and there is no coexistent consistent sleep-related hypoventilation, CPAP may be most appropriate to treat the OSA component. In cases in which there is evidence of any degree of nocturnal hypoventilation in addition to the apneic episodes, bilevel PAP may be more appropriate. Nevertheless, there is no specific evidence in the literature of the superiority of CPAP or bilevel PAP for the treatment of patients with OSA/COPD overlap syndrome regarding long-term outcomes. Supplemental oxygen should be added to the mask or the PAP circuit if the otherwise optimal-appearing PAP regimen (whether CPAP or bilevel PAP) alone fails to provide satisfactory oxygenation. The ideal setting in which to adjust these parameters is the sleep laboratory, and such "titrations" should be conducted by well-trained technicians with the design, guidance, and interpretation of clinicians with sleep breathing expertise.

In most patients with COPD alone, nocturnal hypoxemia, when present, is corrected with supplemental O_2 through a nasal cannula. Nevertheless, alveolar ventilation of such patients is particularly dependent on the peripheral stimulant effect of hypoxemia. Therefore, to minimize the tendency toward CO_2 retention, particularly during sleep hours, such O_2 supplementation should be titrated carefully. The emergence of morning headache after O_2 initiation in patients with

COPD is an indication to perform a PSG study to exclude the coexistence of OSA or to investigate the development of CO_2 retention. In OSA, supplemental oxygen treatment without PAP can eliminate or reduce nocturnal hypoxemia, but it does not reduce the AHI, daytime hypersomnolence,[66] or nocturnal blood pressure.[67] The role of oxygen supplementation as a solo nocturnal therapy in COPD/OSA overlap syndrome has not been sufficiently explored, and at present it is recommended that nocturnal O_2 be used as a complement to NIV in patients with COPD/OSA overlap syndrome.

No specific studies have been conducted on sleep quality, SDB, or long-term clinical outcomes to evaluate the effects of pharmacologic treatment in patients with COPD/OSA overlap syndrome. Potential use of pharmacologic therapy in overlap syndrome can therefore only be extrapolated from limited existing data about such treatment in OSA and COPD alone. There is in fact currently no established role for pharmacologic treatment of OSA alone, whereas patients with COPD alone receive pharmacologic treatment according to current recommendations.[1] The most common drugs currently prescribed in stable COPD, such as long-acting anticholinergics and long-acting beta agonists, have been shown to improve nocturnal O_2 saturation but not quality of sleep.[68,69] Theophylline, potentially useful for patients with COPD and SDB as a central respiratory stimulant with enhancement of the activity of the respiratory muscles,[70] is currently not clearly shown to be efficacious in improving COPD-related sleep breathing disorders or perturbed quality of sleep. Inhaled corticosteroids used in patients with stable COPD have not been specifically linked with either enhanced or decreased sleep continuity. Benzodiazepine sleep aids are typically avoided in patients with COPD and with OSA because of concerns that they may decrease the arousal response to hypercapnia, induce hypoventilation, and decrease upper airway muscle tone. There is evidence that nonbenzodiazepine hypnotics do not decrease respiratory drive and do not cause daytime drowsiness[71]; however, the indications for and contraindications to any type of sleep aid in these conditions, whether OSA or COPD alone or COPD/OSA overlap syndrome, remain to be better established.

The role of surgery in the treatment of COPD/OSA overlap as well as the need for special precautions regarding preoperative and postoperative evaluation and care in such patients undergoing surgery for treatment of their COPD or OSA, including lung transplantation, lung volume reduction, upper airway surgery, and bariatric surgery, also remains to be established.

ASTHMA

According to the Global Strategy for Asthma Management and Prevention of the Global Initiative for Asthma (GINA), asthma is defined by a history of respiratory symptoms such as wheeze, shortness of breath, chest tightness, and cough that vary over time and in intensity, together with variable expiratory airflow limitation.[72] It is typically recognized as a heterogeneous disease, usually characterized by chronic airway inflammation. Current asthma prevalence across all ages in the United States is 8.2%.[73]

Sleep has a deep impact on the morbidity and mortality of patients with asthma. Classical studies linked nocturnal asthma to an increased risk of mortality, with 70% of deaths and 80% of respiratory arrests caused by asthma occurring during nocturnal hours.[74] The normal physiologic changes that affect the lung during sleep and how those changes may contribute to nocturnal asthma have recently been reviewed in depth.[75]

Nocturnal asthma is characterized by coughing, wheezing, or dyspnea that interrupts and disturbs sleep, with such patients complaining of frequent arousals and poor sleep quality.[76] Nocturnal asthma generally indicates poor control of asthma and the need to modify overall asthmatic treatment.[72] Sleep studies done when current asthma treatment was not available showed a lower sleep efficiency, more awakenings, and less stage 3–4 sleep in asthmatics compared with nonasthmatic subjects.[77] Cognitive performance, as tested by psychometric testing, has also been shown to be impaired in patients with nocturnal asthma.[78] Circadian peak expiratory flow variation of 20% or more, a surrogate parameter of asthma instability, has been associated with poorer daytime cognitive performance compared with healthy control subjects.[79] Effective asthma treatment resulted in the recovery of cognitive impairment to a level of performance comparable to that of the healthy control subjects, paralleled by a reduction of circadian peak expiratory flow variation below 10% and by the resolution of nocturnal asthma symptoms.

Asthma and OSA Overlap Syndrome

Epidemiology

In adults, diseases with a known association with asthma include gastroesophageal reflux disease, rhinosinusitis, obesity, mental disorders, and OSA. The GINA initiative recommended investigation for the coexistence of OSA (i.e., asthma/OSA overlap syndrome) in all patients with asthma, especially in those with severe asthma, difficult to control asthma, and asthma with associated obesity.[72]

There are, however, few population-based data to identify the prevalence or severity of OSA in adult asthmatics. In a U.S. academic institution, patients in the asthma clinic and internal medicine clinic were surveyed for OSA risk with the Berlin Questionnaire, a validated instrument with a positive predictive value of 0.89.[80] OSA risk, as determined by the Berlin Questionnaire, was higher in the asthma group (39.5%) than in the internal medicine group (27.2%; $P = .004$). In a Canadian cohort of patients with asthma, whose severity was established in accordance with the American Thoracic Society criteria,[81] OSA as defined by an AHI of 15 or more events per hour of sleep was present in 88% of patients with severe asthma, 58% of patients with moderate asthma, and 31% of controls without asthma.[82] From these limited data and in the absence of robust population-based studies, it appears that the prevalence of asthma/OSA overlap syndrome, defined as the coexistence of both entities in the same patient, likely is high in asthmatics, especially those with the most severe forms of asthma.

In patients with nocturnal asthma whose quality of sleep does not improve with proper antiasthma treatment, the coexistence of OSA (i.e., asthma/OSA overlap syndrome) should be excluded. Whereas there are no specific studies regarding the effect of coexistent OSA on the quality of sleep and daytime function in asthmatics, it is rational to expect an additive adverse effect of OSA on these outcomes.

Pathophysiology and Risk Factors for Asthma/OSA Overlap Syndrome

Numerous pathophysiologic and clinical factors contribute to an increased diathesis for OSA in patients with treated and untreated asthma; similarly, there are many pathophysiologic and clinical factors that increase the diathesis for asthma, including nocturnal asthma, in patients with OSA. Such factors, therefore, not only constitute risk factors for the presence and severity of asthma/OSA overlap syndrome but also thus represent the adverse clinical manifestations of asthma/COPD overlap. Obesity is a risk factor for both asthma and OSA and therefore for asthma/OSA overlap syndrome. There is a "dose response" effect of increasing BMI on increasing risk of incident asthma, especially in women.[83]

Many patients with nonatopic asthma and most atopic asthmatics suffer from nasal obstruction due to rhinitis and chronic sinusitis, which cause nasal congestion and airflow resistance, and nasopharyngeal polyps, which reduce airway caliber. These lead to increasing intrathoracic and pharyngeal negative pressure, which promotes upper airway collapse during inspiration, snoring, and obstructive apnea.[84] Similarly, in patients with chronic asthma, persistent mucosal inflammation affects the upper airway by decreasing cross-sectional area of the pharynx, promoting upper airway collapse.[85]

Inhaled corticosteroids are the most effective and most widely used drugs in asthma. Their long-term effects on the collapsibility of the pharynx remain unknown. However, the effects of oral corticosteroids on the upper airway are well known and are generally adverse, including myopathy of the muscles of the pharynx, fatty infiltration of the pharyngeal wall, and accumulation of liquid in the neck. In asthma clinics, asthmatics requiring frequent bursts or consistent use of oral corticosteroids were found to have a high prevalence of OSA (>90%) after adjustment for BMI and neck circumference.[86]

Factors potentially effective in reducing the risk and severity of OSA in patients with asthma include the same factors as in the case of patients with COPD/OSA overlap: weight loss, sleep in the lateral decubitus position, and smoking cessation. The effect of adjusting asthma medications to improve concomitant OSA has not been studied. In nonasthmatic patients with OSA, there is both molecular and clinical evidence of the ability of inhaled corticosteroids to reduce upper airway inflammation and to improve AHI in a subgroup of patients with concomitant allergic rhinitis.[87] In clinical practice, nasal inhaled corticosteroids and oral antileukotrienes may be beneficial for reducing snoring and obstructive apneas in children with asthma and OSA, but such an effect has not been proved in adults. These noted factors, both predisposing to and protective against OSA in patients with asthma, are shown in schematic form in Figure 29-5.

The potential mechanisms by which OSA may worsen asthma are also multifactorial. Obstructive apneic episodes are associated with repetitive arousals from sleep, perturbations in autonomic activity, and intermittent hypoxemia.[43] Increased vagal tone during obstructive apnea episodes can contribute to nocturnal asthma through stimulation of muscarinic receptors of the central and upper airways. Negative intrathoracic pressure during obstructive events leads to intermittent loss of lower esophageal sphincter tone; associated gastroesophageal reflux is associated with bronchial microaspiration of

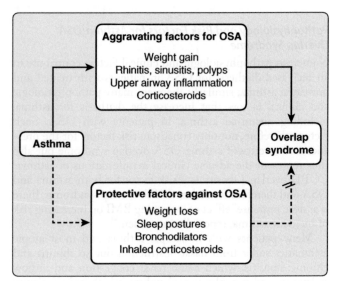

Aggravating factors for OSA

Weight gain
Rhinitis, sinusitis, polyps
Upper airway inflammation
Corticosteroids

Asthma

Overlap
syndrome

Protective factors against OSA

Weight loss
Sleep postures
Bronchodilators
Inhaled corticosteroids

Figure 29-5 Interactions between asthma and obstructive sleep apnea (OSA) contributing to asthma/OSA overlap syndrome.

gastric acid, potentially promoting nocturnal asthma.[88] By stimulation of carotid body receptors, intermittent hypoxia can enhance bronchial responsiveness through vagal pathways.[89] Chronic intermittent hypoxia in OSA may also induce a low-grade systemic inflammation characterized by the elevation of serum proinflammatory cytokines and chemokines. Local inflammatory changes of the upper airways similar to those noted in asthma are also prominent in OSA. Such inflammatory changes may reduce airway caliber and at the same time increase underlying bronchial hyperresponsiveness, thus representing a potential asthma trigger.

Clinical Outcomes and Treatment in Asthma/Overlap Syndrome

In contrast to COPD/OSA overlap syndrome, there are no long-term studies that have evaluated asthma outcomes, either nocturnal or awake, among patients with comorbid untreated OSA or OSA outcomes in OSA patients with comorbid asthma. Consequently, there are currently no guidelines specific to the management of asthma/OSA overlap syndrome. However, in asthma/COPD overlap patients, OSA treatment with CPAP has important potential pathophysiologic beneficial effects for asthmatics, including reducing gastroesophageal reflux, airway and systemic inflammation, and airway smooth muscle contractility.[89] Therefore, CPAP appears to have significant potential clinical benefit in the treatment of the asthma/OSA overlap syndrome, and data do exist documenting that CPAP treatment for comorbid OSA improves asthma symptoms, decreases use of rescue medication, and improves asthma-specific quality of life.[90-93] Further, in a short-term randomized trial, CPAP use decreased airway reactivity in asthmatics without OSA, possibly through reducing bronchial inflammation.[94] Longer term studies are needed to determine the optimal application of CPAP in patients with and without asthma/OSA overlap in improving asthma symptoms, medication need, and overall cardiorespiratory and quality of life outcomes.

Second-line treatments for OSA, such as mandibular advancement devices and upper airway surgery, have not been

prospectively evaluated in patients with asthma/OSA overlap. However, bariatric surgery for patients with OSA and morbid obesity may be effective not only for OSA resolution but also for improving asthma.[95] There are no studies assessing clinical outcomes related to the use of asthma medications in asthma/OSA overlap syndrome. At this time, therefore, it appears that asthma in patients with OSA should be treated according to current asthma treatment guidelines[72] in addition to optimizing treatment of the comorbid OSA.

INTERSTITIAL LUNG DISEASE

Diffuse parenchymal lung disease, also known as interstitial lung disease (ILD), represents more than 200 nonmalignant, noninfectious entities characterized by inflammatory and fibrotic changes affecting alveolar and air spaces. ILD is characterized by progressive dyspnea, hypoxemia, and restrictive-ventilatory limitation. It should be suspected in the appropriate clinical context when there is evidence of impairment of gas exchange or restrictive lung function deficit. Confirmation comes when there is a pattern of usual interstitial pneumonia on lung biopsy or on computed tomography scan.[96] The incidence of ILD appears to be increasing mainly because of improvements in the ability to diagnose the condition due to advances in chest imaging.[97]

Sleep is often disturbed among patients with ILD, which contributes to daytime fatigue in this population.[98] Compared with control subjects, Perez-Padilla et al.[99] reported worse sleep quality in patients with ILD, with more time in stage N1 (33.7% of total sleep time versus 13.5%), less time in REM sleep (11.8% versus 19.9% of total sleep time), and more fragmentation of sleep. In this study, patients with awake hypoxemia (Sao_2 <90%) had greater abnormalities in sleep structure than did those with Sao_2 above 90%. Potential mechanisms that contribute to sleep fragmentation include hypoxemia, hypercapnia, and cough. Most patients report nocturnal cough as an important cause of nocturnal awakenings. Esophageal dysmotility and reflux, also prevalent in ILD, and the pulmonary fibrotic process itself are the main intermediate mechanisms that explain nocturnal cough.[100]

Hypoxemia during sleep is also common and tends to be worse in those with more severe daytime hypoxemia.[99] During REM sleep, O_2 desaturation is often more severe than that occurring during exercise.[101] The role of nocturnal desaturation on health outcomes in patients with ILD has been evaluated retrospectively in a large cohort of patients with ILD.[102] In this study, desaturation index was defined as the number of desaturation events above 4%/hour. Desaturation was present in 37% of patients, and 31% of them had PH on echocardiography. Increased desaturation index was associated with higher mortality independent of age, gender, BMI, and PH. These data indicate the need to conduct sleep studies in patients with ILD. If nocturnal hypoxemia is detected, it is reasonable to treat these patients with oxygen therapy, at least until randomized trials are available.

ILD and Obstructive Sleep Apnea Overlap Syndrome

OSA is prevalent in ILD but clearly underrecognized. In a sample of 50 patients with stable ILD, OSA was confirmed with PSG in 88%.[103] Of those, 68% were moderate to severe (AHI >15 events per hour of sleep). It appears that severity of OSA, as indicated by AHI, inversely correlates with total lung capacity and, interestingly, poorly correlates with BMI.[103] The mechanistic relationship between OSA and ILD and the impact of comorbid OSA on the natural history of ILD remain unknown. Nevertheless, clinicians should evaluate the potential coexistence of SDB in patients with ILD as the appropriate treatment can improve the patient's quality of life and may improve survival.

PULMONARY HYPERTENSION

PH is defined as a mean pulmonary artery pressure higher than 25 mm Hg.[104] The current classification of PH consists of five categories: (1) primary pulmonary arterial hypertension (PAH); (2) PH due to left-sided heart disease; (3) PH associated with chronic pulmonary diseases, such as COPD and OSA; (4) chronic thromboembolic PH; and (5) PH due to various disorders, such as sarcoidosis or systemic vasculitis.[104] The mechanisms by which OSA can lead to the development of PH as a potential long-term complication are reviewed in Chapter 26.

Pulmonary Hypertension and Sleep-Disordered Breathing Overlap Syndrome

SDB overall can be considered a spectrum of ventilatory disorders during sleep that include OSA, central sleep apnea, and sleep-related hypoventilation. The prevalence of SDB/PH overlap is not known. One study conducted to determine the prevalence and significance of nocturnal oxygen desaturation in patients with PH, using home oximetry studies, showed that 69.7% of patients spent more than 10% of sleep time with Sao_2 below 90%.[105] Nocturnal hypoxemia correlates with advanced PH and right ventricular dysfunction. Interestingly, 60% of this subgroup with nocturnal hypoxemia had no exertional hypoxemia. In a small study of patients with idiopathic PH who had full PSG, Schulz et al[106] found that 30% of these patients had periodic breathing, defined as a crescendo-decrescendo pattern of hyperventilatory phases alternating with central apneas or hypopneas of at least three consecutive cycles. Most of these patients, however, had normal nocturnal oximetry. In another study of 38 PH patients who had ambulatory cardiorespiratory sleep studies, 45% had 10 or more apnea-hypopnea events per hour.[107] A subgroup of 22 patients also had in-laboratory PSG. Among patients who underwent both studies, home sleep studies accurately predicted an AHI of 10 events or more during PSG (area under the receiver operating characteristic curve, 0.93; $P = .002$). The corresponding value for pulse oximetry was 0.63 (P = not significant). Therefore, when SDB is suspected among patients with PH, evaluation should include full PSG or modified cardiorespiratory sleep studies rather than pulse oximetry alone.

In the largest series of patients with confirmed PH by right-sided heart catheterization,[108] home cardiorespiratory sleep studies demonstrated that among 169 patients, 26.6% had an AHI above 10 events. Of these, 27 patients (16%) had OSA and 18 patients (10.6%) had central sleep apnea. Despite these limited data, it seems that the prevalence of SDB/PH overlap appears to be higher in PH patients than in the general population.

The extent to which SDB contributes to the PH patient's symptoms and disease progression is unclear. In a retrospective review of 52 consecutive patients with PAH referred for assessment of possible SDB, 71% had SDB (56% of these had primarily OSA and 44% primarily central sleep apnea).[109] There were no differences in cardiopulmonary hemodynamics at baseline assessed by right-sided heart catheterization between patients with PAH only and those with SDB/PH overlap. After a median follow-up of 4.7 years, no differences in survival between those with and without SDB were observed. In this study and in the other studies commented on before,[105,107] there was a lack of subjective daytime sleepiness as assessed by the Epworth Sleepiness Scale in the PAH population with or without coexistent SDB, similar to that found in patients with heart failure with and without SDB; such a phenomenon could be explained by elevated sympathetic nervous activity in both heart failure and PH[110,111] that can act as an adrenergic cortical alerting mechanism. Predictors of SDB in patients with PH do not differ from those of the general population, being mainly older age and BMI.[105-109]

Coexistent OSA may contribute to worsening of underlying PAH. During obstructive events, negative intrathoracic pressures result in right ventricular overload.[112] This is aggravated by intermittent hypoxia and elevated sympathetic nervous activity. Together, these mechanisms contribute to right ventricular hypertrophy and ultimately cardiac failure. Conversely, patients are more predisposed to development of OSA if they accumulate fluid in the neck during sleep.[113] Such rostral shift of fluid from the legs during the daytime to the neck at night has been demonstrated in patients with left ventricular failure[114] (Figure 29-6).

Because of the absence of long-term studies, the prognosis of SDB/PH overlap remains unknown. Similarly, no studies have systematically evaluated the effect of SDB treatment on SDB/PH overlap syndrome outcomes. However, the presence of PH may have prognostic importance in patients with OSA; for example, an observational study of 83 patients with OSA (AHI >5) who underwent pulmonary artery catheterization for unspecified reasons documented 1-, 4-, and 8-year survival rates that were lower among patients with PH (mean pulmonary artery pressure >25 mm Hg at rest) than among those without PH.[115]

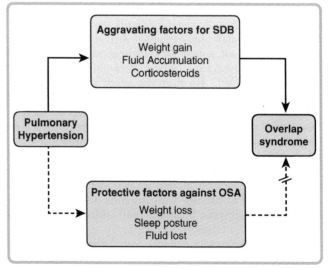

Figure 29-6 Interactions between pulmonary hypertension and sleep disordered breathing (SDB).

We believe that at the present time, patients with PH should be evaluated by PSG when presenting with symptoms that suggest the coexistence of SDB, such as daytime hypoxemia or heart failure. Treatment with CPAP, supplemental oxygen, or both is ideally titrated in the sleep laboratory to customize the treatment as in the other overlap syndromes described before.

INSOMNIA IN PULMONARY DISEASES

Chronic insomnia is a major health problem that leads to worse quality of life and decreased productivity.[116] It is estimated that approximately 10% of the general population is insomniac.[117] There has been little interest in the study of insomnia in pulmonary disorders. Specifically, there are no data on the prevalence and burden of insomnia in patients with PH or ILD. In COPD, relatively older studies reported a high prevalence of self-reported insomnia compared with non-COPD subjects that appears related to the severity of the respiratory symptoms.[118] According to the American Academy of Sleep Medicine, insomnia is defined as history of frequent difficulty in initiating or maintaining sleep and significant disruption of daytime functioning for at least 1 month.[119] Recently, using the American Academy of Sleep Medicine criteria, Budhiraja et al[120] interviewed 183 patients with COPD about sleep complaints. Insomnia was present in 27.3% of participants. Severity of COPD as assessed by pulmonary function test (FEV_1 <50% predicted) or by the Medical Research Council dyspnea scale was not different among participants with insomnia or without insomnia. Interestingly, the presence of insomnia was associated with increased daytime sleepiness and worse quality of life. There are no studies that have evaluated the causality of factors associated with insomnia in patients with COPD or that have evaluated the insomnia as a determinant of health outcomes in COPD.

Because of this high prevalence of insomnia, it is common that COPD patients request medicines to improve their quality of sleep. Benzodiazepines are prescribed for non-COPD insomniacs because they shorten sleep latency, improve sleep efficiency, and decrease arousal frequency. Nevertheless, these agents should be avoided if possible in COPD patients because they reduce alveolar ventilation, diminish arousal response, and increase apnea frequency, and therefore they can worsen hypoxemia and hypercapnia.[121] Some nonbenzodiazepine hypnotics, such as zolpidem,[122] and melatonin receptor antagonists, such as ramelteon,[123] have been reported to have no adverse effects on gas exchange in patients with COPD. Recently, the safety profile of suvorexant, an orexin receptor antagonist approved for treatment of insomnia in the United States, was evaluated in COPD. Suvorexant, at up to twice the maximum recommended dose, did not cause SBDs in a multicenter, randomized, double-blind, placebo-controlled, crossover study in patients with mild to moderate COPD.[124] At the present time and in the absence of comparative studies, we consider that physicians caring for COPD patients with insomnia should preferably use nonbenzodiazepine hypnotics with which they are most familiar.

Sleep disturbances in patients with asthma relate to the occurrence of nocturnal asthmatic crisis. The prevalence of insomnia symptoms was significantly higher among asthmatics than among nonasthmatics (47.3% versus 37.2%) in a postal questionnaire sent to a random sample of 45,000 adults in Sweden.[125] In this study, the risk of insomnia increased with the severity of asthma. In another recent online survey of adolescents from the general community, it was reported that almost twice as many adolescents with severe asthma had clinically significant insomnia than adolescents with mild or no asthma.[126] Daytime sleepiness was frequent in this population, and 28% of its variance was accounted for by insomnia severity, whereas only 2% was accounted for by asthma severity. Insomnia remains a common problem among asthmatics that should be addressed in any patient as part of his or her comprehensive treatment.

CLINICAL PEARLS

- Overlap of OSA with COPD, the COPD/OSA overlap syndrome, affects more than 1% of adults. The prevalence of OSA overlap with asthma, the asthma/OSA overlap syndrome, and the prevalence of SDB overlap with PH, the SDB/PH overlap syndrome, are not well defined. Nevertheless, the coexistence of OSA in asthma and PH increases with increasing severity of both pulmonary disorders.
- Obesity increases the risk of OSA in both COPD and asthma populations.
- Untreated OSA in OSA/COPD overlap is associated with worsened clinical outcomes for both the OSA and the comorbid pulmonary disorder. Conversely, effective identification and treatment of OSA reduce diurnal and nocturnal symptoms and improve clinical outcomes in patients with OSA/COPD.

SUMMARY

OSA and COPD, each a prevalent and clinically important condition in adults, carry numerous common risk factors, including obesity and smoking. It is estimated that the coexistence of OSA and COPD, the COPD/OSA overlap syndrome, affects more than 1% of the general population. The presence of such overlap, when the OSA is untreated, carries a risk of more adverse diurnal and nocturnal physiologic and clinical outcomes, including greater sleep fragmentation, more severe nocturnal hypoxemia, and increased overall mortality, than is documented for COPD alone and OSA alone. Effective identification and treatment of the comorbid OSA and the other features of SDB in the COPD/OSA overlap syndrome improve overall clinical outcomes in the condition.

Asthma, ILD, and PH are also linked with OSA and, in the case of PH, other types of SDB, such as central sleep apnea and sleep-related hypoventilation, by common risk factors and mutually exacerbating pathophysiologic and clinical features. The prevalence of asthma overlap with OSA and PH overlap with SDB is not well defined but increases as the severity of both asthma and PH increases. As with COPD and OSA overlap, effective treatment of the comorbid OSA, using well-established therapy with CPAP, improves asthma-related and overall pathophysiologic and clinical outcomes of the asthma/OSA overlap syndrome, including airway and systemic inflammation, asthma control, and asthma-specific quality of life.

Selected Readings

Gottlieb DJ, Punjabi NM, Mehra R, et al. CPAP versus oxygen in obstructive sleep apnea. *N Engl J Med* 2014;**370**:2276–85.

Greenberg H, Cohen RI. Nocturnal asthma. *Curr Opin Pulm Med* 2012;**18**:57–62.

Konikkara J, Tavella R, Willes L, et al. Early recognition of obstructive sleep apnea in patients hospitalized with COPD exacerbation is associated with reduced readmission. *Hosp Pract (1995)* 2016;**44**:41–7.

Marin JM, Soriano JB, Carrizo SJ, et al. Outcomes in patients with chronic obstructive pulmonary disease and obstructive sleep apnea: the overlap syndrome. *Am J Respir Crit Care Med* 2010;**182**:325–31.

Mohsenin V. Obstructive sleep apnea: a new preventive and therapeutic target for stroke: a new kid on the block. *Am J Med* 2015;**128**:811–16.

Montplaisir J, Walsh J, Malo JL. Nocturnal asthma: features of attacks, sleep and breathing patterns. *Am Rev Respir Dis* 1982;**125**:18–22.

Mulloy E, McNicholas WT. Ventilation and gas exchange during sleep and exercise in severe COPD. *Chest* 1996;**109**:387–94.

Soler X, Gaio E, Powell FL, et al. High prevalence of obstructive sleep apnea in patients with moderate to severe chronic obstructive pulmonary disease. *Ann Am Thorac Soc* 2015;**12**(8):1219–25.

Teodorescu M, Broytman O, Curran-Everett D, et al; National Institutes of Health, NHLBI Severe Asthma Research Program (SARP) Investigators. Obstructive sleep apnea Risk, asthma burden, and lower airway inflammation in adults in the Severe Asthma Research Program (SARP) II. *J Allergy Clin Immunol Pract* 2015;**3**(4):566–75.

Vestbo J, Hurd SS, Agusti AG, et al. Global strategy for the diagnosis, management, and prevention of chronic obstructive pulmonary disease. *Am J Respir Crit Care Med* 2013;**187**:347–65.

A complete reference list can be found online at ExpertConsult.com.

Obesity-Hypoventilation Syndrome

Babak Mokhlesi

Chapter Highlights

- Obesity-hypoventilation syndrome (OHS) has been conventionally and to some extent arbitrarily defined by the combination of obesity and daytime hypercapnia during wakefulness occurring in the absence of an alternative neuromuscular, mechanical, or metabolic explanation for hypoventilation. This syndrome is also invariably accompanied by sleep disordered breathing (e.g., obstructive sleep apnea or sleep hypoventilation), and therefore sleep disordered breathing is included as one of the diagnostic criteria in some definitions of OHS.

- During the last 3 decades, the prevalence of extreme obesity has markedly increased in the United States and other countries. With such a global epidemic of obesity, the prevalence of OHS is likely to increase.

- Patients with OHS have a lower quality of life with increased health care expenses and are at higher risk for development of pulmonary hypertension and early mortality due to cardiopulmonary complications compared with eucapnic patients with obstructive sleep apnea.

- OHS often remains undiagnosed until late in the course of the disease. Early recognition is important as these patients have significant morbidity and mortality if they are left untreated. Effective treatment can lead to significant improvement in patient outcomes, underscoring the importance of early diagnosis.

HISTORICAL PERSPECTIVE

The association between obesity and hypersomnolence has long been recognized. Of historical interest, obesity-hypoventilation syndrome (OHS) was described well before obstructive sleep apnea (OSA) was recognized in 1969.[1-3] In 1955, Auchincloss et al[4] described in detail a case of obesity and hypersomnolence paired with alveolar hypoventilation. One year later, Bickelmann et al[5] described a similar patient who finally sought treatment after his symptoms caused him to fall asleep during a hand of poker, despite having been dealt a full house of aces over kings. Although other clinicians had made the comparison some 50 years earlier,[6] Bickelmann popularized the term *Pickwickian syndrome* in his case report by noting the similarities between his patient and the boy Joe (Figure 30-1), Mr. Wardle's servant in Charles Dickens' *The Posthumous Papers of the Pickwick Club*.

DEFINITION

OHS has been conventionally and to some extent arbitrarily defined by the combination of obesity (body mass index [BMI] ≥ 30 kg/m^2) and daytime hypercapnia (partial pressure of arterial CO_2 [$Paco_2$] ≥ 45 mm Hg at sea level) during wakefulness occurring in the absence of an alternative neuromuscular, mechanical, or metabolic explanation for hypoventilation. This syndrome is also invariably accompanied by a sleep breathing disorder (SBD), and therefore SBD is included as one of the diagnostic criteria in some expert definitions of OHS.[7] Approximately 90% of patients with OHS have OSA, defined by an apnea-hypopnea index (AHI) of 5 events/hour or more. The remaining patients have nonobstructive sleep hypoventilation. The American Academy of Sleep Medicine has arbitrarily defined sleep hypoventilation in adults by the following criteria: the $Paco_2$ (or surrogate, such as end-tidal CO_2 or transcutaneous CO_2) is above 55 mm Hg for more than 10 minutes or there is an increase in the $Paco_2$ (or surrogate) above 10 mm Hg (compared with an awake supine value) to a value exceeding 50 mm Hg for more than 10 minutes.[8] This point is relevant because, although the definition suggests a diurnal pathologic process, overnight polysomnography is required to determine the pattern of nocturnal SBD including hypoventilation (obstructive or nonobstructive) and to individualize therapy, particularly the optimal mode of positive airway pressure (PAP).

OHS is a diagnosis of exclusion and should be distinguished from other conditions that are commonly associated with awake hypercapnia (Box 30-1).

EPIDEMIOLOGY

Nearly 1 of 3 adults in the world are overweight (BMI ≥ 25 kg/m^2), and almost 1 in 10 adults are obese (BMI ≥ 30 kg/m^2). This "obesity epidemic" is associated with myriad comorbidities including OHS. Between 1986 and 2005, the prevalence of morbid obesity (BMI ≥ 40 kg/m^2) increased by fivefold in the United States, affecting 1 in every 33 adults. Similarly, the prevalence of BMI of 50 kg/m^2 and higher has

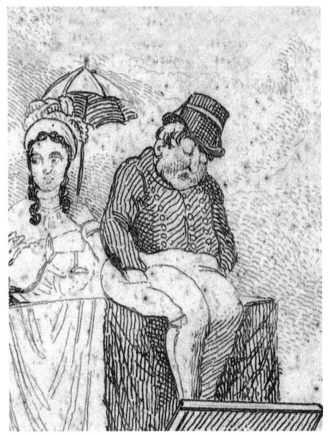

Figure 30-1 Joe the "fat boy." (Detail from "Mr. Pickwick in Chase of His Hat." Illustration by Robert Seymour. In: Dickens C. *The posthumous papers of the Pickwick Club.* Published in serial form. London: Chapman and Hall; 1836. Courtesy The Beinecke Rare Book & Manuscript Library, Yale University.)

Box 30-1 DIAGNOSTIC FEATURES OF OBESITY-HYPOVENTILATION SYNDROME

Obesity
Body mass index $\geq$ 30 kg/m^2

Chronic Hypoventilation
Awake daytime hypercapnia (sea-level arterial $Pco_2 \geq$ 45 mm Hg)
Possible role of serum venous bicarbonate or calculated bicarbonate >27 mEq/L from capillary blood gas

Sleep Breathing Disorder
Obstructive sleep apnea (apnea-hypopnea index [AHI] $\geq$5 events/hour)
Nonobstructive sleep hypoventilation (AHI <5 events/hour, $Paco_2$ above 55 mm Hg for more than 10 minutes or an increase in the $Paco_2$ [or surrogate] above 10 mm Hg [compared with awake supine $Paco_2$] to a value >50 mm Hg for >10 minutes during sleep, or sustained hypoxemia with oxygen saturation $\leq$88% without obstructive respiratory events)

Exclusion of Other Causes of Hypoventilation
Severe obstructive airways disease (e.g., chronic obstructive pulmonary disease)
Severe interstitial lung disease
Severe chest wall disorders (e.g., kyphoscoliosis)
Severe hypothyroidism
Neuromuscular disease
Congenital hypoventilation syndromes

---

increased by 10-fold in the United States, affecting 1 in every 230 adults.[9] With such epidemic obesity, the prevalence of OHS is likely to increase.

Thirteen studies have reported a prevalence of OHS between 8% and 20% in patients referred to sleep centers for evaluation of SBD.[10-12] A meta-analysis of 4250 outpatients with obesity and OSA (mean BMI range between 30 and 44 kg/m^2 and mean AHI range between 40 and 60 events/hour) who did not have chronic obstructive pulmonary disease reported a 19% prevalence of awake hypercapnia.[13] On the basis of these data, approximately 19% of obese patients with OSA have OHS. East Asian populations are known to have OSA at a lower BMI compared with other populations, probably because of cephalometric differences.[14] Therefore, in these populations, OHS may be more prevalent at a lower BMI range than in non-Asian populations.[11,14-16] The prevalence of obesity-associated hypoventilation among consecutive patients with BMI higher than 35 kg/m^2 hospitalized on medical wards (excluding critical care units) has been reported to be 31%.[17] Although it remains unclear why the prevalence of obesity-associated hypoventilation in this hospitalized cohort was higher than the reported prevalence in outpatient obese patients with OSA, it may be related to the facts that the investigators enrolled subjects with a higher BMI (>35 kg/m^2 as opposed to >30 kg/m^2) and there was high prevalence of diuretic use (64% of the patients).

Prevalence estimates for OHS vary significantly across studies, owing partly to differences in sample characteristics, disease definitions, and assessment procedures.[10] In populations of patients with concomitant OSA, as the degree of obesity increases, the prevalence of OHS increases (Figure 30-2).[10] Laaban and Chailleux[18] reported an OHS prevalence of 11% in a cohort of 1141 patients with OSA with a mean BMI of 30 kg/m^2, whereas Mokhlesi et al[19] reported a prevalence of 24% in patients with OSA and a mean BMI of 44 kg/m^2. Among non-Asian populations, the prevalence of OHS is 8% to 11% among patients with OSA with BMI of 30 to 35 kg/m^2 and increases to 18% to 31% among patients with OSA with BMI of 40 kg/m^2 and higher.[18-21] The prevalence of OHS in the general population is unknown but can be estimated. The most recent report from the Centers for Disease Control and Prevention has estimated that approximately 6.4% of the general U.S. adult population has morbid or severe obesity (BMI $\geq$ 40 kg/m^2), and the prevalence is substantially higher at 12.2% amongst non-Hispanic blacks.[22] If we conservatively estimate that half of patients with this degree of obesity have OSA and that approximately 20% of these OSA patients have OHS, the prevalence of OHS can be estimated as roughly 0.6% (approximately 1 in 160 adults in the U.S. population). OHS may be more prevalent in the United States than in other nations because of its obesity epidemic. With such an epidemic, the prevalence of OHS is likely to increase, and therefore there is a need for a high index of suspicion on the part of clinicians to optimize early recognition and treatment of this syndrome.

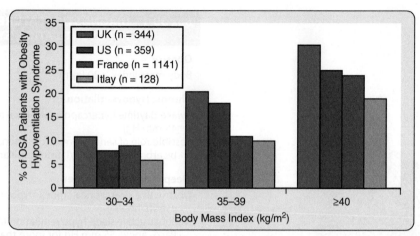

Figure 30-2 Prevalence of obesity-hypoventilation syndrome in patients with obstructive sleep apnea (OSA), sorted by body mass index (BMI). In the U.K. study,[21] the mean BMI was nearly 40 kg/m^2, and 38% of subjects had a BMI higher than 40 kg/m^2. Similarly, in the U.S. study,[19] the mean BMI was 43 kg/m^2, and 60% of subjects had a BMI higher than 40 kg/m^2. In contrast, the mean BMI in the French study[18] was 34 kg/m^2, and only 15% of subjects had a BMI higher than 40 kg/m^2. Italian data[30] were provided by Professor Onofrio Resta (personal communication).

CLINICAL PRESENTATION AND DIAGNOSIS

OHS is typically diagnosed either when an afflicted patient reaches a high state of acuity, in the form of acute-on-chronic hypercapnic respiratory failure,[23] or, alternatively, when ambulatory care is escalated to include evaluation by pulmonary or sleep specialists.[20] Unfortunately, a delay in diagnosis is common; the diagnosis typically occurs during the fifth and sixth decades of life, and during this delay, OHS patients use more health care resources than comparably obese normocapnic patients.[17,23-25] In one study, 8% of all admissions to a general intensive care unit met diagnostic criteria for obesity-associated hypoventilation (BMI >40 kg/m^2; Paco$_2$ >45 mm Hg; and no evidence of musculoskeletal disease, intrinsic lung disease, or smoking history). All of these patients presented with acute-on-chronic hypercapnic respiratory failure.[26] Of these patients, nearly 75% were misdiagnosed and treated for obstructive lung disease (most commonly chronic obstructive pulmonary disease) despite having no evidence of obstructive physiology on pulmonary function testing.

Patients with OHS tend to be morbidly obese (BMI ≥ 40 kg/m^2), have severe OSA (≥30 obstructive respiratory events/hour of sleep), and are typically hypersomnolent. Compared with patients with eucapnic OSA and similar BMI, patients with OHS are more likely to report dyspnea and to manifest cor pulmonale. Box 30-2 provides the typical portrait of an OHS patient based on the clinical features of a large combined cohort of OHS patients reported in the literature.[16-19,25,27-35] Whereas severe obesity (BMI ≥40 kg/m^2) is a predominant risk factor for OHS, not all patients with severe obesity develop OHS. There are significant physiologic differences between obese patients who have OHS and similarly obese patients without OHS as summarized in Box 30-3.[36]

Although the definitive test for alveolar hypoventilation is a room air arterial blood gas analysis, an elevated serum bicarbonate level due to metabolic compensation of respiratory acidosis is supportive of OHS.[19] Mokhlesi et al[19] first demonstrated that a venous serum bicarbonate threshold of

Box 30-2	CLINICAL FEATURES OF PATIENTS WITH OBESITY HYPOVENTILATION SYNDROME*	

Clinical Features	Mean (Range)
Age (years)	52 (42–61)
Male (%)	60 (49–90)
Body mass index (kg/m^2)	44 (35–56)
Neck circumference (cm)	46.5 (45–47)
pH	7.38 (7.34–7.40)
Arterial PCO$_2$ (mm Hg)	53 (47–61)
Arterial PO$_2$ (mm Hg)	56 (46–74)
Serum bicarbonate (mEq/L)	32 (31–33)
Hemoglobin (g/dL)	15
Apnea-hypopnea index	66 (20–100)
SpO$_2$ nadir during sleep (%)	65 (59–76)
Percent sleep time SpO$_2$ <90%	50 (46–56)
FVC (% predicted)	68 (57–102)
FEV$_1$ (% predicted)	64 (53–92)
FEV$_1$/FVC	0.77 (0.74–0.88)
Medical Research Council dyspnea class 3 or 4 (%)	69
Epworth sleepiness scale score	14 (12–16)

*Features are based on aggregated sample of 757 patients from 15 studies.[20]

27 mEq/L, suggestive of chronic respiratory acidosis, could be used for OHS diagnosis in obese patients with diagnosed OSA. Their data demonstrated that among obese patients with OSA and normal renal function, serum bicarbonate level below 27 mEq/L had a 97% negative predictive value for excluding a diagnosis of OHS. Macavei et al[21] assessed ear

Box 30-3 PHYSIOLOGIC DIFFERENCES BETWEEN EUCAPNIC MORBIDLY OBESE PATIENTS AND THOSE WITH OBESITY-HYPOVENTILATION SYNDROME

	Eucapnic Morbid Obesity	Obesity-Hypoventilation Syndrome
Waist:hip ratio	↑	↑↑
FEV_1/FVC	Normal	Normal/↓
Total lung capacity	Normal	Slight ↓
Functional residual capacity	↓	↓
Vital capacity	Normal or ↓	↓↓
Expiratory reserve volume	↓	↓↓
Work of breathing	↑	↑↑
Hypercapnic/hypoxic ventilatory drive	Normal	↓
Inspiratory muscle strength	Normal	↓

FEV_1, Forced expiratory volume in first second; FVC, forced vital capacity.

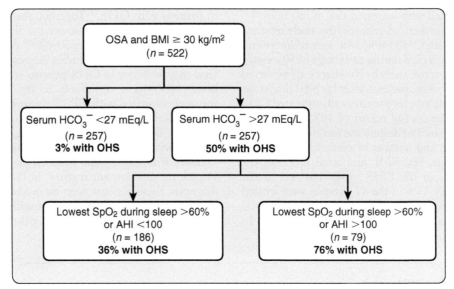

Figure 30-3 Decision tree to screen for obesity-hypoventilation syndrome (OHS) based on observation in 522 obese patients with OSA (BMI ≥30 kg/m² and AHI ≥5). Among those with a venous serum bicarbonate level above 27 mEq/L, OHS was present in 50% of patients. Very severe OSA (AHI >100 events/hour or SpO_2 nadir during sleep <60%) increased the prevalence of OHS to 76%.[19] OSA, Obstructive sleep apnea; AHI, apnea-hypopnea index; BMI, body mass index.

lobe capillary blood gas samples from patients referred to a sleep center and determined that bicarbonate values calculated from the Henderson-Hasselbalch formula have similar predictive values. A calculated serum bicarbonate level of 27 mEq/L and higher had a sensitivity of 85% and a specificity of 89% for the diagnosis of OHS among their patient sample. Two additional studies have confirmed serum bicarbonate to be an independent and reliable predictor of OHS.[12,37] Figure 30-3 shows the prevalence of OHS in obese patients with OSA (BMI ≥30 kg/m² and AHI ≥5) using a serum bicarbonate level combined with other readily available measures, such as severity of OSA.[19] Indeed, several investigators have suggested incorporating serum venous bicarbonate (HCO_3^-) levels into the definition of OHS, particularly because using a single measurement of arterial Pco_2 for OHS diagnosis is susceptible to a number of confounding factors,

including the impact of the patient's periprocedural anxiety leading to hyperventilation.[38]

In addition to blood gas sampling and serum venous bicarbonate assessments, daytime finger pulse oximetry (Spo_2) may be a valuable tool for clinicians in screening for possible OHS.[39] Resting hypoxemia during wakefulness is not a typical feature of either patients with OSA or patients with obesity. Therefore, abnormal resting pulse oximetry during wakefulness should increase the suspicion for OHS among obese OSA patients.[19,40,41] Similarly, significant sleep-associated hypoxemia, defined as oxygen saturation below 85% for more than 10 continuous minutes, in an obese patient with OSA should raise suspicion for presence of sleep hypoventilation and possibly OHS.[42] In a meta-analysis, the mean difference of percentage of total sleep time with Spo_2 spent below 90% was 37.4% (56.2% for OHS, 18.8% for eucapnic obese OSA patients) with very little overlap in the 95% confidence intervals.[13]

Ultimately, a rise in carbon dioxide levels (≥45 mm Hg) during wakefulness is necessary to define hypoventilation. There are a variety of techniques to measure carbon dioxide, such as daytime arterial blood gases, arterialized capillary blood gases, venous blood gases, and end-tidal carbon dioxide and transcutaneous carbon dioxide monitoring. Each of these techniques has its advantages and disadvantages.[43,44] The most reliable and practical method for identifying sleep hypoventilation is to measure carbon dioxide levels continuously during sleep by end-tidal or transcutaneous monitoring.[41] Improving technologies should greatly expand our ability to identify and to quantify nocturnal hypoventilation in sleep laboratories or even at home.

MORBIDITY AND MORTALITY

The majority of OHS patients are severely obese and have severe OSA.[18] Although severe obesity[45] and severe OSA are independently associated with increased risk of mortality,[46-50] OHS may contribute further.[51] A retrospective study reported that 7 of 15 patients with OHS (46%) who refused long-term noninvasive PAP therapy died during an average of 50 months of follow-up.[32] A prospective study by Nowbar et al[17] observed a group of 47 severely obese patients after hospital discharge. The 18-month mortality rate for patients with untreated OHS was higher than for the control cohort of 103 patients with obesity alone (23% versus 9%) despite the fact that the groups had similar BMI, age, and number of comorbid conditions. When adjusted for age, sex, BMI, and renal function, the hazard ratio of death in the OHS group was 4.0 in the 18-month period. Only 13% of the 47 patients were treated for OHS after hospital discharge. The difference in survival was evident as early as 3 months after hospital discharge. In contrast, Budweiser et al[34] conducted a retrospective analysis of 126 patients with OHS who were highly adherent to non-invasive ventilation (NIV) during sleep, with the NIV modality initiated in pressure support mode and after an adaptation period switched to pressure-cycled assist control mode, finding the 1-, 2-, and 5-year survival rates to be 97%, 92%, and 70%, respectively. Similarly, in a large retrospective study, 110 patients with OHS treated with NIV in the form of bilevel PAP (mean inspiratory PAP of 18.5 ± 2.5 cm H_2O and mean expiratory PAP of 8.4 ± 1.9 cm H_2O) were matched with 220 patients with OSA treated with continuous PAP (CPAP; mean pressure of 8.9 ± 1.7 cm H_2O).[51] Despite similar rates of adherence to PAP therapy (mean bilevel PAP use of 6.2 ± 3.0 hours/night vs. mean CPAP use of 5.8 ± 3.2 hours/night; $P = .29$), the 5-year mortality rates were 15.5% in the OHS cohort and 4.5% in the OSA cohort ($P < .05$). Patients with OHS had a twofold increase (odds ratio, 2; 95% confidence interval, 1.11-3.60) in the risk of mortality compared with those with OSA. Using bilevel PAP less than 4 hours/night emerged as the strongest independent predictor of mortality in patients with OHS.[51] Together, these studies suggest that treatment with NIV may lower the short-term mortality of patients with OHS (Figure 30-4).[7,34] Accumulating evidence from prospective cohort studies suggests that long-term survival may be better in OHS patients treated chronically with home NIV (most commonly in the form of bilevel PAP therapy) compared with CPAP therapy.[52]

The morbidity associated with a diagnosis of OHS can be varied, as illustrated by Jennum et al,[53] who evaluated 755 patients with a diagnosis of OHS (using *International Classification of Diseases, Tenth Revision* diagnostic codes) from a Danish national patient registry; in the 3 years before OHS diagnosis, these patients were more likely than age- and sex-matched controls to be diagnosed with a variety of medical conditions, including cellulitis, carpal tunnel syndrome, type

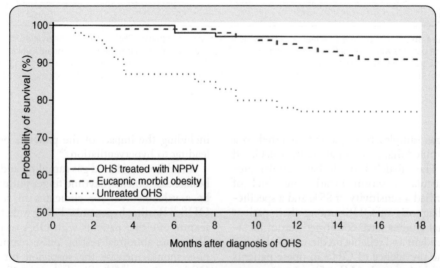

Figure 30-4 Survival curves for patients with untreated obesity-hypoventilation syndrome (OHS; $n = 47$; mean age, 55 ± 14 years; mean body mass index [BMI], 45 ± 9 kg/m²; mean $PaCO_2$, 52 ± 7 mm Hg) and eucapnic obese patients ($n = 103$; mean age, 53 ± 13 years; mean BMI, 42 ± 8 kg/m²) as reported by Nowbar et al[17] compared with patients with OHS treated with nocturnal positive pressure ventilation (NPPV) therapy ($n = 126$; mean age, 55.6 ± 10.6 years; mean BMI, 44.6 ± 7.8 kg/m²; mean baseline $PaCO_2$, 55.5 ± 7.7 mm Hg; mean adherence with NPPV of 6.5 ± 2.3 hours/day). (Data for OHS patients treated with NPPV provided courtesy Stephan Budweiser and colleagues from the University of Regensburg, Germany.[34] Reprinted with permission of the American Thoracic Society. Copyright American Thoracic Society.)

2 diabetes, congestive heart failure, obstructive lung disease, and arthritis of the knee. It remains unclear if these conditions would be more prevalent than in an obese matched cohort with uncomplicated OSA. Furthermore, quality of life ratings among OHS patients appear to be lower than among those with hypoventilatory respiratory disorders such as obstructive lung disease.[54]

Cardiovascular morbidity is of particular concern in OHS.[51] Kessler et al[55] found a pulmonary hypertension prevalence of 58% among a cohort of 34 OHS patients compared with just 9% among a sample of similar OSA patients. Similarly, Berg et al[33] compared 20 OHS patients from a Canadian health registry with obese matched controls. OHS patients in their study were nine times more likely to have a diagnosis of cor pulmonale and nine times more likely to have a diagnosis of congestive heart failure. Moreover, hospitalized patients with obesity-associated hypoventilation are at increased risk of admission to the intensive care unit and need for invasive mechanical ventilation compared with hospitalized patients with eucapnic obesity.[17]

Accordingly, identifying patients with OHS in a timely manner is important, and treatment with PAP therapy should be initiated and monitored without delay to avoid adverse outcomes, such as readmission to the hospital, acute-on-chronic respiratory failure requiring intensive care monitoring, or death. More important, adherence to therapy should be emphasized and monitored objectively.[56]

PATHOPHYSIOLOGY

The partial pressure of CO_2 in the arterial blood ($Paco_2$) is determined by the balance between CO_2 production and elimination. Although the main reason for reduced CO_2 elimination is reduced alveolar ventilation due to an overall decreased level of ventilation (i.e., minute ventilation), maldistribution of ventilation with respect to pulmonary capillary perfusion (i.e., an increase in physiologic dead space) may contribute as well. Further, the rate of CO_2 production in OHS is of particular physiologic concern; severely obese patients, with or without OHS, have increased work of breathing, increased oxygen cost of breathing, and increased CO_2 production compared with lean individuals.[57-59] The majority of individuals with severe obesity maintain homeostasis by increasing alveolar ventilation and associated CO_2 elimination, thereby averting progression to OHS. This is achieved by tight compensatory mechanisms that require an intact integration between respiratory control and acid-base regulatory systems. Ultimately, inadequate elimination of CO_2 relative to CO_2 production leads to chronic hypercapnia in patients with OHS. In addition to the differences as illustrated in Box 30-3, there are a variety of physiologic differences between patients with OHS and those with eucapnic obesity with or without OSA, such as increased upper airway resistance,[60] decreased respiratory system compliance compared with similarly obese subjects without OHS,[61] ventilation-perfusion mismatching secondary to pulmonary edema[62] or low lung volumes/atelectasis,[63] and, most important, impaired central response to hypoxemia and hypercapnia. Although these mechanisms contribute in varying degrees to the gas exchange abnormality observed in patients with OHS, the combination of SBD, a blunted central response to hypercapnia and hypoxia, and renal buffering can explain the

progression from sleep hypoventilation to chronic daytime hypoventilation.[64-67]

Severe obesity (BMI $\geq$40 kg/m^2) increases the work of breathing because of the excess weight on the thoracic wall and abdomen.[61,68] However, it is unclear what role, if any, these altered mechanics have in the pathogenesis of OHS. The lung compliance of OHS patients is less than that of equally obese controls (0.122 versus 0.157 L/cm H_2O). This can be explained by the lower functional residual capacity (1.71 versus 2.20 L). There is an even greater difference in chest wall compliance between the two groups (OHS, 0.079 L/cm H_2O; obese controls, 0.196 L/cm H_2O).[61] Patients with OHS also have a threefold increase in lung resistance that has also been attributed to a low functional residual capacity.[61,69] The changes in lung mechanics are frequently demonstrated on spirometry by a low forced vital capacity (FVC) and forced expiratory volume in 1 second (FEV$_1$) and a normal FEV$_1$/FVC ratio. The spirometric abnormalities may be related to the combination of abnormal respiratory mechanics and weak respiratory muscles.[29,30,70,71] The abnormal respiratory system mechanics in subjects with severe obesity imposes a significant load on the respiratory muscles and leads to a significant increase in the work of breathing, particularly in the supine position.[61,68] As a result, morbidly obese patients dedicate 15% of their oxygen consumption to the work of breathing compared with 3% in nonobese individuals.[58]

The maximal inspiratory and expiratory pressures are normal in eucapnic morbidly obese patients but are typically reduced in patients with OHS.[72-74] Patients with mild OHS, however, may have normal inspiratory and expiratory pressures.[75] Further, the role of diaphragmatic weakness in the pathogenesis of this disorder remains uncertain because patients with OHS can generate similar transdiaphragmatic pressures at any level of diaphragmatic activation compared with eucapnic obese subjects.[73] In a study by Sampson and Grassino,[73] patients with OHS were able to generate equivalent transdiaphragmatic pressures as eucapnic obese patients during hypercapnia-induced hyperventilation, suggesting that respiratory muscle weakness may not play a role in the development of OHS. In addition, the OHS group showed no evidence of acute diaphragmatic fatigue (or neuromuscular uncoupling) throughout the hypercapnic trial when measured by the ratio of peak electrical activity of the diaphragm to peak transdiaphragmatic pressure, which theoretically eliminates the variable of the patient's cooperation. Potentially more accurate assessments of diaphragmatic strength (e.g., by cervical magnetic stimulation) have not been performed in patients with OHS.[76]

Patients with OHS are able to voluntarily hyperventilate to eucapnia,[77] evidence for a defective, "blunted" central respiratory drive. Further, patients with OHS do not hyperventilate to the same degree as eucapnic morbidly obese patients when rebreathing CO_2.[71,73,75] This deficit improves in most patients after PAP therapy.[75,78,79] In addition, patients with OHS do not augment their minute ventilation to the same degree as eucapnic obese OSA patients when breathing a hypoxic gas mixture.[75,79] This blunted hypoxic drive also improves with PAP therapy,[75,79] suggesting that such blunted drive is a secondary effect of the syndrome (and necessary for its persistence) but not the origin of it. Obesity, genetic predisposition, SBD, and leptin resistance have all been proposed as mechanisms for the blunted response to hypercapnia. Such blunted respiratory response to hypercapnia is unlikely to be genetic because the ventilatory response to hypercapnia is similar between first-degree relatives of patients with OHS and control subjects.[80]

Leptin, a satiety hormone produced by adipocytes, stimulates ventilation.[81-84] Obesity leads to an increase in CO_2 production and load.[57,59,81] Therefore, with increasing obesity, the excess adipose tissue leads to increasing levels of leptin to increase ventilation to compensate for the additional CO_2 load. This is likely the reason that most severely obese individuals do not develop awake hypercapnia. Patients with OHS and OSA have significantly higher leptin levels compared with lean or BMI-matched subjects without OSA. Although the independent contribution of OSA or OHS to leptin production remains unclear, the data suggest that excess adiposity is a much more significant contributor to elevated serum leptin levels than the presence of OSA or OHS.[85-88] Patients with OHS, however, have a higher serum leptin level than eucapnic subjects with OSA matched for percentage body fat, and AHI and serum leptin levels each drop after treatment with PAP.[87,89,90] These observations suggest that patients with OHS might be resistant to leptin. For leptin to affect the respiratory center and increase minute ventilation, it has to penetrate the cerebrospinal fluid (CSF). The leptin CSF to serum ratio is fourfold higher in lean individuals compared with obese subjects (0.045 ± 0.01 vs. 0.011 ± 0.002; $P < .05$).[91] Individual differences in leptin CSF penetration may explain why some obese patients with severe OSA develop OHS and others do not.

OSA may well contribute to the ventilatory control defect because treatment with CPAP or bilevel PAP typically improves the response to hypercapnia.[75,78,79] The $P_{0.1}$ response to hypercapnia (a sensitive measure of respiratory drive) improves as early as 2 weeks and reaches normal levels after 6 weeks of therapy with PAP in patients with OHS who demonstrate an awake $Paco_2$ between 46 and 50 mm Hg. The response of minute ventilation to hypercapnia improves by the sixth week of PAP therapy but does not completely normalize,[75] and, although such findings are not universal,[78,92,93] OSA appears well established in the pathophysiologic mechanism of OHS by the resolution of hypercapnia in most patients after treatment with either tracheostomy or PAP therapy.[11,27,32,56,75,94-96]

Norman et al[64] have proposed an elegant mathematical model that explains the transition from acute hypercapnia during OSA to chronic daytime hypercapnia. In most patients with OSA, the hyperventilation after an apnea eliminates all CO_2 accumulated during the apnea.[97] However, if the interapnea hyperventilation is inadequate or the ventilatory response to the accumulated CO_2 is blunted, it could lead to an increase in $Paco_2$ during sleep.[65] Even in this acute setting, during sleep the kidneys can retain small amounts of bicarbonate to buffer the decrease in pH. If the time constant for the excretion of the small amount of accumulated bicarbonate is slow, the patient will have a net gain of bicarbonate, which may blunt the respiratory drive and lead to CO_2 retention during wakefulness to compensate for the retained bicarbonate.[64] Further, the combination of a decreased response to CO_2 and a slow rate of bicarbonate excretion will lead to a blunted respiratory drive for the next sleep cycle. Indeed, obese eucapnic individuals with an elevated serum bicarbonate level exhibit a blunted response to hypercapnic and hypoxic stimulation tests compared with equally obese eucapnic individuals with normal serum bicarbonate level.[39] Further research is needed to elucidate whether these individuals represent a subgroup of "early OHS" and whether they are at increased risk of progressing to overt daytime hypercapnia over time.

Many studies have tried to identify risk factors associated with hypercapnia in patients with OSA, but the results have been mixed.[16,18,19,25,28-31,98] In a large meta-analysis of 15 studies, Kaw et al[13] identified three factors that were significantly associated with chronic hypercapnia in nonchronic obstructive pulmonary disease obese patients with OSA: (1) severity of obesity as measured by the BMI, (2) severity of OSA measured by either the AHI or hypoxemia during sleep, and (3) degree of restrictive chest physiology.

TREATMENT

Treatment modalities for patients with OHS are based on different aspects of the underlying pathophysiologic mechanism of the condition: reversal of SBD (OSA and nonobstructive sleep hypoventilation), weight reduction, and possibly pharmacotherapy. Nocturnal PAP therapies are considered first-line treatment and are effective in improving patient outcomes.[99,100] However, treatment strategies that include weight reduction and physical activity should also be offered to patients with OHS to improve their metabolic and cardiovascular risk profiles.[101-103]

Positive Airway Pressure Therapy

PAP, in the form of continuous PAP (CPAP), was first described in the treatment of OHS in 1982.[94] Whereas subsequent studies confirmed its efficacy, failure of CPAP in some cases has led to uncertainty as to whether CPAP should be attempted initially or if NIV (most commonly in the form of bilevel PAP) is a better modality.[18,56,92,94,104] In one prospective study of outpatients with severe OHS, 57% of patients were successfully titrated with CPAP alone. In these patients, CPAP was titrated to treat OSA, and the mean pressure required was 14 cm H_2O.[42] The remaining 43% of patients failed to respond to CPAP titration because of persistent hypoxemia at therapeutic or near-therapeutic pressures that had successfully treated OSA. In these patients, the oxygen saturation remained below 90% for more than 20% of total sleep time. Because this was a single-night titration study, the question of whether residual hypoxemia would resolve with long-term treatment was not evaluated systematically.[105] Even though several studies have described the efficacy of both NIV and CPAP, only one randomized controlled trial has directly compared the two modes.[106] In this study, 45 consecutive patients with OHS underwent a full night of CPAP titration. Nine patients (20%) had persistent hypoxemia (arbitrarily defined as 10 continuous minutes of Spo_2 <80% without observed apneas) during the CPAP titration and were excluded from the study. The remaining 36 patients who had a successful CPAP titration night with resolution of OSA and hypoxemia were subsequently randomized to either CPAP or NIV (bilevel PAP in the spontaneous mode without a backup respiratory rate). The two groups were well balanced in terms of body habitus, severity of awake hypercapnia, OSA, and nocturnal hypoxemia at baseline. During titration polysomnography, CPAP was increased in increments of 1 cm H_2O with the aim of preventing obstruction, flow limitation, desaturation, and arousal. During the bilevel PAP titration, the expiratory PAP (EPAP) was started at 2 cm H_2O below the pressure needed to abolish obstructive apneas during the CPAP titration or at 5 cm H_2O, whichever was higher. The EPAP was then increased in increments of 1 cm H_2O to resolve obstructive apneas. The inspiratory PAP (IPAP) was initially set 4 cm H_2O higher than EPAP and then increased to eliminate hypopneas and to improve oxygen saturation. After 3 months, there was no significant difference between the groups in terms of adherence to PAP therapy or improvement in daytime sleepiness, hypoxemia, or hypercapnia. However, this relatively small clinical trial found benefits in favor of NIV over CPAP, especially in sleep quality. This study confirms that CPAP can be successful in some patients with OHS as long as OSA and nocturnal hypoxemia are effectively treated. On the other hand, the exclusion of patients with severe nocturnal hypoxemia who were not responsive to CPAP therapy suggests that a subgroup of patients with OHS may need more advanced forms of ventilation. Therefore, NIV is not superior to CPAP a priori; rather, treatment should be individualized to each patient.

The American Academy of Sleep Medicine has proposed guidelines for the titration of NIV in patients with chronic alveolar hypoventilation syndromes, although not specifically for OHS.[107] The most common mode of NIV used in clinical practice is bilevel PAP. During in-laboratory titration, EPAP is increased until obstructive apneas are resolved.[108] If hypoxemia is persistent or estimated tidal volumes are lower than expected for the patient's ideal body weight, pressure support needs to be increased.[107] Pressure support is the difference between IPAP and EPAP. Most patients with OHS require a pressure support level of at least 8 to 12 cm H_2O (i.e., an IPAP pressure setting that is at least 8 to 12 cm H_2O above EPAP) to achieve effective ventilation.[27,32,109,110] Some patients with OHS may experience central apneas during NIV therapy. Central apneas could occur in OHS during CPAP or NIV titration because of decreased respiratory drive, heart failure, or unstable ventilatory control (high loop gain).[111] Advanced modes, such as bilevel PAP with a backup rate, can help alleviate central apneas in OHS. In the spontaneous/timed (S/T) or timed mode, a backup respiratory rate of 10 to 12 breaths/minute should be initiated and titrated upward by one or two increments generally not exceeding 16 breaths/minute. The backup respiratory rate should be initiated when a patient with hypoventilation syndrome manifests central apneas or inappropriately low respiratory rate and consequent low minute ventilation. Therefore, to perform an adequate NIV titration during sleep in patients with OHS, it is important to monitor several parameters during polysomnography, such as mask flow, delivered pressure, air leak, estimated exhaled tidal volume, and triggered backup mechanical breaths.[107] Transcutaneous CO_2 monitoring, if it is available, provides useful information about the effectiveness of NIV or CPAP titration. Scoring of respiratory events during NIV titration can be challenging, and a systematic description of these events has been proposed.[112]

In the minority of patients with OHS who do not have OSA, EPAP can be set at 5 cm H_2O and IPAP can be titrated to improve ventilation.[109,110] Switching to NIV should also be considered if the $Paco_2$ does not normalize after 3 months of CPAP therapy with objective evidence of adherence to prescribed therapy.

There is accumulating evidence suggesting that sleep hypoventilation can be better controlled by NIV settings and modes that optimize delivery of nocturnal ventilation with the use of either a higher mandatory backup respiratory rate of the ventilator[113] or pressure-volume hybrid modes.[114] Two of these hybrid modes are "average" volume-assured pressure support (AVAPS) and "intelligent" volume-assured pressure support. These pressure-volume hybrid modes of pressure support, volume-controlled ventilation deliver a more consistent tidal volume with the comfort of pressure support ventilation. With these hybrid modes, the pressure support or assistance delivered during the inspiratory phase aims to ensure a certain tidal volume that is calculated as a function of predicted body weight (usually 8 to 10 mL/kg ideal body weight or at 110% of the patient's tidal volume). The device assesses the preset tidal volume or minute ventilation during a variable time window of 1 to 5 minutes. The operating IPAP (or pressure assist) level is then allowed to fluctuate between a minimum and maximum pressure support level to ensure the target tidal volume. If a patient's tidal volume or minute ventilation decreases below a certain threshold, the device responds by increasing the IPAP and restores the tidal volume to approximately the preselected target volume. Such devices have an EPAP-minimum and EPAP-maximum range that needs to be preset as well. Although higher inspiratory pressures achieved with volume-targeted hybrid modes may also optimally relieve dyspnea, they may be more disruptive to sleep in some patients.[115] Additional settings may include spontaneous or timed respiratory rate settings, and newer technology has automated the respiratory rate selection on the basis of the patient's minute ventilation and proportion of breaths that are triggered versus spontaneous over a period of time. In a randomized controlled trial of 50 patients with OHS, volume-targeted pressure support mode was compared with fixed bilevel PAP S/T mode (with a backup respiratory rate).[116] In this study, there was no significant difference between the two advanced PAP modes after 3 months of therapy. Both PAP modalities significantly improved daytime $Paco_2$, sleep hypoventilation (as measured by transcutaneous CO_2), hypoxemia during sleep, and quality of life. The lack of such demonstrable difference between AVAPS and fixed bilevel PAP S/T in this trial may be due to the carefully "optimized" bilevel PAP S/T setting in these clinical research conditions. There was no significant difference in the levels of PAP delivered between the two groups. Patients randomized to AVAPS received mean pressures of IPAP 22 ± 5/EPAP 9 ± 1 cm H_2O with a backup rate of 14 breaths/minute versus bilevel PAP S/T mode with mean pressures of IPAP 23 ± 4/EPAP 10 ± 4 cm H_2O with a backup rate of 14 breaths/minute.[116] Despite these high-pressure settings, the mean adherence to therapy was reasonable and not different between the two groups (AVAPS, 4.2 hours/day; bilevel PAP S/T, 5.1 hours/day). Comparative post hoc analysis revealed that patients in whom more than 50% of the breaths were delivered as the backup respiratory rate experienced a greater control of nocturnal carbon dioxide by transcutaneous CO_2 monitoring, improved daytime $Paco_2$, and enhanced health-related quality of life at 3 months,[116] which supports the hypothesis that controlled NIV, which minimizes patient ventilatory effort in sleep, may help unload the respiratory muscles and provide optimal nocturnal ventilatory control and improved patient outcomes. In the largest clinical trial to date, the Spanish Sleep Network investigators performed a randomized controlled trial comparing three treatment strategies in 221 patients with OHS. The treatment strategies consisted of NIV, CPAP, and lifestyle modification (control group). For NIV the 16 centers involved in the study were allowed to use a variety of ventilators all of which were set in the volume targeted pressure support mode (mean IPAP 20 ± 3.3 cm H_2O and mean EPAP 7.7 ± 1.8 cm H_2O; backup respiratory rate of 12–15 breaths per minute and tidal volumes of 550–660 ml). The average CPAP pressure was 11 ± 2.5 cm H_2O. At two months, NIV and CPAP were superior to control group in improving $PaCO_2$, clinical symptoms, and polysomnographic parameters. However, there were no significant differences in the degree of improvement in $PaCO_2$ between NIV and CPAP. Adherence to the PAP modalities was not significantly different (mean adherence to NIV was 5.3 ± 2.3 h/day and CPAP was 5.3 ± 2.1 h/day). Although some health-related quality-of-life assessments, FEV_1, and 6-minute-walk distance improved more with NIV than with CPAP, the long-term significance of these functional improvements requires further investigation. This clinical trial may be able to shed light on the long-term impact of different treatment modalities as the investigators plan to follow these patients for 36 months after randomization.[116a]

There are numerous technical challenges with applying NIV in OHS. Advanced PAP modalities such as volume-targeted pressure support technology rely heavily on and function properly when unintentional air leak from the noninvasive mask remains low.[117] Whereas bench studies have shown that most NIV devices underestimate air leak and exhaled tidal volume, there is significant variability among manufacturers.[118]

The most common reason for persistent hypercapnia and hypoxemia in patients with OHS treated with PAP is lack of adherence to the PAP therapy. In a retrospective study of 75 outpatients with stable OHS, patients who used CPAP or bilevel PAP therapy for more than 4.5 hours/day had a considerably greater improvement in blood gases than less adherent patients ($\Delta PaCO_2$ 7.7 ± 5 vs. 2.4 ± 4 mm Hg, $P < .001$; ΔPaO_2 9.2 ± 11 vs. 1.8 ± 9 mm Hg, $P < .001$).[56] The degree of improvement in ventilation and gas exchange, which can be seen as early as 2 to 4 weeks after therapy,[56,75,119] may allow discontinuation of daytime oxygen supplementation in many patients with OHS.[56] However, the improvement in chronic daytime gas exchange abnormalities (i.e., hypercapnia and hypoxemia) even in patients who are adherent to PAP therapy is neither universal nor complete.[52,102] Other possibilities behind persistent hypercapnia include inadequate CPAP pressure or insufficient NIV support; CPAP failure in OHS patients who do not have significant OSA; other causes of hypercapnia, such as chronic obstructive pulmonary disease; and metabolic alkalosis due to high doses of loop diuretics. In two studies,[56,106] the $PaCO_2$ did not improve significantly in approximately a quarter of patients who had undergone successful PAP titration in the laboratory and were highly adherent (>6 hours/night) with either CPAP or bilevel PAP therapy. It is conceivable that volume-targeted pressure support or higher levels of pressure support with fixed bilevel PAP in the S/T mode would be more effective in normalizing ventilation and gas exchange. Reports of persistent hypoventilation after tracheostomy[27] highlight the need for aggressive nocturnal

mechanical ventilation in addition to support of upper airway patency in at least a subset of OHS patients.

Early follow-up is imperative and should include assessment of adherence to PAP therapy; patients with OSA, although not specifically with OHS, frequently overestimate CPAP adherence.[120-122] Changes in serum bicarbonate level and improvements in resting room air pulse oximetry and end-tidal CO_2 measurements during wakefulness could be used as less invasive surrogates of ventilation if the patient is reluctant to undergo follow-up measurement of arterial blood gases.

Oxygen Therapy

In some patients with OHS, oxygen supplementation is necessary after the resolution of apneas and hypopneas during PAP titration, both CPAP and NIV, to keep SpO_2 above 88% to 90%. In two studies, the percentage of OHS patients requiring supplemental oxygen after adequate CPAP titration (i.e., resolution of obstructive apneas and hypopneas) was as high as 43%.[42,56] In contrast, in a relatively comparable group of patients with OHS, only 12% undergoing aggressive NIV titration with relatively high levels of pressure support (~13 cm H_2O above an average EPAP of 10 cm H_2O) required such oxygen supplementation.[116] This finding suggests that higher levels of pressure support during PAP titration must be considered to achieve adequate oxygenation and ventilation during sleep in a large proportion of patients with OHS. Oxygen supplementation as monotherapy without resolution of upper airway obstruction with CPAP or adequate ventilatory support with NIV is strongly discouraged. Two well-controlled clinical trials have reported that in a significant proportion of patients with OHS who were tested during wakefulness and in steady state, supplemental oxygen at high[123] and medium concentrations[124] worsened hypercapnia (because of a drop in tidal volume and minute ventilation). It is plausible that the risk of CO_2 retention is even higher during acute-on-chronic hypercapnic respiratory failure in OHS.[125]

Weight Reduction

Bariatric surgery has variable long-term efficacy in treating OSA.[126] A meta-analysis that included 12 studies with 342 patients who underwent polysomnography before bariatric surgery and after maximum weight loss reported a 71% reduction in the AHI, from baseline of 55 (95% confidence interval, 49-60) to 16 (95% confidence interval, 13-19).[127] Whereas only 38% achieved cure defined by AHI below 5, this drastic improvement in the severity of SBD would likely be enough to normalize daytime blood gases in most patients with OHS. It is also known that in the 6 to 8 years after weight reduction surgery, patients experience approximately 7% weight gain, which may lead to an increase in the AHI.[128,129] Only one study has examined the impact of bariatric surgery in patients with OHS. One year after surgery in 31 patients with OHS, the PaO_2 increased from an awake baseline on breathing room air of 53 to 73 mm Hg and $PaCO_2$ decreased from 53 to 44 mm Hg after approximately 50 kg of weight loss (baseline BMI, 56 ± 13 kg/m^2; BMI at 1 year, 38 ± 9 kg/m^2). In the 12 patients in whom an arterial blood gas measurement was available 5 years after surgery, values had worsened, with the mean PaO_2 dropping to 68 mm Hg and $PaCO_2$ increasing to 47 mm Hg.[130] The BMI in these 12 patients was 40 ± 10 kg/m^2.

The general perioperative mortality is between 0.5% and 1.0%. Untreated OHS may be associated with higher operative mortality.[131-133] The independent risk factors associated with mortality are intestinal leak, pulmonary embolism, preoperative weight, and hypertension. Depending on the type of surgery, intestinal leak occurs in 2% to 4% of patients and pulmonary embolism occurs in 1% of patients.[132] Ideally, patients with OHS should be treated with PAP therapy before undergoing surgical intervention to decrease perioperative morbidity and mortality. Moreover, PAP therapy using the patient's preoperative settings should be initiated immediately after extubation to avoid postoperative respiratory failure,[133-136] particularly because there is no evidence that PAP therapy initiated postoperatively leads to anastomotic disruption or leakage.[135,137] Such settings, however, may not be optimal for ventilation and/or oxygenation in the immediate postoperative period, particularly with the use of analgesic and/or sedative medication, and must be monitored and adjusted accordingly.

Tracheostomy

Tracheostomy was the first therapy described for the treatment of OHS.[138] In a retrospective study of 13 patients with OHS, tracheostomy was associated with significant improvement in concomitant OSA. However, in seven patients, the AHI remained above 20. Residual respiratory events were associated with persistent respiratory effort, suggesting that disordered breathing was caused by obstructive hypoventilation through an open tracheostomy rather than by central apneas. On occasion, excessive neck skin folds can intermittently obstruct the tracheostomy orifice. However, the overall improvement in the severity of SBD after tracheostomy leads to the resolution of hypercapnia in the majority of the patients with OHS.[139] Currently, tracheostomy is generally reserved for patients who are intolerant of or not adherent to PAP therapy. Patients with tracheostomy may require additional nocturnal ventilation as tracheostomy alone does not treat any central hypoventilation that may be present.[140] Polysomnography with the tracheostomy open is necessary to determine whether nocturnal ventilation is required and to specifically titrate the mode and levels of ventilation necessary.[27]

Respiratory Stimulation

Respiratory stimulants can theoretically increase respiratory drive and improve daytime hypercapnia, but such data in patients with OHS are extremely limited. Medroxyprogesterone acts as a respiratory stimulant at the hypothalamic level.[141] The results of treatment in patients with OHS have been contradictory. In a series of 10 men with OHS who were able to normalize their $Paco_2$ with 1 to 2 minutes of voluntary hyperventilation, treatment with 60 mg/day of oral medroxyprogesterone for 1 month resulted in normalization of the $Paco_2$ (from 51 mm Hg to 38 mm Hg) and improvement in the Pao_2 (49 mm Hg to 62 mm Hg).[142] In contrast, medroxyprogesterone did not improve $Paco_2$, minute ventilation, or ventilatory response to hypercapnia in three OHS patients who remained hypercapnic after tracheostomy.[92] Further, medroxyprogesterone may increase the risk of venous thromboembolism, particularly in this population whose mobility is limited.[143,144] In addition, high doses of medroxyprogesterone can lead to breakthrough uterine bleeding in women and to decreased libido in men.

Acetazolamide induces metabolic acidosis through carbonic anhydrase inhibition, which decreases serum bicarbonate, shifts the CO_2 response to the left, and increases minute ventilation.[92,145] Acetazolamide may also favorably affect OSA by improving loop gain.[146-148]

Most but not all patients with OHS can normalize their $Paco_2$ with 1 minute of voluntary hyperventilation.[77] The inability to eliminate CO_2 with voluntary hyperventilation may be due to mechanical impairment. In one study, the ability to decrease the $Paco_2$ by at least 5 mm Hg with voluntary hyperventilation was the main predictor of a favorable response to respiratory stimulants.[149] Ideally, however, respiratory stimulants should not be used in patients who cannot normalize their $Paco_2$ with voluntary hyperventilation (because of limited ventilation or mechanical impairment); it can lead to an increase in dyspnea or even worsening of acidosis with acetazolamide. Overall, pharmacotherapy with respiratory stimulants cannot be currently recommended as monotherapy in patients with OHS.

Hyperviscosity impairs oxygen delivery and can counteract the beneficial effects of erythrocytosis. Phlebotomy has not been systematically studied in patients with OHS who develop secondary erythrocytosis. In adult patients with congenital cyanotic heart disease, phlebotomy has been recommended if the hematocrit is above 65% only if symptoms of hyperviscosity are present.[150] However, it is difficult to extrapolate this recommendation to patients with OHS because many symptoms of hyperviscosity are similar to the symptoms of OHS. Reversal of hypoventilation and hypoxemia with PAP therapy eventually improves secondary erythrocytosis, and therefore phlebotomy is not needed in patients with OHS.[151]

CLINICAL PEARL

Clinicians should recognize that approximately 8% to 20% of obese patients referred for polysomnography for suspicion of OSA have OHS. The prevalence of OHS is even higher in severely obese patients with OSA. Unfortunately, OHS is typically underrecognized and undertreated. Delay in diagnosis and treatment leads to significant health care resource utilization and increased morbidity and mortality. Therefore, a high index of suspicion is required to diagnose OHS in a timely fashion to improve patient outcomes. Nocturnal PAP therapies are considered first-line treatment and are effective in improving patient outcomes. Whereas significant advances have been made in the delivery of nocturnal PAP therapy, adherence to such therapy remains suboptimal in many patients with OHS. Therefore, comprehensive management should include strategies to improve PAP adherence. Although PAP therapy improves nocturnal and daytime hypoventilation and quality of life, weight reduction and increase in physical activity should be included as part of comprehensive treatment strategies to improve the metabolic and cardiovascular risk profiles of patients with OHS.

SUMMARY

With the current global epidemic of obesity, the prevalence of OHS is likely to increase. Despite the significant morbidity and mortality associated with the syndrome, it is often unrecognized, and treatment is frequently delayed. A high index of suspicion can lead to early recognition of the syndrome and initiation of appropriate therapy. Significant advances have been made in the delivery of PAP therapy and NIV. Clinicians should encourage adherence to PAP therapy to avert the serious adverse outcomes of untreated OHS.

Selected Readings

Berger KI, Rapoport DM, Ayappa I, Goldring RM. Pathophysiology of hypoventilation during sleep. *Sleep Med Clin* 2014;**11**:289–300.

Berry RB, Chediak A, Brown LK, et al. NPPV Titration Task Force of the American Academy of Sleep Medicine. Best clinical practices for the sleep center adjustment of noninvasive positive pressure ventilation (NPPV) in stable chronic alveolar hypoventilation syndromes. *J Clin Sleep Med* 2010;**6**:491–509.

Böing S, Randerath WJ. Chronic hypoventilation syndromes and sleep-related hypoventilation. *J Thorac Dis* 2015;**7**(8):1273–85.

Combs D, Shetty S, Parthasarathy S. Advances in PAP treatment modalities for hypoventilation syndromes. *Sleep Med Clin* 2014;**11**:315–26.

Gonzalez-Bermejo J, Perrin C, Janssens JP, et al. SomnoNIV Group. Proposal for a systematic analysis of polygraphy or polysomnography for identifying and scoring abnormal events occurring during non-invasive ventilation. *Thorax* 2012;**67**:546–52.

Hart N, Mandal S, Manuel A, et al. Obesity hypoventilation syndrome: does the current definition need revisiting? *Thorax* 2014;**69**:83–4.

Huttmann SE, Windisch W, Storre JH. Techniques for the measurement and monitoring of carbon dioxide in the blood. *Ann Am Thorac Soc* 2014;**11**:645–52.

Janssens JP, Borel JC, Pepin JL. Non-PAP treatment modalities in obesity-hypoventilation syndrome: role of exercise, nonsurgical and surgical weight reduction, tracheostomy, respiratory stimulants, and oxygen. *Sleep Med Clin* 2014;**11**:357–64.

Masa JF, Corral J, Alonso ML, et al. Efficacy of different treatment alternatives for obesity hypoventilation syndrome. Pickwick Study. *Am J Respir Crit Care Med* 2015;**192**:86–95.

Mokhlesi B, Tulaimat A, Faibussowitsch I, et al. Obesity hypoventilation syndrome: prevalence and predictors in patients with obstructive sleep apnea. *Sleep Breath* 2007;**11**:117–24.

Murphy PB, Davidson C, Hind MD, et al. Volume targeted versus pressure support non-invasive ventilation in patients with super obesity and chronic respiratory failure: a randomised controlled trial. *Thorax* 2012;**67**:727–34.

Murphy PB, Hart N. Outcomes for obese patients with chronic respiratory failure: results from the observational and randomized controlled trials. *Sleep Med Clin* 2014;**11**:349–56.

Palm A, Midgren B, Janson C, Lindberg E. Gender differences in patients starting long-term home mechanical ventilation due to obesity hypoventilation syndrome. *Respir Med* 2016;**110**:73–8.

Pepin JL, Borel JC, Janssens JP. Obesity hypoventilation syndrome: an underdiagnosed and undertreated condition. *Am J Respir Crit Care Med* 2012;**186**:1205–7.

Piper AJ, Gonzalez-Bermejo J, Janssens JP. Sleep hypoventilation: diagnostic considerations and technological limitations. *Sleep Med Clin* 2014;**9**:301–14.

Piper AJ, Grunstein RR. Obesity hypoventilation syndrome: mechanisms and management. *Am J Respir Crit Care Med* 2011;**183**:292–8.

A complete reference list can be found online at ExpertConsult.com.

Stroke

Claudio L. Bassetti

Chapter Highlights

- Sleep-wake disorders and stroke are common and intertwined neurologic problems; each may cause the other, and they can arise from similar predisposing factors.
- Clinicians who treat patients with sleep-wake disorders or stroke should be aware of this potential comorbidity and its clinical implications.

- In patients with stroke, treatment of sleep-disordered breathing and other sleep-wake disorders can reduce the risk for subsequent stroke and improve short- and long-term outcomes.

Since the 1990s, the link between sleep and stroke, which was suggested already in the nineteenth century, has received increasing attention. This is mainly a result of better recognition of the strong link between sleep-disordered breathing (SDB) and cardiovascular and cerebrovascular diseases, the high incidence of sleep-wake disturbances in stroke victims, and the effect that SDB, sleep-wake disturbances, and their treatment have on the risk for and outcome of stroke.

STROKE

Stroke is a focal neurologic deficit of acute onset and vascular origin. Stroke has an incidence rate of 2 to 3 per 1000 per year and is the most common neurologic cause of hospitalization. Among patients with stroke, about 65% have ischemic strokes, 15% intracerebral hemorrhage, and 20% transient ischemic attacks (TIAs), in which neurologic deficits typically resolve within 1 hour. Risk factors for stroke include atrial fibrillation, arterial hypertension, dyslipidemia, disorders of glucose metabolism, overweight (abnormal waist-to hip ratio), excessive alcohol consumption, cigarette smoking, and physical inactivity.[1] Patients with heart disease, asymptomatic carotid stenosis, history of TIA, depression, psychosocial stress, and age older than 65 years are also at higher risk for stroke.[1]

Primary prevention of stroke includes treatment of risk factors, regular physical exercise, reduction of body mass index to less than 25, anticoagulation for atrial fibrillation, and endarterectomy in patients with at least 70% carotid stenosis.[2] Emergency treatment includes the systemic use of fibrinolytic agents within the first 4.5 hours and endovascular treatment (thrombectomy) within the first 12 hours after onset of symptoms.[3] Management of acute stroke includes placement of patients in a stroke unit, early recognition of medical complications, and prescription of agents that inhibit platelet aggregation. Surgery may be considered in patients with accessible (e.g., cerebellar) hemorrhages and malignant middle cerebral artery strokes. After stroke, therapies for preventing further events includes platelet antiaggregants, blood pressure–lowering medications, statins, treatment of risk factors, and in selected patients anticoagulation and endarterectomy.[2]

SLEEP-DISORDERED BREATHING AND STROKE

Epidemiology

Sleep-Disordered Breathing as a Risk Factor for Stroke

SDB is strongly associated with stroke. Habitual snoring is an independent risk factor for stroke with a pooled risk of about 1.5.[4] A study of 1022 patients showed that obstructive sleep apnea (OSA) is associated with an increased odds ratio (OR) of 2.0 for stroke and death, even after adjusting for multiple cardiovascular risk factors. The risk was even higher (OR = 3.3) in patients with severe OSA (apnea-hypoxia index [AHI] >36/hour).[5] In a single center study of 1387 male patients with OSA followed for up to 10 years, patients with severe OSA (AHI >30/hour) had a significantly higher incidence of fatal and nonfatal cardiovascular events including stroke compared with patients with mild to moderate OSA, OSA patients treated with continuous positive airway pressure (CPAP), 377 simple snorers, and 264 controls.[6] Other studies have confirmed that SDB is associated with an increased risk for stroke.[7,8] A meta-analysis of prospective studies showed that OSA was associated with incident stroke (OR = 2.24, 95% confidence interval [CI] = 1.57 to 3.19), and cardiovascular mortality (OR = 2.09, 95% CI = 1.20 to 3.65), especially in patients with a high AHI.[9]

SDB is also linked with white matter disease on magnetic resonance imaging and silent strokes.[10-12] In a recent study of 503 elderly individuals who were free of previously diagnosed cardiovascular and neurologic diseases, moderate to severe OSA (AHI ≥15) was independently associated with the presence of white matter changes (OR = 2.08, 95% CI = 1.05 to 4.13) compared with no OSA even after adjustment for hypertension.[12]

Sleep-Disordered Breathing in Acute and Postacute Stroke Patients

In the 1990s, three large, systematic studies demonstrated a very high frequency of SDB in patients with stroke and TIA.[13-15] In a meta-analysis of 29 studies with a total of 2343 ischemic or hemorrhagic stroke and TIA patients, the frequency of SDB with AHI greater than 5 was 72% and with AHI greater than 20 was 38%. Males had a higher percentage of SDB (AHI >10) than females (65% vs. 48%; $P = .001$). Patients with recurrent strokes had a higher prevalence of SDB (AHI >10) than those with first strokes (74% vs. 57%).[16] In a literature search until December 31, 2014, we found 54 publications in which SDB frequency was assessed on a total of 4293 stroke patients, solidly confirming these findings.

A few studies have assessed the prevalence of SDB in patients with TIA and have found it to be similar to that of patients with stroke.[16] A few studies have reported a higher frequency of SDB in specific stroke subgroups such as hemorrhagic, brainstem, nocturnal/wake-up, and recurrent strokes.[17-19]

SDB often improves across the acute to the subacute phase.[20-23] In general, central events improve more than obstructive events. One study suggested a greater improvement in SDB in hemorrhagic compared with ischemic strokes.[24]

Clinical Features

Breathing Disturbances During Sleep

The most common form of SDB in stroke patients is OSA (Figure 31-1). Moderate to severe OSA (AHI >30) is found in about 20% to 30% of patients with stroke.[16] Occasionally,

patients may present with both OSA and Cheyne-Stokes breathing (CSB) (Figure 31-2). OSA is often worse in rapid eye movement (REM) sleep, whereas CSB is usually worse in light non–rapid eye movement (NREM) sleep.[13,25] In the first few days after stroke, CSB and other forms of central periodic breathing are present during at least 10% of the recording time in about one third of patients.[20,26-28]

Breathing Disturbances During Wakefulness

Different breathing abnormalities can occur during wakefulness after hemispheric strokes. Abnormalities include selective impairment of behavioral or volitional respiratory control.

Hemispheric strokes in the frontal cortex, basal ganglia, or internal capsule may cause respiratory apraxia, with impaired voluntary modulation of breathing amplitude and frequency, leaving patients unable to take a deep breath or hold the breath.[29,30]

Brainstem strokes can be associated with different forms of abnormal breathing patterns. Sustained respiratory rates above 25 to 30/min in the absence of hypoxemia (neurogenic hyperventilation) were originally described in six comatose patients with ventrotegmental pontine strokes but were subsequently attributed to pulmonary edema (and stimulation of lung and chest wall afferent reflexes).[31] Neurogenic hyperventilation after stroke usually indicates a poor prognosis.[32] Inspiratory breath holding (apneustic breathing), originally described in two patients with bilateral ventrotegmental mediocaudal (infratrigeminal) pontine stroke,[33] is rare and usually secondary to basilar artery occlusion. Erratic variations in breathing frequency and amplitude (ataxic or Biot breathing) and failure of automatic breathing (central sleep apnea or

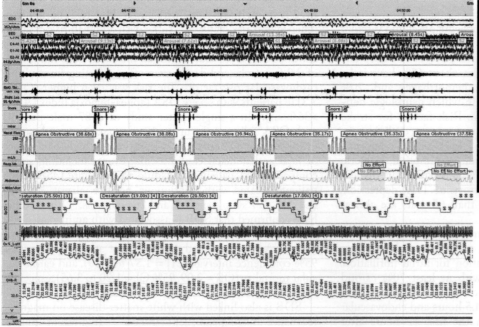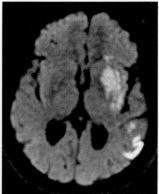

Figure 31-1 Obstructive sleep apnea in acute ischemic stroke. This 70-year-old man has left middle cerebral artery stroke, carotid artery occlusion, and atrial fibrillation. He has habitual snoring but no excessive daytime sleepiness. Aphasia and severe hemiparesis are clinically apparent. National Institutes of Health stroke score is 16, and there are no signs of heart failure. Polysomnography 2 days after stroke onset shows an apnea-hypoxia index (AHI) of 79 and minimum oxygen desaturation of 85%. The AHI normalized (<5/hr) with continuous positive airway pressure. (MRI pictures courtesy Professor A. Valavanis, Institute of Neuroradiology, University Hospital, Zürich, Switzerland.)

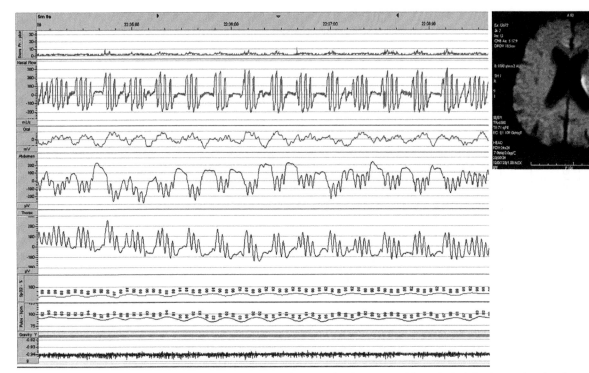

Figure 31-2 Central sleep apnea in acute ischemic stroke. This 63-year-old man had a left subcortical stroke of unknown origin, with arterial hypertension and habitual snoring but no excessive daytime sleepiness. He had a mild hemiparesis, with a National Institutes of Health stroke score of 8 and no signs of heart failure (cardiac ejection fraction, 55%). Polysomnography the first night after stroke onset showed an apnea-hypoxia index (AHI) of 53 (mainly central apneas). The patient spontaneously improved after 1 week (AHI 16). (MRI pictures courtesy Professor G. Schroth, Institute of Neuroradiology, University Hospital, Bern, Switzerland.)

Ondine's curse), usually imply a lateral medullary stroke, often bilateral.[34,35] Damage to the medullary reticular formation and nucleus ambiguous may cause a loss of automatic breathing, whereas a lesion that includes the nucleus of the solitary tract is necessary to cause failure of both automatic and voluntary respiration.[36] Volitional breathing can be impaired by brainstem strokes involving corticobulbar and corticospinal pathways at pontine and medullary levels.[30]

Spinal cord stroke can impair both automatic and voluntary breathing. Anterior spinal artery strokes can affect reticulospinal pathways, located anteriorly in the lateral columns of the first three cervical segments, which are crucial for automatic breathing.[37] In contrast, posterior spinal artery strokes can damage corticospinal pathways in the dorsolateral spinal cord and impair voluntary control of breathing.[38] Strokes that extend up to the C1 level usually cause severe respiratory insufficiency and necessitate ventilatory support.

Repetitive yawning can accompany hypersomnia (e.g., in patients with thalamic or posterior hypothalamus stroke) and can also occur as a release phenomenon in patients with brainstem and supratentorial lesions. Yawning can also occur with insular and caudate lesions.[39]

Pathophysiology

Several acute and chronic consequences of nocturnal respiratory events may explain the link between SDB and increased risk for stroke. Sympathetic hyperactivation, intermittent hypoxemia and oxidative stress, and inflammation likely increase the risk for atherosclerosis and cardiovascular morbidities. However, this link has been difficult to prove because sleep apnea and stroke share many of the same risk factors such as obesity and diabetes.

Sleep-Disordered Breathing as a Risk Factor for Stroke: Acute Effects

Acutely, apneas and hypopneas during sleep can be accompanied by decreased cardiac output, cardiac arrhythmias, systemic hypotension or hypertension, vasodilation due to hypoxia and hypercapnia, and increased intracranial pressure. These factors lead to a roughly 15% to 20% reduction in cerebral blood flow velocities during respiratory events.[40,41] Large fluctuations in cerebral blood velocities (and flow) may be particularly detrimental because patients with SDB have been shown to have diminished vasodilator reserve and impaired cerebral autoregulation.[41]

Type, duration, and timing of respiratory events affect hemodynamic consequences. Near infrared spectroscopy (NIRS) studies have shown that SDB can disrupt autoregulatory mechanisms and cause brain hypoxia, particularly with severe SDB (AHI > 30)[42] (Figure 31-3). These effects may be particularly detrimental to the ischemic region (penumbra) bordering the stroke.[43] Transcranial Doppler studies have shown that obstructive apneas of long duration and occurring during REM sleep may also be particularly detrimental.[44] CSB and central apneas also can alter cerebral blood flow.[44] Paradoxical embolization due to right-to-left shunting in patients with patent foramen ovale during long apneas is another potential mechanism of stroke.[17,45,46]

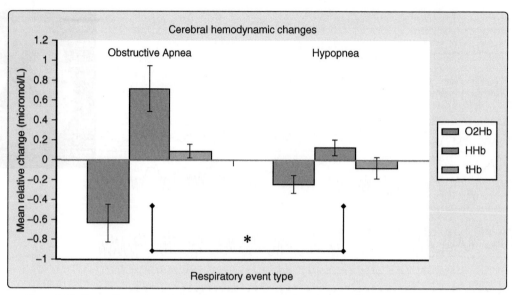

Figure 31-3 Cerebral hemodynamic alterations in patients with sleep-disordered breathing as estimated by near infrared spectroscopy (NIRS). Patients with snoring (*n* = 7, apnea-hypopnea index [AHI] = 2 ± 2/h); mild SDB (*n* = 7, AHI = 14 ± 8/h, range); and severe obstructive sleep apnea syndrome (*n* = 5, AHI = 79 ± 20/h) were studied. NIRS data associated with different respiratory events (obstructive apnea and hypopnea) were averaged for each patient. Subsequently, corresponding cerebral hemodynamic (and peripheral oxygen saturation, SpO₂) relative changes were assessed via integrals adjusted for duration. The relative changes in brain tissue parameters (concentrations of oxyhemoglobin [O₂Hb], deoxyhemoglobin [HHb], and total hemoglobin [tHb]) were significantly larger during obstructive apneas than during hypopneas.[42]

In light of these observations, it is not surprising that snoring and SDB have been associated with the onset of cerebrovascular events at night and strokes that are apparent on awakening (so-called wake-up strokes).[23,46-48]

Sleep-Disordered Breathing as a Risk Factor for Stroke: Chronic Effects

Chronically, SDB and even habitual snoring are associated with hypertension, which is a major risk factor for stroke. In the Wisconsin sleep cohort, an AHI of greater than 15 was independently associated with a threefold increased risk for developing new hypertension within a 4-year period.[49] In a prospective cohort study of 1889 participants without hypertension, Marin and colleagues found an increased risk for incident hypertension within a 12-year period in patients with an AHI of 5 or greater who were ineligible for CPAP therapy (OR = 1.33, 95% CI = 1.01 to 1.75), among those who declined CPAP therapy (1.96; 95% CI = 1.44 to 2.66), and among those nonadherent to CPAP therapy (1.78; 95% CI = 1.23 to 2.58), whereas the risk was lower in patients with AHI of 5 or greater who were treated with CPAP therapy (0.71, 95% CI = 0.53 to 0.94).[50] Importantly, these effects were independent from changes in body weight.

SDB is associated also with coronary heart disease, myocardial infarction, heart failure, and atrial fibrillation, all of which are also risk factors for stroke.[51,52]

Several observations support the hypothesis that SDB worsens atherogenesis. The intima media thickness of the common carotid artery is increased in SDB patients compared with controls matched for age and vascular risk factors.[53] Patients with SDB have increased arterial stiffness, a recognized marker of cardiovascular risk and long-term morbidity.[54]

A few studies have shown that CPAP produces reductions in mean arterial blood pressure. Pepperell and colleagues reported that therapeutic CPAP reduced mean arterial blood pressure by 2.5 mm Hg, whereas subtherapeutic CPAP levels increased blood pressure by 0.8 mm Hg. Such an effect could reduce stroke risk by about 20%.[55] Although the effects of CPAP on hypertension and cardiovascular events are debated, CPAP has been shown to reduce blood pressure in OSA patients with cardiovascular disease or multiple cardiovascular risk factors.[56,57] Treatment with CPAP also can improve other detrimental hemodynamic, neural, and molecular effects of SDB such as factor VII clotting activity, fibrinogen levels, and platelet activation or aggregation.[58]

Sleep-Disordered Breathing as a Consequence of Stroke

Although patients at risk for cerebrovascular disease frequently have SDB before they experience a stroke, some develop SDB as a consequence of stroke. The observation that recovery from stroke may be accompanied by improvement of nocturnal respiratory parameters indirectly supports the hypothesis that SDB can worsen or may even appear de novo after stroke (see earlier). Several factors may be involved.

First, CSB was traditionally attributed to CO_2 hypersensitivity secondary to bilateral and severe strokes with heart failure and a decreased level of consciousness,[59] but subsequent studies have challenged this view.[26,28,60] Changes in ventilatory sensitivity to inhaled CO_2 can also occur in patients with rostrolateral medullary lesions and with unilateral, small strokes of the central autonomic network (including the insula) and without heart failure.[28] Noteworthy, strokes in these areas can also cause acute cardioautonomic changes, including atrial fibrillation.[61] Nonneurogenic factors including older age, left ventricular failure, coronary heart disease, acute caudorostral fluid shifts related to the nocturnal recumbent body position, and carotid stenosis may also contribute to the appearance of CSB.[26,28,62,63] Of note, CSB in the context of asymptomatic carotid stenosis (in 39% of patients in one study) was associated with a shift in sympathicovagal balance secondary to an increased baroreflex and chemoreflex sensitivities in the carotid body.[64]

Second, patients with stroke may have SDB from weak upper airway muscles or poor coordination between upper airway, intercostal, and diaphragmatic muscles due to brainstem or hemispheric lesions that impair cranial nerve function.[65] Accordingly, dysphagia and hypoglossal nerve dysfunction are associated with poststroke SDB.[66,67]

Third, acute brain damage may affect respiratory drive (see earlier).

Finally, other factors such as hypoxemia due to aspiration or respiratory infections, reduction of voluntary chest movements on the paralyzed side, supine position, and sleep fragmentation secondary to stroke or stroke complications can also lead to SDB.

Acute and Chronic Clinical Effects and Consequences

SDB in patients with cerebrovascular disorders can have a variety of detrimental effects. Acutely, SDB detected the first night after brain infarction is associated with early neurologic worsening, longer hospitalization, and detrimental physiologic changes such as higher blood pressure and reductions in cerebral oxygenation[43,47,68,69] Higher blood pressure in the acute phase of stroke is linked with a poorer clinical outcome.

Chronically, habitual snoring and SDB also worsen stroke outcome. A recent systematic review of the effects of SDB on recurrence and death of stroke and TIA patients generally supports a dose-response relationship between severity of SDB and risk for recurrent events and all-cause mortality.[70]

SDB can also worsen functional outcome. Stroke patients with nocturnal oxygen desaturations had a poorer functional outcome than those without desaturations.[71] In 61 patients in a stroke rehabilitation unit, OSA was associated with more functional impairment and longer hospitalization.[72] In a series of 120 stroke patients, those with an AHI of more than 10 within 24 hours of stroke onset had worse functional outcome (as assessed by the Barthel Index) and higher mortality at 6 months.[73] Similarly, in a study of 60 patients, patients with an AHI of more than 15 had a poorer functional outcome at 6 months.[74] More recent studies have shown that SDB may negatively affect clinical outcome within the first weeks after stroke onset.[75-77]

Diagnosis

Based on SDB's impact on stroke outcome and treatability, the American Heart Association and American Stroke Association now recommend that assessment of SDB should be considered in all patients with TIA and stroke.[2] On a practical level, screening and treatment of SDB in stroke patients are also cost-effective.[78]

The suspicion of SDB should be particularly high in obese male patients with a history of habitual snoring, witnessed apneas, hypertension, diabetes mellitus, and sleep-onset/wake-up stroke.[15,23,47] In clinical practice, asking the patients and relatives about sleep-related breathing symptoms (using, e.g., the Berlin Questionnaire) and excessive daytime sleepiness preceding the onset of stroke was shown to be helpful.[79,80]

Bedside assessment of sleep breathing can provide more accurate estimates of SDB. Different forms of unattended respirography or polysomnography (e.g., AutoSet, ApneaLink, and LifeShirt) may be sufficiently accurate to diagnose SDB and estimate its severity even in the acute setting.[19,23,69,81] Full polysomnography is eventually needed only in a minority of patients.

The optimal timing of sleep studies after stroke or TIA is unknown. Although studies within days of a stroke might be less representative of the patient's baseline, treatment of SDB soon after stroke could potentially minimize further brain injury and improve outcome.

Treatment of Sleep-Disordered Breathing

Treatment of SDB in stroke patients can be a clinical, technical, and logistical challenge. Treatment strategies should always include prevention and early treatment of secondary complications (e.g., aspiration, respiratory infections, pain) and cautious use or avoidance of alcohol and sedatives that may worsen breathing during sleep. Patient positioning in the acute phase can improve oxygen saturation and reduce severity of OSA by 20%.[82-84] In heart failure patients, a lateral sleeping position was shown to reduce the severity of central sleep apnea.[85]

The effect of supplemental oxygen in the acute phase after stroke is unclear.[86] Even the most recent guidelines of the European Stroke Organization and American Heart Association/Stroke Association, while pointing to the necessity to keep oxygen saturations above 92% to 94%, do not specify how to measure or correct nocturnal oxygen saturation.[87] In a recent trial of SDB patients, oxygen was found to be inferior to CPAP in reducing blood pressure levels in patients with high cardiovascular risk.[57]

Initial reports questioned the feasibility and utility of treatment with CPAP and other nocturnal ventilator devices in stroke patients. Based on a review of the 26 studies published until December 31, 2014 including a total of 901 treated patients, we recommend a more optimistic approach to treatment (see later).

Treatment of Obstructive Sleep-Disordered Breathing

CPAP is usually the treatment of choice for obstructive SDB, but CPAP compliance can be a challenge because most patients with stroke and SDB lack excessive daytime sleepiness and may not perceive much benefit from CPAP. In addition, stroke patients may have trouble using CPAP if they have dementia, delirium, aphasia, anosognosia, pseudobulbar or bulbar palsy, or severe motor impairment.

Initially, CPAP studies were mainly performed in the subacute phase of stroke (>1 month after onset). In a study of 105 stroke patients treated in a rehabilitation unit, CPAP was accepted by 70%, and poor acceptance was associated with aphasia and severe stroke. CPAP use over 10 days led to an improvement of subjective well-being and lower night-time blood pressure values.[88] CPAP compliance was poor (29%) over the first month of treatment in a series of 51 patients,[89] but over the next 18 months, CPAP use was associated with a five times reduction in vascular events. In a subsequent study, 5-year mortality was reduced in 28 stroke patients with mild to moderate SDB (AHI ≥20) who were treated with CPAP compared with 68 patients with SDB who did not tolerate treatment.[90]

More recently, several studies have examined the feasibility and effects of CPAP treatment started in the acute setting. Sandberg and colleagues reported a good effect on depressive symptoms even when CPAP was started within 2 to 4 weeks from stroke onset.[91] First series emphasized poor CPAP compliance in this clinical setting (ranging from 12% to 22% in patients followed for 2 to 60 months).[22,23,92,93] Recent studies on this topic reported better compliance when CPAP treatment was begun in the first one to three nights after hospitalization. These better results may have arisen from careful selection of patients, the use of new respiratory devices (including adaptive servoventilation [ASV] machines) and headgears, higher motivation and instruction of the treating teams, and frequent contact with patients.[75,94] One randomized trial showed a favorable effect on stroke severity (National Institutes of Health stroke scale) in patients treated with auto-CPAP within 48 hours of hospitalization.[75] In 45 patients with acute TIA, auto-CPAP had acceptable adherence and reduced the risk for recurrent stroke 82% over a treatment period of 90 days.[95] In stroke patients treated within 24 hours with CPAP, stroke severity was improved in those using CPAP more than 4 hours/night.[77] In the largest study thus far, Parra and colleagues reported an improved 1-month neurologic recovery and fewer cardiovascular events by 24 months in 71 patients with moderate to severe SDB (AHI ≥20) started on CPAP within the first 3 to 6 days after stroke onset compared with 69 untreated SDB patients.[81] At 5 years, the treated SDB patients also had better survival than the untreated SDB stroke group.[96]

Treatment of Central Sleep-Disordered Breathing

In patients with mainly central apneas and CSB, breathing disturbances can be improved with oxygen and possibly also lateral sleeping position (see earlier). Clinical experience and a few studies suggest that adaptive ASV may be effective in poststroke CSB and central sleep apnea patients, including those nonresponsive to conventional CPAP.[97]

Tracheostomy and mechanical ventilation may become necessary in patients with central hypoventilation, central apneas, and ataxic breathing.

Hiccups can be treated with neuroleptics or baclofen.

In sum, current data suggest the feasibility of CPAP and ASV treatment in patients with poststroke obstructive and central SDB with an acceptable compliance even when diagnosis and treatment take place in the acute setting. Further studies are needed to better define the best approach in different patient subpopulations according to type and severity of SDB and interval after the acute cerebrovascular event.

SLEEP-WAKE DISTURBANCES AND STROKE

Epidemiology

Sleep-Wake Disturbances and Short Sleep Duration as Risk Factors for Stroke

Several studies have linked insomnia with increased risk for cardiovascular events and death.[98,99] Two meta-analyses have confirmed that short sleep duration (≤6 hours) slightly increases the risk for ischemic stroke (OR = 1.2, 95% CI = 1.0 to 1.3).[100,101] A large study of 21,438 Asian insomniac patients and 64,314 matched noninsomniac patients found a 54% higher risk for stroke over a 4-year follow-up period.[102] Another large study of 30,934 U.S. subjects reported that

short sleep duration (<5 hours) independently increased the risk for stroke 61%.[103] This increase in risk may be due to an increase in sympathetic activity secondary to sleep loss and fragmentation and recurrent arousals with consequent hypertension and impaired glucose metabolism.[104,105]

Conversely, a few studies have suggested an association between long sleep duration or excessive daytime sleepiness and an increased risk for stroke.[100,101,103,106] In a study of 2088 elderly community residents, more than 44% of the cohort reported no daytime dozing, 47% some dozing, and 9% significant daytime dozing. Compared with those reporting no daytime dozing, individuals reporting significant dozing had a 74% increased risk for ischemic stroke.[106]

Restless legs syndrome (RLS) and periodic limb movements during sleep (PLMS) may also increase the risk for cardiovascular diseases, including stroke.[105,107]

Whether shift work increases the risk for stroke remains controversial.[108]

Sleep-Wake Disturbances in Stroke Patients

Clinical experience and a few studies suggest that SWD are frequent after strokes, but few studies have assessed their prevalence and determinants systematically.

In a series of 100 consecutive stroke patients assessed in the acute phase, 22% had an Epworth Sleepiness Scale score of 10 or higher (excessive daytime sleepiness) or increased sleep need (2 or more hours sleep per 24 hours compared with the prestroke situation).[109]

In a series of 235 patients assessed 0.3 to 2 years after stroke, 46% reported abnormal fatigue (fatigue severity scale ≥4.0).[110] Other studies have suggested similarly high frequencies (up to 70% of patients) of poststroke fatigue, making it the most common SWD in stroke survivors.[110-112]

In a series of 277 consecutive patients evaluated 3 months after stroke, insomnia was reported by 38% of patients, and in 18% of these insomnia patients, their insomnia appeared de novo after stroke.[113] In a recent Brazilian study, insomnia was found in 38% of 40 stroke patients.[114]

In a series of 137 patients assessed 1 month after stroke, RLS symptoms were found de novo in 12% of patients.[115]

Other SWD after strokes include an abnormal transition from wakefulness to sleep and vice versa, with dream-reality confusion (oneiric state), dream changes, and an altered perception of time (Zeitgefühl).[116,117]

Clinical Features, Pathophysiology, and Treatment

Hypersomnia and Excessive Daytime Sleepiness

After a stroke, some patients may require more sleep (hypersomnia) and or have excessive daytime sleepiness (EDS). Reduced arousal because of lesions involving the ascending arousal pathways is the most common cause of poststroke hypersomnia.[109] The most severe and persistent hypersomnia occurs in patients with bilateral lesions of the thalamus (Figure 31-4), subthalamic and hypothalamic area, tegmental midbrain, and pons (Figure 31-5), where fibers of the ascending arousal pathways are bundled and can be severely injured even by single small lesions. Hypersomnia after hemispheric stroke (Figure 31-6) usually occurs with large lesions, on the left more than on the right, and anteriorly more than posteriorly.[118-121] In large hemispheric strokes, loss of arousal and coma can occur with injury to the upper brainstem secondary to brain edema and herniation.

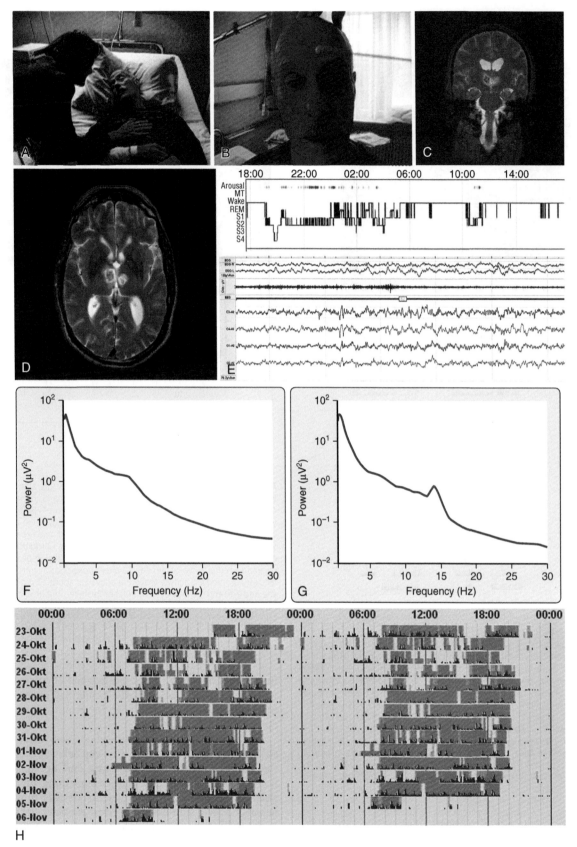

Figure 31-4 Hypersomnia after bilateral paramedian thalamic stroke. This 65-year-old man had initial coma, followed by severe hypersomnia **(A)**, vertical gaze palsy **(B)**, amnesia, and disturbed time perception (Zeitgefühl). Brain magnetic resonance imaging (MRI) showed bilateral paramedian thalamic strokes **(C, D)**. Polysomnography 12 days after stroke onset demonstrated a drastic reduction of sleep spindles **(E)** and loss of spindle peak **(F)** (12 to 14 Hz activity) on spectral analysis (compared with a normal control **[G]**). Severe central apnea (apnea-hypopnea index, 54/hr, >90% central) was observed in the acute phase (in the absence of any signs of cardiac dysfunction) but not on follow-up a few months later. Actigraphy performed in the first month after stroke shows time "asleep" (rest or sleep) was 61% of the recording time (2 weeks) **(H).** One year after stroke, the patient still reported increased sleep need (15 hours per day), apathy (athymormia), and attentional and memory deficits. Modafinil at a dose of 200 mg per day improved his hypersomnia. (MRI pictures courtesy of Professor A. Valavanis, Institute of Neuroradiology, University Hospital, Zürich, Switzerland.) (From Bassetti CL, Hermann DM. Sleep and stroke. In: Vinken PJ, Bruyn GW. *Handbook of Clinical Neurology: Sleep Disorders.* New York: Elsevier; 2010.)

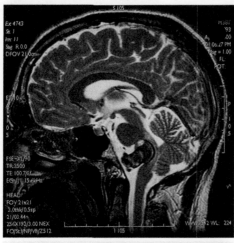

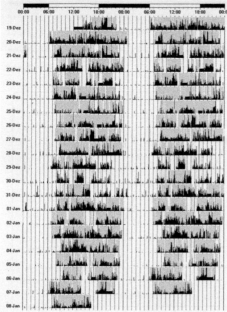

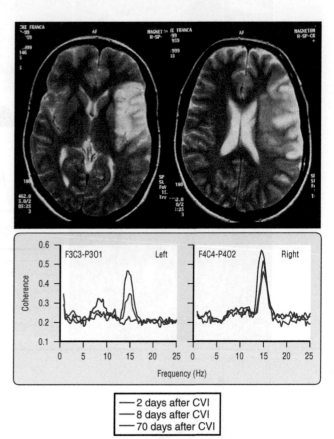

Figure 31-6 Hypersomnia and altered sleep architecture after middle cerebral artery stroke. This 39-year-old woman had aphasia, right hemiparesis, depressed mood, and crying spells. National Institutes of Health stroke score was 16. Before her stroke, the patient slept 7 hours/day, but in the first 1 to 2 weeks after her stroke, she slept 12 hours/day and had mild excessive daytime sleepiness (Epworth Sleepiness Scale score of 12). At 12 months, the patient reported an improvement in sleep need to 10 hours/day. Repeated polysomnograms on day 2, day 8, and day 70 after stroke demonstrated progressive recovery of spindling activity (coherent activity at about 12 Hz) over both the affected (left) and the unaffected (right) hemisphere. CVI, chronic venous insufficiency. (MRI pictures courtesy Professor G. Schroth, Institute of Neuroradiology, University Hospital, Bern, Switzerland.)

Figure 31-5 Hypersomnia and excessive daytime sleepiness after pontomedullary stroke. This 39-year-old man had pontomedullary ischemia following subarachnoid hemorrhage and embolization of a giant aneurysm of the basilar artery. This resulted in a brainstem syndrome with hiccups; left IX, X, XII palsies; dysarthria; gait ataxia; and mild left hemiparesis. Sleep symptoms postintervention were severe excessive daytime sleepiness (Epworth Sleepiness Scale score of 23/24) and increased sleep need (12 to 14 hours/day). Polysomnography showed sleep efficiency 97%, slow wave sleep 8% of total sleep time, no sleep apnea, and no periodic limb movements in sleep. The Multiple Sleep Latency Test showed mean sleep latency of 1 minute and no sleep-onset rapid eye movement periods. Actigraphy showed that time "asleep" (rest or sleep) was 43% of the recording time (2 weeks). Cerebrospinal fluid levels of hypocretin-1 were normal. (MRI pictures courtesy Professor A. Valavanis, Institute of Neuroradiology, University Hospital, Zürich, Switzerland.)

Hypersomnia has occasionally been documented polysomnographically in patients with thalamic, mesencephalic, and pontine strokes.[122-124] Such strokes may cause initial coma or, conversely, manic delirium, hyperalertness, and insomnia before hypersomnia evolves. Mental arousal seems to be affected more severely by medial lesions, whereas motor arousal (including spontaneous motor activities) is impaired more strongly by lateral lesions.[125,126]

In patients with strokes that injure arousal pathways or the paramedian thalamus, hypersomnia may alternate with insomnia (see earlier). For example, one 78-year-old patient with a tegmental mesencephalic infarct had severe, persistent hypersomnia accompanied by an inversion of the sleep-wake cycle with nocturnal agitation.[127]

With deep (subcortical) hemispheric and thalamic strokes, patients may exhibit so-called presleep behavior, during which they yawn, stretch, close their eyes, curl up, and assume a normal sleeping posture, while complaining of a constant sleep urge.[128] Some of these patients are able to control this behavior when stimulated or given explicit, active tasks to perform. This "presleep behavior" may be compulsive in that removal of the patient from bed can result in repeated attempts to lie down and adopt a sleeping posture. However, during what appear to be daytime sleep periods, relatively quick responses to questions or requests suggest wakefulness. For this peculiar dissociation between lack of autoactivation (spontaneous engagement in mental and motor activities) in the presence of preserved heteroactivation (mental and motor activities secondary to external stimulation), Laplane suggested the term *athymormia*, or "pure psychic akinesia."[129]

In some patients, hypersomnia evolves to extreme apathy with lack of spontaneity and initiative, slowness, poverty of movement, and catalepsy, a condition for which the term *akinetic mutism* was coined. Akinetic mutism, and its less severe form—usually referred to as *abulia*—may persist despite normalization of vigilance or even after appearance of insomnia. Some of these patients are eventually diagnosed to have poststroke fatigue (see later) or poststroke depression.

Narcolepsy-like phenotypes (with, however, atypical or questionable cataplexy) are rare with strokes but can occur in the absence of HLA positivity and cerebrospinal fluid hypocretin-1 deficiency. One 23-year-old patient had hypersomnia from bilateral diencephalic strokes; his hypocretin-1 levels were low, suggesting a link between poststroke hypersomnia and deficient hypocretin neurotransmission.[130]

Treatment of poststroke hypersomnia is often difficult, but improvements have been reported with amphetamines, modafinil, methylphenidate, and dopaminergic agents.[109,123] Bromocriptine may improve apathy and presleep behavior.[128] Treatment of an associated depression with stimulating antidepressants may also improve poststroke hypersomnia. It is noteworthy that a favorable influence on early poststroke rehabilitation was reported for both methylphenidate (5–30 mg/day, 3 weeks' trial) and levodopa (100 mg/d, 3 weeks-trial), an effect that may be partially related to improved arousal.[131,132]

Fatigue

A continuum exists among hypersomnia, depression, and fatigue, which is defined as a feeling of physical tiredness, exhaustion with lack of energy accompanied by a strong desire for sleep with usually normal or (paradoxically decreased) sleep propensity. Fatigue may be more common with brainstem strokes.[133] The Epworth sleepiness scale can sometimes help differentiate fatigue from EDS.[134]

An overlap exists between poststroke fatigue and poststroke depression. Psychological stress in coping with stroke probably plays an important role, as suggested by the absence of a correlation between poststroke fatigue and stroke size and site and by a similarly high frequency of fatigue after myocardial infarction (without brain damage).[135] Some have proposed that poststroke fatigue is caused by dysfunction of arousal and attentional circuits.[133] Activating antidepressants and amantadine can be tried for poststroke fatigue.[136] One study reported no benefit with fluoxetine.[137]

Insomnia

On rare occasions, strokes can cause insomnia directly, presumably through disruption of sleep mechanisms. One patient with a pontomesencephalic stroke had almost complete insomnia for more than 2 months.[138] Two patients with locked-in syndrome due to pontomesencephalic or bilateral basal pontine strokes had almost no sleep for more than 1 month.[139,140] Patients with caudate or subcortical (Figure 31-7), thalamic, thalamomesencephalic, and tegmental pontine stroke can have insomnia accompanied by an inversion of the sleep-wake cycle, with insomnia and agitation during the night and hypersomnia during the day.[138,140-142]

Aside from the brain damage, other factors may contribute to poststroke insomnia, including anxiety, dementia, medical disorders (e.g., heart failure, pulmonary disease), SDB, psy-

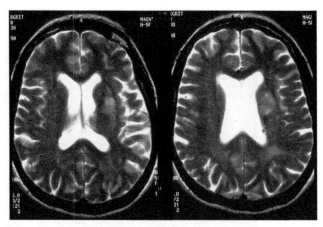

Figure 31-7 Insomnia after subcortical stroke. This 68-year-old woman had a left subcortical stroke in the corona radiata, with mild right motor hemiparesis. National Institutes of Health stroke score was 6. In the first poststroke week, she had almost complete insomnia and excessive daytime sleepiness (EDS). Two weeks later, her EDS was improved and she was sleeping 2 to 3 hours/night. Sleep-wake functions normalized after 4 weeks. (MRI pictures courtesy Professor G. Schroth, Institute of Neuroradiology, University Hospital, Bern, Switzerland.)

chotropic medications, infections and fever, inactivity, environmental disturbances, stress, and depression.[113]

Treatment of poststroke insomnia should focus on behavioral measures such as placing patients in private rooms at night, protection from nocturnal noise and light, and mobilization with exposure to light during the day. If necessary, one could consider temporary use of hypnotics that are relatively free of cognitive side effects, such as zolpidem, zopiclone, and some benzodiazepines.[143,144] Still, these substances should be used cautiously because they can cause delirium and worsen neurologic deficits.[145]

Sleep-Related Movement Disorders and Parasomnias

REM sleep behavior disorder (RBD) has been reported to occur after strokes in the tegmentum of the pons.[146-148]

RLS has been observed de novo after stroke.[149-152] In a recent series of 137 patients with stroke, RLS was found mainly after pontine, thalamic, basal ganglia, and corona radiata strokes.[115] Most commonly, RLS was bilateral, appeared within 1 week after stroke, and was accompanied by PLMS in sleep.

After stroke, PLMS can worsen (and even appear de novo) and lead to insomnia (Figure 31-8). PLMS may also occur after unilateral hemispheric and spinal strokes.[105,153]

Hallucinations and Altered Dreams

Patients with strokes in the pons, midbrain, or paramedian thalamus may experience peduncular hallucinosis, characterized by complex, often colorful, dreamlike visual hallucinations, particularly in the evening and at sleep onset (Figure 31-9).[154-157] Peduncular hallucinosis may represent a release of REM sleep mentation. It can be associated with insomnia and usually resolves spontaneously within a few days.

The Charles Bonnet syndrome generally involves less complex visual hallucinations that also occur in the setting of diminished arousal. These hallucinations maybe limited to a hemianopic field and may be a "release phenomenon" in response to the lack of sensory input.[158,159]

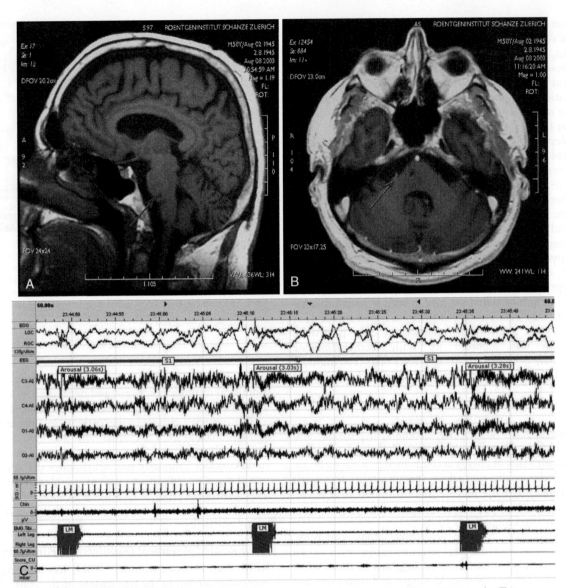

Figure 31-8 Insomnia and left-sided periodic limb movements after right paramedian pontine stroke. This 60-year-old man had a unilateral lacunar stroke in the right paramedian pons (**A** and **B**). He acutely developed severe insomnia, with involuntary, jerky, and tremorlike movements of the left leg and arm appearing intermittently at sleep onset and during sleep (periodic limb movements [LM]) (**C**). The patient denied restless legs symptoms. (MRI pictures courtesy Professor A. Valavanis, Institute of Neuroradiology, University Hospital, Zürich, Switzerland.)

Cessation or reduction of dreaming occurs in the Charcot–Wilbrand syndrome and is occasionally limited to alteration of the visual component of the dream.[160,161] This syndrome can occur in patients with parietooccipital, occipital, or deep frontal strokes, and the lesions are often bilateral.[162-165] Patients frequently show a deficient revisualization (i.e., an impairment to picture again something seen that was previously seen), topographic amnesia, and prosopagnosia. Conversely, REM sleep characteristics may be normal.[164] Severe insomnia and loss of dreaming have been reported with lateral medullary stroke.[142]

Focal (temporal) seizures secondary to stroke can lead to the syndrome of dream-reality confusion or to recurrent nightmares, which may be more frequent with right-sided lesions and can be controlled with antiepileptics.[166]

An increased frequency or vividness of dreaming may occur after stroke, particularly with thalamic, parietal, and occipital strokes.[162]

A few patients with severe motor deficits may report the persistence of seemingly normal motor function within their dreams for up to several years after stroke. Waking up in the morning is a source of great distress in these patients. In other patients, motor handicap may, conversely, be apparent in incorporated in dreams within a few days of stroke onset.

Clinical Significance of Sleep-Wake Disorder after Stroke

Considering the strong evidence that sleep promotes neuroplasticity and the importance of neuroplasticity in recovery after brain damage, it is possible that good quality sleep may

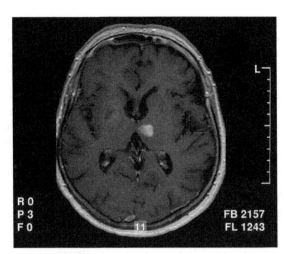

Figure 31-9 Dreamlike hallucinations after unilateral paramedian thalamic stroke. This 62-year-old woman had a left paramedian thalamic stroke and presented with confusion, abulia, anomia, and moderate to severe amnesia in the absence of major sleep-wake disturbances. In the first few days after stroke, the patient had recurrent episodes of visual and acoustic hallucinations in the form of human figures (mostly relatives, partial insight) seen on the right side of the visual field, which the patient described as dreamlike. At 7 months after stroke, the patient had persistent memory problems and reported almost daily episodes of psychic hallucinations ("sensed presence") and a disturbed time perception (Zeitgefühl). On polysomnography, she had no significant changes in rapid eye movement sleep. (MRI pictures courtesy Professor A. Valavanis, Institute of Neuroradiology, University Hospital, Zürich, Switzerland.)

improve outcome after stroke. However, the evidence thus far is only indirect.

Several studies have shown that SWD disturbances after stroke are associated with cognitive and psychiatric (depression, anxiety) disturbances and worse outcome.[113,124,167-169] Fatigue at 2 years after stroke has been found to predict institutionalization and mortality.[170] Poststroke RLS also predicts a worse outcome at 3 and 12 months.[171] In humans, sleep between rehabilitation sessions was recently shown to positively influence motor recovery and learning.[172]

In animal models of stroke, sleep deprivation and fragmentation worsened stroke evolution and outcome, whereas sleep-promoting drugs improved functional outcome.[173-176] Sleep deprivation and disturbance in rats worsens functional recovery from stroke and underlying neuroplasticity processes.[177,178] Although the exact underlying molecular mechanisms remain unclear, axonal sprouting and synaptogenesis were significantly inhibited in rats that underwent sleep deprivation during the acute phase of stroke.[178] Conversely, sleep-promoting drugs such as γ-hydroxybutyrate and baclofen were found in both mice and rats to improve functional outcome and neuroplasticity after stroke.[173]

SLEEP ARCHITECTURE CHANGES

Abnormalities in sleep macrostructure and microstructure are common after acute stroke but result only in part from acute brain damage. Changes in sleep architecture depend on (1) health before the stroke (e.g., age, respiratory disturbances); (2) topography of the lesion; (3) complications of stroke (e.g., SDB, fever, infections, cardiovascular disturbances, depression, anxiety); (4) medications; and (5) time after stroke onset. Even acute myocardial infarction patients without brain damage

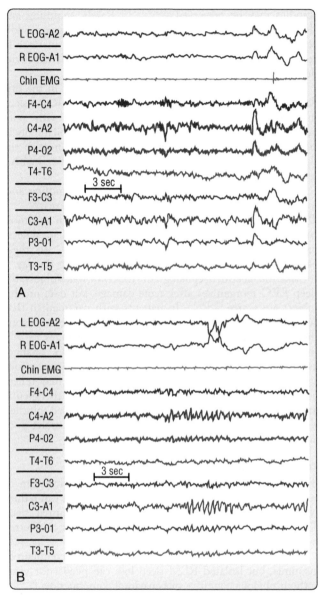

Figure 31-10 Sleep spindles and sawtooth waves after severe middle cerebral artery stroke. This 58-year-old man had a moderately severe left middle cerebral artery stroke (Scandinavian Stroke Scale score, 33/58). Polysomnography 9 days after stroke showed mild obstructive sleep apnea (apnea-hypoxia index = 16). **A,** In NREM sleep, spindling decreased ipsilaterally, with three spindles per hour recorded at C3 and 172 per hour at C4. **B,** In rapid eye movement sleep, sawtooth waves were symmetrical.

who are admitted to an intensive care unit often have decreases in total sleep time, sleep efficiency, REM sleep, and slow wave sleep.[179]

Some changes in sleep architecture are more specifically related to brain damage, such as persistent alterations of spindling and slow wave sleep with supratentorial strokes and REM sleep abnormalities with infratentorial stroke.

Supratentorial Strokes

Reductions in NREM sleep, total sleep time, and sleep efficiency can follow acute supratentorial stroke.[180-186]

Reduced spindling can be observed with thalamic and cortical-subcortical strokes (see Figure 31-4; Figure 31-10).[168,187-190] With unilateral thalamic strokes, sleep spindles may be preserved.[124,168,183,191] Rarely, spindling and slow wave sleep increase in the acute stage of large middle cerebral artery stroke.[182,189,192] In some cases, the increase in scored slow wave sleep may reflect an increase in delta activity during both sleep and wakefulness.[185,193]

Transient reductions in REM sleep can occur in the first days after supratentorial stroke.[183,189] Changes in REM sleep may persist after large hemispheric strokes with poor outcome.[182,186] Sawtooth waves can be decreased bilaterally in large hemispheric strokes, especially those that involve the right side.[183,194] Cortical blindness has been associated with a reduction of rapid eye movements.[195]

Paramedian thalamic strokes often reduce spindling and, to a lesser degree, slow wave activity and K-complexes.[124,168,191] These strokes can produce severe hypersomnia with an almost continuous state of light NREM stage 1 sleep, perhaps reflecting an inability to produce full wakefulness.[124] In these patients, REM sleep can occur at night and during the day.[124]

Like the electroencephalogram (EEG) of wakefulness, the sleep EEG reorganizes after acute damage, but data on this subject are scarce.[186,196,197] In patients with paramedian thalamic stroke, recovery from hypersomnia may occur despite the persistence of significant NREM sleep changes.[124,168,198] In hemispheric stroke, conversely, sleep EEG changes usually recover over time, even in patients with severe stroke (>50 mL in volume).[184] Some of these changes may reflect neuroplasticity during functional recovery and therapeutic interventions.[197,199,200] Low sleep efficiency, decreased spindles, K-complexes, slow wave sleep, and REM sleep predict poor outcome when found after hemispheric strokes.

Infratentorial Strokes

Bilateral, paramedian infarcts in the pontine tegmentum or large bilateral infarcts in the ventrotegmental pons can reduce NREM and, especially, REM sleep.[122,201-206] Normal sleep EEG features such as sleep spindles, K-complexes, and vertex waves may be completely lost.[202,207]

Patients with abnormal sleep architecture may complain of insomnia, but isolated REM sleep loss can persist for years without obvious cognitive or behavioral consequences.[204,208]

Bilateral infarction adjacent to the pontine tegmentum, or unilateral infarction of this area, usually does not alter sleep architecture.[122,207,209]

Occasionally, NREM or REM sleep may be altered selectively. Strokes that affect the pontomesencephalic junction tegmentum and the raphe nucleus can moderately decrease NREM sleep with no major changes in REM sleep.[124,139] Infarctions of the paramedian thalamus and of the lower pons have been associated with absence of slow wave sleep but preservation of REM sleep and appearance of REM sleep at sleep onset.[124,203] In contrast, infarction in the lower pons can cause an almost completely selective decrease in REM sleep.[207] Conversely, midbrain strokes can increase REM sleep.[205,210]

CIRCADIAN ASPECTS AND DISTURBANCES

Ischemic stroke, like myocardial infarction and sudden death, occurs most frequently in the morning hours, particularly after awakening, between 6 AM and noon. A meta-analysis of 31 publications reporting the circadian timing of 11,816 strokes found a 49% increase in stroke of all types (ischemic stroke, hemorrhagic stroke, TIA) between 6 AM and noon.[211] Another study reported that thrombotic, lacunar, and embolic strokes are 20% to 30% more frequent in the morning.[212] Possible explanations for this pattern have focused on circadian or postural changes in platelet aggregation, thrombolysis, blood pressure, heart rate, and catecholamine levels that occur with awakening and resumption of physical and mental activities.[213] In addition, the most prolonged REM sleep period, during which autonomic system instability is known to occur,[214-216] occurs close to awakening. The highest incidence in the early hours of the morning can be overestimated because of patients who awaken with stroke. Treatment with aspirin does not modify the circadian pattern of stroke onset.[217,218]

Whereas intracerebral and subarachnoid hemorrhages rarely occur at night, 20% to 40% of ischemic strokes present at night.[219] This suggests that sleep may represent a vulnerable phase for a subset of patients with cerebrovascular disease, and clinicians should consider evaluation for SDB.

Acute brain infarction—particularly when the right hemisphere and the insula are affected—can disturb normal circadian variation in autonomic functions (e.g., heart rate, blood pressure, temperature control) and breathing and contribute to increased poststroke cardiovascular morbidity.[28,220-226] Acute stroke also may alter other circadian functions such as sleep-related secretion of growth hormone and melatonin.[192,225] A loss of physiologic blood pressure dipping is found in about 50% of patients with acute stroke and predicts a less favorable outcome.[226,227] Hyperthermia can occur with diencephalic strokes and is often associated with a poor prognosis.[228]

CLINICAL PEARLS

- Clinicians should consider SDB and sleep-wake disorders as potential risk factors for stroke as well as modulators of its outcome.
- The study of SDB and sleep-wake functions in poststroke patients offers a unique opportunity to expand our knowledge about the brain mechanisms involved in sleep-wake regulation.

SUMMARY

SDB independently increases the risk for stroke. SDB occurs in 50% to 70% of acute stroke and TIA patients. Although obstructive SDB is more commonly observed, mixed SDB and even central SDB (the latter particularly in the first days after stroke) are also more common in stroke patients than in the general population. In the subacute phase of stroke, SDB (particularly central events) can improve. Treatment of SDB is feasible even in the acute phase and can improve short- and long-term stroke outcome. It remains unclear which treatment should be chosen for which patients, with which severity of SBD, and at which interval after stroke.

Sleep loss or insomnia, EDS, hypersomnia, and RLS are potential risk factors for stroke. These sleep-wake disturbances are also observed in 20% to 50% of stroke victims and negatively affect stroke outcome. Brain damage and stroke complications (e.g., pain, mood changes, immobilization, drugs) are pathophysiologically involved. More systematic data are needed on frequency, characteristics, and management of poststroke sleep-wake disturbances and their effects on stroke outcome.

Sleep EEG changes reflect the topography and severity of stroke but also are influenced by neuroplastic changes during recovery from stroke. High-density sleep EEG may become a sensitive tool not only to monitor brain reorganization after stroke but also the effects of treatment interventions.

Animal experiments support the hypothesis that sleep loss and disturbances negatively affect stroke evolution, and conversely, sleep enhancement (e.g., pharmacologic) may positively influence stroke outcome. The molecular mechanisms involved remain to be elucidated.

Selected Readings

Bassetti C, Aldrich M, Chervin R, Quint D. Sleep apnea in the acute phase of TIA and stroke. *Neurology* 1996;**47**:1167–73.

Bassetti C, Mathis J, Gugger M, et al. Hypersomnia following thalamic stroke. *Ann Neurol* 1996;**39**:471–80.

Birkbak J, Clark AJ, Rod NH. The effect of sleep disordered breathing on the outcome of stroke and transient ischemic attack: a systematic review. *J Clin Sleep Med* 2014;**10**:103–8.

Kim Y, Koo YS, Lee HY, Lee SY. Can Continuous Positive Airway Pressure Reduce the Risk of Stroke in Obstructive Sleep Apnea Patients? A Systematic Review and Meta-Analysis. *PLoS One* 2016;**11**(1):e0146317.

Koo BB, Bravata DM, Tobias LA, et al. Observational Study of Obstructive Sleep Apnea in Wake-Up Stroke: The SLEEP TIGHT Study. *Cerebrovasc Dis* 2016;**41**(5–6):233–41.

Leng Y, Cappuccio FP, Wainwright NW, et al. Sleep duration and risk of fatal and nonfatal stroke. *Neurology* 2015;**84**:1072–9.

Parra O, Arboix A, Bechich S, et al. Time course of sleep-related breathing disorders in first-ever stroke or transient ischemic attack. *Am J Resp Crit Care Med* 2000;**161**:375–80.

Parra O, Sanchez-Armengol A, Capote F, et al. Efficacy of continuous positive airway pressure treatment on 5-year survival in patients with ischaemic stroke and obstructive sleep apnea: a randomized controlled trial. *J Sleep Res* 2015;**24**(1):47–53.

Pearce SC, Stolwyk RJ, New PW, Anderson C. Sleep disturbance and deficits of sustained attention following stroke. *J Clin Exp Neuropsychol* 2016;**38**(1):1–11.

Sarasso S, Santhanam P, Määtta S, et al. Non-fluent aphasia and neural reorganization after speech therapy: insights from human sleep electrophysiology and functional magnetic resonance imaging. *Arch Ital Biol* 2010;**148**:271–8.

Siegsukon CF, Boyd LA. Sleep enhances implicit motor skill learning in individuals poststroke. *Top Stroke Rehabil* 2008;**15**:1–12.

Stone KL, Blackwell TL, Ancoli-Israel S, et al. Sleep Disordered Breathing and Risk of Stroke in Older Community-Dwelling Men. *Sleep* 2016;**39**(3):531–40.

Young T, Finn L, Peppard OE, et al. Sleep disordered breathing and mortality: eighteen-year follow-up of the Wisconsin Sleep Cohort. *Sleep* 2008;**31**:1071–8.

Zunzunegui C, Gao B, Cam E, et al. Sleep disturbance impairs stroke recovery in the rat. *Sleep* 2011;**34**:1261–9.

A complete reference list can be found online at ExpertConsult.com.

Neuromuscular Diseases

Michelle T. Cao; Christian Guilleminault

Chapter Highlights

- Patients with neuromuscular diseases are at risk for sleep-related problems, including sleep-disordered breathing and sleep hypoventilation, and when most severe, diurnal hypoventilation or respiratory insufficiency.
- Many factors can cause poor sleep quantity and quality in neuromuscular disease.

- The greatest advances in medical treatment of neuromuscular disease patients are in respiratory-related sleep disorders. The use of noninvasive ventilatory support devices has improved morbidity and mortality in this patient group.

Neuromuscular disorders are diseases of the motor unit comprising the lower motor neuron, nerve root, peripheral nerve, myoneural junction, and muscle. Any classification of neuromuscular disease may be somewhat arbitrary, and the astute clinician must keep in mind that the pathologic process may involve several segments of the nervous system and muscle. For example, neuropathies can lead to progressive, peripheral motor and sensory impairment along with autonomic dysfunction. Disorders such as amyotrophic lateral sclerosis (ALS) may progress rapidly toward death, whereas certain chronic polyneuropathies such as Charcot-Marie-Tooth disease, or autonomic syndromes such as familial dysautonomia, may have a slower evolution.

Patients with neuromuscular syndromes are at risk for sleep-related problems. Weakness, rigidity, and spasticity limit movement and posture changes during sleep, leading to discomfort, pain, and disrupted sleep. Difficulty maintaining comfortable positions may lead to cramping, abnormal uncontrolled movements, and weakness, which also contribute to poor sleep. Abnormal sphincter control may induce nocturia, incomplete emptying or incontinence, constipation, or painful defecation.

Sleep-related changes in respiration put the patient with a neuromuscular disorder at risk by impairing ventilation. Chronic respiratory muscle failure usually develops over years. It may initially present with sleep-disordered breathing (SDB), followed by progression to nocturnal hypoventilation, then diurnal hypoventilation, cor pulmonale, and eventual respiratory failure and end-stage disease. The slow progression of ventilatory failure in some disorders may go undetected for some time and contribute to increased mortality.

Limited attention is paid to the impact of sleep-related issues in this population, particularly because most clinics see a limited number of patients with neuromuscular disorders. Even in specialized neuromuscular clinics, a minority of patients are asked about their sleep problems or have been given a prior sleep evaluation.[1] Moreover, sleep specialists rarely manage the common problems in this population, such as spasticity, sphincter dysfunction, pain, abnormal movement, confusional arousal that can result in sleep fragmentation, insomnia, parasomnias, daytime fatigue, and hypersomnolence. Thus a multidisciplinary approach to treatment should be the standard of care in patients with neuromuscular disorders.

EPIDEMIOLOGY AND GENETICS

Each neuromuscular syndrome has distinct epidemiology and etiology. For example, ALS affects 0.005% of the U.S. population, and multiple sclerosis, a neurodegenerative disorder, affects 0.11%. There are no cumulative prevalence data that include all neuromuscular disorders. Many neurologic disorders, such as maltase deficiency, myopathy, myotonic dystrophy (MD), Rett syndrome, and familial dysautonomia, have a clear genetic origin. Other neuromuscular disorders can be secondary to traumatic, infectious, vascular, malignant, or degenerative diseases.

Although much research has addressed abnormal sleep and breathing in patients with neuromuscular diseases,[2-5] there are few large studies that examine the prevalence of SDB in these patients. One study from New Mexico[1] attempted to gather information from its entire neuromuscular clinic population. Although complete data were available for only 60 patients (20% of the clinic population), the investigators demonstrated that sleep and breathing abnormalities were present in more than 40% of patients.[1] Such a high prevalence is not surprising given the vulnerability of such patients to sleep-related reductions in muscle tone and overall ventilation. Patients with spinal cord injury (SCI) have been better studied. Compared with the normal population, individuals with SCI have significantly greater difficulties falling asleep and subjectively poor sleep; they also frequently require sleeping pill prescriptions, sleep more hours, take more and longer naps, and snore more.[6]

PATHOPHYSIOLOGY

The diaphragm is the major muscle of respiration during wakefulness and sleep. During non–rapid eye movement (NREM) sleep, there is an overall reduction in ventilation due to altered chemosensation and increased impedance of the respiratory system. However, rib cage activity is maintained (albeit reduced), as is diaphragmatic activity. The importance of the diaphragm is particularly evident during rapid eye movement (REM) sleep. During REM sleep, there is postsynaptic inhibition of somatic motor neurons, causing further reduction or complete loss of tone in the intercostals and other muscles of respiration, but the diaphragm is relatively unaffected. Any process affecting the diaphragm, whether a myopathy or a process involving its innervation, can significantly reduce ventilation and oxygenation during REM sleep. In patients with bilateral diaphragmatic paralysis who are dependent on other respiratory muscles for breathing, marked oxygen desaturations can occur during REM sleep.[7,8] The REM sleep-related inhibition of intercostal and accessory muscles leads to profound hypoventilation during this sleep stage. As noted previously, the suppression of accessory respiratory muscle tone is a normal process of REM sleep and is seen in normal subjects.[9-11]

In some genetic neuromuscular disorders, muscle weakness can begin early in development, interfering with normal development of the skull and facial bones. For example, orofacial muscle weakness can affect growth of the maxilla and mandible, resulting in in the "long face" seen in congenital MD.[12] In rhesus monkeys, experimental reduction of nostril size by ligature with consequent impairment of nasal breathing leads to abnormal facial muscle contraction and secondary abnormal orofacial bone growth.[13,14] Similarly in humans, impaired nasal breathing leads to abnormal masseter contractions, consequently limiting orofacial growth.[15] Narrowing of dental arches, reduction in maxillary arch length, anterior crossbite, maxillary overjet, and overall narrowing of the facial skeleton are a result of changes in muscle contractions. These facial skeletal changes decrease upper airway diameter, consequently increasing its collapsibility during sleep.

Depending on the type of neuromuscular disorder, sleep-related breathing abnormalities may present as central apneas, obstructive apneas, nasal airflow limitation, or periods of prolonged hypoventilation, or there may be a combination that renders the neuromuscular patient at times difficult to treat. Sleep disruption with frequent cortical arousals may be due to discomfort with certain positions, muscle spasm, difficulty in clearing secretions, sphincter control, or increase in upper airway resistance from muscle weakness and secondary craniofacial changes. Periods of hypoventilation can contribute to arousals, reduced sleep time, and sleep deprivation from ventilatory and arousal responses to changes in oxygen and carbon dioxide (CO_2) levels. Although these changes may protect ventilation in the short term, over time ventilatory responses to changes in oxygen and CO_2 levels become blunted. This blunting leads to further worsening of hypoventilation, eventually occurring during both wakefulness and sleep.

CLINICAL FEATURES COMMON TO MOST NEUROMUSCULAR DISORDERS

Nonspecific complaints such as increased fatigue, daytime hypersomnolence, or disrupted sleep can be the initial manifestations of a slowly evolving neuromuscular disease of adult onset.[1] Such nonspecific complaints may also be the sole indication of a progressive neuromuscular disorder. Problems with

clearance such as managing saliva or gastric contents can lead to significant drooling, esophageal reflux, or pulmonary infections from aspiration or retained secretions. Impairment of cough mechanisms may further impair the ability to clear secretions.

Autonomic dysfunction may be present in the form of abnormal sensitivity to temperature or pressure, with discomfort related to the use of sheets and blankets. The disease may psychologically affect individuals, leading to anxiety, depression, and insomnia, as can be seen with many other chronic illnesses. Pharmacologic agents that are prescribed in the evening may have alerting effects, whereas others used in the morning may lead to daytime sleepiness. In all, patients with chronic neuromuscular disorders can have many factors disrupting sleep, consequently worsening daytime function and quality of life. The addition of sleep-related problems complicates their already existing neurologic issues.

Neurodegenerative Diseases Involving the Motor Neuron

ALS is a degenerative motor neuron disease involving upper and lower motor neurons, leading to muscle weakness and atrophy throughout the body. Although ALS has not been shown to directly affect the sleep-regulating areas of the brain, it is likely that indirect effects of the disease contribute to sleep disruption.[16-18] Periodic limb movements associated with arousals and SDB may cause sleep disruption in ALS patients. SDB is reported in 17% to 76% of patients with ALS.[19] ALS patients with normal respiratory function, normal phrenic motor responses, and preserved motor units on electromyography may still have SDB with periodic oxygen desaturations independent of sleep stage (REM or NREM).[20] However, respiratory-related sleep disruption is generally not significant until phrenic motor neurons are involved and the diaphragm becomes weak. When there is involvement of the diaphragm, severe hypoventilation and hypoxemia occur during REM sleep, and nearly all of these patients will need some form of ventilatory support. Some ALS patients without any respiratory disturbance or periodic limb movements still experience sleep fragmentation, independent of age. This suggests that other factors contribute to disturbed sleep, such as anxiety, depression, pain, choking, excessive secretions, fasciculation, cramps, and the inability to find a comfortable position or turn oneself freely in bed. Orthopnea, a frequent complaint in ALS, may also contribute to sleep disruption.[17,18]

Spinal Cord Disease

Poliovirus infection targets the nervous system in several ways by injuring cranial motor nuclei and spinal cord anterior horn cells, resulting in acute paresis. As a result, there are many effects on respiration. Abnormalities in central regulation of breathing in patients with acute and convalescent poliomyelitis were described in 1958 by Plum and Swanson.[21] Subsequently, central, mixed, and obstructive apneas have been noted.[22] Sleep and breathing abnormalities are seen not only in patients who are on respiratory assistance (e.g., rocking beds) during sleep but also before ventilatory assistance is initiated.[23] Sleep abnormalities include decreased sleep efficiency, increased arousal frequency, and varying degrees of apnea and hypopnea. After treatment of sleep and breathing abnormalities, many symptoms frequently attributed to the postpolio syndrome do improve. Although not all symptoms can be explained,[24] excessive daytime sleepiness and fatigue can be explained by poor sleep quality related to abnormal respiration during sleep.[25]

Poliomyelitis can alter central and peripheral respiratory function decades after the acute infection, an important element of postpolio syndrome.[24] Muscle atrophy and immobility can lead to kyphoscoliosis and restricted ventilation. The anatomic deformities resulting from poliomyelitis may cause chronic pain and consequent sleep abnormalities. Also, bulbar involvement may affect upper airway muscles. SDB is reported in 31% of patients with postpolio syndrome.[24] Prolongation of REM sleep latency may result from prolonged recruitment time related to damaged neurons in the pontine tegmentum.[26]

Inherited metabolic diseases such as subacute necrotizing encephalomyelopathy (Leigh disease) typically appear in childhood and may be associated with respiratory disturbance. Rarely, this disease may appear in adulthood with respiratory failure during sleep.[27] Syringomyelia can be associated with central, mixed, and obstructive apneas when it involves the bulbar and high cervical neurons.[28] Malformations of the skull base or high cervical junction (platybasia, Chiari malformations) may cause both central and obstructive types of sleep apnea.[29]

SCI has dramatically increased in frequency over the past 30 years owing to an increase in traffic accidents and military conflicts. Incidence rates are highest in the second to fourth decades of life, and with improvements in long-term supportive care providing longer life expectancy,[30] the prevalence of SCI is destined to grow in the coming years. Overall, morbidity and mortality are higher with cervical and high thoracic spinal cord lesions, especially in ventilator-dependent individuals.[31-33] In a Stockholm, Sweden, epidemiologic survey,[6] muscle spasm, pain, paresthesias, and voiding problems were reported as the most important causes of sleep disturbance.

Gastrointestinal problems related to autonomic dysfunction are more often considered secondary problems. Gastrointestinal motility is also affected, and reflux is common.[32,33] In tetraplegic patients, the higher the spinal cord lesion, the more significant the impairment, not only with diaphragm, intercostal, and abdominal muscle weakness but also with impaired cough and other reflexes for laryngeal and lung clearance.[32,33] All of these elements together can impair breathing, especially during sleep.[33,34] High cord lesions can interrupt pathways to the superior cervical sympathetic ganglion that regulate melatonin secretion.[35,36]

Pharmacologic agents used by patients with SCI (antispasmodic, analgesics, drugs for autonomic dysfunction, psychoactive substances) can also disrupt sleep and wakefulness. An important feature seen in cervical lesions is progressive ventilatory impairment during sleep noted between the 15th day and the 13th week after the injury, often after the patient has been released from an acute care setting. Such worsening may lead to a higher percentage of deaths during sleep, as reported in a cohort of patients with mid to lower cervical SCI during this time period.[37]

Polyneuropathies

The most common polyneuropathy associated with SDB is Charcot-Marie-Tooth disease.[38] It is characterized by chronic degeneration of peripheral nerves and roots, resulting in distal muscle atrophy that begins at the feet and legs and later

involves the hands. SDB can occur in these patients as result of a pharyngeal neuropathy leading to upper airway obstruction (obstructive apnea, upper airway resistance syndrome)[39] or with diaphragmatic dysfunction.[40] Autonomic neuropathy, particularly when secondary to type 1 diabetes, may be associated with impaired chemosensitivity to CO_2, although the effects on sleep and breathing are inconsistent.[41]

Neuromuscular Junction Diseases

Myasthenia gravis (MG) is a disorder of the neuromuscular junction characterized by weakness and fatigability of skeletal muscles. Sleep breathing abnormalities can occur as a result of diaphragmatic or pharyngeal weakness. Risk factors for the development of sleep-related ventilatory problems in patients with MG include age, restrictive pulmonary syndrome, diaphragmatic weakness, and daytime hypoventilation.[42] Younger patients with a shorter duration of illness are less likely to experience sleep-related hypoventilation or hypoxemia,[43] whereas older patients with increased body mass index, abnormal total lung capacity, and abnormal daytime blood gases are more likely to develop hypopneas or apneas, particularly during REM sleep.[44] Sleep apnea was diagnosed in 60% of patients with MG even when the disease was in a clinically stable stage.[45,46] A prospective study by Nicolle and colleagues found that obstructive sleep apnea (OSA) was the predominant abnormality, occurring in 36% of MG patients, with significant associations with older age, male gender, elevated body mass index, and corticosteroid use.[47]

Other neuromuscular disorders that can disturb sleep include congenital myasthenic syndromes,[48] botulism, hypermagnesemia, and tick paralysis. Taking a careful history is extremely helpful in making the diagnosis in these circumstances. Dyspnea that worsens with activity, morning headache, paroxysmal nocturnal dyspnea, fragmented sleep, and daytime somnolence are among the symptoms that suggest SDB in these syndromes.

Muscle Diseases

Myotonic Dystrophy

MD is an autosomal dominant disorder that causes myotonia, muscle weakness, and daytime sleepiness. In this illness, there is consistent involvement of facial, masseter, levator palpebrae, sternocleidomastoid, forearm, hand, and pretibial muscles; MD is, in a sense, a distal myopathy. However, pharyngeal and laryngeal muscles may also be involved, as well as respiratory muscles, in particular the diaphragm.

Central nervous system abnormalities also occur in MD, causing excessive daytime sleepiness by different mechanisms.[12,48-51] For example, neurodegeneration in the dorsomedial nuclei of the thalamus can lead to a medial thalamic syndrome characterized by apathy, memory loss, and mental deterioration. Loss of 5-hydroxytryptamine (serotonin) neurons of the dorsal raphe nucleus and the superior central nucleus,[52] as well as dysfunction of the hypothalamic hypocretin-orexin system,[53] can result in short sleep latencies and sleep-onset REM periods on the Multiple Sleep Latency Test.[49,50] Excessive daytime sleepiness occurs in 33% to 77% of MD patients.[54]

Involvement of the respiratory muscles may result in SDB, including alveolar hypoventilation predominantly in REM sleep,[55-58] obstructive apneas,[59] and central apneas.[60] However, the development of SDB abnormalities in MD is not simply caused by muscle weakness. When patients with MD were compared with patients with nonmyotonic respiratory muscle weakness, periods of hypoventilation and apneas (central and obstructive) occurred at higher frequencies in those with MD than in nonmyotonic patients who had the same degree of muscle weakness (measured by maximal inspiratory and expiratory pressures).[61] This finding suggests that changes in the central nervous system control of respiration contribute to abnormal breathing in patients with MD.

Similarly, decreased ventilatory responses to hypoxia and hypercapnia[62-64] and extreme sensitivity to sedative drugs suggest a central origin of the breathing impairments in MD. The differential diagnosis requires further testing. A standard technique for assessing control of respiration is to study the increase in ventilation as a response to increased arterial CO_2. However, when respiratory muscles are weak, as in MD, it may be difficult to interpret a reduced ventilatory response. That is, chemoreceptor activity and efferent signaling to respiratory muscles may be intact, but weak or inefficient respiratory muscles may not produce a normal ventilatory response to a hypercapnic or hypoxic stimulus. Another method of assessing impairment of respiratory center output is measurement of mouth pressure developed at the beginning of a transiently occluded breath (occlusion pressure, $P_{0.1}$).[65] In patients with MD, $P_{0.1}$ may be as high or higher than that of control subjects at rest and during stimulated breathing, although overall ventilation is lower.[63,66] The finding of a high transdiaphragmatic pressure (P_{di}) despite overall lower ventilation suggests that increased impedance of the respiratory system accounts for incomplete transformation into ventilation of normal or increased respiratory center output.

Magnetic stimulation of the cortex, in conjunction with phrenic nerve recordings, can also be used to test the corticospinal tract to phrenic motor neuron pathways and is a reliable method for diagnosing and monitoring patients with impaired central respiratory drive.[67] The use of transcortical and cervical magnetic stimulation demonstrates that greater than 20% of MD patients have impaired central respiratory drive.[68] The finding of neuronal loss in the dorsal central, ventral central, and subtrigeminal medullary nuclei in MD patients with alveolar hypoventilation[69] and the severe neuronal loss and gliosis in the tegmentum of the brainstem[70] also support a central abnormality.

Another problem in MD patients is orofacial growth impairment early in life. Craniofacial muscle weakness can negatively affect bone growth during development, particularly on orofacial muscles that are involved with stimulation of particular growth areas such as the intermaxillary synchondrosis that usually becomes inactive near 15 years of age. As a result of such muscular weakness, development of craniofacial structures in patients with MD is impaired. They experience more vertical facial growth than normal subjects and have more narrowed maxillary arches and narrow palate as measured between the palatal shelves, with deeper depths. These craniofacial changes may contribute to the development of obstructive sleep apnea owing to a smaller maxilla and mandible, consequently restricting the size of the upper airway and leading to upper airway collapse during sleep.

Other Myopathies

Abnormalities in sleep and breathing have been reported in isolated series of patients with various neuromuscular disorders, such as congenital myopathies (nemaline or congenital fiber-type disproportion myopathy)[71-73] or metabolic myopathies (mitochondrial myopathy such as Kearns-Sayre syndrome[74-77] and acid maltase deficiency[78,79]). In all of these cases, there are various alterations in respiratory control and breathing pattern changes, including hypoventilation, obstructive apneas, and central apneas. All genetic myopathies with orofacial weakness have similar risks for impaired bone growth, particularly on the maxilla and mandible, as in MD.[13-15] Severe central sleep apnea and marked hypoxemia, particularly during REM sleep, resulting in hypoxia-induced pulmonary hypertension, excessive daytime sleepiness, heart failure, morning headaches, and rare nocturnal seizures, may be seen in patients with congenital muscular dystrophy.[80] OSA has also been described in Thomsen disease (myotonia congenita).[81]

Myopathies such as Duchenne muscular dystrophy (DMD) can cause restrictive lung disease and chest wall deformities.[82,83] These changes also contribute to ventilatory impairment, fragmented sleep, hypercapnia and hypoxemia (more profound during REM sleep),[84,85] development of deformities, chronic pain, and discomfort. There is a bimodal presentation of SDB in children with DMD, whereby OSA is more common in younger children in the first decade of life.[86,87] In younger children with DMD, OSA can improve with adenotonsillectomy, whereas in older children who have already developed hypoventilation, OSA is better managed with noninvasive ventilation.

Acid maltase deficiency myopathy can cause SDB, with rapid and significant diaphragmatic impairment noted long before the weakness of other skeletal muscles.[88] In fact, SDB and the secondary daytime fatigue may be presenting symptoms of the myopathy.[88]

Facioscapulohumeral muscular dystrophy (FSHD) is an autosomal dominant disease and the third most frequent form of muscular dystrophy, after DMD and MD. Della Marca and colleagues evaluated FSHD patients and found that impaired sleep quality was directly correlated to the severity of the disease.[89] Among 46 FSHD patients, 27 had snoring and 12 reported respiratory pauses during sleep.[89]

DIAGNOSTIC EVALUATION

The evaluation should consider the type of neurologic disorder, the degree of sensory and motor impairment and the resulting disability, the associated autonomic defects, and the impact of the illness on the patient's mood. Understanding the patient's interaction with society and family is an important factor for subsequent treatment decisions. A detailed sleep history is required to outline the severity and type of sleep-related problems. General assessment should also determine the degree of pain and discomfort (particularly in the supine position and during sleep), the presence or absence of sphincter problems and urinary or digestive dysfunction during wake and sleep, and any evidence of autonomic dysfunction already present during wakefulness and suspected during sleep. A number of additional diagnostic tests may supplement the evaluation of sleep in the patient with neuromuscular disease. These include a disability index scale,[1] a sleep disorder questionnaire, and a sleep log or actigraphy (helpful for the investigation of daily rhythms and sleep-wake disturbances during the 24-hour period). The severe respiratory insufficiency questionnaire, a multidimensional health-related quality-of-life instrument, may be used for patients with neuromuscular disorders on assisted ventilation.[90]

Clinicians should carefully look for craniofacial abnormalities, including high and narrow hard palate, teeth crowding, tongue indentations, and Mallampati or Friedman rating scales[90,91] evaluating the size of upper airway. Routine measures of pulmonary function (spirometry, lung volumes, diffusing capacity) and gas exchange (Pao_2 and $Paco_2$) should be performed in all patients at initial presentation. Static lung volume measurements, both upright and after 15 minutes in supine position, often demonstrate significant changes caused by respiratory muscle weakness, particularly diaphragmatic weakness. A forced expiratory volume in 1 second (FEV_1) or forced vital capacity (FVC) less than 40% of predicted, a $Paco_2$ greater than 45 mm Hg, and a base excess of 4 mmol/L or greater may indicate increased risk for sleep-related hypoventilation, and overnight polysomnography should be performed. Supine inspiratory vital capacity measurements of less than 40%, 25%, and 12% will likely result in hypoventilation during REM sleep, full night, and daytime, respectively.[83,92,93]

Overnight polysomnography is the key to a definitive evaluation of sleep and breathing in these patients. Although it can be done in many settings, including at home, in-laboratory evaluation allows additional measures such as video monitoring. More important, measurement of transcutaneous or end-tidal CO_2 allows continuous tracking of overall ventilation during sleep and can help guide the decision for nocturnal ventilatory assistance.

TREATMENT OF SLEEP ABNORMALITIES IN PATIENTS WITH NEUROMUSCULAR DISEASE

The greatest advances in the medical treatment of neuromuscular disorders have been for sleep-related abnormalities.[51] The goal is restoration of normal sleep architecture, with subsequent improvement of sleep, daytime function, and quality of life. Simple measures such as bedding are often overlooked. Specialized beds and mattresses are available with specifications allowing ease of positional changes, avoidance of skin lesions at pressure points, and segmental inflation or deflation (e.g., air mattresses), thus improving autonomic dysfunction, cramps, spastic contraction, and rigidity. Great efforts should be made to diminish pain and discomfort of any type. Treatment of abnormal behavior and confusional arousals may necessitate use of sedatives such as benzodiazepines, but such therapy should be considered only after careful evaluation of ventilatory function and risk for worsening the sleep-related abnormal breathing.

Judicious use of wake-promoting drugs, such as modafinil or armodafinil, can improve daytime alertness without nocturnal sleep disruption. Prior reports of patients with MD and ALS have shown beneficial effects of modafinil in improving daytime fatigue.[94-104] Baclofen can reduce muscle spasms and help nocturnal sleep but may worsen daytime sleepiness. Treatment of pain with opioids can complicate treatment of SDB by inducing sleep hypoventilation or central sleep apnea. Treatment of abnormal breathing during sleep should be based on polysomnographic findings and should be adjusted with regular follow-up considering clinical symptoms and polysomnographic studies. Various therapies may improve nocturnal hypoventilation or offset the attendant oxygen desaturation.

Supplemental oxygen has been used to alleviate the REM sleep–related oxygen desaturation in patients with DMD but does not clearly improve sleep.[105] Repeated nocturnal hypoxia may worsen muscle weakness, which begets further oxygen desaturation, and reversal of the hypoxemia may arrest the muscle weakness. In one patient with acid maltase deficiency treated with nocturnal oxygen, hypoxemia and muscle weakness did not progress over an 8-year period.[106] Because most of the hypoventilation occurs during REM sleep, pharmacologic suppression of REM sleep with a tricyclic antidepressant is a theoretical option. In a small study of patients with DMD, protriptyline markedly improved the nocturnal oxygen saturation profile.[107,108] However, anticholinergic side effects limit the widespread use of such therapy. Inspiratory muscle training has improved waking respiration in one patient with acid maltase deficiency,[88] with major improvement in the nocturnal oxygen saturation. In general, muscle training is often helpful in neuromuscular patients.[109]

In children, two syndromes have a high prevalence of sleep hypoventilation: DMD and spinal muscular atrophy. Both conditions can cause progressive hypoventilation during sleep and, as the disease progresses, hypoventilation during wakefulness. In this young age group, the appropriate time to begin airway clearance and to introduce noninvasive ventilatory support that can preserve or enhance lung growth and chest wall mobility must be carefully assessed. The presence of an imbalance between mechanical load and the capacity of the respiratory muscles must be evaluated because fatigue may occur, leading to respiratory failure. Inspiratory muscle training can significantly improve respiratory parameters after 1 month of training.[110-112] Children with impaired orofacial bone development as a consequence of abnormal muscle contractions secondary to the genetically induced generalized muscle dystrophy may benefit from myofunctional reeducation (i.e., orofacial muscle exercises aiming at improving suction, mastication, swallowing, and nasal breathing).[113-115]

Noninvasive Positive Airway Pressure

Mechanical ventilation has been a mainstay in supporting ventilation since the days of the poliomyelitis epidemic. Rocking beds, negative-pressure tank ventilators, positive-pressure ventilation through tracheostomy, and cuirass ventilation have been long-term options in the past.[116] However, all of these options are cumbersome, severely limit the mobility of patients, and in the case of tracheostomy, may have unwanted complications. Therefore other forms of assisted ventilation have been developed, including phrenic nerve pacing,[117] and noninvasive positive-pressure ventilation devices.[118,119]

Positive airway pressure devices, including continuous positive airway pressure, bilevel positive airway pressure with or without backup respiratory rate (a noninvasive positive-pressure ventilation device), and the advanced devices targeting minute ventilation by way of pressure support have been used to treat hypoventilation of various causes. Treatment of hypoventilation requires adequate delivery of tidal volume and maintaining minute ventilation to effectively eliminate CO_2, therefore illustrating the limitations of continuous positive airway pressure in treating hypoventilation. Because bilevel positive airway pressure acts as a noninvasive ventilator and supports ventilation, it also treats CO_2 retention, which is commonly seen in patients with advanced neuromuscular disorders. Low-flow oxygen can be bled into the nasal mask during nocturnal sleep to maintain adequate oxygenation if needed.

In the past two decades, noninvasive positive-pressure ventilation has improved the natural course of neuromuscular disorders, and it is often the treatment of choice. Noninvasive positive-pressure ventilation has been shown to improve quality of life and increase survival in neuromuscular disorders.[120-128] In postpolio syndrome, the median time for prolongation of life expectancy is more than 20 years. In patients with spinal muscular dystrophy types 2 and 3, DMD, and acid maltase deficiency, the median improvement in life expectancy is 10 years. In MD, the median improvement in life expectancy is 4 years, and in ALS it is 1 year.[120,121,124] Compared with ventilation through tracheostomy, noninvasive positive-pressure ventilation through nasal interfaces and portable ventilators is becoming the preferred means of assisting ventilation because it is much simpler to administer, is more comfortable, and reduces costs.

Nocturnal noninvasive positive-pressure ventilation had been used predominantly for patients with postpoliomyelitis and other neuromuscular disorders. With eradication of poliomyelitis in most of the world, ALS has become the most common neuromuscular disorder for which noninvasive positive-pressure ventilation is used. In ALS patients with orthopnea, maximum inspiratory pressure less than 60% of predicted, or symptomatic daytime hypercapnia, noninvasive positive-pressure ventilation significantly improved quality of life, sleep-related symptoms, and survival in those without severe bulbar dysfunction.[120] These improvements were greater than those achievable with any currently available pharmacotherapy. Therefore a trial of noninvasive positive-pressure ventilation in ALS patients is warranted even in those with severe bulbar dysfunction for palliative reasons.

Bilevel positive airway pressure therapy is an effective treatment for a number of neuromuscular diseases and in early stages of the disease may be as effective as an invasive conventional ventilator. However, patients may need better control of their hypoventilation during sleep and require more ventilatory support, particularly with progressive muscle weakness. Advanced noninvasive positive-pressure ventilation devices are available specifically for treatment of hypoventilation during sleep by targeting tidal volume or minute ventilation (e.g., average volume assured pressure support [AVAPS] and intelligent volume assured pressure support [iVAPS]).[129] Because the AVAPS and iVAPS devices adjust pressure support based on the patient's respiratory cycle breath by breath, they adapt to changes in severity of disease and therefore are ideal for sleep hypoventilation or respiratory insufficiency. Adaptive servoventilation, an anticyclic positive airway pressure device, has been considered when opioid intake complicates the clinical presentation because of a high number of central apneas, provided that hypoventilation is not significant.[130,131]

The choice of settings when choosing noninvasive positive-pressure ventilation can influence sleep architecture and quality in patients with various neuromuscular diseases. Tailoring the settings (options available depending on portable ventilator used) to the individual's respiratory effort rather than the usual or default parameters is associated with better nighttime gas exchange, percentage of REM sleep, and sleep quality.[132] The AVAPS mode, for example, requires predetermined tidal volume that is calculated from the patient's ideal body weight, with a recommended 6- to 8-mL/kg of ideal body weight used instead of actual body weight. However, if rib cage and abdominal muscles are weak, the recommended volume setting for the patient may be too high, and pain may develop during chest expansion; in these cases we recommend decreasing the predetermined tidal volume to 6 to 7 mL/kg.

Another parameter that is an important component in the patient's comfort and compliance is the "rise time" (i.e., the speed at which airflow is delivered from expiration to inspiration in 10ths of a second). It should be adjusted based on the severity of thoracic muscle weakness, lung inflation capabilities, and amount of secretion accumulated in the airway. This adjustment may be critical because the patient may not tolerate noninvasive positive-pressure ventilation if the rise time is inadequate for the condition.

In endotracheally intubated patients or those with a tracheostomy, the differential between inspiratory and expiratory positive airway pressure on the ventilator can be wide. However, unlike an endotracheal or tracheostomy tube, the upper airway is not rigid, and as a result there is variability in airway dilator contraction during inspiration due to multiple factors: the degree of local muscle impairment, sleep stage, sleep state, neck position, and narrowing because of anatomic factors (deviated septum, enlargement of nasal turbinates, presence of adenoids and tonsils). If the bilevel "pressure differential" becomes too wide, in the presence of nonlinear flow (turbulence) there will be a greater tendency for upper airway obstruction that translates into airflow limitation (visible when studying nasal flow during polysomnography).[133] We generally keep a differential of 6 cm H_2O to avoid induction of variable abnormal upper airway resistance. Besides determination of appropriate inspiratory and expiratory pressures during overnight polysomnography, the need for a backup respiratory rate may also be assessed if central sleep apnea complicates the picture. The backup rate is commonly set at about 8 to 10 breaths/min but will need adjustment over time based on the severity and evolution of the syndrome. In all, the use of noninvasive positive-pressure ventilation allows patients to return to work and even travel, something previously impossible when constrained by reliance on a rocking bed or the complications of tracheostomy for nocturnal ventilatory support.

Decision to Assist Nocturnal Ventilation

When patients present with disrupted sleep, snoring, excessive daytime sleepiness, and unexplained development of peripheral edema or polycythemia, sleep studies can help characterize a breathing disorder, and the decision to assist with ventilation is generally straightforward, with addition of low-flow oxygen bled into mask if needed. The American Academy of Sleep Medicine has published guidelines for noninvasive ventilation.[134]

Nocturnal noninvasive positive-pressure ventilation should be started when nocturnal hypoventilation is present. Clinical symptoms and physiologic markers of hypoventilation assess disease severity and assist in the decision to initiate nocturnal noninvasive positive-pressure ventilation. Patients usually first develop nocturnal hypoventilation followed by diurnal hypoventilation with associated clinical symptoms, which can lead to acute respiratory failure. Continuous monitoring of arterial CO_2 by end-tidal CO_2 or transcutaneous CO_2

during an overnight sleep study is necessary to document nocturnal hypoventilation, which may occur exclusively during REM sleep. Arterial blood gas and serum chemistry can document daytime hypoventilation with elevated arterial CO_2 ($Paco_2$), low arterial oxygen (Pao_2), relatively normal pH, and high serum bicarbonate. Many clinicians consider starting noninvasive positive-pressure ventilation with an arterial Pco_2 greater than 45 mm Hg and an arterial Po_2 less than 70 mm Hg. An isolated change in nocturnal oxygen saturation alone is insufficient for deciding whether the patient needs ventilatory assistance. However, sustained nocturnal oxygen desaturations may be an indicator of nocturnal hypoventilation.

In summary, there is long-standing consensus[134-136] on the management of severe progressive neuromuscular disorders in which respiratory failure plays a significant part of the natural history of the disease. The positive impact of noninvasive ventilatory support in neuromuscular disease patients has become clear in the past two decades. The most effective time to introduce noninvasive positive-pressure ventilation is when SDB develops, including nocturnal hypoventilation. Issues such as quality of life must be taken into account. Each patient must be assessed in detail, and the clinician must bear in mind that nocturnal (and later, 24-hour) ventilation will treat only one (albeit important) aspect of the disorder.

CLINICAL PEARLS

- Sleep is a vulnerable state for patients with neuromuscular disorders because normal REM sleep–related changes in ventilation are magnified as a result of muscle weakness, resulting in hypoventilation and oxygen desaturation.
- In addition to SDB, sleep may also be disturbed by spasticity, poor secretion clearance, sphincter dysfunction, inability to turn, pain, and autonomic dysfunction. All of these factors can impair sleep and worsen daytime disability.
- Noninvasive ventilation can aid neuromuscular disease patients by reducing morbidity and improving life expectancy.
- The most effective time to introduce noninvasive ventilatory support is when SDB develops, including nocturnal hypoventilation.
- New advanced noninvasive ventilatory equipment, such as AVAPS or iVAPS, is ideal for ventilatory insufficiency in neuromuscular patients because it targets tidal volume or minute ventilation and therefore treats hypoventilation and CO_2 retention.

SUMMARY

Neuromuscular disorders consist of central and peripheral neurologic disorders with impairment of the motor system.

The disability of patients with a neuromuscular disorder worsens during sleep, and the abnormal sleep and secondary impairment of daytime function further degrade quality of life. Nocturnal sleep disruption can result from pain and discomfort related to weakness, rigidity, or spasticity that limits movement and posture. Sleep disruption may also be caused by autonomic dysfunction, poor sphincter control, problems with clearance of secretions, and abnormal movements and behaviors during sleep. Most important, sleep-related hypoventilation is common with neuromuscular disorders, and overlooking this may lead to death. Daytime evaluation will determine the severity of the disability but may not identify the presence and severity of an associated sleep-related disorder. Nonspecific symptoms of daytime fatigue and sleepiness can indicate poor sleep in these patients. Polysomnography with continuous monitoring of CO_2 is the only test that can objectively identify and evaluate the severity of sleep-related disorders as well as ventilatory impairment. By recognizing and treating sleep-related problems, these patients can enjoy improved survival and better quality of life.

Selected Readings

Aboussouan LS. Sleep-disordered breathing in neuromuscular disease. *Am J Respir Crit Care Med* 2015;**191**:979–89.

Alves RSC, Resende MBD, Skomro RP, et al. Sleep and neuromuscular disorders in children. *Respir Physiol Neurobiol* 2009;**169**:165–70.

Begin R, Bureau MA, Lupien L, et al. Pathogenesis of respiratory insufficiency in myotonic dystrophy. *Am Rev Respir Dis* 1982;**125**:312–18.

Berry RB, Chediak A, Brown LK, et al. NPPV Titration Task Force of the American Academy of Sleep Medicine. Best clinical practices for the sleep center adjustment of noninvasive positive pressure ventilation (NPPV) in stable chronic alveolar hypoventilation syndromes. *J Clin Sleep Med* 2010;**6**:491–509.

Bourke SC, Gibson GJ. Sleep and breathing in neuromuscular disease. *Eur Respir J* 2002;**19**:1194–201.

Camacho M, Certal V, Abdullatif J, et al. Myofunctional therapy to treat obstructive sleep apnea: a systematic review and meta-analysis. *Sleep* 2015;**38**:669–75.

Contal O, Janssens JP, Dury M, et al. Sleep in ventilator failure in restrictive thoracic disorders. Effects of treatment with non invasive ventilation. *Sleep Med* 2011;**12**:373–7.

Fermin AM, Afzal U, Culebras A. Sleep in Neuromuscular Diseases. *Sleep Med Clin* 2016;**11**(1):53–64.

Finder JD, Birnkrant D, Carl J, et al. Respiratory care of the patient with Duchenne muscular dystrophy: ATS consensus statement. *Am J Respir Crit Care Med* 2004;**170**:456–65.

Hukins CA, Hillman DR. Daytime predictors of sleep hypoventilation in Duchenne muscular dystrophy. *Am J Respir Crit Care Med* 2000;**161**:166–70.

Selim B, Junna M, Morgenthaler T. Therapy for sleep hypoventilation and central apnea syndromes. *Curr Treat Options Neurol* 2012;**14**:427–37.

Shneerson JM, Simonds AK. Noninvasive ventilation for chest wall and neuromuscular disorders. *Eur Respir J* 2002;**20**:480–7.

Udd B, Krahe R. The myotonic dystrophies: molecular, clinical, and therapeutic challenges. *Lancet Neurol* 2012;**11**:891–905.

A complete reference list can be found online at ExpertConsult.com.

Obstructive Sleep Apnea in Older Adults

Barbara A. Phillips

Chapter Highlights

- The prevalence of obstructive sleep apnea (OSA) increases with age, but the peak prevalence of clinically diagnosed OSA is in middle age. Differences in the clinical presentation, severity, and manifestations of obstructive sleep-disordered breathing between older and younger persons probably account for much of the gap in diagnosis.

- More than half of older adults report sleeping difficulty.[1-5] Because sleep complaints are common in the older age group, clinicians may discount them. Sleep complaints in seniors, however, correlate with health complaints, depression, and mortality.[1-6] Undiagnosed OSA probably accounts for some of the sleep complaints voiced by older adults. Indeed, OSA leads both to sleep disturbance and to increased mortality and is likely to account for much of the association between sleep complaints and adverse outcomes in older people. Despite this, sleep-disordered breathing is woefully underdiagnosed and undertreated in the older adult population.

- Accumulating data indicate that continuous positive airway pressure use is associated with reduced cardiovascular morbidity, cognitive dysfunction, and all-cause mortality in seniors; clinicians caring for geriatric patients should consider sleep-disordered breathing in the older adult with sleep complaints. This chapter focuses on OSA in the older patient. For discussion of central sleep apnea, see Chapters 12 and 15.

EPIDEMIOLOGY AND DEFINITIONS

Although studies of clinical populations identify peak prevalence of clinically significant sleep-disordered breathing in middle age, population-based studies have shown that sleep-disordered breathing increases with age.[7,8] Longitudinal and cross-sectional studies also have shown that the prevalence of sleep apnea increases with increasing age[9-13] (Table 33-1).

Estimates of the prevalence of obstructive sleep apnea (OSA) in older people depend on how it is defined, so prevalence estimates for OSA in older people are moving targets. Indeed, there has been considerable variation in the definitions and measurements of respiratory events (such as apneas, hypopneas, and respiratory effort–related arousals used to identify sleep-disordered breathing, even since the last edition of this text. Furthermore, which respiratory events to "count" toward the threshold used to define "sleep apnea" has also varied. The apnea-hypopnea index (AHI) typically includes only apneas and hypopneas, but the respiratory disturbance index (RDI) may include other events, such as respiratory effort–related arousals, or may be defined on the basis of recording time rather than sleep time. Finally, the demarcation between "normal" and "abnormal" also has been somewhat fluid. In population-based studies, approximately one third of those older than 65 years of age have AHIs of 5 or more events per hour of sleep,[14,15] and some two thirds have RDIs of 10 or more events per hour.[15,16] Although measures of sleep-disordered breathing events alone do not establish a diagnosis of OSA, the classically associated symptoms of the disorder—sleepiness, hypertension, cognitive dysfunction—increase in prevalence with aging. Thus a majority of older persons who meet laboratory-defined numeric criteria for OSA also will have a clinical symptom that is commonly associated with the syndrome; for this reason, defining clear-cut criteria for sleep apnea in older persons is difficult. However, the Centers for Medicare and Medicaid Services, the primary provider of health care coverage for people older than 65 in the United States, defines OSA as an AHI 15 or greater, or an AHI of greater than 5 plus hypertension, stroke, sleepiness, ischemic heart disease, or mood disorder.[17] The Centers for Medicare and Medicaid Services now covers continuous positive arway pressure (CPAP) therapy as indicated by results of portable monitor testing and requires objective documentation of use for payment beyond the first 90 days.

Regardless of how sleep apnea is defined, its prevalence increases progressively from age 18 to approximately 70, when it may plateau.[18] On the basis of these findings, it is likely that the underdiagnosis of sleep apnea in older people is even more common than in younger people, and this may be especially true in minority populations[18]

Diagnosis of sleep-disordered breathing is evolving rapidly, with revised, more liberal diagnostic criteria[19] and the

Table 33-1	Differences between Younger (<60 years) and Older Patients with Obstructive Sleep Apnea (OSA)	
Risk Factor	Older Patients	Younger Patients
Male gender	1:1	2:1
Obesity	Unimportant	Very important
Clinical features		
Witnessed apneas	Witnessed apneas rarely reported	Witnessed apneas strongly predictive
Snoring	Infrequently reported	Frequently reported
Prevalence		
AHI >5	30%-40%	9% for women, 24% for men
RDI >10	62%	10%
Consequences	Death, cardiovascular disease, stroke, nocturia, impaired cognition, atrial fibrillation	Death, ischemic cardiac disease, hypertension, cerebrovascular disease, depression, metabolic disturbances
Treatment	May require lower CPAP pressures	May require higher CPAP pressures
	No difference in tolerance or adherence	No difference in tolerance or adherence

AHI, Apnea-hypopnea index; CPAP, positive airway pressure; RDI, respiratory disturbance index.

recognition that oximetry alone can be quite predictive of important outcomes. For example, in a study of 100 patients with a mean age of 62 years, Ohmura and associates reported that sleep-disordered breathing, as determined by predischarge pulse oximetry (based on oxygen desaturation index of 4% [i.e., ODI = 4]), was associated with significantly increased risks for necessity for readmission and death, independent of other risk factors.[20] In a study of patients with OSA and matched control subjects, oxygen saturation predicted cognitive function, but AHI did not.[21] In the Spanish Sleep Network study, oxygen desaturation predicted cancer risk, but again, AHI did not.[22] Similarly, time elapsed with oxygen saturation below 90% predicted 3-year mortality in older persons with cardiovascular disease. It also predicted self-reported insomnia.[23] These and other findings are likely to change, yet again, the diagnostic criteria for significant sleep apnea, at least for third-party payers, who are increasingly data-driven.

CLINICAL MANIFESTATIONS AND PRESENTATION

Most studies of the clinical presentation and manifestations of OSA have focused on the middle-aged. Reports derived from clinical populations tend to include people whose mean age is approximately 50. As more data accumulate about sleep-disordered breathing in older people, it is becoming increasingly clear that the phenotype of OSA can be quite different in younger and in older populations.

Perhaps most striking is the change in gender as a risk factor for sleep-disordered breathing with aging. Prospective

data from the Wisconsin Sleep Cohort have demonstrated male sex is no longer an important risk factor for OSA after the age of approximately 50 years,[24] confirming work from other studies.[8] At least part of the reason for this phenomenon is that the prevalence of OSA rises strikingly for women as they go through menopause, which occurs at approximately age 50.[25-27] As a consequence, some investigators have reported a male-to-female ratio of 1:1 for older people.[24]

In addition to the loss of effect of male gender as a risk for OSA with aging, there is reduced importance of obesity as a risk factor. Beginning at approximately 60 years of age, obesity is no longer a statistically significant risk factor for sleep-disordered breathing.[24,26] These observation are of particular interest, in view of known decreases in obesity with increasing age.[28] Some data suggest that obesity is a more important risk factor for men than for women, but that aging, perhaps specifically achieving menopause, is a more important risk factor for women than for men.[24-27,29,30] However, in an 18-year follow-up study of 427 community-dwelling elderly persons, Ancoli-Israel and associates found that observed changes in RDI were associated only with changes in BMI and were independent of age[31]; they pointed out that this finding underscores the importance of managing weight for older adults, particularly those with hypertension.

In a study of nearly 100 community-dwelling adults aged 62 to 91 years, Endeshaw found that almost one third (equally divided between men and women) had an AHI of 15 or more events per hour of sleep, and that the "traditional" risk factors such as snoring, body mass index, and neck circumference were not significantly associated with OSA in this group.[32] Rather, those with an AHI of at least 15 were more likely to report not feeling well rested in the morning and to have higher Epworth Sleepiness Scale scores and a greater frequency of nocturia.[32] These findings confirm earlier work from the Sleep Heart Health Study, which reported that witnessed apneas are much less frequently reported in older patients than in younger ones.[33]

Studies of OSA in older people have tended to report "milder" disease, with lower AHIs, and better-preserved oxygen saturation than in younger adults.[9,14,26]

In short, the "classic" clinical presentation of OSA is uncommon in older adults, which may account in part for the reduced prevalence of clinical diagnosis of the disorder in this population.

PATHOPHYSIOLOGY

The pathophysiology of OSA may be different in older persons from that in younger people. Chapter 13 outlines the pathophysiology of OSA in adults. With aging, loss of tissue elasticity also may contribute to airway collapse. For older women, declining levels of sex hormones appear to be partly responsible for increased collapsibility of the posterior oropharynx.[34,35]

CLINICAL CONSEQUENCES

Overview

A majority of studies of the consequences of OSA have been undertaken in clinical samples of middle-aged people. Data specifically focusing on the consequences of OSA in older persons are limited. OSA has long been associated with increases in the risk of death in younger populations, but early studies suggested that it was not associated with increased mortality in older groups.[36,37] A recent well-done study from the Spanish Sleep Network, however, clearly demonstrated a twofold increase in risk of death in a group of patients with severe OSA (AHI of 30 or greater) whose mean age was 71 years over that in the control group, after initiation of controls for age, body mass index, preexisting cardiovascular disease, smoking, diabetes, sleepiness, gender, dyslipidemia, and/or respiratory failure. Furthermore, CPAP use reduced risk of all-cause mortality, as well as cardiovascular death and death from stroke and heart failure, but did not reduce the risk of death from ischemic disease in this cohort. Indeed, even those seniors 75 years of age and older had reduced risk of cardiovascular death with CPAP use, and continuous adherence was associated with reduced risk of cardiovascular death as a continuous variable.[38] The inclusion of a large cohort with severe sleep apnea (AHI of 30 or higher) probably partly accounts for the ability of this study to demonstrate a mortality effect with sleep apnea and with CPAP. In a meta-analysis of prospective cohort studies of OSA and risk of cardiovascular disease, Wang and colleagues demonstrated a "dose-response" relationship between OSA severity and cardiovascular outcomes and calculated a 17% greater risk of cardiovascular disease for each 10-unit increase in AHI.[39] It is possible that older people tolerate milder degrees of sleep-disordered breathing better than do their younger counterparts, and that part of the past difficulty in demonstrating an association between OSA and adverse outcomes in older patients was because few patients with moderate to severe disease were included in earlier studies.

Other plausible explanations have been proposed for the inability to readily demonstrate the impact of sleep-disordered breathing on cardiovascular outcomes in older people. Lavie and Lavie, for example, speculated that the reduced effect of OSA on mortality in older people is because of ischemic preconditioning resulting from the nocturnal cycles of hypoxia-reoxygenation and pointed out that in patients with sleep-disordered breathing, there is an association of ischemic preconditioning with increased levels of vascular endothelial growth factor and increased production of oxygen reactive species, heat shock proteins, adenosine, and tumor necrosis factor alpha.[40]

Among the most striking manifestations of sleep-disordered breathing in aging populations are nocturia, cognitive dysfunction, and cardiac disease.

Nocturia

Nocturia is a particularly troublesome symptom of aging and appears to be related to the severity of sleep-disordered breathing. Because older adults with significant sleep-disordered breathing may not manifest classic symptoms of OSA, the presence of nocturia in the older patient should heighten clinical suspicion for OSA. Indeed, nocturnal urination more than three times nightly had positive and negative predictive values of 0.71 and 0.62, respectively, for severe OSA in one study.[41]

The postulated mechanism of nocturia in OSA is that the negative intrathoracic pressures resulting from occluded breaths cause distention of the right atrium and ventricle. This right-sided cardiac distention results in release of atrial natriuretic peptide, which inhibits the secretion of antidiuretic hormone and aldosterone and causes diuresis through its effect on glomerular filtration of sodium and water.[42] Several studies have demonstrated symptomatic improvement in patients with nocturia with use of CPAP.[43-45] The mechanism of CPAP-related improvement may involve promoting the normal nocturnal rise in antidiuretic hormone, resulting in increased resorption of sodium and water from the collecting tubules and production of lower volumes of more concentrated urine.[46] In a retrospective review of data on 196 patients whose mean age was 49 years, predictors of nocturia included increasing age and diabetes mellitus. Although a complaint of nocturia was equally likely to occur in patients with and without OSA, nocturic frequency was significantly related to age, diabetes, and severity of sleep-disordered breathing in those patients who had OSA. Furthermore, patients with OSA and nocturia who were treated with CPAP experienced significant reductions in the frequency of nocturnal voiding.[47] In a study of 21 women with a mean age of 65 years, the same group of investigators reported that OSA is present in a majority of women with nocturia, and that the presence of diluted nighttime urine in a patient with nocturia is a sensitive marker for OSA.[48]

Impaired Cognition

Impaired cognition, including sleepiness, impaired vigilance, worsened executive function, and dementia, increases in prevalence with aging. Neuropsychological assessment of patients with OSA demonstrates decline in cognition similar to that with aging. For example, patients with OSA experience sleepiness[49] and demonstrate impaired executive function,[50] working memory,[51] alertness,[52] and attention.[53] In general, the association between sleep-disordered breathing and impaired cognition has been best studied in middle-aged patients. Because of the association with aging itself on impaired cognition, the effects of OSA on cognitive function in older people have been difficult to tease out. In a small study with subjects older than 55 years of age who had OSA, Aloia and associates found that the degree of sleep-disordered breathing, especially oxygen desaturation, was associated with delayed verbal recall and impaired constructional abilities. After 3 months, subjects who were compliant with CPAP showed greater improvements in attention, psychomotor speed, executive functioning, and nonverbal delayed recall than in those who were not compliant.[54] Despite the logical notion that cognitive impairment associated with OSA in older people might be more severe than in younger people because of cumulative effects of age and sleep-disordered breathing, Mathieu and colleagues were unable to demonstrate any group-by-age interaction for any neuropsychological variable; in a study of matched older and younger patients both with and without OSA, they found that performance on most tasks deteriorated with advancing age in both control subjects and patients with OSA without evidence of a compounded effect.[55] Persons at high risk for OSA based on Berlin questionnaire scores (57% of whom were female) had lower cognitive function scores than those without, but the risk was most pronounced during middle age and was attenuated after age 70.[56]

The evidence indicates age- and gender-dependent relationships as well. In a large study of patients with OSA who were at least 40 years old, the risk of developing dementia within 5 years of diagnosis was 1.70 times greater than in age- and sex-matched subjects who did not have OSA, after appropriate adjustment for some potential confounders. In this study, men aged 50 to 59 had a sixfold increased risk of developing dementia compared with matched control subjects, but women 70 years of age or older had a threefold increased risk of developing dementia. One large study reported that sleep-disordered breathing severity was not associated with indices of sleep-related symptoms or sleep-related quality of life in community-dwelling older women, suggesting that this group may be resistant to the adverse effects of OSA on cognition.[57]

In addition to age and gender differences in susceptibility to dementia in patients with OSA, genetic predispositions also are likely. Data from the Wisconsin Sleep Cohort suggest that apolipoprotein E epsilon 4 genotype (APOE4)-positive persons with sleep apnea of moderate severity have impairment of cognition and executive function comparable to that in persons without this genotype.[58] Preliminary work suggests an association between sleep-disordered breathing and Alzheimer disease biomarker in the cerebrospinal fluid of cognitively normal persons.[59] These early data point to genetic influences on the propensity to develop dementia in patients with SDB.

It is likely that many other factors affect susceptibility to cognitive dysfunction in patients with OSA. For example, Alchantis and coworkers have proposed that high intelligence may protect against cognitive decline caused by sleep-disordered breathing, perhaps as a consequence of increased cognitive reserve.[60]

The mechanism by which sleep-disordered breathing impairs neurocognitive function remains incompletely understood. Some investigators have suggested that sleep fragmentation is the primary culprit,[61] whereas others maintain that hypoxemia is the primary cause. It is likely that the functions are affected by hypoxemia differ from those affected by sleep deprivation. As suggested by Sateia, "Disturbances in general intellectual function and executive function show strongest correlations with measures of hypoxemia. Not unexpectedly, alterations in vigilance, alertness, and, to some extent, memory seem to correlate more with measures of sleep disruption."[62] However, in a small study of matched patients with OSA, AHI did not predict or correlate with cognition, but mean oxygen saturation correlated with executive functioning and access to long-term memory.[21]

Kim and associates demonstrated that moderate to severe OSA is an independent risk factor for white matter change in more than 500 people (mean age 59 ± 7.48 years) and presented an excellent discussion of potential mechanisms, including hypoxemia and hypercapnia during apneic events, which activate arousal- and chemoreflex-mediated increases in the cerebral circulation and activation of oxidative and imflammatory processes.[63]

Information about the effects of CPAP treatment on cognition in older people is limited, and data about CPAP's effects on cognition in older persons even more so. In a small group of patients whose mean age was 56 years, CPAP resulted in normalization in attentive, visuospatial learning and in motor performances after 15 days, but no further improvement was observed after 4 months of treatment. CPAP did not improve performance on tests evaluating executive functions and constructional abilities.[64] A meta-analysis

of randomized, placebo-controlled crossover studies of CPAP treatment involving 98 patients with sleep apnea demonstrated mostly trends for better performance on CPAP than on placebo.[65] In a group of middle-aged adults with significant OSA, Zimmerman and associates demonstrated that memory normalized for the group that used CPAP at least 6 hours a night[66] but did not improve in those who were not adherent to CPAP treatment. In a review of CPAP adherence and benefits among older people, Weaver and Chasens noted that in general, older adults demonstrate increased alertness; improved neurobehavioral outcomes in cognition, memory, and executive function; and decreased sleep disruption.[67] These investigators also noted that older persons may require lower CPAP pressures than younger ones and tolerate CPAP well, with similar rates of adherence. Thus despite differences in the clinical presentation and impact of sleep apnea in the elderly population, CPAP treatment is likely to be well tolerated and beneficial in symptomatic patients.[68,69]

With regard specifically to Alzheimer disease, the prevalence of OSA is higher among patients with this disorder than among nondemented seniors, and sleep-disordered breathing is believed to contribute to cognitive dysfunction in those with Alzheimer disease. A randomized double-blind, placebo-controlled crossover trial of CPAP in patients with OSA and Alzheimer disease demonstrated a significant improvement in cognition after 3 weeks of CPAP.[70] In addition to improving cognition, CPAP treatment may reduce sleepiness in patients with Alzheimer disease and OSA.[71]

In view of the facts that improvement in cognition is likely to depend on CPAP adherence, that gender, age, genetic, and intelligence are probable influences on susceptibility to impaired cognition, and that most studies addressing this issue have not included geriatric patients with OSA or objectively measured adherence, firm conclusions about the reversibility of cognitive deficits in older patients woth OSA are impossible at present.

Cardiovascular Disease

In addition to nocturia and cognitive impairment, sleep-disordered breathing also is strongly linked to *cardiovascular disease*, including hypertension, congestive heart failure, stroke, cardiac arrhythmias, ischemic events, and pulmonary artery hypertension.[72] Few studies of the relationship between OSA and cardiovascular disease are prospective and control for confounding variables such as obesity. Even fewer studies have been conducted in older adults. Hypertension, atrial fibrillation, and stroke, however, are particularly relevant comorbid conditions associated with OSA in older patients, because of their higher prevalence and clinical importance in that population.

Hypertension

That sleep-disordered breathing causes *hypertension* has been demonstrated by multiple studies, including prospective and CPAP sham–controlled work.[73-79] Recent data also have established that severe sleep apnea (AHI of 30 events or more per hour) is an independent risk factor for incident hypertension in older people (mean age, 68.2 years).[80] In general, CPAP has modest effects on blood pressure in patients with OSA but is most effective in those who have significant hypertension and are most adherent with its use.[73,81,82]

Atrial Fibrillation

Atrial fibrillation is strongly associated both with aging and with OSA.[72,83] The Sleep Heart Health Study investigators found that persons with severe sleep-disordered breathing had double or quadruple the risk of complex cardiac arrhythmias compared with those with no sleep-disordered breathing, after institution of controls for multiple relevant confounders.[83] In this study, atrial fibrillation was the arrhythmia most strongly associated with sleep-disordered breathing. Gami and coworkers reported that both obesity and nocturnal oxygen desaturation were independent predictors of incident atrial fibrillation, but only in subjects younger than 65 years of age.[84] However, Ganga's group noted that the presence of overlap syndrome (OSA combined with chronic obstructive pulmonary disease) is associated with a marked increase in new-onset atrial fibrillation in elderly patients over that associated with the presence of either OSA or chronic obstructive pulmonary disease alone.[85]

In a small, retrospective study of patients with atrial fibrillation, some of whom had either treated or untreated sleep apnea and some of whom did not have sleep apnea, the patients with untreated OSA had a higher recurrence of atrial fibrillation after cardioversion than that for the patients without sleep apnea.[86] Furthermore, treatment with CPAP in the sleep apnea group was associated with lower recurrence of atrial fibrillation at 1-year follow-up evaluation. This study is particularly relevant for the management of older patients because the mean age of the study population was approximately 66 years. A study of patients undergoing pulmonary vein isolation reported that the 32 patients who had OSA and used CPAP were less likely to have atrial tachyarrhythmias, use of antiarrhythmic drugs, and need for repeat ablations were compared to the 30 patients who did not use CPAP during a follow-up period of 12 months; the difference in atrial fibrillation–free survival rate was 71.9% versus 36.7% ($P = .01$).[87]

As in younger adults, sleep-disordered breathing is associated with subtle measures of myocardial injury. In a large study of patients whose mean age was 62.5 years, OSA severity correlated with measures of high-sensitivity troponin T and N-terminal pro–B-type natriuretic peptide, and high-sensitivity troponin was related to risk of death or heart failure in all categories.[88] Elderly patients with OSA exhibit cardiac structural changes and diminished left ventricular function compared with that in control subjects who do not have OSA.[89] In a nonrandomized, retrospective review of data on 130 patients aged 65 to 86 years, Nishihata and associates demonstrated that those with untreated sleep apnea had increased likelihood of cardiovascular death and hospitalization due to cardiovascular disease, including heart failure, over a follow-up period of approximtely 3 months. Furthermore, adequate CPAP treatment improved the cardiovascular outcomes in this cohort.[90]

Stroke

The prevalence of stroke increases with age, but untreated sleep apnea appears to impose an additive risk. In a 6-year follow-up study of more than 1000 patients whose mean age at enrollment was approximately 60, Yaggi and coworkers found that OSA was a risk factor for stroke, controlling for other important variables.[91] Treatment did not affect the risk of either stroke or death in this study.

A review of the findings in 10 reports that included 1203 patients who had experienced stroke or transient ischemic attacks noted a dose-response relationship between severity of sleep-disordered breathing and the risk of recurrent events and all-cause mortality; 3 of the studies included information about patients who received CPAP, but the data were too limited for a compelling argument that CPAP improves outcome in patients with stroke/transient ischemic attack.[92] In a study of patients with acute cerebral ischemia who underwent polysomnography, Kepplinger and colleagues showed that sleep apnea is associated with clinically silent microvascular brain tissue changes such as leukoaraiosis (white matter hyperintensities) and lacunar infarcts.[93]

In summary, OSA is strongly associated with cardiovascular disease in middle-aged populations, and the accumulating evidence suggests that sleep-disordered breathing increases the risk of cardiovascular disease and stroke in the elderly population. The best-proven association and evidence for benefit is with hypertension, for which the data are derived largely from middle-aged populations.

Other Effects

Sleep-disordered breathing is a systemic problem with systemic consequences. In addition to the adverse outcomes already noted, OSA in elderly persons is associated with multiple potential consequences.

In middle-aged men, OSA is associated with increased health care costs that decrease after treatment. CPAP treatment is cost-effective for treatment for severe sleep apnea in middle-aged people.[94] Within the sleep apnea population, expenditures for health care in older patients are approximately twice as high as they are in middle-aged patients. After adjustments for age, body mass index, and AHI, cardiovascular disease and use of psychoactive drugs were important determinants of health care costs for older patients with sleep apnea in one study.[95] An enormous study of elderly veterans documented that 4.4% (in all likelihood, representing only the "tip of the iceberg") were diagnosed with OSA, and these patients had many more comorbid conditions and much higher health care utilization than those who did not carry the diagnosis.[96]

Sleep apnea also was associated with an increased risk of pneumonia (the "old man's friend") in a large study.[97]

Nocturnal hypoxemia also is associated with increased risk of falls in older men[98] but paradoxically is associated with preserved bone mineral density in elderly men and women, even after adjustment for sex, BMI, metabolic values, and hypertension.[99]

Gender is likely to influence the effects of sleep-disordered breathing in older people, just as it does for younger persons. For example, a significant relationship between sleep-disordered breathing and hypertension, history of diabetes, and low high-density lipoprotein cholesterol has been reported in women older than 65 years of age, but these effects were not demonstrable in older men.[100]

TREATMENT OF OBSTRUCTIVE SLEEP APNEA IN OLDER ADULTS

Continuous Positive Airway Pressure

As with younger adults, CPAP is the treatment of choice in older patients. Because most studies of effects of CPAP have been done in clinical (e.g, middle-aged) populations, evidence for the benefits of CPAP in older persons is not yet robust.

Complex sleep apnea appears to be more prevalent in older than in younger people. *Complex sleep apnea* is characterized as OSA in which central apneas and periodic breathing develop when CPAP is applied.[101,102] This phenomenon appears to be more prevalent in older men with congestive heart failure, and its clinical significance is unclear. In many cases of these "treatment-emergent central apneas," the central apneas will simply resolve over time. In a convenience sample of a variety of sleep-disordered breathing syndromes resistant to CPAP, the mean age of 72 years was much higher than typically observed in clinical populations of sleep apnea patients. In that cohort, adaptive servoventilation appeared to be effective and well tolerated in approximately half.[103] Because complex or treatment-emergent central apnea appears to be more prevalent in older adultss, formal, in-lab titrations may be more important for this group. (For a more detailed discussion of complex sleep apnea, see Chapter 15.) Adherence to CPAP therapy in older patients may be impaired by factors such as cognitive impairment, medical and mood disturbances, nocturia, lack of a supportive partner, and impaired manual dexterity. Older age in itself, however, does not affect adherence to CPAP treatment,[67,104,105] and behavioral interventions can improve CPAP adherence in the elderly.[106] The major predictors of CPAP nonadherence in older patients with sleep apnea are nocturia, current cigarette smoking, lack of symptom resolution, and advanced age at time of diagnosis.[107] Older men with nocturia may find CPAP particularly confining and may be particularly likely to have difficulty with its use, although CPAP may actually help with the nocturia.[104,107]

Patients with OSA who have dementia, including Alzheimer disease, have been demonstrated to tolerate CPAP, although depressive symptoms appear to predict worsened adherence in demented seniors with sleep apnea.[108]

Oral Appliances

Oral appliances are effective in treating snoring and mild to moderate OSA.[109-112] Although not as effective as CPAP, these agents improve sleep-disordered breathing, sleepiness, nocturnal oxygen saturation, and blood pressure. There are two basic types of oral appliances:

1. Mandibular repositioners, which pull the mandible (and with it, the tongue) forward
2. Tongue-retaining devices, which adhere to the tongue by suction and pull it forward. Because these are not approved by the U.S. Food and Drug Administration for treatment of sleep apnea, they are used much less commonly in clinical practice.

See Chapter 19 for a detailed discussion of the use of oral appliances.

Common side effects of oral appliances include dry mouth, increased salivation, tooth soreness, and jaw muscle or jaw joint discomfort. Pain occasionally can be severe enough that patients discontinue the use of the appliance.[112] Bite changes (e.g., the inability to close on the back teeth) combined with heavy contact of the front teeth on removal of the appliance in the morning also are reported, but these changes generally resolve on removal of the device.

Oral appliances can be made to fit over false teeth, although this is not optimal. The use of oral appliances in people who are edentulous may be attempted with a tongue-retaining

device, but these devices are not U.S. Food and Drug Administration-approved, and the efficacy of this approach is unknown. A small prospective study of factors associated with efficacy of oral appliances has suggested that age older than 55 years may be associated with reduced efficacy.[113]

Surgery

As with younger adults, upper airway surgery is not particularly effective treatment for OSA for older patients and may be associated with especially high morbidity in the elderly.[114] However, as in younger patients with significant sleep-disordered breathing in the context of obesity, bariatric surgery, specifically laparoscopic-adjustable gastric banding, has been shown to be well tolerated and reasonably effective in resolving or reducing sleep apnea in people older than 70.[115]

Pharmacologic Treatment

Several medications have been applied to the treatment of sleep-disordered breathing. In general, no drug is effective enough to recommend for use in first-line treatment. Antidepressants, nasal steroids, hormone replacement therapy (HRT), and modafinil all have been studied in younger patients.

More than two decades ago, protriptyline was demonstrated to show modest efficacy in treating apnea, probably because it reduces REM sleep, when apnea is worst.[116] There is some early experimental work with the selective serotonin reuptake inhibitors (SSRIs) in the treatment of sleep apnea, but results have not been promising in humans.[117] SSRIs can suppress REM sleep, but not as much as that seen with the tricyclic antidepressants.

Nasal steroids have been demonstrated to have modest efficacy in the treatment of sleep-disordered breathing.[118]

In the Sleep Heart Health Study, women who were on HRT were less likely to have sleep apnea, but overall lifestyle and health care are significant confounders in drawing conclusions about the efficacy of HRT for OSA.[119] Although estrogen is an option to consider, it would need to be discussed carefully with the patient because of subsequently recognized complications of HRT.

Body Position

The supine position predisposes the sleeper to airway collapse and to reduced lung volume and has long been known to exacerbate OSA; indeed, some affected persons experience obstructive events exclusively when sleeping on their backs.[120-122] Upper airway size decreases with increasing age in both men and women, and upper airway collapsibility with supine positioning increases with age.[122]

In my own clinical experience, position-related obstructive apnea is relatively common among older individuals. Position therapy has not been well studied for any group of patients but shows promise as treatment for the older patient with mild disease.[123]

DRIVING AND THE OLDER PATIENT WITH OBSTRUCTIVE SLEEP APNEA

Untreated OSA is a well-established risk factor for involvement of drivers in motor vehicle crashes (see Chapter 16) and might be expected to affect older drivers as well. In a review of conditions increasing crash risk in older drivers,

Marshall found that several conditions were believed to be associated with increased risk of crash in older persons, including alcohol abuse and dependence, cardiovascular disease, cerebrovascular disease, depression, dementia, diabetes mellitus, epilepsy, use of certain medications, musculoskeletal disorders, schizophrenia, vision disorders, and, finally, OSA. He noted that these "conditions can serve as potential warnings for reduced fitness to drive, but many persons with these medical conditions would still be considered safe to continue driving."[124]

CLINICAL PEARLS

- The clinical presentation of OSA in older adults differs from that in their middle-aged counterparts, so the disorder may be overlooked by clinicians when it manifests in this age group.
- Female gender and obesity are less important risk factors in older people than in younger people.
- Symptoms of sleep apnea change with aging: Whereas the classic symptoms of OSA are witnessed apneas and sleepiness, older patients are more likely to present with sleep complaints, nocturia, and cognitive dysfunction.
- Moderate to severe OSA is associated with increased risk of cardiovascular morbidity and mortality as well as cognitive dysfunction, and CPAP treatment is associated with reduced risk.

SUMMARY

OSA is prevalent and potentially deadly in older people and may be overlooked by clinicians because the clinical presentation is different from that in younger people. Seniors with OSA tend to be "thinner" and are more likely to be female and less likely to report classic symptoms of witnessed apnea, snoring, and fatigue. Because CPAP use is associated with reduced morbidity and mortality in older (as well as younger) people, clinicians need to consider the possibility of OSA in older patients with sleep complaints.

Selected Readings

Ancoli-Israel S, Gehrman P, Kripke DF, et al. Long-term follow-up of sleep disordered breathing in older adults. *Sleep Med* 2001;**2**:511–16.

Chang WP, Liu ME, Chang WC, et al. Sleep apnea and the risk of dementia: a population-based 5-year follow-up study in Taiwan. *PLoS ONE* 2013; **8**:e78655.

Guillot M, Sforza E, Achour-Crawford E, et al. Association between severe obstructive sleep apnea and incident arterial hypertension in the older people population. *Sleep Med* 2013;**14**:838–42.

Holmqvist F, Guan N, Zhu Z, the ORBIT-AF Investigators. Impact of obstructive sleep apnea and continuous positive airway pressure therapy on outcomes in patients with atrial fibrillation-Results from the Outcomes Registry for Better Informed Treatment of Atrial Fibrillation (ORBIT-AF). *Am Heart J* 2015;**169**:647–54.

Jennum P, Tønnesen P, Ibsen R, Kjellberg J. All-cause mortality from obstructive sleep apnea in male and female patients with and without continuous positive airway pressure treatment: a registry study with 10 years of follow-up. *Nat Sci Sleep* 2015;**7**:43–50.

Kushida C, Nichols DA, Holmes TH, et al. Effects of continuous positive airway pressure on neurocognitive function in obstructive sleep apnea patients: The Apnea Positive Pressure Long-term Efficacy Study (APPLES). *Sleep* 2012;**35**:1593–602.

Martinez-Garcian MA, Campos-Rodruigez F, Catalan-Serra P, et al. Cardiovascular mortality in obstructive sleep apnea in the elderly: role of long-term continuous positive airway pressure treatment. *Am J Respir Crit Care Med* 2012;**186**:909–16.

McMillan A, Bratton DJ, Faria R, et al. A multicentre randomised controlled trial and economic evaluation of continuous positive airway pressure for the treatment of obstructive sleep apnoea syndrome in older people: PREDICT. *Health Technol Assess* 2015;**19**(40):1–188.

Peppard PE, Young T, Barnet JH, et al. Increased prevalence of sleep-disordered breathing in adults. *Am J Epidemiol* 2013;**177**:1006–14.

Russo-Magno P, O'Brien A, Panciera T, et al. Compliance with CPAP therapy in older men with obstructive sleep apnea. *J Am Geriatr Soc* 2001;**49**:1205–11.

Stone KL, Blackwell TL, Ancoli-Israel S, et al. Sleep Disordered Breathing and Risk of Stroke in Older Community-Dwelling Men. *Sleep* 2016;**39**(3): 531–40.

A complete reference list can be found online at ExpertConsult.com.

Sleep-Disordered Breathing in Pregnancy

Francesca Facco; Judette Louis; Melissa Pauline Knauert; Bilgay Izci Balserak

Chapter Highlights

- Pregnant women may be particularly predisposed to obstructive sleep apnea and other major sleep-related breathing disorders as a consequence of the physiologic changes associated with the gravid state.
- Sleep-disordered breathing (SDB) symptoms are common during pregnancy and worsen as the pregnancy progresses.
- Outcomes that have been linked to SDB in the nonpregnant population, such as hypertension and insulin-resistant diabetes, have correlates in pregnancy (e.g., gestational hypertension, preeclampsia, gestational diabetes).
- This chapter reviews the physiology that may influence SDB prevalence and severity in pregnancy, the epidemiology of SDB in pregnancy, the possible link between SDB and adverse pregnancy outcomes, and special considerations in screening for and treating SDB in pregnancy.

PREGNANCY PHYSIOLOGY AND SLEEP-DISORDERED BREATHING

The many changes that occur during pregnancy are accompanied by certain alterations in physiology secondary to hormonal, mechanical, and circulatory changes characteristic of the gravid state. A Clinician who examines a pregnant woman for potential sleep-disordered breathing (SDB) needs to be familiar with these pregnancy adaptations; while some changes predispose to SDB, others may protect from it.

Respiratory System Changes that Predispose Pregnant Women to Sleep-Disordered Breathing

Multiple mechanisms lead to anatomic narrowing and increased resistance within the respiratory system during pregnancy. Increased levels of estrogen and progesterone induce capillary engorgement, hypersecretion, and mucosal edema of the upper airway.[1-3] These changes begin early in the first trimester and increase progressively throughout pregnancy. They may lead to a reduction in dimensions of the nasopharynx, oropharynx, and larynx, with consequent increased airflow resistance and an increase in the Mallampati score as pregnancy progresses.[4-6] Furthermore, pregnancy rhinitis is nasal congestion of pregnancy without other signs of respiratory tract infection and with no known allergic cause. This rhinitis results in difficulty breathing and resolves within 2 weeks after delivery. It occurs in up to 42% of women by the third trimester of pregnancy.[1,3]

Increased nasal congestion also may cause increased nasopharyngeal resistance and produce more intrapharyngeal pressure during inspiration. Elevated intrapharyngeal pressure during inspiration contributes to pharyngeal airway narrowing during sleep.[7] The narrowed airway results in snoring and obstructed breathing during sleep. Thus pregnant women are more likely to snore than nonpregnant women, and the prevalence of habitual snoring (on 3 or more nights/week) increases

from the first to the third trimester.[5,8,9] Increased fat deposition within the soft tissue regions of the neck with weight gain of pregnancy also could cause pharyngeal narrowing and predispose affected women to snoring and SDB.[4,5,10,11] Pregnant women with a larger neck circumference and higher baseline body mass index (BMI) report more symptoms of SDB than other women.[4,5,10,12]

In addition, maternal blood volume peaks at 40% to 50% greater over baseline by third trimester. The combination of increased blood volume, interstitial fluid, and recumbent position during sleep displaces fluid, which could adversely affect upper airway patency.[2] Evidence regarding nocturnal displacement of fluid is conflicting. Whereas some studies indicated that nocturnal fluid shifting from the legs into the neck increases susceptibility to or severity of pharyngeal obstruction,[13,14] others reported that such rostral fluid shifts do not increase the frequency of obstructed breathing events.[15]

A compensatory increase in the anterior-posterior diameter of the chest and elevated diaphragm caused by the enlarging uterus result in tracheal shortening and progressive functional residual capacity reductions by 20% to 25%, expiratory reserve volume by 15% to 20%, and residual volume by 22%.[2,16] These alterations can lead to the closure of small airways during normal tidal breathing.[4,5,17] In late pregnancy, airway closure results in ventilation-perfusion mismatch and reduced gas exchange,[18,19] especially in the supine position, owing to gravity, increased intraabdominal pressure, and loss of muscle tone during sleep.[2,4,17,20]

Oxygen consumption and minute ventilation progressively increase during pregnancy by 20% and 30% to 50%, respectively.[2] The increased ventilatory drive may induce obstructive respiratory events by increasing diaphragmatic effort that creates negative inspiratory (suction) pressure on the hyperemic upper airway.[7] Furthermore, higher ventilatory drive, along with resultant respiratory alkalosis, may cause instability in respiratory control pathways, potentially increasing the likelihood of central apnea episodes at sleep onset and during sleep.[2,20,21] However, findings from one recent study suggest that pregnancy does not increase risk for central apnea.[22]

Finally, frequent awakenings due to pregnancy-related discomfort may cause respiratory instability and periodic breathing at sleep onset.[21] The resulting sleep deprivation also can increase arousal threshold, impair upper airway muscle activity, and increase upper airway collapsibility.

Respiratory and Circulatory System Changes that May Protect against Sleep-Disordered Breathing

Several mechanisms that influence respiratory and cardiovascular changes in pregnancy may also lessen risk of apnea or hypopnea episodes. High circulating progesterone during pregnancy may protect the upper airway from obstruction by increasing upper airway dilator muscle (genioglossal) activity and its responsiveness to chemical stimuli (carbon dioxide) during sleep.[23] Pregnancy-related increases in heart rate, stroke volume, and cardiac output with reductions in peripheral vascular may diminish the impact of apneic episodes.[23] Furthermore, as pregnancy advances, women tend to spend less time in the supine position during sleep.[10,24] This may decrease the rate of adverse respiratory events during sleep, as the supine position is frequently associated with increased event rates.[9] However, a recent study reported that 82% of women spend some time sleeping in the supine position in the second and third trimesters of pregnancy.[25]

EPIDEMIOLOGY OF SLEEP-DISORDERED BREATHING IN PREGNANCY

A majority of studies evaluating the prevalence of SDB have been carried out in middle-aged nonpregnant women populations. General population studies have estimated that obstructive sleep apnea (OSA), occurs in 2% to 25% of middle-aged adults in the community, but certain populations are at greater risk,[26,27] particularly the obese and morbidly obese.[28-30] Among reproductive-age women, epidemiologic studies suggest a 2% to 13% prevalence of SDB, with higher rates in certain populations of women.[30,31] For example, among 420 premenopausal women with sleep complaints who were referred for polysomnography (PSG) sleep studies, SDB was present in 70% of those younger than 30 years and in 83% of those older than 30 years of age. Their apnea-hypopnea index (AHI) indicated that younger women had less severe SDB (AHI of 15.5 ± 22) than women older than 30 years of age (AHI of 22.4 ± 34.6).[32] Findings also suggested that SDB is common in pregnancy and worsens as pregnancy progresses.[9,33-35]

Frequent snoring during pregnancy has been well characterized, and studies have consistently demonstrated that SDB symptoms, including snoring, increase as pregnancy progresses.[8,36,37] The prevalence of pre-pregnancy snoring has been reported to be 7% to 11%.[8,36,37] By the third trimester, frequent snoring ranges from 16% to 25%.[8,36-38] Using the apnea symptom score from the Multivariable Apnea Prediction Index, one study found that SDB symptoms increased significantly from the first trimester to the month of delivery, and the increase in symptoms was not limited to snoring but included gasping, choking, difficulty breathing, and apneic events.[9] In this study, 11.4% of the participants reported an apnea symptom score increase of 2 units or more, consistent with a clinically significant increase in symptoms; these

women also experienced a significant increase in subjective sleepiness compared with other women.[9]

Epidemiologic data on the prevalence of objectively assessed SDB are more limited. Olivarez and colleagues[39] performed sleep studies in 100 hospitalized pregnant women, admitted for a variety of obstetric and nonobstetric complications. The mean gestational age at the time of the sleep study was 32 weeks, and these investigators reported a 20% incidence of SDB (AHI of 5 or greater).[39] Louis and associates[40] used ambulatory sleep monitoring to assess SDB in 175 obese women at an average of 21 weeks' gestation. The prevalence of SDB was 15.4%, and most cases were mild (AHI of 5.0 to 14.9).[40]

Two studies have reported serial assessments of SDB across pregnancy.[12,41] Pien and colleagues[12] studied 105 women (28% normal weight, 24% overweight, and 50% obese). SDB was present in 10.5% of their subjects during the first trimester (median, 12 weeks). By the third trimester (median, 33.6 weeks), 26.7% had SDB.[12] Facco and associates[41] studied 128 high-risk pregnant women with one or more of the following risk factors: obesity, chronic hypertension, presentational diabetes, previous preeclampsia, and twin pregnancies.[41] Early SDB assessments were performed at 6 to 20 weeks of gestation (mean, 17 weeks) and late-pregnancy SDB assessments were performed at 28 to 37 weeks of gestation (mean, 33 weeks). In early pregnancy the frequency of mild, moderate, and severe SDB was 12%, 6%, and 3%, respectively, and these rates increased to 35%, 7%, and 5% in late pregnancy (Figure 34-1). Of the 128 women, 34 (27%) experienced a worsening of SDB during pregnancy; of the women so affected, 26 had new-onset SDB, and the other 8 had SDB in early pregnancy that became more severe. The incidence of new-onset SDB was 20%, and most of these new-onset cases were mild.[41]

Of note, all of the studies objectively assessing SDB in early or late pregnancy reported that most cases are mild

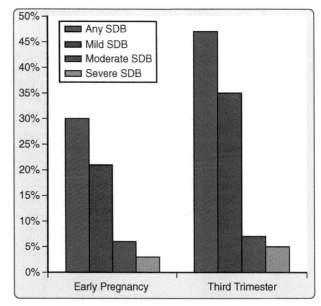

Figure 34-1 Trends in sleep-disordered breathing (SDB) across pregnancy in a high-risk cohort: early pregnancy (6 to 20 weeks), third trimester (32 to 37 weeks). (From Facco FL, Ouyang DW, Zee PC, Grobman WA. Sleep disordered breathing in a high-risk cohort: prevalence and severity across pregnancy. *Am J Perinatol* 2014;31:899–904.)

forms of SDB. Generalizability from these studies is limited, however, because they all studied high-risk populations. Pien et al attempted to correct for this limitation by using BMI distribution for all women screened for their study to estimate SDB among the general obstetrical population from which their subjects were recruited.[12] These investigators then estimated SDB prevalence in their sample at 8.4% (95% CI, 5.6% to 11.9%) in early pregnancy and 19.7% (95% CI, 15.6% to 24.4%) in the third trimester.

Risk factors for SDB in pregnancy have not been well characterized. Pre-pregnancy BMI, age, and chronic hypertension are known risk factors for SDB outside of pregnancy and are also associated with SDB in early pregnancy.[12,41] Excessive gestational weight gain is theorized to be a risk factor for developing new-onset SDB in pregnancy, but epidemiologic data supporting this theory are lacking. Facco and colleagues[41] reported that twin gestation is associated with increased risk of developing new-onset SDB in pregnancy. Although women with twin pregnancies in their cohort, as expected, had greater weight gain, weight gain did not significantly differ between women who developed new-onset SDB and women who did not. Similarly, Pien and colleagues[12] also reported that gestational weight gain was not associated with third-trimester SDB. Maternal weight gain and weight distribution may play a role in incident SDB in pregnancy, but assessing this variable by merely measuring total weight gain may be inadequate. Other measures such as changes in neck circumference, body fat composition, and trajectory of weight gain in relation to baseline BMI warrant further study as risk factors for incident SDB in pregnancy.

SLEEP-DISORDERED BREATHING AND ADVERSE MATERNAL OUTCOMES

Potential Mechanisms for Adverse Maternal Outcomes

Any underlying mechanistic pathway linking sleep disturbances and adverse outcomes for the mother is likely to be multifactorial.[42] Dysregulation of pregnancy adaptations to the cardiovascular, metabolic, and immune systems can make women vulnerable to complications.[43,44] Even small changes in sleep parameters and subtle obstructive respiratory events could exacerbate these adaptations and increase risk for adverse outcomes. SDB causes oxidative stress, autonomic dysfunction, inflammation, and altered hormonal regulation of energy expenditure.[45] These same pathways are associated with adverse pregnancy outcomes.[46,47] Figure 34-2 is a conceptual model depicting potential pathways linking SDB and pregnancy complications.

Oxidative stress, a consequence of intermittent hypoxia-reoxygenation cycles in SDB, plays a pivotal role in development of hypertensive disorders of pregnancy, inducing proinflammatory cytokines that trigger further oxidative stress, sympathetic activation, and endothelial dysfunction.[48] Increased oxidative stress also is linked to development of gestational diabetes.[49] In an animal model of SDB, gestational exposure to hypoxia was associated with increased pancreatic beta cell proliferation, cell death, impaired fetal growth, and hyperlipidemia.[50,51]

SDB leads to sympathetic nervous system and hypothalamic-pituitary axis activation.[52-54] Disproportionate sympathetic

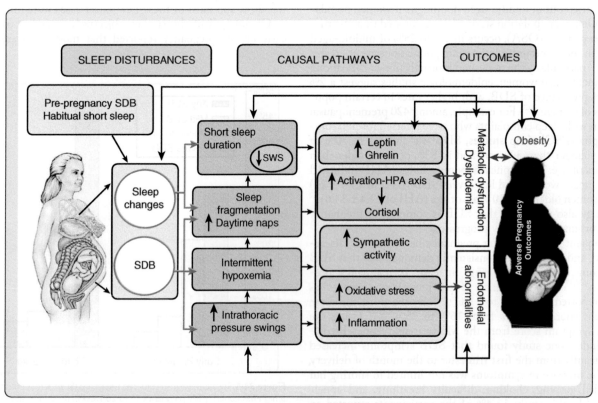

Figure 34-2 Schematic illustration of potential causal pathways linking sleep disturbances during pregnancy with adverse pregnancy outcomes. HPA, Hypothalamic-pituitary-adrenal; SDB, sleep-disordered breathing; SWS, slow wave sleep.

activation persists into the daytime, leading to increased peripheral vascular reactivity and catecholamine production, blunted baroreflex sensitivity, hindered pancreatic insulin secretion, and altered hepatic glucose release.[55] All of these downstream SDB effects have been linked to processes seen in preeclampsia: endothelial dysfunction, elevated systemic arterial blood pressure, and decreased cardiac output.[56-58] SDB also has been strongly linked to systemic inflammation, as evidenced by markers including elevated interleukin-6 (IL-6), tumor necrosis factor alpha (TNF-α), and C-reactive protein levels and leukocyte counts.[59-61] Increased inflammation in early pregnancy is associated with adverse outcomes, particularly preeclampsia and preterm birth.[46,62,63]

Slow wave delta sleep (N3 sleep) is disrupted as a consequence of SDB, and this effect may be the mechanism for adverse pregnancy outcomes. Experimental studies in healthy subjects have demonstrated that disruption of N3 sleep can adversely alter insulin and glucose metabolism, sympathovagal balance, and cortisol levels.[64-66] Sleep loss and intermittent hypoxia also have been reported to induce changes in leptin and ghrelin hormones that regulate appetite, satiety, and energy metabolism.[67-69] Recent data suggest that dysregulation of leptin and ghrelin may contribute to the pathophysiology of gestational diabetes and preeclampsia.[70,71]

Impact of Sleep-Disordered Breathing on Pregnancy

Considerable heterogeneity in the definition of SDB is apparent among the studies examining pregnancy outcomes. In some of the largest cohorts, SDB was defined on the basis of symptoms such as self-reported habitual snoring. The method of ascertainment of those symptoms varied, with some using interviews and others using questionnaires. Among studies using objective testing, both in-laboratory and portable PSG, there is variation types of devices used, AHI criteria for establishing a SDB diagnosis, and timing of assessment (prospective-longitudinal versus cross-sectional). These differences lead to difficulty in summarizing the research data and in determining significance for clinical practice.

Sleep-Disordered Breathing and Hypertensive Disorders of Pregnancy

Hypertensive disease complicates 5% to 10% of all pregnancies[72] and can be classified into subtypes according to clinical features: gestational hypertension, preeclampsia-eclampsia, and preeclampsia superimposed on chronic hypertension.[73] The risk factors include obesity and increased maternal age, which overlap with risk factors for SDB. This overlap makes it difficult to investigate potential links between the diseases. Substantial evidence, however, suggests a link between SDB and pregnancy-related hypertension, with most studies demonstrating a two-fold increase in odds of gestational hypertension and preeclampsia.[36,40,74,75]

In two of the largest epidemiologic studies to date, OSA diagnosis was associated with preeclampsia (adjusted odds ratio [OR], 1.60 and 1.89, respectively).[74,76] Although the two studies have been criticized for limitations in the quality of assessment for SDB and pregnancy outcomes, smaller studies using symptoms based on PSG-diagnosed OSA show similar findings of a two-fold increase in the likelihood of preeclampsia in pregnancies complicated by SDB.[77,78] Other studies, however, have failed to confirm this increased risk.[12,79]

Sleep-Disordered Breathing and Diabetes in Pregnancy

Gestational diabetes, a condition characterized by carbohydrate intolerance with onset or recognition during pregnancy, is a common complication, affecting 5% to 8% of pregnant women.[72,80] The incidence of gestational diabetes has increased in recent years, paralleling the increase in maternal obesity.[81] Recognized complications of diabetes include gestational hypertension, preterm birth, malformations, fetal growth restriction or macrosomia, and stillbirth.[79] Studies of gestational diabetes have included SDB as an outcome and as a predictor. The relationship between SDB and diabetes in the general population is well established. Although a causal link has not been demonstrated, SDB has been noted to precede the onset of diabetes, and initiating treatment of SDB with continuous positive airway pressure (CPAP) improves glucose control in nonpregnant populations.[82,83]

Independent of other risk factors, all patients with SDB are at increased risk for development of type 2 diabetes (see Chapter 24). Emerging data indicate that this relationship also may also occur in pregnant women specifically as it relates to gestational diabetes. A systematic review of five observational studies noted that pregnant women with SDB were at increased risk for development of gestational diabetes (adjusted OR, 1.86; 95% CI, 1.30 to 2.42).[78] The presence of SDB was ascertained with questionnaires in four studies and with PSG in one study. A prospective study using longitudinal, objective assessment of SDB demonstrated a dose-response relationship between SDB and gestational diabetes. The prevalence rates of gestational diabetes with no SDB, mild SDB, and moderate to severe SDB were 25%, 43%, and 63%, respectively.[79] Conclusions drawn from these data must consider that not all studies were able to demonstrate a relationship between SDB and gestational diabetes that was independent of BMI.

Sleep-Disordered Breathing and Severe Maternal Morbidity

Severe maternal morbidity refers to conditions or events that if uninterrupted are proximal causes of maternal death. After significant gains in reducing maternal mortality, recent years have been plagued by plateaus and slight increases in maternal death rates in even developed countries.[84] Although most studies regarding SDB and pregnancy have been underpowered to detect severe morbidity, data from a large database of delivery-related hospital discharges are compelling: Among 55,781,965 women, OSA was associated with increased risk of hospital death (adjusted OR, 5.28), pulmonary embolism (adjusted OR, 4.47), and cardiomyopathy (adjusted OR, 9.01).[74] These relationships persisted and were exacerbated by obesity.

Implications of Sleep-Disordered Breathing for Cesarean Delivery

In a large cohort study, pregnant women who snored were more likely to undergo elective cesarean (OR, 2.25; 95% CI, 1.22 to 4.18) or emergency cesarean delivery (OR, 1.68; 95% CI, 1.22 to 2.30).[85] This relationship also has been reported by other smaller, observational studies that have used both symptom-based and PSG-diagnosed SDB.[38,40,75] Although the reason for this association is not immediately clear, it is postulated to be secondary to the high prevalence of obesity, hypertension, and diabetes among women with SDB. These conditions increase the rate of pregnancy complications and promote induction of labor, which in turn can result in a higher rate of cesarean births.

Sleep-Disordered Breathing and Adverse Fetal Outcomes

To date, the potential effects of SDB on the fetus have received limited attention. Effects may be exerted directly or indirectly by exacerbation of the underlying comorbid conditions that often track with SDB. Initial reports of fetal complications came from case reports of fetal growth restriction and fetal heart rate decelerations.[77] In many of those cases, however, confounding comorbid conditions such as hypertensive disease and diabetes coexisted and associations could not be assumed. More recent studies have attempted to examine that relationship more closely.

Stillbirth

Stillbirth is a fetal death at or beyond 20 weeks of gestation.[72] No large-scale studies have been conducted to examine the role of SDB in stillbirth. Risk factors for stillbirth overlap with SDB risk factors and include advancing age, African American ancestry, smoking, maternal conditions such obesity, diabetes or hypertension, fetal growth restriction, and previous adverse pregnancy outcomes.[86] These correlations provide biologic plausibility for an association between stillbirth and maternal SDB, but such an association has not yet been demonstrated.

Miscarriage

Miscarriage or spontaneous abortion involves the loss of a pregnancy, usually within the first 3 months of conception. The estimated frequency of spontaneous abortion is between 12% and 24% of all clinically identified pregnancies. The risk factors for miscarriage include extremes of age, smoking history, obesity, previous miscarriage, hypertension, and diabetes. All of these are also overlapping risk factors for SDB. Data linking SDB and miscarriage are limited, and any discussions are mostly theoretical in nature. In a retrospective review of sequential clinic charts of 147 premenopausal women who had been referred to a sleep disorders clinic for an evaluation of sleep complaints, an association between SDB and number of miscarriages was demonstrated. In that review, overweight or obese women with SDB, especially those with moderate to severe SDB, were more likely to have had a miscarriage than women without SDB.[87]

Preterm Delivery

Preterm births are births that occur before 37 weeks of gestation. Although preterm birth occurs in 11.6% of births, it is responsible for a significant amount of neonatal morbidity and mortality. Preterm birth may be classified as spontaneous or medically indicated if it was precipitated by obstetric intervention for maternal or fetal benefit.[72] Data on preterm birth and SDB have been inconsistent. Large cross-sectional studies of SDB in pregnancy have reported higher risk of preterm delivery.[74,88] However, these studies were unable to differentiate spontaneous from medically indicated preterm birth. One smaller retrospective study noted an increase in medically indicated preterm delivery associated with preeclampsia among women with SDB[75] and a higher rate of preterm birth

among pregnant women with SDB (29.8%) compared with control subjects of normal weight (12.3%).

Fetal Heart Rate Abnormalities

The fetal nonstress test was introduced in 1975 to describe fetal heart rate acceleration in response to fetal movement as a sign of fetal health.[72] It currently is the most common form of fetal assessment in obstetrics. A few studies have attempted to examine fetal well-being in response to nocturnal desaturations and results are conflicting. In a small study, 3 of the 4 women with snoring had fetal heart decelerations that accompanied maternal desaturation, but types of decelerations were not characterized.[89] In larger prospective studies with sample sizes of 20 women with PSG evidence of SDB, findings have not been replicated.[90,91] In these studies, despite episodes of oxygen desaturation, no fetal heart rate decelerations were noted during apneic events. In summary, it is unclear whether fetal hypoxia during maternal apnea occurs and, moreover, whether it is a primary contributor to adverse pregnancy outcomes associated with SDB.

Fetal Growth Abnormalities

Intrauterine growth restriction (IUGR) is defined as retardation of fetal development resulting in small size in relation to gestational age, with most studies using less than the tenth percentile as a cutoff growth criterion.[72] Findings from retrospective and observational studies of SDB and IUGR are mixed, with some failing to show any association. However, studies point to an increased likelihood of fetal growth restriction among pregnant women with moderate to severe SDB (OR, 1.44; 95% CI, 1.22 to 1.71).[92]

Low birth weight is an important cause of neonatal morbidity and is defined as birth weight less than 2500 g. Two potential mechanisms for low birth weight are well documented: preterm delivery and growth restriction. Regardless of the etiology, low birth weight is associated with higher rates of short- and long-term morbidity[72] and with maternal SDB among pooled studies (unadjusted OR, 1.39; 95% CI, 1.14 to 1.65).[78] Most studies have not found a difference between mothers with and without SDB when birth weight is assessed as a continuous value.[78] Two large studies found significant differences in birth weight, with maternal SDB–exposed neonates weighing 100 g less than unexposed neonates. However, this difference is of questionable clinical significance.[75,93]

Most of the focus on growth abnormalities and SDB has been on growth restriction. However, it is also important to consider that there may also be an association with large for gestational age (LGA) neonates due to the increased prevalence of obesity and diabetes among women with SDB. LGA neonates have higher rates of birth trauma, respiratory complications, and short- and long-term morbidity.[72] One study found more LGA infants born to women with SDB than to obese and normal-weight control subjects (17% vs. 8% and 2.6%, respectively).[75]

SCREENING FOR SLEEP-DISORDERED BREATHING IN PREGNANCY

Despite the growing prevalence of SDB and risk factors for SDB in pregnancy, obstetric providers generally remain unaware of this important sleep disorder. In a survey of practitioners and patients regarding prenatal sleep assessment, less than 3% of clinicians reported routinely asking patients about snoring. Yet 32% of women reported that they snored, and only 5% reported being asked about snoring during a prenatal visit.[94]

Investigators have struggled to identify the most appropriate screening tools for SDB in pregnancy. As with all screening tools, questionnaires need to be easily implemented, inexpensive, and useful in the clinical setting for identifying patients requiring referral for more definitive diagnostic testing. Canonical symptoms of SDB include excessive daytime sleepiness, snoring, and witnessed pauses during sleep. Excessive daytime sleepiness most typically has been assessed with the Epworth Sleepiness Scale (ESS). However, because daytime sleepiness is so prevalent in pregnancy, the ESS does not seem to inform risk assessment of pregnant patients for OSA.[95,96]

Pre-pregnancy BMI and maternal age are inconsistent predictors of SDB. Older women and those entering pregnancy with higher baseline BMI, however, are at high risk for pregnancy-onset SDB.[36] In a study using PSG to assess for SDB in the first and third trimesters, maternal weight before pregnancy and maternal age were major predictors of SDB risk.[97]

Snoring may be one of the most useful single symptoms to identify at initial clinical assessment. In nonpregnant patients, habitual snoring has good correlation with PSG.[98,99] For example, for women who say they "often" snore, the PSG odds ratio is 3.8 higher than for nonsnoring peers. Similarly, for women who say they usually (always or almost always) snore, the PSG odds ratio is 16.3 higher than that for nonsnoring peers.[98] Thus in the first trimester, habitual pre-pregnancy snoring may be a useful indicator of *preexisting* OSA. The Berlin questionnaire is widely used for SDB screening in nonobstetric populations, and a high-risk Berlin score has a sensitivity ranging from 68% to 86% and a specificity ranging from 46% to 95% for OSA.[100] In pregnancy, however, the Berlin score has poor predictive capacity (sensitivity of 35% to 39%, specificity of 64% to 68%).[39,96] By contrast, a pregnancy-specific tool that includes frequent snoring ("yes or no"), chronic hypertension ("yes or no"), and maternal age and baseline BMI as continuous variables performed well in predicting SDB in early pregnancy.[96]

In summary, habitual snoring, chronic hypertension, baseline BMI greater than 25 to 30 kg/m², and older maternal age are easily ascertained assessment elements that can effectively indicate the risk for either preexisting SDB or pregnancy-onset SDB.

DIAGNOSING SLEEP-DISORDERED BREATHING IN PREGNANCY

The available evidence is insufficient to guide diagnostic evaluation of SDB specific to pregnant patients. Accordingly, pregnant women in whom SDB is suspected should be evaluated in line with standard guidelines that recommend evaluation by a sleep specialist for a sleep-directed history and physical examination and sleep testing.[101] Sleep testing can be reasonably accomplished by laboratory PSG,[97] or home testing can be performed using type 3 portable monitors.[40] Validation of home monitors for pregnant women is limited, but the convenience makes it a viable option for women who are unable to spend a night away from home for a PSG study. The usual caveats regarding decreased negative predictive value associated with home monitoring apply to pregnant patients, and the need for laboratory PSG for sleep testing in patients with comorbid cardiac, pulmonary, psychiatric, or neurologic disease also applies to pregnant women.[102]

TREATMENT OF SLEEP-DISORDERED BREATHING IN PREGNANCY

Women with a preexisting SDB diagnosis and an established treatment regimen should continue that treatment during pregnancy. CPAP is considered to be safe and effective during pregnancy.[103,104] AHI increases appear to be relatively modest for most women,[9] and a pressure setting increase of 1 to 3 cm H_2O during the second trimester usually is needed.[103,104] CPAP settings are now more easily monitored because devices function in an autoset mode that adjusts pressures within a designated range and reports compliance and residual AHI data. Pregnancy-induced nasal congestion and increased BMI may necessitate adjustments in mask fit and humidification.

Use of a mandibular advancement device (MAD) with previously documented efficacy could be continued during early pregnancy. One study, however, demonstrated autoset CPAP superiority over MAD plus nasal strip in treating SDB in pregnant women.[105] At the very least, effectiveness of MAD should be monitored and a sleep study should be done early in the third trimester, when women are likely to have a higher AHI and require increased CPAP support.[103,104] Positional therapy can be recommended as an adjuvant, in the absence of extenuating circumstances, because most women have a positional component to their SDB, and nonsupine sleep generally is preferred during pregnancy.[106] Postpartum AHI values can be expected to return to pre-pregnancy levels.[107]

In women with known preexisting SDB not already undergoing treatment, immediate initiation of a CPAP therapy regimen is indicated. Autoset CPAP with data download is appropriate for these women and allows for rapid treatment, tracking, and adjustment as pregnancy progresses. MAD treatment is not recommended, because it generally takes several weeks to months to fit, adjust, and test the device. In the absence of a preexisting SDB diagnosis, data are lacking to support a strategy of universal screening for SDB in pregnancy. It is important to recognize, however, that as the general population is becoming more obese, clinicians are likely to encounter more women with symptomatic SDB in pregnancy. Obstetric care providers should refer any patient with suspected SDB to a sleep specialist for diagnosis and possible treatment.

To date, studies examining the effect of CPAP treatment on pregnancy end points have been insufficiently powered or limited in the scope of the end points.[103,104,108-110] The largest of these trials followed women already diagnosed with pre-eclampsia who were treated with CPAP and used improvements in fetal movement and cardiac output as primary clinical end points.[108,109]

In caring for obstetric patients with SDB, it is important to consider increased risk of perioperative complications associated with SDB.[111,112] An analgesic strategy that minimizes the need for systemic opioids should be considered. If used, opioids should be prescribed as single doses rather than by standing order. Monitoring maternal oxygen saturation should be considered if systemic opioids are administered, and women should wear their CPAP device while in the hospital recovering from labor and delivery, as well as after discharge to home. Predelivery consultation with an anesthesiologist to plan intrapartum and postpartum pain management also should be considered.

CLINICAL PEARLS

- SDB prevalence and severity increase from the first to the third trimester of pregnancy.
- Risk factors for SDB in pregnancy have not been well characterized. Habitual snoring, chronic hypertension, maternal baseline BMI greater than 25 to 30 kg/m², and older maternal age are easily obtained information that may effectively indicate risk of either preexisting SDB or pregnancy-onset SDB.
- Data suggest that SDB during pregnancy may increase the incidence of adverse pregnancy outcomes such as gestational hypertension, preeclampsia, and gestational diabetes. Many studies, however, did not control for obesity, a strong risk factor for both SDB and adverse outcomes, nor did they clearly define a temporal relationship between SDB and the subsequent development of adverse outcomes.
- In pregnant women with a preexisting SDB diagnosis and an established treatment protocol, treatment should be continued during the pregnancy and the AHI evaluated for an increase in the early third trimester.
- In pregnant women without preexisting SDB, data are currently lacking to recommend a strategy of universal screening for SDB in pregnancy.

SUMMARY

SDB in pregnancy is an ongoing area of research. It is clear that SDB prevalence and severity increase as pregnancy progresses, especially among high-risk obese women. Data also suggest that SDB during pregnancy may increase the incidence of adverse pregnancy outcomes such as gestational hypertension, preeclampsia, and gestational diabetes. Many of the reported studies, however, did not control for obesity, a strong risk factor for both SDB and adverse pregnancy outcomes, nor did they clearly define a temporal relationship between SDB and subsequent development of adverse outcomes. The optimal way to screen for SDB during pregnancy has yet to be determined, but data suggest that instruments used in nonpregnant populations (e.g., Berlin questionnaire, ESS) perform poorly in pregnancy. Pregnant women in whom SDB is suspected should be evaluated and treated using standard guidelines; however, the available evidence currently is too limited to suggest that treatment of SDB during pregnancy can alter pregnancy outcomes.

Selected Readings

Chen YH, Kang JH, Lin CC, et al. Obstructive sleep apnea and the risk of adverse pregnancy outcomes. *Am J Obstet Gynecol* 2012;**206**(2):136 e131–5.

Facco FL, Ouyang DW, Zee PC, Grobman WA. Development of a pregnancy-specific screening tool for sleep apnea. *J Clin Sleep Med* 2012;**8**(4):389–94.

Izci-Balserak B, Pien GW. Sleep-disordered breathing and pregnancy: potential mechanisms and evidence for maternal and fetal morbidity. *Curr Opin Pulm Med* 2010;**16**(6):574–82.

Lockhart EM, Ben Abdallah A, Tuuli MG, Leighton BL. Obstructive sleep apnea in pregnancy: assessment of current screening tools. *Obstet Gynecol* 2015;**126**(1):93–102.

Louis J, Auckley D, Bolden N. Management of obstructive sleep apnea in pregnant women. *Obstet Gynecol* 2012;**119**(4):864–8.

Louis J, Auckley D, Miladinovic B, et al. Perinatal outcomes associated with obstructive sleep apnea in obese pregnant women. *Obstet Gynecol* 2012;**120**(5):1085–92.

O'Brien LM, Bullough AS, Owusu JT, et al. Pregnancy-onset habitual snoring, gestational hypertension, and preeclampsia: prospective cohort study. *Am J Obstet Gynecol* 2012;**207**(6):487 e481–9.

Pamidi S, Pinto LM, Marc I, et al. Maternal sleep-disordered breathing and adverse pregnancy outcomes: a systematic review and metaanalysis. *Am J Obstet Gynecol* 2014;**210**(1):52.e1–14.

Rice JR, Larrabure-Torrealva GT, Luque Fernandez MA, et al. High risk for obstructive sleep apnea and other sleep disorders among overweight and obese pregnant women. *BMC Pregnancy Childbirth* 2015;**15**:198.

Romero R, Badr MS. A role for sleep disorders in pregnancy complications: challenges and opportunities. *Am J Obstet Gynecol* 2014;**210**(1):3–11.

Sharma SK, Nehra A, Sinha S, et al. Sleep disorders in pregnancy and their association with pregnancy outcomes: a prospective observational study. *Sleep Breath* 2016;**20**(1):87–93.

A complete reference list can be found online at ExpertConsult.com.

Obstructive Sleep Apnea in the Workplace

Chunbai Zhang; Mark B. Berger; Albert Rielly; Atul Malhotra; Stefanos N. Kales

Chapter Highlights

- Obstructive sleep apnea (OSA) is highly prevalent among workers and a common cause of excessive daytime sleepiness at work.
- Untreated OSA negatively affects occupational health, safety, and productivity.
- Untreated OSA increases the risk of transportation accidents.

- Clinicians are likely to encounter employees in several situations for evaluation for possible OSA.
- In the occupational setting, subjective symptom reports are unreliable for screening and diagnosis of OSA.

OVERVIEW AND BACKGROUND

Obstructive sleep apnea (OSA) is characterized by repetitive cessations of or decrements in airflow through the upper airway during sleep, resulting in a variety of physiologic and metabolic disturbances, including frequent arousals from sleep.[1] Untreated OSA has been linked to excessive health, safety, and lost productivity costs in the range of $65 billion to $165 billion per year in the United States alone.[2] Motor vehicle accidents and other workplace injuries in safety-sensitive occupations are increased owing to the resulting excessive daytime sleepiness and decreased vigilance/attention associated with OSA.[3-6] In addition to lost productivity and increased absenteeism, individual and public health costs attributable to the cardiovascular and metabolic comorbidity associated with OSA have been well documented.[7,8]

OSA remains underdiagnosed and often goes untreated. Accordingly, sleep specialists and occupational physicians can expect to encounter several typical workplace referral scenarios in which patients or employees with potential OSA will require evaluation. One of the most common scenarios is that in which an employee is observed to be sleeping at work (as with an employee in an unsupervised position that requires close attention to the assigned task) or falling asleep repeatedly during group meetings. Supervisors may mistake such behavior for laziness or may recognize the possibility of a medical problem. In such cases, the employee may agree to be medically assessed or may be in denial regarding his or her impairment. A more urgent referral scenario is that in which the employee is required to present to the sleep clinic after falling asleep and causing an accident during performance of a safety-sensitive job (e.g., professional driver, airline pilot, health care worker, nuclear plant employee, public safety officer). In keeping with the increased public awareness of transportation accident risk associated with OSA, sleep professionals can expect to see occupational medicine professionals and employers refer transportation operator-employees who deny all symptoms of OSA yet are found to have objective risk factors (e.g., obesity, increased neck circumference

and/or hypertension). These employees may be referred for evaluation to rule out OSA as a condition of employment or to medically qualify for an operating license. In all of these scenarios, the determination of a diagnosis of OSA and reports of treatment compliance data will have medicolegal relevance for the clinician and potential job security implications for the referred employee.

CONSEQUENCES OF OBSTRUCTIVE SLEEP APNEA IN TRANSPORTATION WORKERS

Experts estimate that between 7%[9] and 20%[10] of all large truck crashes are due to drowsy or fatigued driving.[11] As reported over the past decade (2003-2012), between 3454 and 9528 deaths and between 84,000 and 224,000 serious injuries (mostly among the traveling public) are likely attributable to sleep-related impairment in commercial motor vehicle (CMV) drivers in the United States alone.[9,10,12] OSA is the most common medical cause of excessive daytime sleepiness.[13] Not surprisingly, therefore, several high-profile transportation accidents related to insufficient sleep and OSA have been reported.[14] In one such accident, a pilot of an oil tankship collided with a general cargo vessel, which led to a spill of crude oil. The volume of the spill was estimated at 1000 to 11,000 barrels. The official investigation concluded that contributing to the accident was the pilot's fatigue caused by his untreated obstructive sleep apnea and his work schedule.[15] In 2008, a tour bus carrying passengers returning from a weekend ski trip crashed and killed nine people and injured 43 others. The driver was found to be suffering from OSA that was inadequately treated in the days before the accident. In 2009, two airline pilots on a flight in Hawaii dozed for at least 18 minutes during a midmorning flight, initially overshooting the specified destination. The captain subsequently was diagnosed with OSA. In December 2013, a southbound New York Metro-North Railroad train derailed as a consequence of excessive speed, killing four passengers and injuring 59 others. A diagnostic evaluation of the train's engineer as part of the accident investigation revealed that he was suffering from untreated severe OSA.[16]

PRINCIPLES OF OBSTRUCTIVE SLEEP APNEA MANAGEMENT IN THE WORKPLACE

Occupational medical programs that address OSA screening, diagnosis, and management should be accompanied by administrative controls related to hours of service, shift work, and other factors that affect worker fatigue. Taken together, these factors are referred to as *fatigue risk management systems* (FRMSs). In 2012, the American College of Occupational and Environmental Medicine (ACOEM) Presidential Task Force on fatigue risk management published a guidance statement to assist in the design and implementation of FRMSs.[17] A successful FRMS should be science-based, data-driven (with decisions based on collection and objective analysis of data), cooperative (designed together by all stakeholders), fully implemented (systemwide use of tools, systems, policies, and procedures), integrated (built into existing corporate safety and health management systems), continuously improved (for progressive reduction of risk using feedback, evaluation, and modification), adequately budgeted (justified by an accurate return-on-investment business model), and "owned" (responsibility accepted by senior corporate leadership).[17] For an FRMS to function efficiently, a senior manager must be assigned accountability for the program. Active engagement from everyone employed will make the program more successful, as will a culture of mutual trust between management and employees.

Sleep Disorder Management

The principles of fatigue management apply to OSA management and require a proactive approach rather than a reactive approach. In safety-sensitive positions, minimizing fatigue by actively screening, diagnosing, and managing OSA in advance, with implementation of corrective actions when necessary to address noncompliance with prescribed treatment, is expected to be more cost-effective than responding to a fatigue-related incident after it occurs. For most workplaces, the sleep disorder management program need not be extensive. A screening questionnaire that encourages follow-up evaluation with personal physicians for response profiles suggestive of sleep disorders may be adequate. In safety-sensitive occupations, however, objective physical assessments may be required because they are much more sensitive and reliable screening tools than most self-report questionnaires (as discussed further on).

Screening and Risk Factors

Nonmodifiable risk factors for OSA include older age, male gender, postmenopausal status in females, and ethnicity (Asian American or African American descent). Obesity/adiposity is the most significant risk factor and is modifiable.[18-21] Results from studies have shown that OSA is closely associated with higher body mass index (BMI) and larger neck and waist circumference.[21-24] These findings make the foregoing parameters key objective elements for OSA screening in an occupational setting. Visceral fat is significantly correlated with increasing OSA severity.[23,25-27] Higher waist-to-hip ratio also has been shown in some studies to be more predictive of OSA than is obesity in general. Among morbidly obese patients with a BMI of 40 kg/m² or higher, OSA is nearly universal. Among men with BMI of 32 kg/m² or higher, the prevalence of OSA is approximately 75%.[28] Persons with large neck

circumferences (in men, greater than 17 inches; in women, greater than 16 inches) should raise clinical suspicion for presence of OSA.[29]

Women with OSA tend to report fewer "classic" daytime symptoms of OSA—for example, instead of reporting daytime sleepiness, they may report fatigue and lack of energy. In addition, women have different anatomic and functional upper airway properties and differences in control of breathing compared with men.[30,31] These diagnostic and biologic differences between men and women contribute to lower rates of sleep apnea diagnosis in women.

Among different races, obesity plays a variable degree of importance. For example, adult African Americans younger than 25 years or older than 65 years have higher prevalence of OSA than others.[20,32] In the East Asian population, although the prevalence of obesity is lower, the prevalence of OSA is similar to that for Western populations.[33,34] Ethnic differences in adipose tissue distribution (i.e., peripheral versus visceral) and predisposing craniofacial profiles such as crowded posterior oropharynx, shorter cranial base, and more acute cranial base flexure may be important in explaining the pathogenesis of OSA among certain nonobese populations.[18,30,35]

Finally, smoking and use of alcohol and other sedatives are important modifiable risk factors.

OBSTRUCTIVE SLEEP APNEA SCREENING METHODS IN THE WORKPLACE

Screening is defined in this chapter as risk assessment or stratification before referral for a diagnostic test. Employer screening refers to the use of questionnaires (such as the STOP-Bang questionnaire; for further information, see www.stopbang.ca), anthropometric measures, and other subjective and objective criteria applied to all employees to identify those who should be referred to a sleep disorders specialist, who will then confirm or exclude the diagnosis of OSA. "Diagnosis" and "diagnostic procedures" for OSA refer to sleep studies that measure or estimate the presence of sleep apnea (see later text). OSA screening modalities include (1) subjective/self-identified reports of perceived sleep disorders, daytime sleepiness, and sleep-related symptoms; (2) objective measures such as BMI and neck circumference, with cutoff values, and blood pressure; (3) guidelines that combine subjective and objective criteria; and (4) functional performance screens designed to detect impairment related to fatigue or sleepiness. Table 35-1 summarizes a number of these screening methods regarding characteristics of workplace performance (in this case, transportation operators) and effectiveness in detecting OSA.

Subjective Measures

Subjective screening modalities depend on the individual employee's self-report of previous OSA or daytime sleepiness. However, this approach to OSA screening in an occupational setting creates multiple challenges.[36-39] Unlike in a sleep clinic, where patients with undiagnosed OSA typically are actively seeking diagnosis and treatment for inadequate sleep, snoring, and/or excessive daytime sleepiness, employees in safety-sensitive positions (e.g., truck drivers, pilots, mariners) wish to avoid incurring an OSA diagnosis because of its potential negative economic and occupational consequences.[40] In fact,

Table 35-1 Comparison of Various Obstructive Sleep Apnea (OSA) Screening Strategies in a Typical Population of Transportation Operators

Screening Criterion	Estimated Performance during Occupational Medical Examinations of Transportation Operators				
	Prevalence of Positive Screens (%)	OSA Case Yield* (%)	Sensitivity (%)	Positive Predictive Value (%)	Mean AHI in Cases Detected
U.S. Federal Commercial Drivers' License Exam Driver Sleep Question	0-3	0-2	0-7	—	—
ESS score >10	3.4	1.4	4	—	37± 28
SomniSage Questionnaire	30	21	75	68	40 ± 28
BMI ≥30 kg/m²	50	19	68-70	38	41 ± 29
Joint Task Force Guidelines	12-13	10-12	36-46	79-≥95	42-49
BMI ≥ 40 kg/m²	6-7	6-7	23	>95	51 ± 32

*Percent of commercial drivers who will screen positive and then be diagnosed with OSA (defined as AHI >10) by polysomnography.
AHI, Apnea-hypopnea index; BMI, body mass index; ESS, Epworth Sleepiness Scale.
Modified from Kales SN, Straubel MG. Obstructive sleep apnea in North American commercial drivers. *Ind Health* 2014;52:13-24.

data from diverse sources confirm that commercial drivers generally do not report their symptoms and diagnoses because of the negative economic and occupational consequences (perceived or real) of an OSA diagnosis. These concerns range from the inconvenience of having to submit to a diagnostic workup after a positive screening result, to the negative impact on employee pay resulting from being pulled out of service during a medical evaluation, to potential loss of a job and/or medical certification for employment.[9,14,41] In view of this reluctance of employees to self-report symptoms of OSA, it is especially important that occupational medicine physicians take the time to implement objective measures (described further on) as well as to ask supplementary questions in evaluating high-risk drivers.

In the United States, commercial vehicle drivers are required to complete a federal medical form that contains the single yes-or-no question "Do you have sleep disorders, pauses in breathing while asleep, daytime sleepiness, loud snoring?" Among those drivers identified as being at high risk for OSA, as many as 85% answered "No" to this question.[38]

The Epworth Sleepiness Scale (ESS) is a widely used questionnaire designed to identify persons with excessive daytime sleepiness due to either lifestyle circumstances (e.g., chronic sleep deprivation stemming from demanding work or social schedules) or a sleep disorder.[42] Unfortunately, among commercial drivers, the ESS questionnaire may produce a high rate of false-negative results. Most commercial vehicle operators report very low ESS scores at driver certification examinations (ESS scores in the range of 2 to 4 indicate a low likelihood of abnormal sleepiness), lower than ESS scores from the general community.[40] Similarly, results from an anonymous survey of transportation operators conducted by the National Sleep Foundation revealed a mean ESS score of 5.2 among professional truck drivers assessed.[43] By contrast, in another anonymous survey of U.S. truck drivers, more than 20% reported falling asleep at traffic lights.[39]

Somni-Sage is a questionnaire that incorporates weighted values for BMI, neck circumference, hypertension, and other medical comorbid conditions, as well as heavy snoring,

witnessed apneic episodes, and other manifestations of excessive daytime sleepiness, and calculates categories of relative OSA risk.[44] Results from a retrospective assessment of SomniSage Questionnaire validity in more than 19,000 drivers showed that almost 6000 of the respondents (30%) were at higher risk for OSA. Of more than 2000 higher-risk drivers who underwent PSG, 68% were diagnosed with definite OSA (AHI greater than 10) and 80% had at least probable OSA (AHI of 5 or greater). A conservative prevalence estimate for definite OSA (AHI greater than 10) was 21% among commercial drivers in the population studied.[44]

Although evidence-based data are lacking, our own clinical experience supports the practice of a more probing interview of higher-risk commercial drivers by an experienced physician to obtain critical information. Drivers who deny symptoms and diagnoses on questionnaires and self-report forms often divulge more information when skilled physicians ask repetitive and additional questions regarding sleep hygiene, symptoms of daytime sleepiness, comorbid conditions, and findings on previous evaluations.[40]

Objective Measures

Objective screening tools have the advantage over questionnaires that they are less subject to manipulation, deception, and underreporting by drivers. Therefore application of such tools to obtain objective physical findings (e.g., BMI cutoff values) should be the screening modality of choice for OSA evaluation of employees who are in safety-sensitive positions.

At least four groups have generated recommendations for objectively screening CMV operators: (1) Dagan and colleagues,[45] (2) the U.S. Department of Transportation's Federal Motor Carrier Safety Administration (FMCSA) Medical Review Board (MRB),[46] (3) the FMCSA Medical Expert Panel (MEP),[47] and (4) the Joint Task Force (JTF) of the American College of Chest Physicians, the ACOEM, and the National Sleep Foundation.[48,49] Dagan's group showed that 78% of commercial drivers with a BMI of 32 kg/m² or greater had polysomnography (PSG)-confirmed

OSA, and almost 50% also had objectively confirmed excessive daytime sleepiness as measured by a Multiple Sleep Latency Test. Confirming our review finding (see earlier) that subjective measures may yield a high number of false negatives, Dagan and colleagues also found that 100% of these affected drivers denied symptoms of OSA or excessive daytime sleepiness.[45]

The FMCSA MEP consisted of experienced clinicians and researchers knowledgeable in evidence-based medicine. In its 2008 report, the panel recommended referral of all CMV operators with BMI of 33 kg/m^2 or greater for a sleep study.[47] The MEP took feasibility of implementation into consideration by aiming to identify those CMV operators who were most likely to have severe OSA. After reviewing all of the negative long-term medical outcomes from untreated OSA, the FMCSA MRB recommended that a lower BMI criterion (BMI of 30 kg/m^2 or higher) be used for referral.[46] Neither set of recommendations from the MEP and the MRB have been implemented by the FMCSA as requirements. Barriers to a federal mandate include political, financial, liability, and legal concerns.[36,38]

The 2006 JTF issued recommendations for OSA screening of commercial drivers at certification examinations performed by commercial driver medical examiners (CDMEs).[48,49] Their screening recommendations include self-reported historical findings and the ESS, but they emphasized objective physical examination findings such as BMI, neck circumference, and hypertension criteria. The JTF guidelines recommended a higher BMI threshold (BMI of 35 km/m^2 or higher) for sleep study referral compared with that issued by either the MEP or the MRB of the FMCSA. This threshold was designed to have a high positive predictive value and to identify more severe OSA cases while not removing too many drivers from service. In the absence of a clear federal mandate for OSA screening of commercial drivers, the JTF guidelines are viewed by many occupational medicine professionals as representing a minimum standard for OSA screening to be implemented by the occupational medicine community.

Functional Screening

Functional or performance-based screening is an emerging approach for OSA screening at work sites using techniques such as psychomotor vigilance testing (PVT) and driving simulation. PVT is attractive as an adjunct to screen for OSA[50]: This testing modality has been shown to detect decrements in performance due to sleep deprivation, and it requires only a few minutes to administer. However, PVT performance cutoff criteria and correlation with accident or safety risks associated with OSA have not yet been established. Likewise, results from studies of driving simulation consistently demonstrate decrements in performance among subjects with OSA and other sleep disorders, as well as in subjects who have been sleep-deprived. At present, however, robust evidence associating simulator performance with on-road driving performance is lacking.[48] Additionally, performance criteria for identifying operators with OSA have not been established, and testing generally takes at least 30 minutes to complete. The latter characteristic makes use of simulators less attractive as an addition to occupational medical examinations.[40]

DIAGNOSIS OF OBSTRUCTIVE SLEEP APNEA IN OCCUPATIONAL SETTINGS

A "diagnosis" of OSA incorporates the results obtained from different types of sleep studies. Sleep studies may be performed using portable monitors (PMs) or full-channel PSG to measure (or estimate) the subject's sleep-disordered breathing (if present) via the AHI, respiratory disturbance index (RDI), or other means.[1] Although the current gold standard for diagnosing OSA is a laboratory-based PSG study, in-laboratory PSG is more expensive, time-consuming, and frequently of limited availability. The high prevalence of obesity means that more employees will have a positive result on screening and require follow-up sleep studies; consequently, the up-front costs of performing sleep studies has become a challenge to more widespread OSA screening and detection.[51-56] Using laboratory-based PSG as the diagnostic standard is less feasible because U.S. health insurers have placed increasing restrictions on reimbursement for the use of such studies. For all of these reasons, there has been an increasing interest in and push for use of PMs for diagnosing OSA in occupational settings, and this topic recently has been reviewed in depth.[51] To date, comparative effectiveness studies in safety-sensitive occupations (e.g., truck drivers, pilots) are lacking.

In the occupational setting, the major concern regarding the use of PMs is that transportation operators may actively avoid incurring an OSA diagnosis because of its economic and occupational implications (as discussed previously).[51] It is therefore imperative that clinicians be aware of scenarios whereby employees could alter PM results. They may stay awake to avoid sleep-disordered breathing events, which would go undetected if the PM does not record or estimate sleep stages, or the device may be placed on a healthier family member to avoid diagnosis. Accordingly, occupational medicine experts advocate using PM devices with a so-called chain-of-custody feature (such as a bracelet or other identifier placed on the driver by a professional technician), which deactivates the PM if it is removed. The best diagnostic use of PMs in an occupational context is to confirm the presence of OSA in an employee who already has been deemed to be at high risk for the disorder on the basis of symptoms or other screening techniques. When OSA is confirmed using the PM, treatment can be recommended and implemented without further testing. On the other hand, a negative or indeterminate result from a PM should not be considered sufficient evidence to exclude OSA, particularly in a high-risk employee working in a safety-sensitive position (e.g., transportation).[51]

Other unique considerations have emerged as important in interpreting diagnostic sleep tests in the occupational setting. Unlike in the nonoccupational setting (where the presence of symptoms can be used to make the diagnosis or decide on the necessity of treatment in cases in which the AHI or RDI is relatively low), the absence of symptoms should not be used to rule out OSA or accident risk.[38,40,45] Second, no clear thresholds of OSA severity (i.e., based on AHI/RDI, oxygen desaturation, or other measures) below which OSA-affected employees are *not* at an increased risk for accidents have been established.[4] Accordingly, in cases of mild OSA, the bias should be toward treating the OSA in affected employees who work in safety-sensitive positions (e.g., transportation operators).

TREATMENT OPTIONS AND COMPLIANCE MONITORING

As in the nonoccupational setting, continuous positive airway pressure (CPAP) is the first-line and best treatment for OSA in an occupational context. For employees in non–safety-sensitive positions, other OSA treatments may be considered. For transportation operators, however, CPAP is the only non-surgical therapy for which the effectiveness of treatment and compliance can be objectively monitored. All employees in safety-sensitive positions (including transportation operators who receive surgical treatment) should undergo follow-up PSG to document improvement.

For safety-sensitive workers, once CPAP is instituted, compliance should be documented for at least 2 to 4 weeks and then reassessed at least yearly. Compliance is based on objective measures using data downloads or printouts from the CPAP device. Most practitioners regard minimum adequate compliance to consist of at least 4 hours of CPAP use per sleep period (or nightly) on at least 70% of nights.[48]

Adjunctive treatment with prescription stimulants for residual excessive daytime sleepiness in safety-sensitive workers should be undertaken only after consultation with the company medical director and after review of applicable federal rules. Failure to successfully respond to CPAP therapy should be a red flag regarding overall fitness for duty (particularly among transportation operators). Furthermore, some federal agencies may prohibit stimulant use or advise caution (see further on).

FEDERAL REGULATIONS AND RECOMMENDATIONS

Transportation operators with known diagnoses of OSA generally should be disqualified when their condition is untreated. However, despite various calls from the National Transportation Safety Board (NTSB), expert panels, and other bodies, regulating agencies under the Department of Transportation do not contain explicit objective requirements for OSA screening. Selected relevant regulations and recommendations are summarized in Table 35-2.

In April 2012, the FMCSA published a request for public comments on its proposed recommendations on regulatory guidance for diagnosis and management of obstructive sleep apnea.[57] The proposed guidance was based on MRB recommendations, as reviewed previously. A final ruling is still pending—and subsequent legislation forbids the FMCSA from using guidance alone to mandate sleep apnea screening for drivers before formal federal rulemaking.[58] On the other hand, since May 2014, medical examiners (i.e., CDMEs) providing screening examinations must belong to a Federal Registry of Certified Medical Examiners, which requires meeting certain licensing, continuing education, and testing requirements. Previously, such screening could be conducted by almost any health care practitioner, and these assessments often were performed by providers with little knowledge of occupational medicine, sleep disorders, and fitness for driving.[59] It is now expected that more drivers will be subject to examinations conducted in a stringent manner by persons with training in objective OSA screening as part of their practice standards.

The Federal Aviation Administration (FAA) regulates pilots and air traffic controllers. Pilots who are identified by an aviation medical examiner as being at risk for OSA are granted a medical certificate but are then required to undergo OSA evaluation within 90 days.[60] Examiners may reissue an airman medical certificate under the provisions of an Authorization, if the applicant provides the following: a current report (performed within the last 90 days) from the treating physician that references the present treatment, whether the treatment has eliminated any symptoms—with specific comments regarding daytime sleepiness. If any question arises regarding response to or compliance with treatment or if the applicant has developed some associated illness (e.g., right-sided heart failure), then examiners must defer to the Aerospace Medical Certification Division or the Regional Flight Surgeon.[61]

For the U.S. Coast Guard, the Mariner Medical Standards apply for OSA screening. No objective screening criteria are required or recommended, but the mariner is asked to disclose voluntarily an OSA diagnosis, if present.[62] To be considered for a waiver for sleep disorders, the mariner must demonstrate compliance with and efficacy of OSA treatment. In the case of OSA treatment with dental devices or positional therapy, the mariner must undergo PSG while using a dental device or positional therapy to demonstrate efficacy. If the condition was treated with surgery, then a postoperative sleep study is requested to document resolution of the condition. Once the initial information has been reviewed and a determination made that a mariner qualifies for a sleep disorder waiver, then the mariner is required to submit to periodic evaluations that include compliance information.[62]

The Federal Railroad Administration does not have any specific regulations regarding OSA; however, it has issued a safety advisory, which is summarized in Table 35-2.[63]

The FAA disqualifies pilots using prescription stimulants.[64] The FMCSA does not disqualify drivers using modafinil but advises monitoring and other precautions.[65] The U.S. Coast Guard Mariner Medical Standards do not routinely allow use of stimulants for OSA treatment, and waivers are granted on a case-by case-basis.[62]

RISK FACTOR REDUCTION

Beyond screening, diagnosis, and treatment of OSA in the workplace, other risk factor reduction measures can further mitigate OSA-related sleepiness and its consequences (see also the earlier discussion of FRMSs).

Because obesity is a primary risk factor for OSA, effective employee fitness and wellness programs can produce a return on investment for the transportation industry. Such programs fall within the realm of productivity and health management, where employee health and employer costs are viewed from a holistic perspective—with the ultimate goal of reducing costs by improving health.

Shift work is another risk factor for accidents, and shift work is likely to produce synergistic impairment with OSA. Therefore we do not recommend rotating shifts or night shift driving or night operations for OSA-affected employees even when they are compliant with CPAP treatment. This is particularly true for OSA-affected transportation operators.[40]

When possible, the work environment can be modified to allow for short but frequent breaks and strategically timed

Table 35-2   Summary of Selected Federal Regulations* or Recommendations for Medical Examiners Regarding Obstructive Sleep Apnea (OSA)

Federal Agency	Regulation/Recommendation	Required/Recommended Reporting Specifically Related to OSA	BMI Threshold for PSG Referral
FMCSA	*Regulation(s)*: No established medical history or clinical diagnosis of respiratory or neurologic dysfunction likely to interfere with the ability to control and drive a commercial motor vehicle safely[a]	*Required*: "Do you have sleep disorders, pauses in breathing while asleep, daytime sleepiness, loud snoring?"[b]	*Required*: None
FRA	*Regulation(s)*: With the exception of examinations and minimum standards for vision and hearing, U.S. commercial railroad companies have discretion as to the content, frequency and extent of their medical screening programs.[c] *Recommended*: That railroads and representatives of employees working together, develop and implement policies such that, "when a railroad becomes aware that an employee in a safety sensitive position has an incapacitating or performance-impairing medical condition related to sleep, the railroad prohibits that employee from performing any safety-sensitive duties until that medical condition appropriately responds to treatment."[d]	*Required*: None *Recommended*: That "employees' medical examinations include assessment and screening for possible sleep disorders and other associated medical conditions"[d]	*Required*: None
FAA	*Regulation(s)*: Untreated OSA is a disqualifying medical condition. "If a pilot is diagnosed with OSA, an AME must submit all pertinent medical information and a current status report, a sleep study with a polysomnogram, and use of medications and titration study results to the FAA. The FAA will then decide whether a special issuance medial certificate is appropriate."[f]	*Required*: None	*Recommended*: BMI >40 (high BMI not disqualifying by itself)[e]
U.S. Coast Guard	*Regulation(s)*: "Are of sound health; have no physical limitations that would hinder or prevent performance of duties; and are free from any medical conditions that pose a risk of sudden incapacitation, which would affect operating, or working on vessels."[g]	*Required*: None— relies on self-disclosure of a sleep apnea diagnosis[h]	*Required*: None
NTSB	*Recommended*: Elicit preexisting diagnoses of OSA; screen for OSA risk factors; and ensure operators with sleep apnea are effectively treated before granting unrestricted medical certification.[i]	*Recommended*: Develop standard medical examination forms to elicit diagnoses of sleep disorders and to screen for sleep disorders; require use of these forms[j]	*Recommended*: Not specified

*As of 2014. Data from cited sources.
[a]Qualifications of drivers and longer combination vehicle (LCV) driver instructors. *CFR* 2012;49, §391.41.
[b]Federal Motor Carrier Safety Administration. *Medical examination report for commercial driver fitness determination.* Form 649-F (6045). Washington (D.C.): Federal Motor Carrier Safety Administration; March 19, 2014. <http://www.fmcsa.dot.gov/regulations/medical/medical-examination-report-commercial-driver-fitness-determination>; 2014.
[c]U.S. Department of Transportation, Federal Railroad Administration. *Medical standards for railroad workers.* Final report.Washington (D.C.): Office of Safety; January 2005.
[d]Notice of Safety Advisory 2004-04; Effect of sleep disorders on safety of railroad operations. *Fed Reg* 2004;69(190):58995-6.
[e]Federal Aviation Administration. *Fact sheet—sleep apnea in aviation* [press release]. <http://www.faa.gov/news/fact_sheets/news_story.cfm?newsid=15994>; 2014.
[f]Federal Aviation Administration. *Fact sheet—sleep apnea in aviation* [press release]. <http://www.faa.gov/news/fact_sheets/news_story.cfm?newsId=15474>; 2013.
[g]U.S. Department of Homeland Security, U.S. Coast Guard. *Merchant Mariner credential medical evaluation report.* Form CG-719K Rev. (01-09). <http://www.uscg.mil/forms/cg/cg_719k.pdf>; 2009.
[h]U.S. Department of Homeland Security, U.S. Coast Guard. *Medical and physical evaluation guidelines for Merchant Mariner credentials.* NVIC 04-08, COMDTPUB 16700.4. Washington (D.C.): June 7, 2013.
[i]National Transportation Safety Board. *Safety recommendation (M-09-14 through -16).* Washington (D.C.): October 20, 2009. <http://www.ntsb.gov/doclib/recletters/2009/M09_14_16.pdf>; 2009.
[j]National Transportation Safety Board. *Safety recommendation (A-09-61 through -66).* Washington (D.C.): August 7, 2009. <http://www.ntsb.gov/doclib/recletters/2009/a09_61_66.pdf>; 2009.
BMI, Body mass index; FAA, Federal Aviation Administration; FMCSA, Federal Motor Carrier Safety Administration; FRA, Federal Railroad Administration; NTSB, National Transportation Safety Board; PSG, polysomnography.

naps. It has been shown that naps decrease subjective fatigue and improve objective alertness and performance.

CLINICAL PEARLS

- Employees in safety-sensitive positions (e.g., truck drivers, pilots, mariners) may specifically deny or underreport symptoms to avoid incurring an OSA diagnosis because of its potential negative economic and occupational consequences.
- Screening for OSA should include BMI, neck circumference, and other easily obtained objective criteria. Negative subjective symptom reports should be considered unreliable. A more probing interview performed by an experienced physician to obtain critical information often is required.
- Monitoring with portable devices can be used to confirm the presence of OSA so that appropriate treatment can be initiated. Negative or inconclusive PM-based findings warrant a follow-up evaluation with full in-laboratory PSG, particularly for high-risk employees working in safety-sensitive positions.
- CPAP remains the first-line treatment for OSA, and minimum adequate compliance consists of at least 4 hours of CPAP use per sleep period on at least 70% of nights.

SUMMARY

OSA is common in the workplace and often goes undiagnosed and thus untreated, with negative consequences for health, safety, and productivity. Transportation accidents constitute a particular concern. Sleep and occupational medicine professionals are likely to encounter a number of patients in several workplace referral scenarios that trigger evaluation for possible OSA, including falling asleep at work, on-the-job accidents, and screening or diagnostic assessment for safety-sensitive positions (especially in transportation). Because employees may be reluctant to disclose OSA-related symptoms, clinicians cannot depend on symptom reports for screening or diagnosis and must rely primarily on objective measures, tests, and demonstration of treatment compliance. Screening can be accomplished objectively through use of BMI and neck circumference, for which thresholds can be set for referring employees to a sleep medicine specialist.

Selected Readings

Berger M, Varvarigou V, Rielly A, et al. Employer-mandated sleep apnea screening and diagnosis in drivers. *J Occup Environ Med* 2012;**54**(8): 1017–25.

Colvin LJ, Collop N. Commercial motor vehicle driver obstructive sleep apnea screening and treatment in the United States: an update and recommendation overview. *J Clin Sleep Med* 2016;**12**(1):113–25.

Kales SN, Straubel M. Obstructive sleep apnea in North American commercial drivers. *Ind Health* 2014;**52**(1):13–24.

Perlman S. Sleep apnea and workplace safety. *BCMJ* 2014;**56**(2):94–6.

Tregear S, Reston J, Schoelles K, Phillips B. Obstructive sleep apnea and risk of motor vehicle crash: systematic review and meta-analysis. *J Clin Sleep Med* 2009;**5**(6):573–81.

Zhang C, Berger M, Malhotra A, Kales SN. Portable diagnostic devices for identifying obstructive sleep apnea among commercial motor vehicle drivers: considerations and unanswered questions. *Sleep* 2012;**35**: 1481–9.

A complete reference list can be found online at ExpertConsult.com.

Index

Page numbers followed by "*f*" indicate figures, "*t*" indicate tables, and "*b*" indicate boxes.

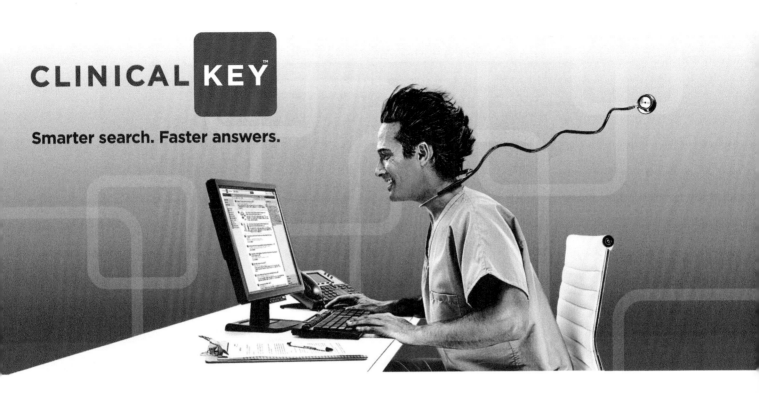